INTERACTIVE PHENOMENA IN THE CARDIAC SYSTEM

ADVANCES IN EXPERIMENTAL MEDICINE AND BIOLOGY

Recent Volumes in this Series

Volume 338
CHEMISTRY AND BIOLOGY OF PTERIDINES AND FOLATES
Edited by June E. Ayling, M. Gopal Nair, and Charles M. Baugh

Volume 339
NOVEL APPROACHES TO SELECTIVE TREATMENTS OF HUMAN SOLID TUMORS: Laboratory and Clinical Correlation
Edited by Youcef M. Rustum

Volume 340
THE DESIGN OF SYNTHETIC INHIBITORS OF THROMBIN
Edited by G. Claeson, M. F. Scully, Vijay V. Kakkar, and J. Deadman

Volume 341
CIRRHOSIS, HYPERAMMONEMIA, AND HEPATIC ENCEPHALOPATHY
Edited by Santiago Grisolía and Vicente Felipo

Volume 342
CORONAVIRUSES: Molecular Biology and Virus–Host Interactions
Edited by Hubert Laude and Jean-François Vautherot

Volume 343
CURRENT DIRECTIONS IN INSULIN-LIKE GROWTH FACTOR RESEARCH
Edited by Derek LeRoith and Mohan K. Raizada

Volume 344
MECHANISMS OF PLATELET ACTIVATION AND CONTROL
Edited by Kalwant S. Authi, Steve P. Watson, and Vijay V. Kakkar

Volume 345
OXYGEN TRANSPORT TO TISSUE XV
Edited by Peter Vaupel, Rolf Zander, and Duane F. Bruley

Volume 346
INTERACTIVE PHENOMENA IN THE CARDIAC SYSTEM
Edited by Samuel Sideman and Rafael Beyar

A Continuation Order Plan is available for this series. A continuation order will bring delivery of each new volume immediately upon publication. Volumes are billed only upon actual shipment. For further information please contact the publisher.

INTERACTIVE PHENOMENA IN THE CARDIAC SYSTEM

Edited by

Samuel Sideman and Rafael Beyar

Technion-Israel Institute of Technology
Haifa, Israel

PLENUM PRESS • NEW YORK AND LONDON

Library of Congress Cataloging-in-Publication Data

Interactive phenomena in the cardiac system / edited by Samuel Sideman and Rafael Beyar.
p. cm. -- (Advances in experimental medicine and biology ; v. 346)
"Proceedings of the Eighth Henry Goldberg Workshop on Interactive Phenomena in the Cardiac System, held December 6-10, 1992, in Bethesda, Maryland"--T.p. verso.
Includes bibliographical references and index.
ISBN 0-306-44637-5
1. Heart--Physiology--Congresses. 2. Myocardium--Congresses. 3. Heart conduction system--Congresses. 4. Microcirculation--Congresses. 5. Coronary arteries--Congresses. I. Sideman, S. II. Beyar, Rafael. III. Henry Goldberg Workshop (8th : 1992 : Bethesda, Md. IV. Series.
[DNLM: 1. Cardiovascular System--physiology--congresses. 2. Microcirculation--physiology--congresses. 3. Electrophysiology--congresses. W1 AD559 v. 346 1993 / WG 102 I586 1992]
QP111.2.I54
612.1'7--dc20
DNLM/DLC
for Library of Congress 93-41097
CIP

Proceedings of the Eighth Henry Goldberg Workshop on Interactive Phenomena in the Cardiac System, held December 6–10, 1992, in Bethesda, Maryland

ISBN 0-306-44637-5

A Division of Plenum Publishing Corporation
233 Spring Street, New York, N.Y. 10013

Printed in the United States of America

In Memory

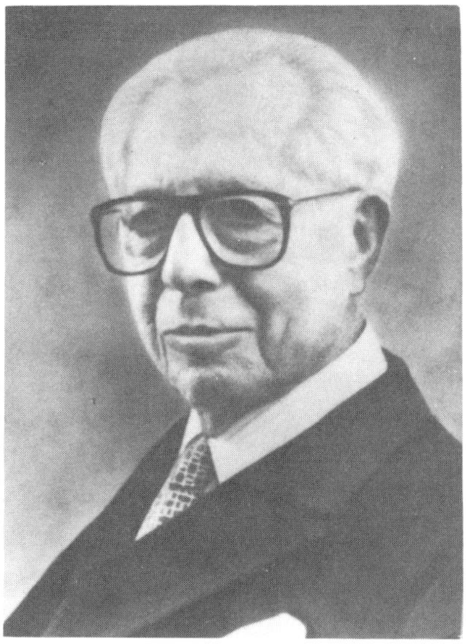

Henry Goldberg
1899 - 1991

Henry Goldberg was born in New York. Starting at 14 as an errand boy on Wall Street, he bought a seat on the New York Stock Exchange at the age of 21 and started a lifelong journey of living well and giving much to others. A self-made man, he had a life-long rule "to associate with people who know more than I do, so that I can always learn." Intelligent and bright, he was well read and extremely knowledgeable. His inquisitive mind knew no satisfaction. He supported the arts and saw every Broadway show, ballet and opera in New York City. He was on the Board of the Beth-Israel Hospital and took great interest in medical research and great pride when his support showed some promising results.

His contacts with the Technion-Israel Institute of Technology started when he established the Henry Goldberg Chair for a Visiting Professor in Biomedical Engineering and continued with the establishment of the Henry Goldberg Workshop series. He was most delighted with "his private library," the published proceedings of the workshops, and enjoyed the fact that he had been instrumental in building bridges between scientists from many different disciplines coming form different countries around the globe. New interactions between this extended Goldberg family gave him the greatest satisfaction, and the interplay between theoretical models, physiological reality and clinical practice, which was highlighted in the Henry Goldberg Workshops, gave him an intellectual charge. He believed that challenging the unknown in the cardiac system is a conscious intellectual task that requires great effort from cardiac scientists and practicing cardiologists around the globe. It is in this multidiscipline/multinational group that he helped bring together that we proudly and thankfully remember him, resolved to continue the international multidisciplined persuit to uncover the multilayered secrets of the cardiac system. May his soul rest in peace.

תנצב"ה

The 8th Henry Goldberg Workshop on
INTERACTIVE PHENOMENA IN THE CARDIAC SYSTEM

Sponsored by

MR. HENRY GOLDBERG
THE NATIONAL INSTITUTES OF HEALTH (NIH), USA
THE TECHNION–ISRAEL INSTITUTE OF TECHNOLOGY
THE ISRAEL CARDIOLOGY SOCIETY

Dedicated to

Our families – for their infinite patience and love
Our sponsors – for their trust and support
Our students and collaborators – for their intellectual stimulation
Our colleagues – for their competitive friendship

The 8th Henry Goldberg Workshop
on Interactive Phenomena in the Cardiac System

December 6–10, 1992
NIH - Bethesda, Maryland

Organizing Committee

Professor J. Bassingthwaighte
Director, Center of Biomedical Engineering, University of Washington, Seattle, WA, USA

Associate Professor R. Beyar, Co–Chairman
Department of Biomedical Engineering, Technion–Israel Institute of Technology, Haifa, 32000, Israel

Professor S. Sideman, Chairman
Chair, Department of Biomedical Engineering, Technion–Israel Institute of Technology, Haifa, 32000, Israel

Professor R. Reneman
Department of Physiology, University of Limburg, Rijksuniv, Limburg, The Netherlands

Professor E.L. Ritman
Biodynamics Laboratory, Mayo Medical School, Roshester, MN, USA

Professor W. Welkowitz
Department of Biomedical Engineering, Rutgers University, Piscataway, NJ, USA

Scientific Advisory Committee

Professor M. Gotsman
Director, Cardiology Department, Hadassah Medical Organization, Jerusalem, Israel

Professor J.I.E. Hoffman
Cardiovascular Research Institute, School of Medicine, University of California, San Francisco, CA, USA

Professor M. L. Weisfeldt, Chairman
Chair, Department of Medicine, Columbia Presbyterian Medical Center, New York, NY, USA

Professor A.L. Wit
Chair, Pharmacology Department, Columbia University, College of Physicians & Surgeons, New York, NY, USA

PREFACE

The cardiac system represents one of the most exciting challenges to human ingenuity. Critical to our survival, it consists of a tantalizing array of interacting phenomena, from ionic transport, membrane channels and receptors through cellular metabolism, energy production to fiber mechanics, microcirculation, electrical activation to the global, clinically observed, function, which is measured by pressure, volume, coronary flow, heart rate, shape changes and responds to imposed loads and pharmaceutical challenges. It is a complex interdisciplinary system requiring the joint efforts of the life sciences, the exact sciences, engineering and technology to understand and control the pathologies involved. The Henry Goldberg Workshops were set up to address these multivariable, multidisciplinary challenges. Briefly, our goals are: To encourage international cooperation and foster interdisciplinary interaction between scientists from the different areas of cardiology; to relate microscale cellular phenomena to the global, clinically manifested cardiac function; to relate conceptual modeling and quantitative analysis to experimental and clinical data; to gain an integrated view of the various interacting parameters, identify missing links, catalyze new questions, and lead to better understanding of the cardiac system.

The outstanding success of past workshops has encouraged their continuation. The first Henry Goldberg Workshop, held in Haifa in 1984, introduced the concept of interaction between mechanics, electrical activation, perfusion and metabolism, emphasizing imaging in the clinical environment. The second Workshop, in 1985, discussed the same parameters with a slant towards the control aspects. The Third Henry Goldberg Workshop, held in the USA at Rutgers University in 1986, highlighted the transformation of the microscale activation phenomena to macroscale activity and performance, relating electrophysiology, energy metabolism and cardiac mechanics. The Fourth Henry Goldberg Workshop in 1987 continued the effort to elucidate the interactions between the various parameters affecting cardiac performance, with emphasis on the ischemic heart. The Fifth Workshop, held in Cambridge, UK, in 1988, dwelt on the effects of inhomogeneity of the cardiac muscle on its performance in health and disease. The Sixth Workshop, aimed to highlight the role of new modern imaging techniques, which allow us to gain more insight into local and global cardiac performance in cardiac research and clinical practice. The seventh Workshop aimed at in–depth exploration of the basic microlevel phenomena that affect the cardiac system in health and disease. The present Workshop aims at highlighting some of the basic interactions which affect the activation and performance of the cardiac system.

The present volume represents our eighth attempt to bring together diversified expertise in the various fields of science, engineering and medicine, and to relate the numerous interactive parameters and disciplines involved in the performance of the heart. This gathering of outstanding scientists from all over the world is a testimonial to international cooperation and highlights the pleasure of joining hands in the pursuit of the secrets of life.

It is with great pleasure that we acknowledge here those who have helped make this meeting a reality. Special thanks are due to Mr. Julius Silver and Ms. Dinny Winslow (Silver) of New York, for their personal support and continued friendship which inspired and shaped our goals and made it all possible. Thanks are also due to the Women's Division of the American Society for the Technion, who encouraged us with their unshakable trust and provided the means to start the Heart System Research Center. Personal thanks go to the Scientific Advisory Committe, and the Organizing Committee. Particular thanks go to our hosts of the NIH, Drs. Murray Eden and Richard Chadwick, who set the environment to make this meeting a most enjoyable encounter. Our warmhearted thanks go to the late Mr. Henry Goldberg and his wife Viola, for their generosity and kindness, which made these Henry Goldberg Workshops significant milestones in cardiac research. Last, we acknowledge with pleasure and many thanks the secretarial and editorial work of Ms. Deborah Shapiro, who made this book what it is.

Samuel Sideman
Rafael Beyar

The cardiac system and cardiac interactions involve both engineering and medicine. Medicine and engineering are two great ancient professions, both dedicated to the betterment of the human condition. Medicine helps men and women cope with the wellbeing of their bodies and minds, whereas engineering helps man cope with his environment by providing food and shelter and improving the standard of living. Both are crucial in man's struggle for survival. To a large extent, these two professions have made us the only animal that does not fit into an evolutionary niche destined for it by nature; man creates his own niche and makes his own unique physical, mental and cultural environment.

Medicine and engineering have come from *practice* and *not* from *theory*. They have both *preceded* science by hundreds of centuries but they have both been enormously enriched by the permeation of the sciences. The central task of the natural sciences is to make the wonderful commonplace, to show that complexity correctly viewed is only a mask for simplicity. Indeed, dissecting medicine and engineering by the scientific tools of analysis uncovers not only the simplicity behind the complexity, and makes it understandable to humans, but also enables the recombination, the synthesis of the components into magnificent new controllable and *understandable* complexities.

The greater the decomposition down to the cell, the molecule, the atomic levels, the greater the potential for reassembling, creating and synthesizing novel and immensely important healing solutions, properties and products.

It is science that weaves medicine and engineering together. This is why you find them both on the Technion campus; this is the essence of the work carried out by Prof. Sideman and his colleagues at the Julius Silver Institute of Biomedical Engineering at the Technion. Fusing together medicine and engineering, both permeated by the sciences, creates a synergistic amalgam of enormous potential for the betterment of the human condition.

It is in this spirit of scientific progress that I wish you successful deliberations.

Professor Zeev Tadmor
President, Technion–Israel Institute of Technology

GREETINGS

On behalf of the Office of the Director and in particular Dr. Healey, who you know is a cardiologist, I would like to welcome all of you to the 8th Henry Goldberg Workshop on Interactive Phenomenon in the Cardiac System. This is the latest in a series of what I believe to be a very successful and extremely innovative Workshops that have been held in the USA only once before. The purpose of this Workshop is to bring together internationally renowned cardiac scientists from a variety of disciplines and, through cross–fertilization of ideas and insights, develop an integrated approach to the science of the cardiac system. These meetings are a catalyst for multi–institutional and international collaboration. The area of focus is molecular cardiology today and tomorrow, with an emphasis on regulation, cross–communication, and remodeling, going from the individual signaling molecules in the myocardial cell to cell–cell interactions at the chemical, electrical and mechanical level, all the way to remodeling phenomena and system dynamics. One overall theme is control through molecular communication. As Norbert Weiner, an American engineer and an inspirational mathematician stated, "the theory of control of engineering, whether human, or animal, or mechanical, is a chapter in the theory of messages."

In this Workshop we will be examining the messages themselves at the molecular, cellular and system level. We are grateful to the co–sponsors of this meeting, the National Center for Research Resources–NIH, the Technion–Israel Institute of Technology and the Israeli Cardiology Society. I extend my congratulations to Sam Sideman, Rafael Beyar, Murray Eden, Richard Chadwick and the others, and all the terrific speakers, for what promises to be a landmark conference. Henry Goldberg would have been very proud.

Lance Liotta, M.D., Ph.D.
Deputy Director for Intramural Research–NIH
Co–Director, Anatomic Pathology Residency Program, National Cancer Institute

I am happy to welcome all of you to Bethesda and look forward to this very important Workshop. I want to thank the Henry Goldberg Family for their generous support for this Workshop, and Dr. Sideman and Dr. Beyar for the time and energy that they have spent organizing this important Workshop. The National Center for Research Resources is happy to be a co–sponsor with Technion. Technion is Israel's oldest university and the only institute of higher education devoted solely to the education of engineers, architects, scientists and physicians. At this Workshop, NCRR's Biomedical Engineering and Instrumentation Program as well as its Biomedical Research Technology and Cardiac Medicine Programs are represented. This is a fine example of how the national set–up for research resources carries out its broad mission to develop and support critical research technologies, to maintain and improve our nation's health, and specifically, in the context of this Workshop, cardiac related research.

The 8th Henry Goldberg Workshop promotes an integrated approach to the study of the cardiac system. This paradigm provides for an exciting exchange of ideas by bringing together investigators from a wide variety of disciplines to stimulate new collaborations and catalyze new research areas. Dr. Liotta has spoken of the electricity and cross–fertilization that comes from the diverse ideas and proximity of excellence. I believe that the same electricity will spark a lively interchange here today, to include a broad spectrum of research throughout the academic communities everywhere.

Dr. Judith L. Vaitukaitis, M.D.
Director, National Center for Research Resources (NCRR)–NIH

CONTENTS

Cell to Organ: Electromechanical Activation

Chapter 1
Regulation of Intracellular Calcium in Cardiac Muscle
Peter H. Backx, Wei Dong Gao, Michelle D. Azan-Backx, and Eduardo Marban 3

Chapter 2
Neuromodulation of Calcium Current by Extracellular ATP in Isolated Ventricular Myocytes
Yusheng Qu, Donald L. Campbell, Herbert H. Himmel and Harold C. Strauss 11

Chapter 3
Intracellular Calcium and Myocardial Function during Ischemia
David G. Allen, Simeon P. Cairns, Stuart E. Turvey and John A. Lee 19

Chapter 4
Intracellular Signaling in Vascular Smooth Muscle
Avril V. Somlyo and Andrew P. Somlyo 31

Chapter 5
Myocardial Energetics
Lincoln E. Ford 39

Chapter 6
Mechanisms of Endocardial Endothelium Modulation of Myocardial Performance
Stanislas U. Sys, Luc J. Andries, Thierry C. Gillebert, and Dirk L. Brutsaert 51

Chapter 7
Calcium Kinetic and Mechanical Regulation of the Cardiac Muscle
Amir Landesberg and Samuel Sideman 59

Chapter 8
Cellular Responses to Electrical Stimulation: A Study Using a Model of the Ventricular Cardiac Action Potential
Yoram Rudy and Ching-hsing Luo 79

Chapter 9
Excitation-Contraction Coupling and Contractile Protein Function in Failing and Nonfailing Human Myocardium
Gerd Hasenfuss, Burkert Pieske, Christian Holubarsch, Norman R. Alpert and Hanjörg Just 91

Mechanics and Microcirculation

Chapter 10
Estimation of Myocardial Mechanical Properties with Dynamic Transverse Stiffness
Henry R. Halperin, Joshua E. Tsitlik, Barry K. Rayburn, Jon R. Resar, Julie Z. Livingston, and Frank C.P. Yin 103

Chapter 11
Intramyocardial Mechanical States: Vessel–Interstitium–Muscle Interface
J. Yasha Kresh 113

Chapter 12
Myocardial Mechanics and Coronary Flow Dynamics
Rafael Beyar, Dan Manor and Samuel Sideman 125

Chapter 13
Modeling of Coronary Capillary Flow
Gadi Fibich, Yoram Lanir, Nadav Liron, and Mark Abovsky 137

Microstructure: Mechanics and Microcirculation

Chapter 14
Models for Coronary Pressure–Flow Relationships
Robert E. Mates and Robert M. Judd 153

Chapter 15
In Vivo Myocardial Microcirculation: Evaluation with a Whole–Body X–Ray CT Method
Erik L. Ritman 163

Chapter 16
Endocardial Coronary Microcirculation of the Beating Heart
Fumihiko Kajiya, Toyotaka Yada, Akihiro Kimura, Osamu Hiramatsu, Masami Goto, Yasuo Ogasawara, and Katsuhiko Tsujioka 173

Chapter 17
Distribution and Control of Coronary Microvascular Resistance
Christopher J. H. Jones, Lih Kuo, Michael J. Davis, and William M. Chilian 181

Chapter 18
Theoretical Analysis of Coronary Blood Flow and Tissue Oxygen Pressure–Control
Jos A.E. Spaan and Jenny Dankelman 189

Microcirculation and Metabolic Transport

Chapter 19
Adenosine Coronary Vasodilation during Hypoxia Depends on Adrenergic Receptor Activation
Eric O. Feigl 199

Chapter 20
Chaos in Cardiac Signals
James B. Bassingthwaighte 207

Chapter 21
Intramyocardial Fluid Transport Effects on Coronary Flow and Left Ventricular Mechanics
Daniel Zinemanas, Rafael Beyar and Samuel Sideman 219
Chapter 22
Metabolic Protection of Post–Ischemic Phosphorylation Potential and Ventricular Performance
Robert T. Mallet and Rolf Bünger 233
Chapter 23
Metabolic and Mechanical Control of the Microcirculation
Uri Dinnar 243

Remodeling of Muscle and Vessels

Chapter 24
Asymmetrical Changes in Ventricular Wall Mass by Asynchronous Electrical Activation of the Heart
Frits W. Prinzen, Tammo Delhaas, Theo Arts, and Robert S. Reneman 257
Chapter 25
Ventricular Remodeling after Myocardial Infarction
Gary F. Mitchell, Gervasio A. Lamas, and Marc A. Pfeffer 265
Chapter 26
Arterial Remodelling after Percutaneous Transluminal Balloon Angioplasty
Yoseph Rozenman, Chaim Lotan, Dan Gilon, Morris Mosseri, Dan Sapoznikov, Sima Welber, and Mervyn S. Gotsman 277
Chapter 27
Structural and Functional Remodeling of Poststenotic Arteries in the Rat
Jo G.R. De Mey, Harry Van Der Heijden, Ger Janssen, and Gregorio Fazzi 283
Chapter 28
Myocardial Collagen and Its Functional Role
Joseph S. Janicki, Beatriz B. Matsubara, and Ameer Kabour 291

Cardiac Function and Circulation

Chapter 29
Ventricular–Arterial Interaction: Cardiac Effects of Mean versus Pulsatile Arterial Load
David A. Kass 301
Chapter 30
The Veins and Ventricular Preload
John V. Tyberg, Nairne W. Scott–Douglas, Yudi Wang, and Dante E. Manyari 313
Chapter 31
Why Smaller Animals Have Higher Heart Rates
Nicolaas Westerhof and Gijs Elzinga 319

Chapter 32
Feedback Effects in Heart–Arterial System Interaction
John K–J. Li . . . 325

Integrated Analysis

Chapter 33
The Relationship between Altered Load and Impaired Diastolic Function in Conscious Dogs with Pacing Induced Heart Failure
Richard P. Shannon . . . 337

Chapter 34
Interactions: The Integrated Functioning of Heart and Lungs
Eric A. Hoffman . . . 347

Chapter 35
Carotid–Cardiac Interaction: Heart Rate Variability during the Unblocking of the Carotid Artery
Metin Akay, Giora Landesberg, Walter Welkowitz, Yasemin M. Akay, and Dan Sapoznikov . . . 365

Chapter 36
Right and Left Ventricle Interaction and Remodeling in Congenital Heart Disease
Richard S. Chadwick, Annabelle Azancot–Benisty, Jacques Ohayon, and Yuho Ito . . . 373

Chapter 37
Macroscopic Three–Dimensional Motion Patterns of the Left Ventricle
Theo Arts, William C. Hunter, Andrew S. Douglas, Arno M.M. Muijtjens, Jan W. Corsel, and Robert S. Reneman . . . 383

Chapter 38
Cardiovascular Flow Velocity Measurements by 2D Doppler Imaging for Assessment of Vascular Function
Dan R. Adam, Kenneth M. Kempner, Mark A. Vivino, Eben E. Tucker and Michael Jones . . . 393

Closing Discussion: *A View into the Future* . . . 401

The Editors . . . 407

Contributors . . . 409

Index . . . 415

Cell to Organ:

Electromechanical Activation

CHAPTER 1

REGULATION OF INTRACELLULAR CALCIUM IN CARDIAC MUSCLE

Peter H. Backx, Wei Dong Gao, Michelle D. Azan–Backx, and Eduardo Marban[1]

ABSTRACT

We have investigated the regulation of intracellular free calcium in heart muscle using the free acid form of the Ca^{2+} indicator fura–2 iontophoretically microinjected into rat cardiac trabeculae or ferret papillary muscles. This method shows great promise in elucidating a number of crucial questions in cardiac excitation–contraction coupling.

INTRODUCTION

Ionized free calcium (Ca^{2+}) is 1,000– to 10,000–fold lower in the cytosol than it is in the extracellular space. The maintenance of this enormous transmembrane gradient for Ca^{2+} consumes much of the cardiac cell's energy, either directly or indirectly. Such tight regulation is crucial because Ca^{2+} plays a central role in the transduction mechanism linking excitation to contraction in cardiac muscle. As intracellular free Ca^{2+} concentration ($[Ca^{2+}]_i$) begins to exceed 100–200 nM, Ca^{2+} binds to troponin–C, initiating the cascade of crossbridge cycling and force generation. Using a variety of different calcium indicators in preparations ranging from isolated cells to intact hearts, much has been learned regarding the control of $[Ca^{2+}]_i$ in the myocardium. Nevertheless, important questions remain unresolved. One crucial area of deficiency has arisen from our inability to measure $[Ca^{2+}]_i$ reliably in small multicellular preparations in which force and sarcomere length can also be measured. Recently, Backx and TerKeurs [1] have described a novel method which fills this gap. We have adapted this method for use in our laboratory; the preliminary results described here illustrate the potential utility of this new methodology.

[1]Division of Cardiology, Department of Medicine, The Johns Hopkins University, 844 Ross Building, Baltimore MD 21205, USA.

Interactive Phenomena in the Cardiac System, Edited by
S. Sideman and R. Beyar, Plenum Press, New York, 1993

METHODS, MATERIALS AND PROCEDURES

Two types of myocardial preparations were used: rat trabeculae, or ferret papillary muscles. Trabeculae (approx. 3 mm long, 0.04 mm thick and 0.14 mm wide) were dissected from the right ventricle of 2–6 month–old Sprague–Dawley rats. Papillary muscles (approx. 4 mm long and 0.3 mm in diameter) were dissected from the right ventricles of ferrets (7 – 10 weeks old). The muscles were mounted in a perfusion bath (25 x 2 x 5 mm^3) on the stage of an inverted microscope (Nikon Diaphot, Tokyo, Japan) between a platinum wire attached to the silicon beam of a force transducer (AE801, AME, Sensonor, Norway) and a stainless steel needle attached to a micromanipulator. Muscles were superfused with a solution composed of (in mM) NaCl 120, $NaHCO_3$ 20, $MgCl_2$ 1, NaH_2PO_4 1, KCl 4.5, glucose 10, $CaCl_2$ 0.5 (unless otherwise indicated); pH was adjusted to 7.4 (22°C). Stimulation at 1 Hz was accomplished across two platinum electrodes running down either side of the bath.

Fura–2 salt was loaded into the muscle by intracellular iontophoresis, as described previously [1]. Briefly, fura–2 (K salt, 1 mM; Molecular Probes, Eugene, OR) was used to fill the tip of a microelectrode (˜0.2 μm tip diameter) while the remainder of the micropipette was back–filled with a solution containing 140 mM KCl and 10 mM HEPES buffered to a pH of 7.0. Following impalement of a superficial cell in the unstimulated muscle (as verified by membrane potential recordings), 4–10 nA of negative current was passed for about 10 – 20 minutes. The process of loading was followed visually by occasional ultraviolet illumination. Fura–2 was initially concentrated at the impalement site, then gradually spread to adjacent regions, consistent with the prediction that the molecule is sufficiently small (M.W. = 831) to cross gap junctions. The preparation was then stimulated at 1 Hz for about 1 hour, which appeared to enhance the rate of spread of fura–2 from the injected site. After this period of rapid stimulation, the preparation was uniformly loaded with the indicator.

To measure epifluorescence of fura–2, excitation ultraviolet (UV) light from a 75 W Xenon lamp (Oriel, Stanford CT), bandpass–filtered (Omega Optical, Brattleboro, VT) at 340 nm, 360 nm or 380 nm, was projected onto the muscle via a 10x objective (10x Fluor, Nikon, Tokyo, Japan) using a dichroic mirror (400DPLC, Nikon, Tokyo, Japan). The UV excitation light illuminates an area about 1.2 mm in diameter in the focal plane which contains the papillary muscle. The use of a large field of view minimizes movement artifacts and also reduces the amount of excitation light required to measure Ca^{2+}–dependent changes in fluorescence. In fact, the excitation light intensity was reduced by a factor of 10–100 (usually 50) by the interposition of fused silica neutral density filters (Omega Optical, Brattleboro, VT) in the light path. The fluorescent light is collected by the objective and transmitted through a bandpass filter at 510 nm (10 nm bandwidth) to a photomultiplier tube (R1527, Hamamatsu, Bridgeport NJ) attached to the camera port of the microscope. The photomultiplier output was filtered at 100 Hz (3dB), collected via an A/D converter (2801A Data–Translation, MA) and stored in the computer for later analysis. To avoid photobleaching, a manual shutter was used to restrict illumination to selected sampling intervals during the protocol (see below).

Intracellular Ca^{2+} concentration was given by the following equation [1]:

$$[Ca^{2+}]_i = K\,(R - R_{min})/(R_{max} - R) \qquad (1)$$

where R = observed ratio of fluorescence at 340 nm to that at 380 nm; K = apparent dissociation constant; R_{max} = the ratio of the fluorescence at 340 nm to that at 380 nm at a saturating $[Ca^{2+}]$; and R_{min} = the ratio of the fluorescence at 340 nm to that at 380 nm at a zero $[Ca^{2+}]$.

In this study, we used the following values for K, R_{min}, and R_{max} which were obtained in previous studies [1]: K = 3.3 μM, R_{min} = 0.3, R_{max} = 12. R_{min} and R_{max} were determined in situ by applying 140 mM KCl solution with 1 mM or zero [Ca^{2+}] in the presence of 20 μM 4–Br–A23187, 4 mM NaCN and 2 mM iodoacetate. K was determined by similar method using calibration solutions with known [Ca^{2+}]'s. End–systolic sarcomere length, measured using laser diffraction, was set at 2.1–2.2 microns in these studies.

RESULTS

The utility of our novel methodology for measuring intracellular [Ca^{2+}] along with force in cardiac muscle is illustrated in Fig. 1. The top panel shows the fluorescence at 380 nm (left) and 340 nm (right) excitation prior to ("back") and after placing ("auto") a muscle in the perfusion chamber. The difference between these fluorescence levels at either wavelength is a measure of the autofluorescence of the trabecula. The preparation was then loaded with fura–2 by passing 6 nAmps of current for a period of 17 minutes; this resulted in a two–fold increase in fluorescence of the trabecula above the autofluorescence level. After fura–2 loading, characteristic changes in fluorescence ("fluor") can be observed

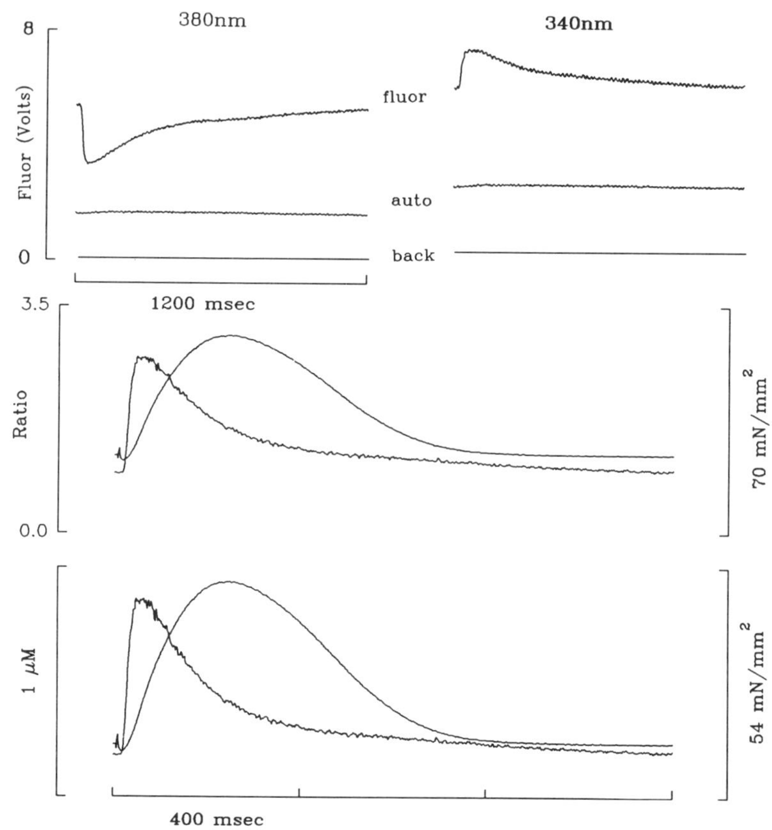

Figure 1. Single–wavelength signals at 340 nm and 380 nm excitation, as well as the 340/380 ratio and calculated $[Ca^{2+}]_i$ with force superimposed.

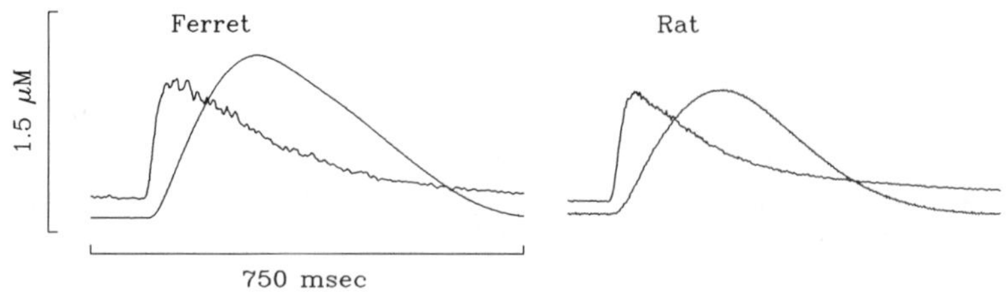

Figure 2. Calcium transients in ferret and rat ventricular muscle preparations.

during twitch contractions: the 380 nm signal decreases transiently, while 340 nm fluorescence increases transiently. The ratio of the background–subtracted fluorescence (340/380) is shown in the middle panel along with the force during a twitch. The bottom panel illustrates the [Ca^{2+}] transient estimated from the ratio in the middle panels using Eq. (1) above. Note that the rate of rise and the rate of relaxation of the [Ca^{2+}] transient are significantly greater than for the fluorescence ratio. This is a consequence of the non–linear relationship between the fluorescence ratio and the [Ca^{2+}] as given by equation (1). From this observation it is clear that accurate estimates of the kinetics of the [Ca^{2+}] transient cannot be determined from examination of either the raw fluorescence signals or the fluorescence ratio.

Despite well–recognized phylogenetic divergence, [Ca^{2+}] transients in rat and ferret ventricular muscle look remarkably similar when recorded under similar conditions. Figure 2 shows a side–by–side comparison of intracellular [Ca^{2+}] and force in a ferret papillary muscle (left) and in a rat trabecula (right). Both the [Ca^{2+}] transients and the twitches last somewhat longer in the ferret, consistent with known differences in action potential duration in the two species.

Elevations in the extracellular [Ca^{2+}] elevate the peak force generated by cardiac muscle. The direct dependence of this elevation of force on the [Ca^{2+}] transients is illustrated in Fig. 3, which shows twitch force and [Ca^{2+}] transients at three different

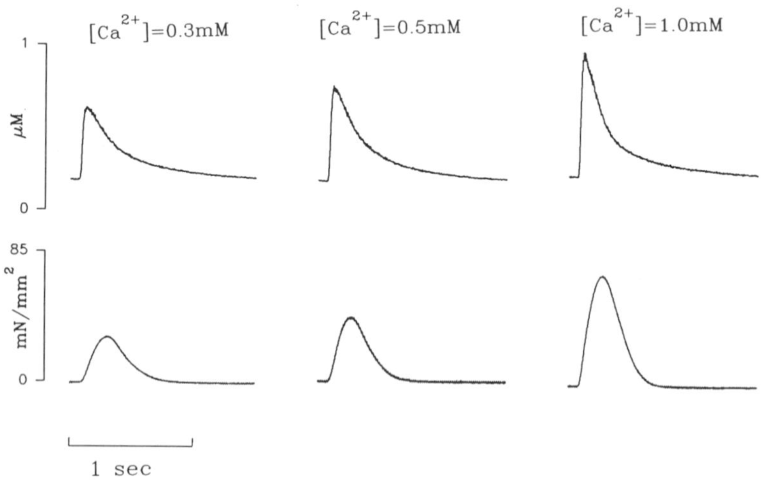

Figure 3. Calcium transients at three extracellular Ca concentrations in rat.

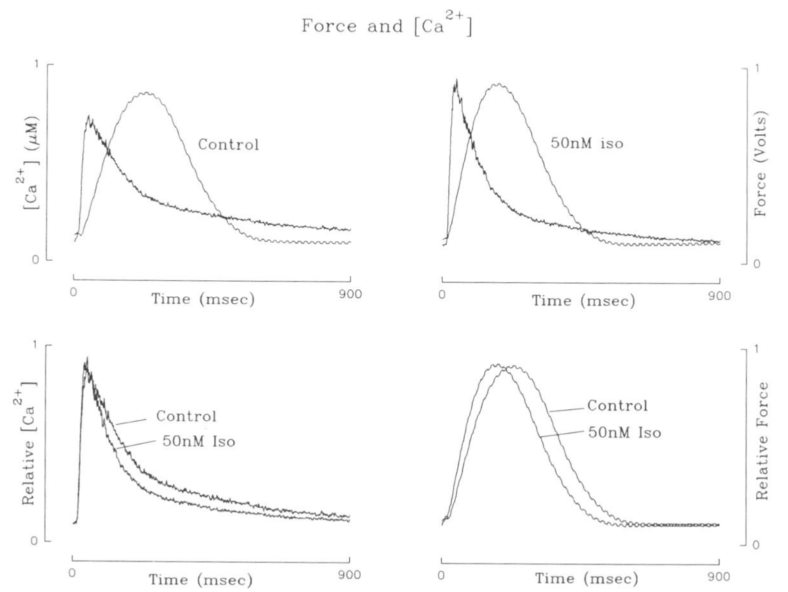

Figure 4. Effects of isoproterenol on $[Ca^{2+}]_i$ and force, absolute (top) and normalized (bottom).

$[Ca^{2+}]_o$s in a rat preparation. Interestingly, the rate of relaxation of the $[Ca^{2+}]$ transientincreases significantly as the peak increases. This may result from the known $[Ca^{2+}]$-dependence of the rate of activity of the SR–$[Ca^{2+}]$–ATPase and the Na^+/Ca^{2+} exchanger, which are primarily responsible for Ca^{2+} sequestration from the cytosol.

As a result of the strong direct dependence of force on $[Ca^{2+}]_i$, regulation of contraction in the heart occurs predominately by regulation of Ca^{2+} availability. Agents such as isoproterenol are commonly used to modulate the inotropic state of the heart and act at least partially by altering the availability of activator Ca^{2+}. Figure 4 illustrates the effects of a relatively low concentration of isoproterenol (50 nM) on $[Ca^{2+}]$ transients and force in a rat trabecula. The $[Ca^{2+}]$ transients are higher and decay more rapidly during exposure to isoproterenol. Interestingly, accelerated relaxation dominates the effects on force; the positive inotropic effect is surprisingly modest, perhaps because of myofilament desensitization related to cyclic–AMP–dependent phosphorylation.

DISCUSSION AND CONCLUSIONS

The present results illustrate the potential utility of this important new method. Compared to other available techniques, this is perhaps the best–suited for simultaneous measurement of Ca^{2+} transients and force in preparations in which sarcomere length can also be determined. Intracellular iontophoresis enables us to load fura–2 free acid throughout the myocardial syncytium whilst limiting the mechanical trauma of microelectrode penetration to only one cell. The use of the free acid form rather than the popular acetoxymethyl ester derivative obviates the complications of loading into organelles and of the accumulation of calcium–insensitive but fluorescent intermediates. Aequorin–injected papillary muscles have yielded much useful data, but the results are limited by a low signal–to–noise ratio and by the insensitivity of aequorin to changes of $[Ca^{2+}]_i$ in the diastolic range. While fura–2 or indo–1 are routinely applied in single cardiac cells, unloaded cell length rather than force has been utilized to index contraction, with potentially misleading results.

Despite its strong points, the present method has its own set of limitations, the most notable of which is the potential uncertainty introduced by possible changes in fura–2's calcium–binding properties within the cytosol. Fura–2 can bind to proteins in solution such that the dye becomes less calcium–sensitive. To the extent that this occurs within the cell, $[Ca^{2+}]_i$ may be underestimated. We have calibrated fura–2 within the cytosol using the approach of Li et al. [2]; the values for $[Ca^{2+}]_i$ so obtained are not very different from those estimated using techniques with quite complementary errors, such as aequorin, Ca–selective microelectrodes or the NMR–detectable indicator 5F–BAPTA. While such agreement is generally reassuring, specific conclusions reached with one indicator should be confirmed using another before being taken at face value. The more controversial the finding, the more important that it be validated with multiple methods. Thus, our next major effort will be directed at re–examining the controversial observation of Yue, Marban and Wier [3] that myofilament Ca^{2+} sensitivity is much greater in intact cells than in skinned fibers.

DISCUSSION

Dr. D. Allen: Clearly, the intact fiber is the gold standard and the question is why the skinned fiber is different. My favorite explanation is that intact fibers are now known to have endogenous sensitizers such as imidazole compounds which are washed out when you skin them; another possibility is the influence of ionic strength. We do not know what the ionic strength is inside a fiber and if you vary the ionic strength of a skinned fiber you can vary Ca^{2+} sensitivity over a wide range.

Dr. E. Marban: I completely agree. I like the idea that there are endogenous sensitizers and this preparation puts us in a position to try and reconcile the two sets of data by readdition of different substances. That is one thing we would like to try. As far as ionic strength is concerned, we have taken a rather conventional skinning solution and applied it just to try to reproduce the discrepancy, but varying ionic strength is another thing that we would like to do. The other thing worth testing is myofilament lattice expansion, and we need to do things like addition of dextrans.

Dr. A. Somlyo: There are some new methods for permeabilizing cells which have been successfully used in smooth muscle. Instead of using glycerol, saponin, digitonin, or mechanically removing the membrane, you can use staphlyococcal–alpha–toxin. The protein actually incorporates into the membrane and forms a pore of about 2 nanometers with a cut–off of about 1000 Dalton molecular weight, so that what happens is you retain all the kinases, phosphatases, calmodulin and possibly, the sensitizing factors, the receptor–G–protein coupling remains intact. This approach might be another interesting way to probe your preparations.

Dr. E. Marban: Staphlyococcal–alpha–toxin is expensive and does not work very well in heart muscle, I've been told, but we have not used it yet. Did you use that in vascular smooth muscle or in heart cells?

Dr. A. Somlyo: Predominately in vascular smooth muscle. I have heard that it permeabilizes cardiac muscle.

Dr. E. Marban: That would be useful; that is something we have on our menu. We heard from Yale Goldman that you use beta–escin, and I would like to discuss the relative advantages of those two methods with you.

Dr. A. Somlyo: Yes, beta–escin basically makes larger holes yet retains the receptor–G protein coupling, as we reported *[Kobayashi et al., J Biol Chem 1984; 264: 17997–18004]*.

Dr. A. Landesberg: You have shown that there is a difference in calcium sensitivity in the intact cell compared with the skinned cell. Kentish et al. *[Circ Res 1986; 58: 755–768]* measured force–length relationship in the intact cell and the skin cell and they show that you can get the same curves of the force–length relationship for the skin cell and for the intact cell. Thus, although there is a difference in calcium transient, the mechanism may be the same. This means that calcium affinity has an adaptive mechanism. Calcium binding to troponin can change at different conditions, but the mechanism that regulates the mechanical property and dictates the length–force and free calcium relationship is the same for the intact cell and the skin cell.

Dr. E. Marban: The known dependence of calcium transients on length works in the wrong direction to explain this discrepancy. First of all we have measured sarcomere length in these preparations and set them to a place where the force–calcium relation is maximally sensitized; at about 2.2 microns end–systolic sarcomere length. In the intact cell there is a bit of internal shortening which is less predominant during a steady activation after skinning. But if there were some shortening deactivation occurring in the intact cell, it would help desensitize rather than sensitize the intact relative to the skinned cell.

Dr. A. Landesberg: In your measurements of the force–length relationship in the intact cell, did you get a different relationship and curvilinearity from these for skinned cell, except for the difference in calcium concentration.

Dr. E. Marban: We have actually done it, and we get some differences. We have compared intact and skinned cells; they both were qualitatively the same, but the calcium–force curves exhibited less cooperativity in the skinned cells.

Dr. G. Hasenfuss: How do you load your cells with fura–2? Do you use a pipette to micro–inject it? what is the procedure?

Dr. E. Marban: We penetrate a single cell in this preparation. We then verify that we are intracellular by measuring membrane potential. At that point we pass current which hyperpolarizes the membrane; since fura–2 free acid is a negative molecule, we get the fura–2 into the cell by iontophoresis. Essentially fura–2 is the charge carrier. One cell gets injected and its neighbors get loaded via the gap junctions.

Dr. S. Sys: How does the mechanical performance of the very thin trabeculae compare to the mechanical performance of the papillary muscle?

Dr. E. Marban: The trabeculae are somewhat more robust, not surprisingly, because they are thinner and more homogenous but in retrospect, the early papillary muscles were actually not that bad.

Dr. D. Kass: What is known about the ultra–structure of sarcomeres after skinning? Is there any change in the registration of sarcomeres, as has been described in some failure models, where there is disruption of the registration of sarcomeres.

Dr. E. Marban: You can sometimes see gross sarcomere inhomogeneity after skinning and we discard those data. The ones that we like to use are those that, even after skinning, preserve sarcomere homogeneity; you get a very nice diffraction pattern and that diffraction pattern is conserved along the area of observation.

REFERENCES

1. Backx PH, terKeurs, HEDJ. Fluorescent properties of rat cardiac trabeculae microinjected with fura–2 salt. *Am J Physiol* 1993; in press.
2. Li Q, Altschuld RA, Stokes BT. Quantitation of intracellular free calcium in single cardiomyocytes by fura–2 fluorescence microscopy. *Biochem Biophys Res Commun* 1987; 147:120–126.
3. Yue DT, Marban E, Wier WG. Relationship between force and intracellular [Ca^{2+}] in tetanized mammalian heart muscle. *J Gen Physiol* 1986; 87:223–242.

CHAPTER 2

Neuromodulation of Calcium Current by Extracellular ATP in Isolated Ventricular Myocytes

Yusheng Qu[1], Donald L. Campbell[1], Herbert H. Himmel[1] and Harold C. Strauss[1,2]

ABSTRACT

The effects of extracellular ATP on the L-type Ca^{2+} current (I_{Ca}), action potential, and resting and intracellular Ca^{2+} levels were examined in enzymatically isolated myocytes from the right ventricles of ferrets. Extracellular ATP decreased the peak amplitude of I_{Ca} in a time- and concentration-dependent manner. The concentration-response relationship for ATP inhibition of I_{Ca} was well described by a conventional Michaelis-Menten relationship with a half maximal inhibitory concentration of 1μM and a maximal effect of 50%. Extracellular ATP did not change the resting myoplasmic Ca^{2+} levels; however, it did decrease the Ca^{2+} transient. The effects of extracellular ATP were mediated independently of adenosine A_1 receptors and a pertussis-toxin sensitive G protein. Pharmacological characterization of receptor subtype using ATP analogs was consistent with ATP binding to a P_{2Y} type receptor.

INTRODUCTION

The autonomic nervous system is recognized to play an important role in post-infarction arrhythmias in man [1, 2]. Studies in dogs have demonstrated that transmural myocardial infarction causes denervation sensitivity apical to the infarct region in the left ventricle, making the heart more vulnerable to electrical induction of ventricular arrhythmias during stimulation of the ansae subclaviae than in these animals with denervation or infarction alone [3]. The protective effect exhibited by propranolol in this animal model suggests that this arrhythmogenic mechanism is mediated in part via ß-adrenergic recep-

Departments of [1]Medicine and [2]Pharmacology, Duke University Med. Center, Durham, NC 27710, USA.

Interactive Phenomena in the Cardiac System, Edited by
S. Sideman and R. Beyar, Plenum Press, New York, 1993

tors, although other contributing factors were not evaluated [4]. One additional possibility that should be considered is that cotransmitters released from sympathetic nerve terminals may play an important contributing role in the generation of post–infarction arrhythmias.

ATP has been reported to be a cotransmitter released with NE from sympathetic nerve terminals [5]. ATP has been demonstrated to have arrhythmogenic properties in rat ventricular myocytes by virtue of its ability to increase resting myoplasmic $[Ca^{2+}]_i$ and to activate a non–selective cation current [6–9]. Such ATP–activated nonselective currents produce cellular depolarization to action potential threshold, leading to the opening of voltage–gated, L–type Ca channels [8–11]. However, results concerning the effects of ATP on both the intracellular calcium transient and other cation currents appear controversial [12–14], with the excitatory effects of ATP reported only in rat ventricular myocytes thus far. In addition, information about the signalling pathway underlying these electrophysiologic actions is limited. Thus, we initiated a combined electrophysiologic and biochemical study of ATP's neuromodulatory effects on ferret single ventricular myocytes.

METHODS

Single myocytes were isolated from ferret right ventricles via the Langendorff perfusion method, as previously described [14,15]. Action potentials and I_{Ca} were recorded using the single microelectrode "gigaseal" patch clamp technique in the whole–cell recording configuration as previously described [14–17]. Intracellular Ca^{2+} ($[Ca^{2+}]_i$) and cell shortening were measured using a microfluorimetry system as previously described [15]. Changes in $[Ca^{2+}]_i$ were measured using either the salt or base form of fura–2.

RESULTS

Extracellular ATP reversibly inhibited voltage–activated L–type I_{Ca} in isolated ferret ventricular myocytes in a concentration–dependent manner. Effects of low and high concentrations (10^{-7}, 10^{-5} M) of ATP were also examined on the current–voltage relationship for I_{Ca} (Figs. 1 and 2). ATP reduced the peak I_{Ca} I–V relationship without significantly altering either the apparent reversal potential for I_{Ca} or the holding current (Fig. 2). The concentration–response relationship measured at 0 mV could be described by a conventional Michaelis–Menten relationship with maximal inhibition of I_{Ca} (0 mV) of 45.9 ± 11.0% (n=10) and half–maximal inhibitory concentration (IC_{50}) of ~1 μM (Fig. 3).

Since ATP reduced the amplitude of I_{Ca}, one would predict that it would decrease action potential duration consistent with its effect on I_{Ca}. ATP (0.5 μM) hyperpolarized the plateau phase of the action potential and accelerated early repolarization, thereby shortening action potential duration. To exclude the possibility that Na free solutions might modify the effects of extracellular ATP, ATP (10 μM) was also examined in physiologic salt solutions, where it reduced the peak net inward current by 35 ± 3.0%.

Because $[Ca^{2+}]_i$ has been reported to increase during ATP exposure in rat ventricular myocytes, we examined the effects of ATP on quiescent ferret ventricular myocytes loaded with fura–2. No consistent change in fluorescence ratio was seen during exposure to 10 μM ATP (Fig. 4). As extracellular ATP decreased I_{Ca}, we also examined its effects on the $[Ca^{2+}]_i$ transient using K_5–fura–2 (Fig. 5). ATP (10 μM) markedly attenuated the amplitude of the $[Ca^{2+}]_i$ transient, which was partially reversible on washout. On average, ATP (10 μM) reduced the $[Ca^{2+}]_i$ transient by 37.5 ± 3.8% (n=8), while the amplitude of peak net inward current concomitantly decreased by 35.2 ± 2.9%.

To establish that the effects of ATP were distinguishable from those produced by adenosine and A_1 receptors, we performed the following series of experiments. A non-hydrolyzable form of ATP, ATPγs (10 μM), produced a reversible inhibition of I_{Ca} similar to that produced by ATP (40.3 ± 12.8%). Exposure to the A_1 receptor antagonist CPDX (50 μM) did not block the inhibitory effect of ATP (41.5 ± 7.6%). Finally, the inhibitory effects of supramaximal concentrations of adenosine and ATP on I_{Ca} were additive. In the

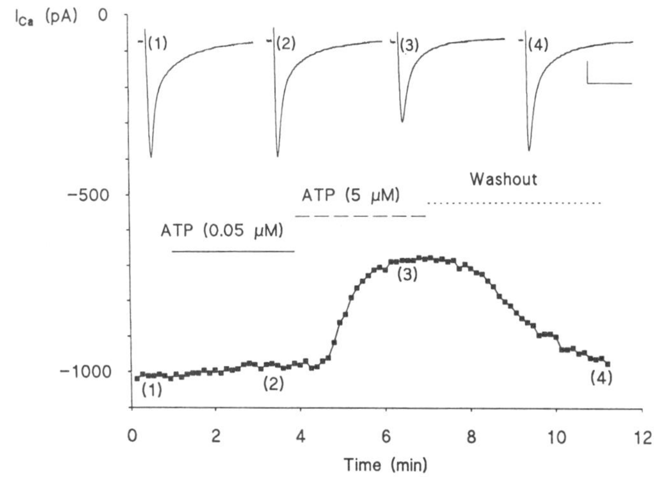

Figure 1. Effects of extracellular ATP on L-type Ca^{2+} current (I_{Ca}) in an isolated ferret right ventricular myocyte. The holding potential was – 70 mV and a 500 msec test pulse to 0 mV was introduced every 8 s. Current traces 1 to 4 correspond to control (1), 0.05 μM ATP (2), 5.0 μM ATP (3), and washout (4). Note that the inhibitory effects of ATP on I_{Ca} are concentration dependent and reversible. Calibration: 200 pA, 100 ms (from [15], with permission of the American Physiological Society).

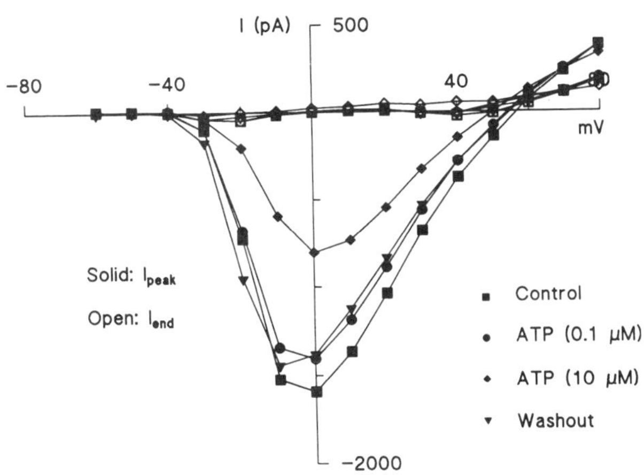

Figure 2. Effects of ATP on current-voltage (I–V) relationship of I_{Ca} in isolated ferret right ventricular myocytes. I–V relationship was measured using a holding potential of –70 mV and 500 ms depolarizing pulses ranging between –70 to +80 mV in 10 mV steps. Peak difference ($I_{Ca,peak}$ – $I_{Ca,500ms}$) and isochronal (500 ms) I–V relationship are illustrated for control, 0.1 μM ATP, 10 μM ATP, and washout (from [15], with permission of the American Physiological Society).

presence of 1 mM adenosine, subsequent addition of 1 mM ATP caused an additional inhibition of I_{Ca} of 36.6 ± 6.4%. These data support the view that adenosine and ATP inhibit I_{Ca} by different pharmacological mechanisms.

Pharmacological characterization of the P_2 receptor subtype revealed a potency order among ATP analogs as follows: 2-methylthio ATP (IC_{50}=0.05 μM) > ATP (IC_{50} = 1 μM) > α,ß-methylene-ATP (inhibition minimal at 1 mM), which is consistent for ATP analogs binding to a P_{2Y} type receptor.

To evaluate whether or not a pertussis toxin sensitive G protein was involved in the receptor coupling process, isolated ventricular myocytes were incubated in PTX for 4 hr at 37°C, which produced greater than 90% ribosylation of PTX-sensitive G proteins. PTX pretreatment abolished the inhibitory effect of adenosine on basal I_{Ca} without attenuating the effect of 5 μM ATP on I_{Ca} (PTX, 33.4±2.6% inhibition; control, 36.6±4.3% inhibition).

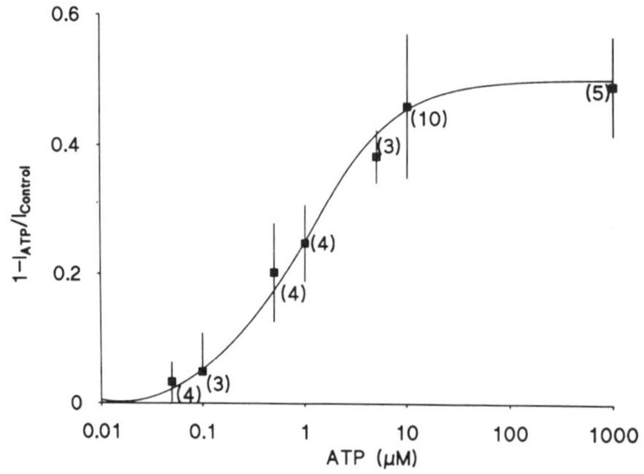

Figure 3. Concentration-response relationship for ATP effect on I_{Ca} using protocol illustrated in Fig. 1. Numbers in parentheses indicate mean number of cells studied at each concentration. Data were fit by a Michaelis–Menten relationship [$E = E_{max} \times [ATP]/(IC_{50} + [ATP])$]. E_{max} = maximal effect and IC_{50} = half-maximal inhibitory concentration (from [15], with permission of the American Physiological Society).

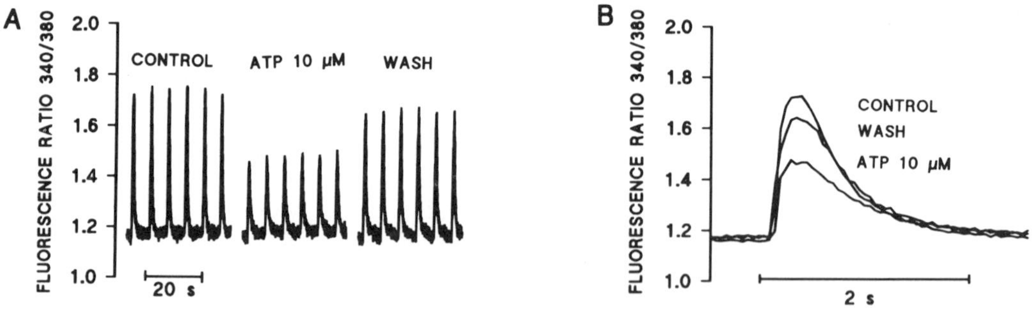

Figure 4. Effect of 10μM ATP on resting cytosolic [Ca^{2+}] in resting ferret ventricular myocytes loaded with fura-2/AM. **A:** time course of the fluorescence ratio (340/380 nm) in 5 different individual resting myocytes. Myocytes were exposed to ATP for 5 min; interruption at the beginning of the washout period represents 5 min. **B:** average fluorescence ratio (mean ± SD, n = 12) measured prior, during, and following exposure to ATP (7 min washout) (from [15], with permission of the American Physiological Society).

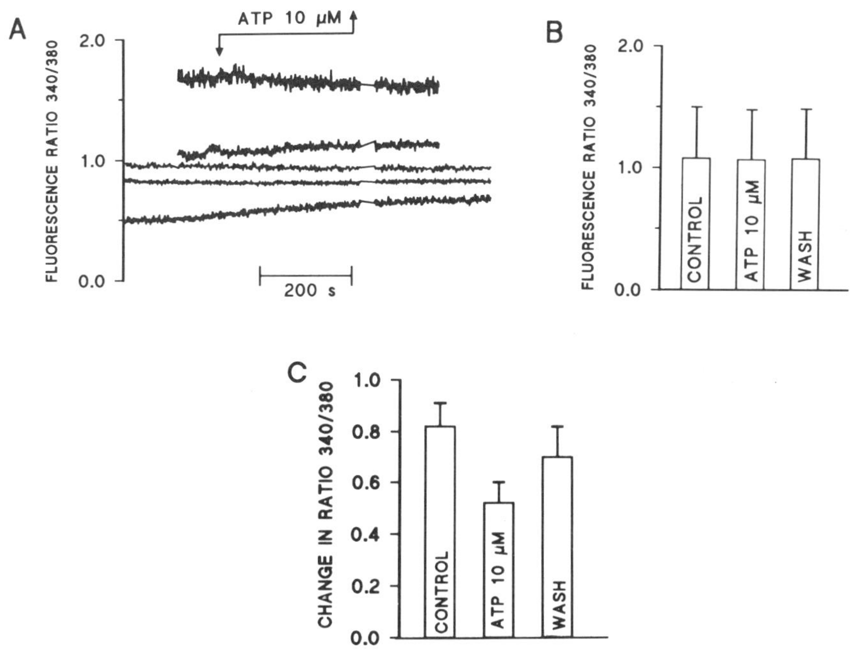

Figure 5. Effect of ATP (10μM) on amplitude of $[Ca^{2+}]_i$ transient in voltage-clamped isolated ferret ventricular myocytes loaded with K_5-fura-2. **A:** successive $[Ca^{2+}]_i$ transients during control, ATP, and washout. $[Ca^{2+}]_i$ transients illustrated were elicited by test potentials to +5mV from a holding potential of −40mV (pulse duration, 300 ms) every 6 s. At intervening times holding potential was −80mV. **B:** superimposition of 3 individual $[Ca^{2+}]_i$ transients from A. **C:** average amplitude of $[Ca^{2+}]_i$ transients (mean ± SD, n = 8) under control, ATP exposure and after 7 min of washout (from [15], with permission of the American Physiological Society).

To determine if ATP inhibits I_{Ca} by activating intracellular second messengers, single Ca channel activity was recorded using the cell-attached patch-clamp configuration, and ATP was applied to the solution perfusing the myocyte surface outside of the patch pipettes. If ATP were exerting its effects on Ca channels by activating diffusible second messengers, these effects should be evident in Ca channels inside the patch. An inhibitory effect of bath-applied ATP (10 μM) on ensemble average currents was seen in 3 patches (each containing at least 3 Ca channels). These data suggest that ATP modulation of I_{Ca} involves diffusible cytosolic second messengers generated following P_{2Y} receptor activation. However, using intracellular dialysis techniques, we were able to show that changes in $[Ca^{2+}]_i$, inositol phosphates, protein kinase A and protein kinase C were not involved in mediating the reduction of L-type I_{Ca} in isolated ferret right ventricular myocytes [17], indicating that some other second messenger system must be involved.

DISCUSSION AND CONCLUSIONS

The responses to extracellular ATP are diverse and variable among different cell types [18]. It is well documented that extracellular ATP increases $[Ca^{2+}]_i$ levels in a variety of cell types [8,19]. In isolated mammalian cardiac myocytes, the effects of extracellular

ATP have up until now only been studied in rat ventricular myocytes, with variability in the reported results. In this preparation, extracellular ATP has been reported to activate a non–specific cation current, which in turn depolarized the membrane and elicited an action potential [9]. However, while there does seem to be a consensus that extracellular ATP increases resting myoplasmic $[Ca^{2+}]_i$ in rat ventricular myocytes, both extracellular ATP–mediated increases and decreases in I_{Ca} have been reported [20], as well as both increases [7] and decreases [8] in the $[Ca^{2+}]_i$ transient. As a result, the effects of extracellular ATP on Ca^{2+} homeostatic mechanisms in rat ventricular myocytes appear to be complicated and not entirely agreed upon.

Our results are the first to demonstrate that ATP inhibits basal L–type I_{Ca} in isolated ferret ventricular myocytes via a mechanism that is independent of the A_1 adenosine receptor signalling pathway, and that a PTX–insensitive G protein is involved in coupling activation of the P_{2Y} receptor to inhibition of I_{Ca}. Finally, although we have not identified the second messenger pathways, our results indicate that $[Ca^{2+}]_i$, protein kinase C, protein kinase A, and inositol phosphates are not primarily involved in mediating the inhibitory effect of ATP on I_{Ca} in these myocytes.

In contrast to the results obtained in rat ventricular myocytes, we consistently failed to observe any increases in resting $[Ca^{2+}]_i$ in ferret ventricular myocytes upon application of micromolar levels of extracellular ATP [15]. Furthermore, we failed to find any consistent evidence that non–selective cation channels activated by extracellular ATP are present in ferret ventricular myocytes, as evidenced by the lack of any consistent changes in holding current or the apparent E_{rev} of I_{Ca} (in either NMDG or normal Na^+, K^+ solution: see 19). Such non–selective cation channels appear to be the main mechanism by which ATP increases $[Ca^{2+}]_i$ levels in rat ventricular myocytes [9].

The "single–channel, second messenger test" experiments demonstrated that extracellular ATP decreased the ensemble average current of single L–type Ca channels recorded in the cell–attached patch configuration, i.e. even though the patch itself was not exposed to extracellular ATP. These data would argue that some intracellular diffusible second messenger(s) are produced on exposure to extracellular ATP. Our data exclude $[Ca^{2+}]_i$, protein kinase A, protein kinase C, and inositol phosphates (IP_3 and IP_4) as primary candidates. One group of potential second messengers is arachidonic acid and its metabolites, namely prostaglandins, leukotrienes, and thromboxanes. Sequential activation of phospholipase C and diacylglycerol release arachidonate [21]. It has been reported in a number of organs that ATP stimulates the production of prostaglandin I_2 [22].

The single–channel experiments demonstrating the reduction of L–type Ca channel activity during extracellular perfusion of ATP suggest involvement of diffusible second messengers instead of direct G protein modulation of channel activity. However, it is now recognized that single α subunits may be released from the membrane as soluble proteins following activation of G proteins. Therefore, the results from the cell–attached, single–channel experiments do not allow us to convincingly distinguish between direct G–protein modulation of I_{Ca} and second messenger participation.

In addition to being released as a cotransmitter from nerve terminals [5], ATP can also be released from endothelial cells, aggregating platelets, and hypoxic myocardium [18,23]. The amount of ATP in the coronary circulation can approach several micromoles per liter [24], and higher levels can be reached under ischemic conditions [23]. The inhibitory effects that extracellular ATP produces on the basal action potential, $[Ca^{2+}]_i$ transients, and cell–length shortening in these myocytes [15] suggest that in ferret ventricular myocardium extracellular ATP could serve a cardioprotective role by being potentially antiarrhythmic. In contrast, in isolated rat ventricular myocytes, extracellular ATP, by activating non–specific cation channels [9], is potentially arrhythmogenic.

Therefore, both the effects and the functional role of extracellular ATP appear to be fundamentally different between the two species. It will be interesting to examine the effects of extracellular ATP on I_{Ca} in myocytes isolated from other mammalian species, especially from human myocardium, so as to determine the generality of the effects of extracellular ATP on the heart.

Acknowledgement

This work was supported in part by National Heart, Lung and Blood Institute Grants HL 17670, HL 19216, and HL 45132.

DISCUSSION

Dr. J. De Mey: One of the reasons for using ATP in this study is a possibility of access of neurotransmitter. Do you have evidence that P_{2Y} receptors that you believe are involved actually mediate the effects of neurogenically released ATP? Or, to put it differently, are these receptors solely responsible for mediating the effects of ATP released from nerve terminals or are they responsible for mediating the effects of extracellular ATP released from other sites?

Dr. H. Strauss: I do not believe that the P_{2Y} receptor distribution is primarily around nerve terminals. We have no data that establish the density and distribution of P_{2Y} receptors in ventricular myocytes. I have also alluded to the fact that ATP is also released from platelets, hypoxic or ischemic endothelium and myocardium in addition to the nervous system. Establishing the relative importance of these sources will need to be addressed in future studies.

Dr. E. Marban: I seem to remember that in the surgical literature there was some interest for a while in ATP as a positive inotropic agent. Your effects would be in the wrong direction. Is there in fact a positive inotropic effect of exogenously applied ATP or a negative one? Have you checked that?

Dr. H. Strauss: In ferret ventricular myocytes, extracellular ATP acts as a negative inotropic agent. In rat ventricular myocytes, a positive inotropic effect is seen. Whether a positive inotropic effect occurs in man is uncertain. Receptor subtype and/or G protein isoforms may be different in ferret ventricular myocytes then in other mammalian systems. For example, acetylcholine appears to have a greater effect on repolarizing currents in ferret ventricular myocytes than in other mammalian species. As a result, I am unsure how applicable are our data to other mammalian systems. However, the ferret heart has been used to investigate the effects of hypoxia on calcium metabolism and contraction. Our data suggest that release of intracellular ATP into the extracellular space could contribute to the negative inotropic effect of hypoxia or ischemia in the ferret ventricle. At this point it appears premature to speculate about such effects in other mammalian species.

Dr. F. Prinzen: I want to comment that our measurements with ATP in anesthetized dogs show an increased contractility.

Dr. A. Somlyo: Do phosphatase inhibitors affect your current?

Dr. H. Strauss: We have no data that answer this question.

Dr. A. Landesberg: Can you estimate the amount of change in the ATP concentration during one cardiac cycle?

Dr. H. Strauss: No. We have no data that address this question.

REFERENCES

1. Zipes DP. Autonomic innervation of the heart: Role in arrhythmic development during ishcemia and in the Long QT Syndrome, in Fozzard HA, Haber E, Jennings RB, Katz AM, Morgan HE (eds): *The Heart and Cardiovascular System. Scientific Foundations.* (second edition). New York, Raven Press, 1991, pp 2059–2112.
2. Wharton JM, Coleman RE, Strauss HC. The role of the autonomic nervous system in sudden cardiac death. *Trends Cardiovasc Med* 1992; 2: 65–71.
3. Inoue H, Zipes DP. Results of sympathetic denervation in the canine heart: supersensitivity that may be arrhythmogenic. *Circulation* 1987; 75: 877–887.
4. Herre JM, Welstein L, Lin Y–L. Effect of transmural versus non–transmural myocardial infarction on inducibility of ventricular arrhythmias during sympathetic stimulation in dogs. *J Am Coll Cardiol* 1988; 11: 414–421.
5. Burnstock G. Purines as cotransmitters in adrenergic and cholinergic neurones. *Prog Brain Res* 1987; 68: 193–203.
6. DeYong MB, Scarpa A. Extracellular ATP induces Ca^{2+} transients in cardiac myocytes which are potentiated by norepinephrine. *FEBS Letters* 1987; 223: 53–58.
7. Danziger RS, Raffaeli S, Moreno–Sanchez R, Sakai M, Capogrossi MC, Spurgeon HA, Hansford RG, Lakatta EG. Extracellular ATP has a potent effect to enhance cytosolic calcium and contractility in single ventricular myocytes. *Cell Calcium* 1988; 9: 193–199.
8. Bjornsson OG, Monck JR, Williamson JR. Identification of P_{2Y} purinoceptors associated with voltage–activated cation channels in cardiac ventricular myocytes of the rat. *Eur J Biochem* 1989; 186: 395–404.
9. Christie A, Sharma VK, Sheu SS. Mechanism of extracellular ATP–induced increase of cytosolic Ca^{2+} concentration in isolated rat ventricular myocytes. *J Physiol* 1992; 445: 369–388.
10. Friel DD, Bean BP. Two ATP–activated conductances in bullfrog atrial cells. *J Gen Physiol* 1988; 9: 1–27.
11. Scamps F, Vassort G. Mechanism of extracellular ATP–induced depolarization in rat isolated ventricular cardiomyocytes. *Pflugers Archiv* 1990; 417: 309–316.
12. Alvarez JL, Mongo K, Scamps F, Vassort G. Effects of purinergic stimulation on the Ca current in single frog cardiac cells. *Pflugers Archiv* 1990; 416: 189–195.
13. Scamps F, Legseyer A, Marjoux E, Vassort G. The mechanism of positive inotropy induced by adenosine triphosphate in rat heart. *Circ Res* 1990; 67: 1007–1016.
14. Qu Y. Modulation of L–type Ca–current by adenosine and ATP in isolated ferret right ventricular myocytes. *Ph.D. Thesis*, Duke University. 1992.
15. Qu Y, Himmel HM, Campbell DL, Strauss HC. Effects of extracellular ATP on I_{Ca}, $[Ca^{2+}]_i$, and contraction in isolated ferret ventricular myocytes. *Am J Physiol (Cell Physiol)* 1993; in press.
16. Qu Y, Campbell DL, Whorton AR, Strauss HC. Modulation of basal L–type Ca–current by adenosine in isolated ferret right ventricular myocytes. *J Physiol (London)* 1993; in press.
17. Qu Y, Campbell DL, Strauss, HC. A PTX–insensitive G–protein couples P_{2Y} purinergic receptors to inhibition of L–type Ca channels in ferret right ventricular myocytes. *J Physiol (London)*, (In review).
18. Gordon JL. Extracellular ATP: Effects, sources, and fate. *Biochem J* 1986; 233: 309–319.
19. Schneider P, Hopp HH, Isenberg G. Ca^{2+} influx through ATP–gated channels increment $[Ca^{2+}]$ and inactivate I_{Ca} in myocytes from guinea pig urinary bladder. *J Physiol* 1991; 440: 479–496.
20. Scamps F, Rybin U, Puceat M, Tzachuk V, Vassort G. A Gs protein couples P_2–purinergic stimulation to cardiac Ca channels without cyclic AMP production. *J Gen Physiol* 1992; 100: 675–701.
21. Rana RS, Hokin LE. Role of phosphoinositides in transmembrane signalling. *Physiol Rev* 1990; 70: 115–164.
22. Needleman P, Minkes MS, Douglas JR. Stimulation of prostaglandin biosynthesis by adenine nucleotides. *Circ Res* 1974; 34: 455–460.
23. Clemens MG, Forrester T. Appearance of adenosine triphosphate in the coronary sinus effluent from isolated working rat heart in response to hypoxia. *J Physiol* 1980; 312: 143–158.
24. Born GV, Kratzer MA. Source and concentration of extracellular adenosine triphosphate during homeostasis in rats, rabbit and man. *J Physiol* 1984; 354: 419–429.

CHAPTER 3

INTRACELLULAR CALCIUM AND MYOCARDIAL FUNCTION DURING ISCHEMIA

David G. Allen[1], Simeon P. Cairns[1], Stuart E. Turvey[1] and John A. Lee[2]

ABSTRACT

Cardiac ischemia causes a rapid decline in mechanical performance and, if prolonged, myocardial cell death occurs on reperfusion. The early decline in mechanical performance could, in principle, be caused either by reduced intracellular calcium release or by reduced responsiveness of the myofibrillar proteins to calcium. It is now known that intracellular calcium rises during ischemia and that the early decline in mechanical performance is caused largely by the inhibitory effects of phosphate and protons on the myofibrillar proteins. The rise of intracellular calcium during ischemia is related to the acidosis and is probably caused by calcium influx on the Na/Ca exchanger. This is triggered by a rise in intracellular sodium which enter the cell in exchange for protons on the Na/H exchanger. Intracellular calcium rises still further on reperfusion and the elevation of calcium and the degree of muscle damage are closely correlated.

INTRODUCTION

Ischemic heart disease remains a common cause of disability and early death. A wide range of clinical syndromes can be produced including reduced exercise performance, angina, life–threatening arrhythmias and terminal cardiac failure. As a reflection of its clinical importance, a variety of new methods of treatment have been developed including bypass or dilation of atheromatous coronary arteries, early treatment of coronary thrombi with thrombolytic agents, and transplantation of the heart. A common feature of all these treatments is that the myocardium, which has been subject to acute or chronic restriction of coronary flow, has its flow suddenly increased. Implicit in these therapies is the

[1]Department of Physiology, University of Sydney, NSW 2006, Australia and [2]Department of Pathology, University of Sheffield Medical School, Sheffield S10 2UL, U.K.

Interactive Phenomena in the Cardiac System, Edited by
S. Sideman and R. Beyar, Plenum Press, New York, 1993

assumption that restoration of flow to the ischemic myocardium will produce at least some functional recovery. However, it has been recognized from the earliest days of cardiac surgery that the moment of reperfusion may be associated with rapid and terminal damage to the heart (the stone heart [1]). Much of the early investigative work concentrated on defining the maximum safe ischemic period and determining the conditions which prolonged this safe period. Over this same period understanding of ionic regulation in the myocyte has increased dramatically and there is good evidence that ionic changes in the ischemic and reperfused myocardium have an important role in the functional and pathological changes [2, 3].

The effects of ischemia on contractile performance have been reviewed previously [4, 5]. The Langendorff–perfused heart is a suitable preparation for many investigations and can be rendered globally ischemic by simply stopping the perfusate flow. Global ischemia causes a rapid decline in developed pressure. This decrease in force production is apparent within one minute and is generally complete, with little or no developed force, after 5–10 minutes. After 10–20 minutes of ischemia, a gradual rise in diastolic pressure becomes apparent (the ischemic contracture), and increases in size as ischemia progresses. If reperfusion is started before or during the early stages of ischemic contracture, eventual recovery of contractile function can be virtually complete. However, there is often a prolonged period of impaired mechanical performance even after short exposures (i.e. myocardial stunning [6]). If reperfusion is delayed until the contracture is well established (0.5–1 hr), muscle damage is accelerated and recovery is poor. Long periods of ischemia (> 2 hr) show no developed force on reperfusion (e.g. Fig. 2) and immediately following reperfusion there is rapid loss of cell proteins, cell swelling and gross structural signs of damage. In addition to the mechanical changes noted above, electrophysiological changes and arrhythmias are common both in the early period of ischemia and during reperfusion [7].

This chapter reviews intracellular calcium ($[Ca^{2+}]_i$) regulation in the heart during ischemia and discusses the role of $[Ca^{2+}]_i$ in the early decline of mechanical performance and in the tissue damage observed on reperfusion.

THE MECHANISM OF THE EARLY ISCHEMIC DECLINE OF FORCE

The early ischemic decline of force is a dramatic phenomenon of great clinical importance so there have been many attempts to understand its mechanism. Early theories were often based on the intracellular acidosis which accompanies the accelerated anaerobic glycolysis [8]. It is well established that acidosis reduces the sensitivity of the myofibrillar proteins to Ca^{2+} and also causes a small reduction in maximum developed force [9]. While acidosis contributes to the decline of force it was shown clearly by Jacobus and colleagues [10] that it cannot explain all the fall in force in ischemia. The idea that a decline in ATP would inhibit crossbridge cycling has been made less likely by the demonstration that ATP falls rather little during the early part of ischemia [11]. Another important class of possibilities is that intracellular Ca^{2+} release is impaired in ischemia. For instance the action potential shortens during ischemia but many studies have shown that over the period in which force declines (5–10 min) the changes in the action potential are very small [11, 12]. Ca^{2+} release could fail for other reason e.g. a metabolite which closes the sarcoplasmic reticulum Ca^{2+} channel, and for this reason a number of groups have measured the Ca^{2+} transient during ischemia. Such results are discussed in the next section but it is generally agreed that the Ca^{2+} transient increases rather than decreases in early ischemia.

The discovery that Ca^{2+} transients increase during early ischemia means that the decline of force production must be caused by reduced myofibrillar responsiveness to

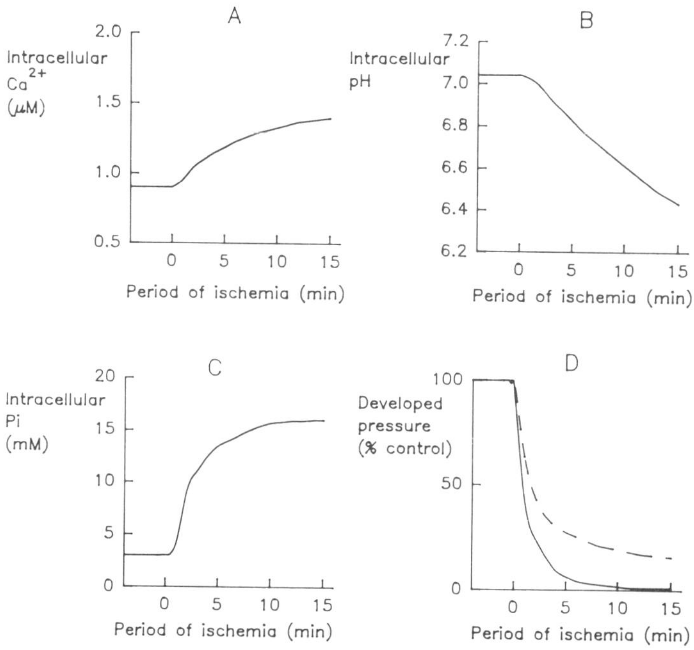

Figure 1. Changes in intracellular Ca^{2+}, pH, Pi and developed pressure during global ischemia. All data are taken from experiments on ferret hearts at 30°C. Panel **A** shows changes in peak systolic $[Ca^{2+}]_i$ estimated from [18,19]. Panels **B** and **C** show measurements of pH and Pi using phosphorus NMR [11]. Panel **D** (solid line) shows left ventricular developed pressure during ischemia [11]. The dotted line in Panel **D** is a theoretical curve calculated from the data in Panels **A, B** and **C** as described in text. See [4] for details. Reproduced from [4] by copyright permission of the American Society for Clinical Investigation.

$[Ca^{2+}]_i$, presumably as a consequence of metabolites. Systematic studies on skinned fibers have shown that of the metabolites which accumulate during ischemia, phosphate (Pi) and protons, have the most significant inhibitory effect [13, 14]. By combining the inhibitory effects of Pi and pH on the myofibrillar proteins, as determined by skinned fibre studies with measurements of the changes in Pi, pH and Ca^{2+} transients during ischemia, it is possible to predict the fall of pressure during ischemia. Fig. 1 shows the result of this exercise. In Panel D the dashed line is the result of this prediction while the full line is the experimentally measured pressure. While the inhibitory effects of Pi and pH appear to explain much of the decline of pressure, there is an additional component which may be a result of the changing pressure or flow in the coronary arteries [4, 12, 15]. This view is reinforced by observations of another model of ischemia (application of cyanide and cinnamate, to block oxidative phosphorylation and the lactate transporter) in which the changes of pH and Pi are indistinguishable from ischemia but the decline of force is somewhat less [11].

INTRACELLULAR CALCIUM DURING ISCHEMIA

In the last few years a number of methods have been developed which are capable of measuring $[Ca^{2+}]_i$ during ischemia. These methods include NMR using a fluorine labelled Ca^{2+} detector [16], fluorescent Ca^{2+} indicators[17], and the luminescent Ca^{2+} indicator aequorin [18–20]. The results of these different approaches are reasonable similar and have been recently reviewed [4]. Here we describe representative results from our own work. Figure 2 shows the tension and $[Ca^{2+}]_i$ (estimated from aequorin light) from a papillary muscle in which ischemia was modelled using N_2 gas perfusion [19, 20]. Note that tension falls to zero within 10 minutes and that over the same period the Ca^{2+} transients show first a small fall but then a very striking rise which peaks at about 20 min. Subsequently the Ca^{2+} transients decline but random increases of $[Ca^{2+}]_i$ are visible which are terminated by a very large increase of $[Ca^{2+}]_i$ at one hour. Thereafter resting $[Ca^{2+}]_i$ is elevated (hardly visible on this scale) but changes little over one hour. When perfusion is restarted there is a very large increase in $[Ca^{2+}]_i$ (which consumes much of the aequorin in the preparation) but, when this consumption is corrected for, a very large increase of $[Ca^{2+}]_i$ persists. As expected after two hours of ischemia, there is no recovery of developed force and it has been shown in many studies that there is an inverse correlation between elevation of $[Ca^{2+}]_i$ and recovery of function after periods of metabolic inhibition or ischemia [2, 4, 21, 22].

The changes in $[Ca^{2+}]_i$ in Fig. 2 are complex and it is easiest to consider them in various phases. During the first 30 min the main changes are a large rise in the Ca^{2+} transients and an accompanying rise in diastolic $[Ca^{2+}]_i$. This is the period over which a substantial intracellular acidosis develops [11] and it seems possible that the acidosis and the increase in $[Ca^{2+}]_i$ are related. A number of lines of evidence support this view [19]. (i). If glycolysis is inhibited, by glycogen depletion and removal of external glucose, then the rise in Ca^{2+} transients is eliminated. (ii). Intracellular acidosis induced by other manoeuvres produces a similar rise in Ca^{2+} transients. (iii). During both ischemia and acidosis there is prolongation of the Ca^{2+} transients and abbreviation of the timecourse of the tension response. Possible mechanisms whereby intracellular acidosis elevates $[Ca^{2+}]_i$ will be considered in the next section.

In the second phase of ischemia, Ca^{2+} transients gradually decline in amplitude and spontaneous Ca^{2+} release becomes increasingly frequent; these are the cause of the irregular Ca^{2+} signals between 30 min and 1 hour in Fig. 2. It is well known that the over this period the membrane potential becomes depolarized, conduction velocity is reduced and the action potentials become very abbreviated [7]. These changes are observed in the present preparation [19] and in addition the stimulus threshold starts to rise. These abbreviated

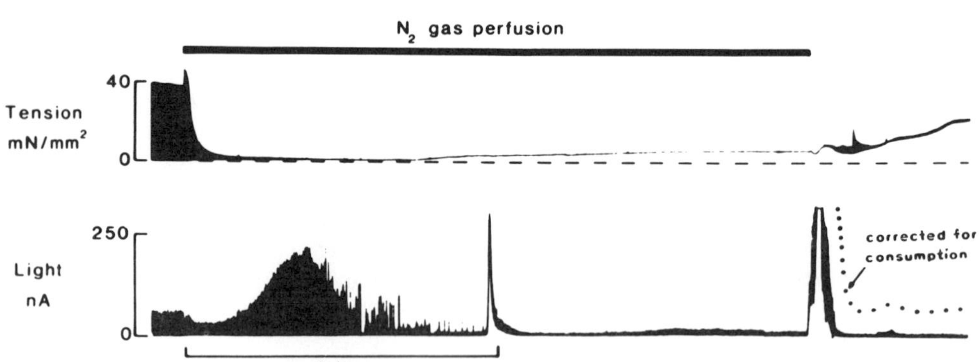

Figure 2. Records of tension (above) and aequorin light (below; a function of $[Ca^{2+}]_i$) from an isolated ferret papillary muscle during a 2 hr period of simulated ischemia followed by reperfusion. Ischemia was simulated by N_2 gas perfusion (37°C, 1 Hz stimulation rate). See [19, 20] for details. Reproduced from [4] by copyright permission of the American Society for Clinical Investigation.

action potentials will eventually fail to propagate and will be much less effective at stimulating Ca^{2+} release and this is the likely cause of the gradual decline of the Ca^{2+} transients over this period. The continued presence of spontaneous Ca^{2+} release shows that the sarcoplasmic reticulum (SR) is loaded with Ca^{2+} and this spontaneous Ca^{2+} release probably contributes to the arrhythmias which occur in this period [4, 7]. In support of this possibility it has been shown that drugs, such as caffeine and ryanodine, which deplete the SR of Ca^{2+} and therefore prevent spontaneous Ca^{2+} release, reduce the incidence of arrhythmias over this period [23].

The very large but temporary increase in $[Ca^{2+}]_i$ which occurs at one hour heralds the end of spontaneous Ca^{2+} release and seems likely to be cause by the decline of [ATP] (or the free energy of ATP hydrolysis) to the point at which the SR can no longer accumulated Ca^{2+}. Surprisingly the resting $[Ca^{2+}]_i$ is not elevated immediately after this period which suggests that some other intracellular Ca^{2+} store can still accumulated Ca^{2+} or there is an efflux pathway from the cell which can still function, at least for a short time, under these conditions.

In the second hour of ischemia, the resting $[Ca^{2+}]_i$ increases to a moderately elevated level (˜1.3 μM) and remains at that level. The final rise is unlikely to be caused by acidosis, which is relatively constant over this period; it seems more likely to be caused by reduced Ca^{2+} efflux across the surface membrane as energy levels in the cell and ionic gradients across the surface membrane decline. For instance, if [ATP] falls to the point at which the Na pump ceases to function, $[Na^+]_i$ will gradually increase. Provided the Na/Ca exchanger is still operative this will lead to a rise in $[Ca^{2+}]_i$. The rise in $[Ca^{2+}]_i$ is substantially lower than the level achieved in complete metabolic blockade [21] and the difference could represent better preservation of metabolic levels in ischemia or perhaps a reduction of the extracellular $[Ca^{2+}]_o$ in ischemia.

During reperfusion there is a striking further increase in $[Ca^{2+}]_i$ often associated with oscillatory Ca^{2+} signals. Both the magnitude and the form of the $[Ca^{2+}]_i$ on reperfusion depend on the duration of the preceding period of ischemia [19, 20]. Short periods of ischemia (10–20 min) were associated with elevated Ca^{2+} transients on reperfusion [18,19]. Intermediate periods of ischemia (<1 hr) were associated with large, oscillatory increases in $[Ca^{2+}]_i$ which recovered to more or less normal Ca^{2+} transients in time. Such oscillatory increases in $[Ca^{2+}]_i$ are most likely to be associated with arrhythmias [7, 23]. Long periods of ischemia (>2 hr) showed the largest increases in $[Ca^{2+}]_i$ which were maintained and non-oscillatory (Fig. 2). This elevation of $[Ca^{2+}]_i$ was associated with complete failure of mechanical recovery.

ROLE OF Na/H AND Na/Ca EXCHANGE DURING ISCHEMIA

Evidence has already been presented that acidosis has a key role in producing the increased $[Ca^{2+}]_i$ in the early part of ischemia. One well established mechanism by which this could occur involves the coupled activity of the Na/H and the Na/Ca exchanger. Deitmer and Ellis [24] first showed that intracellular acidosis in cardiac muscle activated the Na/H exchanger and caused a coupled H+ efflux and Na^+ influx. It is also established that the resulting increase in $[Na^+]_i$ causes an increase in $[Ca^{2+}]_i$ by means of a reduced Ca^{2+} efflux on the Na/Ca exchanger [25]. The question which then arises is whether this mechanism operates during ischemia? We have approached this question by applying lactate to isolated cardiac myocytes to mimic some of the effects of ischemia [26]. Lactic acid rapidly enters the cell, both as undissociated lactic acid and also by means of the lactate transporter [27]. Figure 3 shows the contraction of the cell on stimulation (shortening shown downwards) and the intracellular pH (pH_i) when Na lactate (pH_o 7.4) is applied to an isolated cardiac myocytes. Contraction shows a sudden reduction caused by the inhibitory effect of intracellular acidosis on the myofibrillar proteins but then there is a recovery of contraction in the continuing presence of lactate. The pH_i trace shows the expected acidosis when lactate is applied but there is then a substantial recovery of pH_i over the 10 min of exposure. The middle trace shows selected Ca^{2+} transients during the exposure. There is an increase in both diastolic and systolic $[Ca^{2+}]_i$ immediately after the application of lactate and then a secondary increase in diastolic and systolic $[Ca^{2+}]_i$ during the continuing exposure to lactate. To establish which of these phenomena are linked to operation of the Na/H exchanger, Fig. 4 shows the same experiment in the presence of ethylisopropylamiloride (EIPA), a potent inhibitor of the Na/H exchanger [28]. The slow increase in contraction after application of lactate, the slow recovery pH_i and the slow increase in $[Ca^{2+}]_i$ are all eliminated in the presence of EIPA. Thus these experiments support the interpretation given at the beginning of this section; namely that acidosis caused by intracellular lactate causes H+ extrusion and causes the pH_i recovery. Associated with this is an increase in diastolic and systolic $[Ca^{2+}]_i$ of which the slow component seems to be linked to the Na/H exchanger. The most obvious link would be via a rise in $[Na^+]_i$ and similar experiments in perfused hearts but using the Na^+ indicator benzofuran isophthalate [29] (SBFI), show that such rise in $[Na^+]_i$ does occur (Fig. 5).

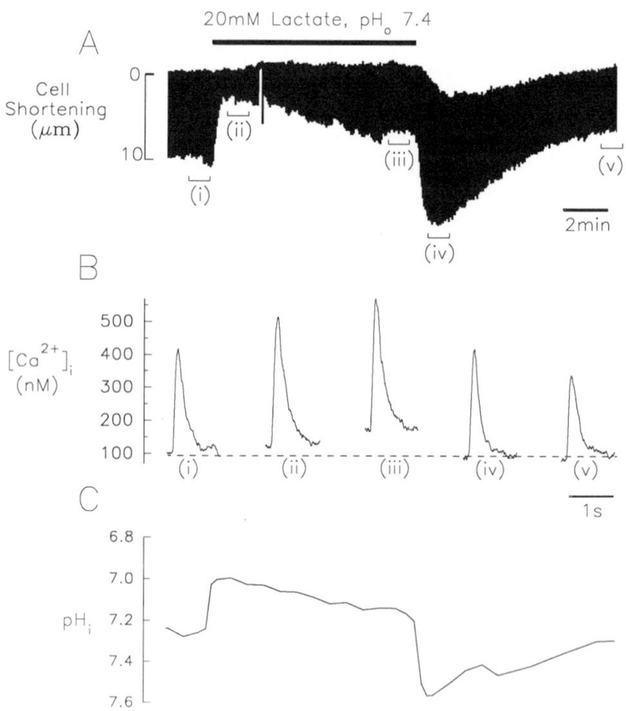

Figure 3. Effect of extracellular lactate (20 mM, pH_o 7.4 throughout) on rat ventricular myocyte. **A:** Shortening trace; the myocyte was stimulated to contract at 0.4 Hz (30°C) and shortening produces a downward deflection (individual contractions are fused on this time base). **B:** Averaged (n=8) Ca^{2+} transients from the times shown in Panel A. **C:** Intracellular pH (measured in a separate experiment). Modified from [26].

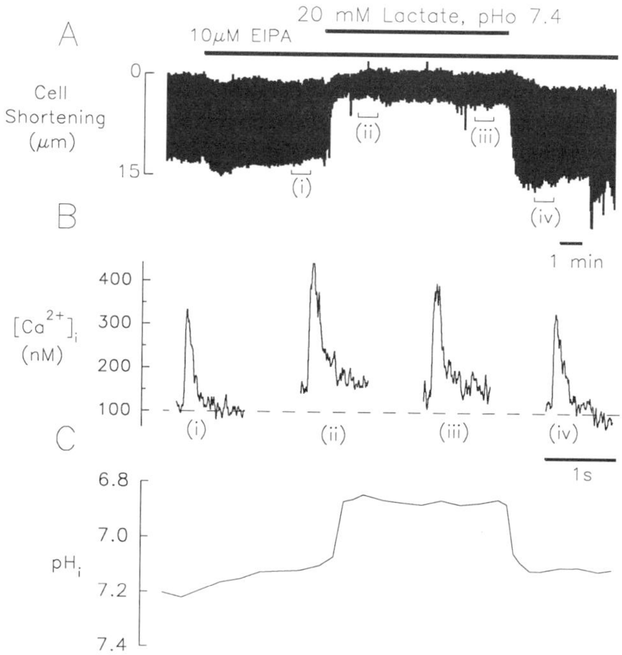

Figure 4. Effect of extracellular lactate on a rat ventricular myocyte during inhibition of the Na/H exchange with EIPA (10 mM, present during bar). Format identical to Fig. 3. Modified from [26].

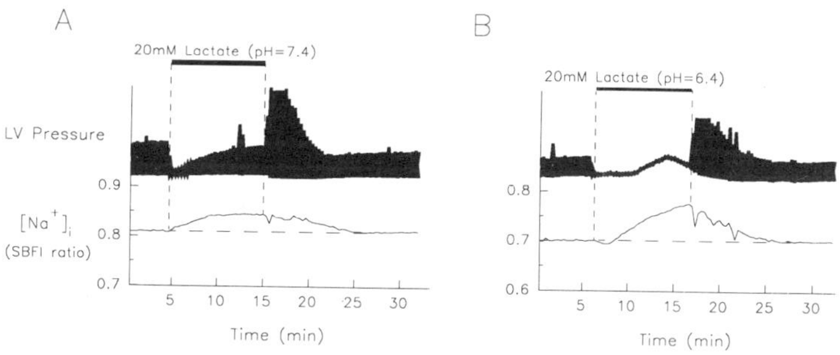

Figure 5. Effect of lactate on intracellular $[Na^+]$. Upper trace shows pressure record from a perfused rat heart. Development of pressure produces an upward deflection (30°C, heart spontaneously contracting at about 1 Hz). Lower trace shows fluorescence ratio signal from SBFI representing $[Na^+]_i$. **A:** Lactate (20 mM applied without osmotic compensation) applied with pH_o 7.4 throughout. **B:** Lactate applied at pH_o 6.4 (pH_o otherwise 7.4). Same heart and same format as Panel **A**. See [37] for details.

These experiments clearly show that the coupled operation of the Na/H and the Na/Ca exchanger can lead to an increase in $[Ca^{2+}]_i$ when lactic acid accumulates in the myocardial cell. However there is conflicting evidence as to whether this mechanism operates in ischemia. (i). On the basis of this hypothesis one would expect a rise in $[Na^+]_i$ during the early part of ischemia which could be (at least in part) inhibited by Na/H exchange blockers. However the evidence on this point is equivocal. In support of the theory, several studies have found substantial rise in $[Na^+]_i$ during ischemia [22, 30, 31] which was reduced by pretreatment with amiloride [22, 30]. However measurements with microelectrodes [32, 33] have generally found little change in $[Na^+]_i$ during early ischemia. (ii). It is known that the Na/H exchanger is inhibited by extracellular acidosis and this has led to the suggestion that the extracellular acidosis which is known to occur in ischemia [34] might prevent this mechanism operating. We have investigated this point by measuring the changes in pH_i, $[Na^+]_i$, and $[Ca^{2+}]_i$ in a ventricular cell when lactate is applied is in a more acid extracellular solution (pH_o 6.4). If acid extracellular conditions inhibited the exchanger one might predict a result rather like that in Fig. 4 in which the exchanger was inhibited by EIPA. However, in fact, the slow pH_i recovery, the slow increase in $[Ca^{2+}]_i$ and the increase in $[Na^+]_i$ were all found to be bigger than in the corresponding experiments at pH_o 7.4. Figure 5 illustrates this result for $[Na^+]_i$. This result suggests that while extracellular acidosis may inhibit the exchanger, the effect can be more than offset by the increased changes in pH_i which occur under these conditions [26]. This conclusion is also consistent with the systematic studies of the activity of the exchanger at a wide range of pH_o and pH_i [35, 36].

The very large influx of Ca^{2+} during reperfusion was explained by Lazdunski and colleagues [34] as a consequence of reactivation of the Na/H exchanger as the extracellular acidosis rapidly recovered on reperfusion. On this hypothesis there should be little rise in $[Na^+]_i$ during ischemia (at least due to operation of the exchanger) but there should be a large rise of $[Na^+]_i$ on reperfusion which drives the Ca^{2+} influx. Again the experimental evidence is equivocal. Tani and Neely [22] observed a large rise in $[Na^+]_i$ during ischemia followed by a further small increase on reperfusion. However Van Heel et al. [32] observed little change in $[Na^+]_i$ during simulated ischemia and also failed to record an increase on reperfusion.

In summary, there is good evidence that acidosis in isolated myocytes leads to rise in $[Na^+]_i$ and $[Ca^{2+}]_i$ caused by the coupled operation of the Na/H and the Na/Ca exchangers. However the extent to which this mechanism explains the ionic changes in ischemia and reperfusion remains uncertain.

CONCLUSIONS

The recent development of methods for measuring $[Ca^{2+}]_i$, $[Na^+]_i$, and pH_i in perfused hearts offers the potential to test hypotheses for the ionic changes in ischemia and reperfusion. It has already been demonstrated [30] that inhibition of the Na/H exchanger improves recovery after ischemia and it seems likely that inhibition of the Na/Ca exchanger might also be valuable. Increasing understanding of the mechanisms involved and of the molecular structure of the exchangers will offer new approaches to the design of inhibitors and to the minimization of ischemic damage.

Acknowledgements

Recent experimental work was supported by National Heart Foundation of Australia.

DISCUSSION

Dr. H. Strauss: I relate to your attempt to tease out the pH component responsibile for the decline in tension during ischemia. The method you are using to analyze the problem, in addition to modulating the calcium dependence of the contractile process, also presumably has an effect upon repolarization of the action potential, either through change in the hydrogen ion *per se* and/or lactate effect on the ATP sensitive potassium channel. Have you looked at action potential duration in these myocytes during the course of these experiments to try and establish whether a change in repolarization is occurring and compounding the interpretation of your interventions.

Dr. D. Allen: Yes we have. Action potential duration measured in papillary muscles was hardly affected by the concentrations of lactate that we used.

Dr. Y. Rudy: Have you tried to compare the behavior that you see with the behavior that you obtain when you directly block the sodium–calcium exchanger?

Dr. D. Allen: The big problem in this field is that there is no specific blocker of the sodium and calcium exchanger. Nickel certainly blocks it, but of course it also does many other things, e.g. it blocks calcium channels. It is obviously not a useful clinical drug. None of the available sodium–calcium blockers are specific for the sodium–calcium exchanger. We just can not do the experiments we would like to do with a clean sodium–calcium exchange blocker. There is now an antibody available that blocks sodium–calcium exchange, but it has to be applied inside the cell so it is only applicable to single cell studies for the moment.

Dr. E. Marban: Your conclusions are very reasonable, but I notice that you were careful to present the sodium data in terms of a ratio rather than concentration. SBFI has known complications in cells, where it changes its calibration properties. Could you comment on that?

Dr. D. Allen: We have performed *in vivo* calibration of the SBFI ratio and this works well. We follow the method David Eisner described using gramicidin and low divalent cations to calibrate SBFI inside the cell and it is indeed different to its calibration outside the cell. But, provided one calibrates it in the correct environment, that is not a real problem.

Dr. E. Marban: In that case, I wonder how your 6% ratio changes and 12% ratio changes translate to actual sodium numbers.

Dr. D. Allen: The 6% represents an increase of about 1 mM [Na^+] and the 12% almost 2 mM [Na^+]. The real reason we started the SBFI is to look at ischemia. One would not really choose to study sodium in a whole heart unless you are interested in ischemia. We are just starting the experiments. We find very little change of sodium early in ischemia, which is surprising. Very likely, ion sensitive electrode results are quite different from your results with NMR and the people who try to measure total sodium. It is interesting that the two techniques that measure free sodium, namely SBFI and the micro–electrode, find no change, whereas the other techniques that find big increases in sodium measure total sodium (NMR and tissue homogenization). It may be that what you are seeing is an artifact of swelling of the cells in sodium accumulation rather than a genuine change in sodium, but that is a preliminary feeling.

Dr. G. Hasenfuss: During ischemia you see a fall in tension and a rise in intracellular calcium. What is the underlying mechanism of this uncoupling? Is it a decrease in calcium sensitivity or is it a direct effect of pH on crossbridges?

Dr. D. Allen: It is a mixture of both effects; the pH reduces the sensitivity and the phosphate reduces the force.

Dr. G. Hassenfuss: The increase in the intracellular calcium signal might also be due to decreased sensitivity which liberates more calcium from the troponin C.

Dr. D. Allen: That is why I showed the result (Figs. 3 and 4) which show calcium transients in the early part of lactate exposure. There is a step increase of calcium when you make the cell acid inside which cannot be due to the sodium–hydrogen exchange coupled to sodium–calcium exchange because it has had no time to work. That may be a straight forward effect of acidosis on sensitivity. Acidosis will reduce the effecitve number of Ca^{2+} binding sites and the same release of Ca^{2+} will give a bigger myoplasmic [Ca^{2+}].

Dr. J. De Mey: You elaborated on the possible interaction between sodium–hydrogen exchange and sodium–calcium exchange. You suggest an increase in intracellular sodium. If that is true, why does increased activity of the sodium–potassium ATPase not compensate for that? Is there a possible explanation?

Dr. D. Allen: There are two things to say about that. Obviously when you just apply lactate, as we show in Fig. 5, there will be an increase in sodium and that will be in competition with the pump which is trying to pump it out. Later in ischemia, when the ATP is as close to zero, the sodium pump will stop, and then you have an additional mechanism for sodium rise. But most sodium measurements are in the very early period so far. As you go longer and longer into ischemia, you have more and more problems with cell integrity and many possible mechanisms may operate.

Dr. W.M. Chilian: Since the myocardium is composed of almost 20% non–muscle cells, how do you know the calcium signal is coming from muscle. How do you know it is not coming from the endothelium and the fibroblasts?

Dr. D. Allen: Twenty years ago that was a difficult question to answer. Now that isolated myocytes have been studied one can compare one's results with what happens in an isolated myocyte. All the things that I have shown here can also be seen in isolated myocytes. Of course, when you load a whole heart with the SBFI, you have a responsibility to prove to the world that your signal is coming from the myocytes rather than from the endothelial cells. There are various tricks to try and do that. One possibility would be to perfuse the heart very briefly with a detergent, such as Triton–X, which should damage endothelial cells but not myocytes.

REFERENCES

1. Cooley DA, Reul J, Wukash DC. Ischemic contracture of the heart: stone heart. *Am J Cardiol* 1972; 29: 575–577.
2. Shen AC, Jennings RB. Myocardial calcium and magnesium in acute ischemic injury. *Am J Path* 1972; 67: 417–440.
3. Tani M. Mechanisms of Ca^{2+} overload in reperfused ischemic myocardium. *Ann Rev Physiol* 1990; 52: 543–559.
4. Lee JA, Allen DG. Mechanisms of acute ischemic contractile failure of the heart: role of intracellular calcium. *J Clin Inves* 1991; 88: 361–367.
5. Kléber AG, Oetliker H. Cellular aspects of early contractile failure in ischemia. In: Fozzard HA, et al (eds) *The Heart and Cardiovascular System*; 2nd Ed.; Raven Press, New York, 1992.
6. Kusuoka H, Marban E. Cellular mechanisms of myocardial stunning. *Ann Rev Physiol* 1992; 54: 243–256.
7. Janse MJ, Wit AL. Electrophysiological mechanisms of ventricular arrhythmias resulting from myocardial ischemia and infarction. *Physiol Rev* 1989; 69: 1049–1169.
8. Katz AM, Hecht HH. The early "pump" failure of the ischemic heart. *Am J Med* 1969; 47: 497–502.
9. Fabiato A, Fabiato F. Effects of pH on the myofilaments and the sarcoplasmic reticulum of skinned cells from cardiac and skeletal muscles. *J Physiol (Lond)* 1978; 276: 233–255.
10. Jacobus WE, Pores IH, Lucas SK, Kallman CH, Weisfeldt ML, Flaherty JT. The role of intrcellular pH in the control of normal and ischemic myocardial contractility: a 31P nuclear magnetic resonance and mass spectroscopy study. In Nuccitelli R, Deamer DW (eds): *Intracellular pH: Its Measurement, Regulation and Utilisation in Cellular Function*, New York, Alan R Liss Inc, 1982.

11. Elliott AC, Smith GL, Eisner DA, Allen DG. Metabolic changes during ischemia and their role in contractile failure in isolated ferret hearts. *J Physiol (Lond)* 1992; 454: 467–490.
12. Koretsune Y, Corretti M, Kusuoka H, Marban E. Mechanism of early ischemic contractile failure: inexitability, metabolite accumulation or vascular collapse? *Circ Res* 1991; 68: 255–262.
13. Godt RE, Nosek TM. Changes of intracellular milieu with fatigue or hypoxia depress contraction of skinned rabbit skeletal and cardiac muscle. *J Physiol (Lond)* 1989; 412: 155–180.
14. Kentish JC. The effects of inorganic phosphate and creatine phosphate on force production in skinned muscles from rat ventricle. *J Physiol (Lond)* 1986; 370: 585–604.
15. Kitakaze M, Marban E. Cellular mechanism of the modulation of contractile function by coronary perfusion pressure in ferret hearts. *J Physiol (Lond)* 1989; 414: 455–472.
16. Steenbergen C, Murphy E, Levy L, London RE. Elevation in cytosolic free Ca concentration early in myocardial ischemia in perfused rat heart. *Circ Res* 1987; 60: 700–707.
17. Lee H–C, Mohabir R, Smith N, Franz MR, Clusin WT. Effect of ischemia on Ca–dependent fluorescence transients in rabbit hearts containing indo–1. *Circulation* 1988; 78: 1047–1059.
18. Kihara Y, Grossman W, Morgan JP. Direct measurement of changes in intracellular Ca transients during hypoxia, ischemia and reperfusion of the intact mammalian heart. *Circ Res* 1989; 65: 1029–1044.
19. Allen DG, Lee JA, Smith GL. The consequences of simulated ischemia on intracellular Ca^{2+} and tension in isolated ferret ventricular muscle. *J Physiol (Lond)* 1989; 410: 297–323.
20. Lee JA, Allen DG. Changes in intracellular free calcium concentration during long exposures to simulated ischemia in isolated mammalian ventricular muscle. *Circ Res* 1992; 71: 58–69.
21. Smith GL, Allen DG. The effects of metabolic blockade on intracellular calcium concentration in isolated ferret ventricular muscle. *Circ Res* 1988; 62: 1223–1236.
22. Tani M, Neely JR. Role of intracellular Na^+ in Ca^{2+} overload and depressed recovery of ventricular function of reperfused ischemic rat hearts. Possible involvement of H^+–Ca^{2+} and Na^+–Ca^{2+} exchange. *Circ Res* 1990; 65: 1045–1056.
23. Thandroyen FT, McCarthy J, Burton KP, Opie LH. Ryanodine and caffeine prevent ventricular arrhy–thmias during acute myocardial ischemia and reperfusion in rat heart. *Circ Res* 1988; 62: 306–314.
24. Deitmer JW, Ellis D. Interactions between the regulation of the intracellular pH and sodium activity of sheep cardiac Purkinje fibres. *J Physiol (Lond)* 1980; 304: 471–488.
25. Allen DG, Eisner DA, Orchard CH. Factors influencing free intracellular calcium concentration in quiescent ferret ventricular muscle. *J Physiol (Lond)* 1984; 350: 615–630.
26. Cairns SP, Westerblad H, Allen DG. Changes of myoplasmic pH and calcium concentration during exposure to lactate in isolated rat ventricular myocytes. *J Physiol (Lond)* 1993 (in press).
27. De Hemptine A, Marrannes R, Vanheel B. Influence of organic acids on intracellular pH. *Am J Physiol* 1983; 245: C178–C183.
28. Kleyman TR, Cragoe EJ Jr. Amiloride and its analogs as tools in the study of ion transport. *J Memb Biol* 1988; 105: 1–21.
29. Minta A, Tsien RY. Fluorescent indicators for cytosolic sodium. *J Biol Chem* 1989; 264: 19449–19457.
30. Murphy E, Perlman M, London RE, Steenbergen C. Amiloride delays the ischemia–induced rise in cytosolic free calcium. *Circ Res* 1991; 68: 1250–1258.
31. Pike MM, Kitakaze M, Marban E. 23Na–NMR measurements of intracellular sodium in intact perfused ferret hearts during ischemia and reperfusion. *Am J Physiol* 1990; 259: H1767–H1773.
32. Wilde AAM, Kléber AG. the combined effects of hypoxia, high K+, and acidosis on the intracellular sodium activity and resting potential in guinea pig papillary muscle. *Circ Res* 1986; 58: 249–256.
33. Vanheel B, De Hemptine A, Leusen I. Acidification and intracellular sodium ion activity during simulated myocardial ischemia. *Am J Physiol* 1990; 259: C169–C179.
34. Lazdunski M, Frelin C, Vigne P. The sodium/hydrogen exchange system in cardiac cells: its biochemical and pharmacological properties and its role in regulating internal concentrations of sodium and internal pH. *J Mol Cell Cardiol* 1985; 17: 1029–1042.
35. Vaughan–Jones RD, Wu M–L. Extracellular H+ inactivation of Na^+–H+ exchange in the sheep cardiac Purkinje fibre. *J Physiol (Lond)* 428: 441–466.
36. Kaila K, Vaughan–Jones RD. Influence of sodium–hydrogen exchange on intracellular pH, sodium and tension in sheep cardiac Purkinje fibres. *J Physiol (Lond)* 1987; 390: 93–118.
37. Turvey SE, Allen DG. The use of SBFI to measure intracellular sodium in Langendorff perfused rat hearts. *Proc Australian Physiol Pharmacol Soc* 1992; 23: 143P.

CHAPTER 4

INTRACELLULAR SIGNALING IN VASCULAR SMOOTH MUSCLE

Avril V. Somlyo[1] and Andrew P. Somlyo[2]

ABSTRACT

The two major modalities of pharmacomechanical coupling, inositol 1,4,5 trisphosphate induced Ca^{2+} release and modulation of Ca^{2+}–sensitivity, are reviewed. Recent studies show that although changes in cytoplasmic Ca^{2+} play the major role in regulating smooth muscle contraction, agonists can also significantly affect the contractile state by modifying Ca^{2+}–sensitivity. Inhibition of myosin light chain kinase or myosin light chain phosphatase leads to, respectively, desensitization or sensitization of the contractile apparatus to Ca^{2+}. G–protein linked inhibition of myosin light chain phosphatase and Ca^{2+} release mediated by the phosphatidylinol cascade are the two major pharmacomechanical coupling mechanisms.

INTRODUCTION

Excitation–contraction coupling in smooth muscle is mediated by two pathways: a voltage–dependent mechanism termed "electromechanical coupling," which is the dominant mode in skeletal and cardiac muscles, and voltage–independent processes termed "pharmacomechanical coupling" [1]. Although both mechanisms can work in concert and contribute to the contractility of smooth muscle, this review will place an emphasis on pharmacomechanical coupling, reflecting recent major advances in our understanding of its molecular mechanisms. Pharmacomechanical coupling encompasses voltage–independent intracellular Ca^{2+} release and modulation of the Ca^{2+}–sensitivity of the contractile regulatory apparatus [2]. Modulation may also occur at the level of the myosin crossbridge, where the lifetime

[1]Department of Pathology and Molecular Physiology and Biological Physics, and [2]Department of Molecular Physiology and Biological Physics, and the Department of Medicine (Cardiology), University of Virginia, Charlottesville, VA 22908, USA.

Interactive Phenomena in the Cardiac System, Edited by
S. Sideman and R. Beyar, Plenum Press, New York, 1993

of force–generating states may be altered by changes in the ADP concentration in the vicinity of the myosin heads [3].

METHODS

Small strips (100–200 μm wide and 1–2 mm long) of guinea pig or rabbit blood vessels or ileum longitudinal smooth muscle were dissected and isometric tension was measured with a force transducer in a well on a "bubble" plate, as reported previously [4]. Vessels were permeabilized with staphylococcal α–toxin (GIBCO/BRL or List Biological Laboratories, Inc.). Channels formed by the α–toxin in the surface membrane are 2–3 nm and permit the passage of low (e.g., ATP, inorganic ions) but not high molecular weight (M_r > 1,000) solutes [5]. β–escin (Sigma) was used when larger holes were required to introduce higher molecular weight solutes of biological interest, such as heparin and calmodulin. Both methods retain coupled receptors. Measurements of myosin light chain phosphorylation were carried out on the same muscle strips used for force measurements using methods previously described [6]. Measurements of myosin light chain phosphatase (MLCP) and kinase activities [7] have been previously published. Details of the use of osmium ferrocyanide have also been described [8].

RESULTS AND DISCUSSION

Intracellular Ca^{2+} Stores and Pharmacomechanical Ca^{2+} Release

The sarcoplasmic reticulum (SR) is an anastomosing network of tubules and sheets with specialized regions that form surface couplings with the plasma membrane (Fig. 1). The volume and distribution of the SR varies in different types of smooth muscle, but both peripheral and central SR can sequester Ca^{2+}. The total SR Ca has been directly measured *in situ* by electron probe microanalysis and shown to decrease with agonist stimulation [9, 10]. Unlike the SR, mitochondria, studied in a large variety of cells, do not regulate cytoplasmic Ca^{2+} under physiological conditions, but are capable of accumulating molar concentrations of Ca phosphate when cytoplasmic Ca rises to pathological levels [11].

Smooth muscles contain both the inositol 1,4,5–trisphosphate ($InsP_3$) and the ryanodine Ca–release receptor/channels. Both $InsP_3$ and ryanodine will release Ca in permeabilized fibers in which the SR has been Ca^{2+}–loaded. The physiological significance of $InsP_3$ as the messenger for pharmacomechanical coupling was tested in systems approaching the physiological state by permeabilization with staphylococcal α–toxin or by using a reverse permeabilization technique [4, 5]. Permeabilization with α–toxin offers the major advantage that the 2 nm–diameter pores formed by the toxin molecules preclude passage of molecules greater than 1,000 daltons, and thus retain the intracellular proteins and enzymes, while allowing precise control of Ca^{2+} concentrations and introduction of low molecular weight molecules, such as $InsP_3$. Agonists in the presence of GTP cause Ca^{2+} release and contraction that can be blocked by prior exposure to GDPβS, reflecting the coupling of the receptor via a G–protein to the effector (phospholipase C) [5]. Similar receptor coupling was maintained in smooth muscles permeabilized with β–escin. This method allows the transmembrane passage of larger molecules, such as heparin, a blocker of $InsP_3$ binding to its receptor and a specific inhibitor of $InsP_3$–induced Ca^{2+} release in smooth muscles. Heparin blocked both the agonist–GTP and the $InsP_3$–induced contrac–

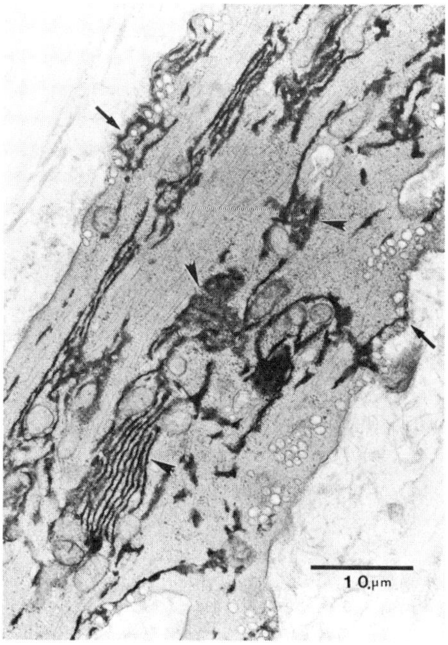

Figure 1. Longitudinal view through the center of a portion of a rabbit pulmonary artery smooth muscle cell. The network of sarcoplasmic reticulum has been selectively stained with osmium ferrocyanide. The network forms tubules which approach the plasma membrane (arrows) at regions called "surface couplings," and stacks of tubules which, when viewed in three dimensions, are sheets of reticulum with fenestrations (arrow heads) similar to the fenestrated collar of the sarcoplasmic reticulum found in striated muscles. The reticulum is continuous with the nuclear envelope (not shown). This tonic type of smooth muscle has a more extensive network of reticulum than phasic muscles such as the portal vein or taenia coli, in which the reticulum is predominantly at the periphery of the cell.

tions, but not the responses to caffeine. Neomycin, an inhibitor of phospholipase C, blocked Ca release induced by carbachol, but not by caffeine. These studies were extended to reversibly permeabilized ileum smooth muscle cells in which heparin and Fura–2 acid were introduced. Ca and force responses to high potassium were normal, but intracellular heparin inhibited carbachol–induced Ca^{2+} release and contraction in Ca^{2+}–free high K^+ solution [4]. These results provide strong evidence that $InsP_3$ is the major physiological messenger of the Ca^{2+}–release component of pharmacomechanical coupling. The kinetics of Ca^{2+} release, recorded with fluo–3, and force development following photolytic release of $InsP_3$ from caged $InsP_3$, to circumvent diffusional delays, further support this hypothesis [12]. The cascade of events and the timing of the Ca^{2+}–release component of pharmacomechanical coupling are shown in Fig. 2. The two major components of the long 1–1.5 second delay between photolysis of caged phenylephrine and force development are the pre–$InsP_3$ steps of the phosphatidylinositol cascade (0.5–1.0 sec) [13–15] and the pre–phosphorylation and phosphorylation reactions of myosin light chain phosphorylation (0.2–0.3 sec) [16, 17]. If the 20,000 dalton light chains are pre–phosphorylated with ATPγS followed by photolysis of caged ATP, the delay to force development is less than 50 milliseconds. Thus the kinetics of $InsP_3$–induced Ca release and contraction are consistent with the major physiological role of $InsP_3$ as the messenger of pharmacomechanical Ca^{2+} release in smooth muscle [18].

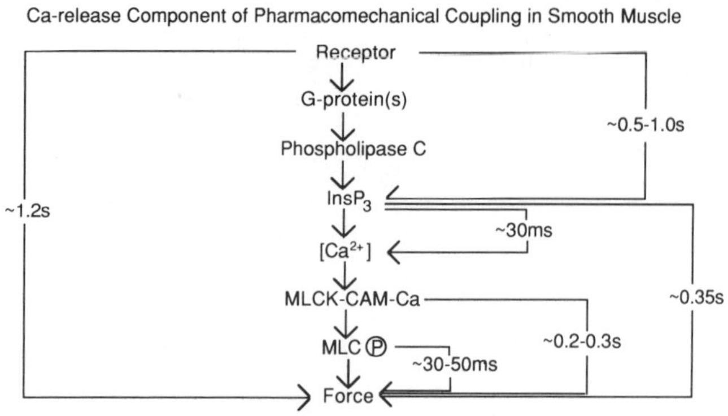

Figure 2. The cascade of events and kinetics of events between the binding of an agonist and the onset of force development triggered by the Ca^{2+}–release component of pharmacomechanical coupling in smooth muscle. Caged phenylephrine and caged Ins(1,4,5)P_3 were used to measure two of the delays [12, 18]. The time course of the increase in $InsP_3$ (0.5–1.0 sec) has been measured in tracheal smooth muscle [13–15]. Photolytic release of saturating concentrations of Ins(1,4,5)P_3 in permeabilized smooth muscle leads to an increase in Ca^{2+}–Fluo–3 signal in less than 10 msec, whereas at more " physiological" concentrations of Ins(1,4,5)P_3, Ca^{2+} rises with a delay of approximately 30 msec [26]. Photolysis of caged ATP in portal vein smooth muscle in the rigor state, with and without phosphorylation of myosin light chains, leads to significantly different delays and rates of force development (data from [12, 16, 18, 30, 31]). Modified from [31].

Ca^{2+} Sensitization

Ca^{2+} sensitization is another mode of pharmacomechanical coupling that, like $InsP_3$–induced Ca release, is G–protein coupled to excitatory receptors. Although the two processes can be dissociated [19], it is not known whether they are coupled through the same G–protein nor has the G–protein (s) been identified. Ca sensitization can be observed in intact muscles in which the ratio of force developed to cytoplasmic [Ca^{2+}] can be much greater in response to agonist stimulation than following depolarization with high K^+ [20–22]. In permeabilized smooth muscles, agonists or GTPγS cause a marked shift to the left of the Ca force curve under conditions where $[Ca^{2+}]_i$ is accurately clamped with EGTA and all intracellularly releasable Ca^{2+} is removed with A23187 [5, 21, 23, 24]. GDPβS blocks the agonist–induced Ca^{2+} sensitizing effects, indicative of coupling via a G–protein. This Ca^{2+}–sensitizing effect of agonists on force development is secondary to increased myosin light chain 20 (MLC_{20}) phosphorylation [5, 23].

Contraction in smooth muscle is switched on by the rise in intracellular Ca^{2+}, which activates the Ca^{2+}–calmodulin–dependent enzyme, myosin light chain kinase, leading to phosphorylation of MLC_{20}, which turns on actomyosin ATPase activity and crossbridge cycling leading to force development and shortening. The muscle relaxes when cytoplasmic Ca^{2+} falls and MLC_{20} is dephosphorylated by myosin light chain phosphatase (MLCP). Thus, force could be modulated through changes in either kinase or phosphatase activity. The agonist– or GTPγS–induced increase in force and MLC_{20} phosphorylation at constant [Ca^{2+}] could reflect a decrease in MLC_{20} phosphatase activity. Dephosphorylation was markedly slowed in the presence of GTPγS or GTP plus phenylephrine when Ca^{2+} and ATP were removed and an inhibitor of myosin light chain kinase was added to contracted muscles [25], consistent with the original hypothesis of Somlyo and colleagues [26], that G–protein mediated Ca^{2+}–sensitization is due to inhibition of MLCP.

Myosin phosphatase is thought to be bound to the myosin filaments and, therefore, it is necessary to invoke a messenger or cascade of messengers to couple the receptor G–protein activation to the inhibition of MLCP. Arachidonic acid (AA) is a potential candidate, as in permeabilized smooth muscle preparations it induces Ca sensitization, MLC_{20} phosphorylation, and it inhibits dephosphorylation [27]. This effect of AA is not due to products of AA metabolism, as it can be mimicked by a non–metabolizable analogue (5,8,11,14–eicosatetraynoic acid) and is not inhibited by inhibitors of AA metabolism. A purified, oligomeric MLC_{20} phosphatase isolated from gizzard smooth muscle can be dissociated into subunits by AA, and the activity of the dissociated enzyme is inhibited towards heavy meromyosin, but not phosphorylase. Therefore, AA may act as a messenger, promoting protein phosphorylation through direct inhibition of the form of protein phosphatase (s) that dephosphorylate MLC_{20} *in vivo* [27]. It is quite likely that such G–protein coupled modulation of phosphatase activity also operates in other cell systems. AA can be produced in eukaryotic cells through several mechanisms, and has been proposed to act as a cellular messenger [28, 29]. However, whether AA has the specific role of a messenger of agonist–induced Ca^{2+}–sensitization in intact smooth muscle remains to be determined.

Myosin Light Chain Kinase and Phosphatase Activities in Phasic and Tonic Smooth Muscles

The kinetics of contraction of phasic and tonic smooth muscles were measured in permeabilized muscles activated by laser flash photolysis of caged adenosine triphosphate in the presence of Ca^{2+} with or without pre–thiophosphorylation of MLC_{20} with ATPγS prior to photolysis. When not prephosphorylated, the half–time of force development at 20°C was four to five times faster in the phasic than in tonic muscles. Thiophosphorylation of MLC_{20} to fully activate that contractile regulating system prior to initiating the cross–bridge cycle with ATP reduced the half–time for force development fivefold in the tonic trachealis and by eightfold in the phasic ileum smooth muscles. Even following thiophosphorylation of MLC_{20} the rate of force development ($t_{1/2}$) was three to four times faster in phasic than in tonic smooth muscles [16]. These results indicate that both the regulatory and the contractile mechanisms are faster in phasic than in tonic smooth muscles.

The slow tonic smooth muscles were also significantly more sensitive to the phosphatase inhibitors microcystin–LR, tautomycin, and okadaic acid. The half–times of relaxation and dephosphorylation were 4–6 times longer and the HMM phosphatase and myosin light chain kinase activity per smooth muscle cell weight was 2.0– and 1.9–fold lower in the tonic, femoral artery, than in the phasic, ileum or portal vein, smooth muscle. The higher kinase and phosphatase activities would account for the higher initial rates of force development, with the rate constant of activation reflecting the sum of the forward (phosphorylation) and backward (dephosphorylation) rate constants. On the other hand, the higher phosphatase activity is consistent with the lower steady–state value of force and phosphorylation in the phasic smooth muscles and would account for their more rapid relaxation upon removal of Ca. Thus the combination of higher myosin light chain kinase and phosphatase activities probably plays a major role in the higher rate of both force development and relaxation of the fast, phasic smooth muscles. In addition, differences in the rates of crossbridge cycling, perhaps due to different affinities of myosin for ADP and isozymic variability of the contractile or thin filament–associated proteins, may modulate contractility and contribute to the different contractile properties of phasic and tonic smooth muscles.

CONCLUSIONS

It is now apparent that contractility in smooth muscle is controlled not solely by changes in cytoplasmic [Ca^{2+}]. Modulation of MLC phosphatase and possibly kinase activities through receptor–G–protein coupled processes, as well as differences in the amounts and ratio of these enzymes, can have marked effects on contractility. It will be important to determine whether smooth muscle disease states such as hypertension and asthma have defects in the pathways leading to pharmacomechanical Ca^{2+} release and/or Ca–sensitization.

Acknowledgements

We gratefully acknowledge the contributions of our collaborators who co–authored the publications reviewed in this communication. We thank Ms. Barbara Nordin for preparation of the manuscript. This work has been supported by PO–HL19242 and 1–PO–1HL48807 from the National Institutes of Health.

DISCUSSION

Dr. F. Prinzen: You showed the effect of heparin on the coupling with IP3. What concentration is that? Is it in the same range of the anticoagulative effect of heparin?

Dr. A. Somlyo: We determined the inhibitory concentration of heparin (IC_{50} = 5 μg/ml) and found it was identical to the concentration which inhibited $InsP_3$ binding to the $InsP_3$ receptor. I am aware that heparin does other things when applied to whole cells, but in this case we are using it to evaluate the contribution of the $InsP_3$ releasable Ca^{2+} store to pharmacomechanical coupling.

Dr. F. Prinzen: If heparin in these concentrations also acts in the whole body, then adding heparin just as an anticoagulative agent might affect testing drugs acting through the IP3.

Dr. A. Somlyo: In the experiments I reported, heparin was applied to permeabilized fibers in order to bind to intracellular $InsP_3$ receptors. I would not expect that it would cross the cell membrane of intact cells.

Dr. D. Allen: You have shown very nicely that IP3 plays an important role in vascular smooth muscle and it turns out that in the heart there is a surprisingly high density in myocardial cells of IP3 receptors. In that case they are like receptors looking for a function. I am not aware of a very clear cut physiological or pharmacomechanical role for IP3 in heart muscle. Can you comment on the possible role of IP3 mediated mechanisms in the heart muscle?

Dr. A. Somlyo: There is a very interesting recent paper by P. Volpe and colleagues of Padova, where they report localization of $InsP_3$ receptors to the conduction system with much less signal in the myocardial wall. They suggest that alpha 1–adrenergic stimulation of $InsP_3$ induced Ca^{2+} release could be the mechanism of increased automaticity of Purkinje cells. Incidently, there are extremely high concentrations of $InsP_3$ receptors in the brain, which apart from being a wonderful source for biochemists, is also in search of a function.

Dr. C. Holloway: I am very interested in the arachidonic acid as a possible factor in the dissociation of the catalytic and regulatory subunits. What concentrations of arachidonic acid does one expect in the cell?

Dr. A. Somlyo: There have been studies done on pancreatic islet cells and cardiac cells where concentrations are on the order of 50 μM.

Dr. C. Holloway: What do you think are the effects of the arachidonic acid metabolites?

Dr. A. Somlyo: The Ca^{2+}-sensitizing effect of AA is not inhibited by inhibitors of AA metabolism (indomethacin, nordihydroguaiaretic acid or propyl gallate) and was abolished by oxidation of AA in air. A non-metabolizable analogue, ETYA, also had Ca^{2+} sensitizing effects. Therefore, the AA metabolites are not mediating Ca^{2+} sensitization.

Dr. D. Kass: Do you know of changes that occur at the level of phosphatase-kinase control of phosphorylation of myosin light chain. In chronic conditions in which blood-pressure is increased, vessels see high stress or high levels of circulating catecholamines. This also occurs with chronic vascular adaptations in heart failure patients.

Dr. A. Somlyo: Both concentration and regulation of phosphatases and kinases may be a very interesting and fruitful area to explore in pathological states of smooth muscle. I am not aware of any information to date.

Dr. D. Kass: What do you know about the role of this kind of regulation of myosin phosphorylation in myocytes.

Dr. A. Somlyo: I expect that this type of sensitization and desensitization may very well be present in other cells. I doubt if it is exclusive to smooth muscle.

Dr. D. Allen: In one cell you could get an apparent change in sensitivity with different agonists and you attribute that to phosphorylation of the myosin-light chain. I wonder if in addition to that there might be changes in distribution of calcium within the cell. I know there are some suggestions that calcium distribution in smooth muscle cells can differ with different agonists and that can lead to changes in apparent sensitivity under some circumstances. Is there much evidence on that point?

Dr. A. Somlyo: The different magnitudes of Ca^{2+} sensitization observed with different agonists in intact smooth muscle were retained in permeabilized cells where the Ca^{2+} concentration was clamped with 10 mM EGTA and Ca stores were depleted with A23187. Under these conditions it is highly unlikely that gradients of Ca^{2+} exist in the cells.

REFERENCES

1. Somlyo AP, Somlyo AV. Electromechanical and pharmacomechanical coupling in vascular smooth muscle. *J Pharmacol Exp Therap* 1968; 59: 129–145.
2. Somlyo AP, Kitazawa T, Kobayashi G, Somlyo AV. Pharmacomechanical coupling: the membranes talk to the cross-bridges. In: Moreland RS (ed), *Regulation of Smooth Muscle*. Raven Press Publishers: New York, 1991: 185-208.
3. Nishiye E, Somlyo AV, Török K, Somlyo AP. The effects of MgADP on cross-bridge kinetics: a laser flash photolysis study of guinea-pig smooth muscle. *J Physiol* 1993; 260: 247–271.
4. Kobayashi S, Kitazawa T, Somlyo AV, Somlyo AP. Cytosolic heparin inhibits muscarinic and α-adrenergic Ca^{2+}-release in smooth muscle. *J Biol Chem* 1989; 264: 17997–18004.
5. Kitazawa T, Kobayashi S, Horiuti T, Somlyo AV, Somlyo AP. Receptor-coupled, permeabilized smooth muscle: Role of the phosphatidylinositol cascade, G-proteins, and modulation of the contractile response to Ca^{2+}. *J Biol Chem* 1989; 264: 5339-5342.
6. Kitazawa T, Gaylinn BD, Denney GH, Somlyo AP. G-protein-mediated Ca^{2+}-sensitization of smooth muscle contraction through myosin light chain phosphorylation. *J Biol Chem* 1991; 266: 1708-1715.
7. Gong MC, Cohen P, Kitazawa T, Ikebe M, Masuo M, Somlyo AP, Somlyo AV. MLCP activities and the effects of phosphatase inhibitors in tonic and phasic smooth muscle. *J Biol Chem* 1992; 267: 14662-14668.

8. Lesh RE, Marks AR, Somlyo AV, Fleisher S, Somlyo AP. Anti–ryanodine receptor antibody binding sites in aortic and endocardial endothelium. *Circ Res* 1993; 72: 481–488.
9. Bond M, Kitazawa T, Somlyo AP, Somlyo AV. Release and recycling of calcium by the sarcoplasmic reticulum in guinea pig portal vein smooth muscle. *J Physiol* 1984; 355: 677–695.
10. Kowarski D, Shuman H, Somlyo AP, Somlyo AV. Calcium–release by noreadrenaline from cenral sarcoplasmic reticulum in rabbit main pulmonary artery smooth muscle. *J Physiol* 1985; 366: 153–175.
11. Somlyo AP, Somlyo AV, Bond M, Broderick R, Goldman YE, Shuman H, Walker JW, Trentham DR. Calcium and magnesium movements in cells and the role of inositol trisphosphate in muscle. In: Eaton DC, Mandel LJ (eds), *Cell Calcium and the Control of Membrane Support*. Rockefeller University Press: New York, 1987; 42: 77–92.
12. Somlyo AV, Horiuti K, Trentham DR, Kitazawa T, Somlyo AP. Kinetics of Ca^{2+}–release and contraction induced by photolysis of caged D–myo–inositol 1,4,5–trisphosphate in smooth muscle: The effects of heparin, procaine and adenine nucleotides. *J Biol Chem* 1992; 267: 22316–22322.
13. Duncan RA, Kryzanowski JJ, Davis JS, Polson JB, Coffey RG, Shimoda T, Szentivanyi A. Polyphosphoinositide metabolism in canine tracheal smooth muscle (CTSM) in response to a cholinergic stimulus. *Biochem Pharmacol* 1987; 36: 307–310.
14. Miller–Hance WC, Miller JR, Wells JN, Stull JT, Kamm KE. Biochemical events associated with activation of smooth muscle contraction. *J Biol Chem* 1988; 263(28): 13979–13982.
15. Chilvers ER, Challis RAJ, Barnes PJ, Nahorski SR. Mass changes of inositol (1,4,5)–trisphosphate in trachealis muscle following agonist stimulation. *Eur J Pharmacol* 1989; 164: 587–590.
16. Horiuti K, Somlyo AV, Goldman YE, Somlyo AP. Kinetics of contraction initiated by flash photolysis of caged adenosine trisphosphate in tonic and phasic smooth muscle. *J Gen Physiol* 1989; 94: 769–781.
17. Somlyo AV, Goldman YE, Fujimori T, Trentham DR, Somlyo AP. Cross–bridge kinetics, cooperativity, and negatively stained crossbridges in vertebrate smooth muscle: A laser flash photolysis study. *J Gen Physiol* 1988; 91: 165–192.
18. Somlyo AP, Walker JW, Goldman YE, Trentham DR, Kobayashi S, Kitazawa T, Somlyo AV. Inositol trisphosphate, calcium and muscle contraction. *Phil Trans R Soc Lond B* 1988; 329: 399–414.
19. Kobayashi S, Gong MC, Somlyo AV, Somlyo AP. Ca^{2+} channel blockers distinguish between G–protein–mediated pharmacomechanical Ca^{2+}–release and Ca^{2+}–sensitization. *Am J Physiol* 1991; 260: C364–C370.
20. Rembold CM, Murphy RA. Myoplasmic [Ca^{2+}] determines myosin phosphorylation in agonist–stimulated swine arterial smooth muscle. *Circ Res* 1988; 63: 593–603.
21. Himpens B, Kitazawa T, Somlyo AP. Agonist–dependent modulation of Ca^{2+}–sensitivity in rabbit pulmonary artery smooth muscle. *Pflugers Arch* 1990; 417: 21–28.
22. Morgan JP, Morgan KG. Stimulus–specific patterns of intracellular calcium levels in smooth muscle of ferret portal vein. *J Physiol (Lond)* 1984; 351: 155–167.
23. Fujiwara T, Itoh T, Kubota Y, Kuriyama H. Effects of guanosine nucleotides on skinned smooth muscle tissue of the rabbit mesenteric artery. *J Physiol* 1989; 408: 535–547.
24. Nishimura J, Kobler M, van Breemen C. Norepinephrine and GTP–gamma–S increase myofilament Ca^{2+}–sensitivity in alpha–toxin permeabilized arterial smooth muscle. *Biochem Biophys Res Commun* 1988; 157: 677–683.
25. Kitazawa T, Masuo M, Somlyo AP. G–protein–mediated inhibition of MLCP in vascular smooth muscle. *Proc Natl Acad Sci USA* 1991; 88: 9307–9310.
26. Somlyo AP, Kitazawa T, Himpens B, Matthijs G, Horiuti T, Kobayashi S, Goldman YE, Somlyo AV. Modulation of Ca^{2+}–sensitivity and of the time course of contraction in smooth muscle: a major role of protein phosphatases? *Adv Prot Phosp* 1989; 5: 181–195.
27. Gong MC, Fuglsang A, Alessi D, Kobayashi S, Cohen P, Somlyo AV, Somlyo AP. Arachidonic acid inhibits MLCP and sensitizes smooth muscle to calcium. *J Biol Chem* 1992; 267: 22316–22322.
28. Axelrod J. Receptor–mediated activation of phospholipase A_2 and arachidonic acid in signal transduction. *Biochem Soc Trans* 1990; 18: 503–507.
29. Burch RM. G protein regulation of phospholipase A2. *Mol Neurobiol* 1989; 3: 155–171.
30. Somlyo AP, Somlyo AV. Flash photolysis studies of excitation contraction coupling, regulation, and contraction in smooth muscle. *Ann Rev Physiol* 1990; 52: 857–874.
31. Somlyo AP, Somlyo AV. Smooth muscle structure and function. *The Heart and Cardiovascular System*, Second Edition. Fozzard HA, Jenning RB, Haber E, Katz AM, Morgan HE (eds). New York, NY: Raven Press Ltd., 1991; pp 1295–1324.

CHAPTER 5

Myocardial Energetics

Lincoln E. Ford[1]

ABSTRACT

Inotropic alterations may alter contractile efficiency. Positive inotropic agents act mainly, if not exclusively, by increasing activation, which has very little effect on contractile efficiency. The metabolic effects of hypoxia may depress the contractile machinery directly. Acidosis is likely to decrease efficiency while an elevated phosphate, by itself, is likely to have little effect on efficiency.

INTRODUCTION

The main interest of my laboratory is discovering the basic mechanisms by which the heart varies the strength of its beat. This interest frequently leads to studies which may seem far removed from our main interest, and one purpose of this presentation is to relate our apparently disparate studies to the common theme of basic inotropic mechanisms. As will be explained, at least half of our experimental work is done in skeletal muscle, not because of any divergence of our interests, but because the greater simplicity of this preparation allows us to draw less equivocal conclusions. Another purpose of this presentation is to explain some of our thinking regarding the energetics of contraction that underlies our present line of investigation.

A useful but sometimes overlooked consideration regarding systems that vary their output is that they have a maximum capability which is not attained under normal working conditions. Such systems increase their output by decreasing the normal inhibition to maximum output rather than by some increase in their maximum capability. This concept of varying inhibition is epitomized by the single word "valve" used by the British to denote a vacuum tube amplifier. Variations in electronic output are achieved by regulating the flow of power through the valves in the circuit. Similarly, the power output of muscle is regulated by the modulation of the transduction processes that convert chemical energy into

[1]Cardiology Section, University of Chicago, Chicago, IL 60637, USA.

Interactive Phenomena in the Cardiac System, Edited by
S. Sideman and R. Beyar, Plenum Press, New York, 1993

mechanical force and work. In the short term, this regulation is provided mainly, if not exclusively, by the activating system. Over very long periods, muscle power output can be regulated by alterations in the type of myosin in the muscle. Our present efforts are directed at determining whether, over intermediate periods, the power output of muscle can be regulated by direct effects on the contractile elements, independent of variations in activation. Before discussing the background to these efforts, I will describe some of our work on the activating system.

MECHANICAL MANIFESTATIONS OF ACTIVATION

When the troponin–tropomyosin system of muscle was discovered, a question arose as to whether this activating system acted solely as a switch, or whether it had some other interaction with the contractile proteins. The switch-like mechanism is summarized schematically in Fig. 1. The troponin–tropomyosin complexes are shown in Fig. 1C as providing a stearic hinderance to the attachment of the myosin crossbridges to their thin filament sites. If the bridges act independently, reducing the number of activated bridges (Fig. 1C) should have the same effect as decreasing the number of bridges by some other means, such as reducing the cross-section of the muscle (Fig. 1B). In assessing the effects of these changes on the force–velocity curves (Figs. 1 D and E) it is helpful to think of velocity as the independent variable and of force as being determined by the velocity.

If the crossbridges act independently, maximum velocity will be an intrinsic property of the population of bridges, independent of their number. At all velocities less than the maximum the force generated will be proportional to the number of bridges available to carry the load (Fig. 1D). The curves can be made to superimpose if they are scaled in proportion to the number of active bridges. Since isometric force is assumed to

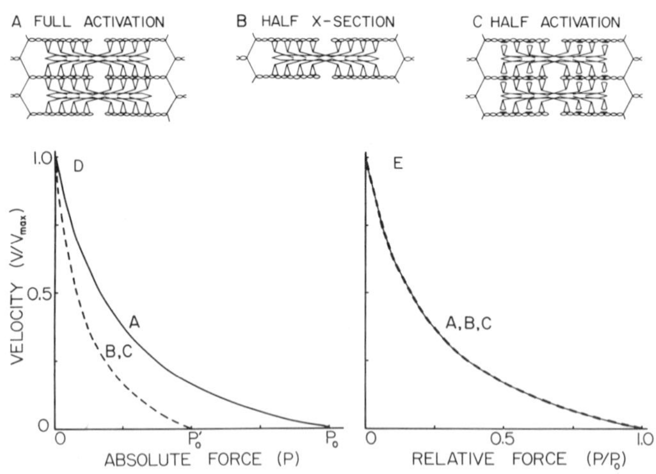

Figure 1. Schematic representation of the postulate that crossbridges function independently. Reducing the number of bridges in parallel from the fully activated state, **A**, by stearic hinderance of the thin filament attachment sites, **C**, is no different than reducing the cross-sectional area of the muscle, **B**. Both interventions decrease force at each velocity in proportion to the decrease in parallel bridges, **D**. The curves can be made to superimpose by normalizing the force to its isometric value, **E**.

be proportional to the number of activated bridges, it has become conventional to scale the isotonic forces in proportion to the isometric force, i.e. to plot the isotonic force as a fraction of the isometric, as in Fig. 1E. As shown in that figure, the assumptions that the bridges act independently and that the activating system acts as a simple switch, predict that plots of velocity against relative force should superimpose exactly, and that maximum velocity should be independent of the level of activation. Although the concept is simple, determining how the muscle behaves has been more problematic. Before describing these problems, I should point out that my own interest in this issue arose from the practical question of how direct effects of inotropic interventions on the contractile elements could be distinguished from changes in calcium activation. Quite apart from any theoretical questions of crossbridge mechanisms, it was imperative to know the influence of calcium when assessing the effects of other interventions.

Skinned Skeletal Muscle

Among the many controversies that characterized the 1970s was that which clouded the issue of calcium activation. Two laboratories known for careful work used skinned skeletal muscle fibers to address the question posed in Fig. 1 and arrived at exactly opposite conclusions [1]. When such controversies arise, other laboratories are well advised to investigate something else until they are resolved, but the questions posed by these results were so central to the issue of inotropic mechanisms that they could not be ignored. For reasons described below, the results obtained in intact cardiac muscle are complicated by several extraneous factors, so investigation of the basic effects of calcium activation required a simpler system, such as the skinned skeletal fiber. Before setting out to investigate this question for ourselves, we published a fairly comprehensive review of the history of this issue [1].

Our own results [2] are summarized in Fig. 2. Force–velocity curves were obtained in skinned fibers activated at both full activation and at a level of partial activation that produced 45% of maximum force. As shown, the two curves superimpose almost exactly, as expected on the basis of the assumptions made in Fig. 1. We take this as strong evidence that the crossbridges act independently and that the function of the bridges that attach in partially activated fibers is not altered by the lack of activation of neighboring attachment sites. I should also point out that Moss [3] has shown that velocity is more reduced by extensive shortening in partially as compared with fully activated fibers, so that the results shown in Fig. 2 would not be obtained if the measurements were not made shortly after a release to an isotonic load. There are, however, several reasonable explanations of this additional finding that are not inconsistent with the basic interpretation proposed here.

Intact Cardiac Muscle

Activation in cardiac muscle appears to vary continuously throughout the twitch, so that changes in activation can be assessed by studying the muscle at different times in the twitch. In addition, peak force can be increased conveniently by interpolating an extra-systole. Since the response to this intervention is almost immediate, it is reasonable to assume that its only effect is to increase the amount of activating calcium, without any other chemical alteration in the contractile proteins. By varying time in the twitch and by using post–extrasystolic potentiation we were able to study force–velocity curves over a 6–fold range of activation [4]. In this study, maximum velocity was not the same at different levels of activation (Fig. 3), as it is in skinned fibers (Fig. 2), and the force–velocity curves could not be made to superimpose by a simple scaling of the isotonic force. They

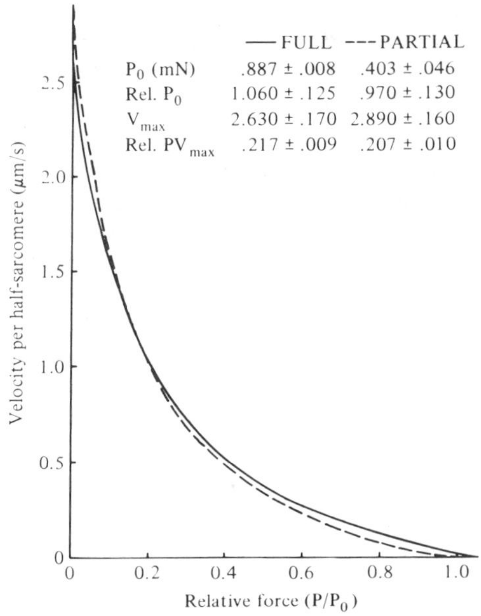

Figure 2. Force–velocity curves fit to the data obtained in skinned skeletal fibers at full activation (solid curve) and at a level of partial activation which produced a 55% reduction in isometric force (interrupted curve). (From Podolin and Ford [2].)

could, however, be made to superimpose quite closely if there is added to each value of force a constant load equivalent to about 4% of the isometric force produced at the peak of the twitch (Fig. 3B). This coincidence does not, by itself, prove that the small activation dependence of maximum velocity in cardiac muscle is due to an internal load. However, when combined with the finding that maximum velocity of a simpler, single-cell preparation is independent of activation (Fig. 2), it provides strong evidence that the activation dependence of maximum velocity in cardiac muscle is due to a small internal load provided by passive elements in this multicellular preparation.

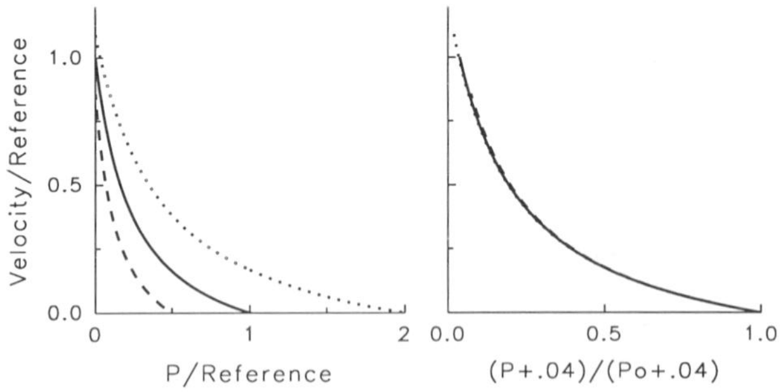

Figure 3. Force–velocity curves obtained at three levels of activation: peak of a normal twitch (solid curve), when activation had achieved half of this value (dashed curve), and at the peak of a potentiated twitch (dotted curve). The curves superimpose when a load equivalent to 4% of unpotentiated twitch force is added to all forces and the isotonic force is scaled to the isometric force.

EFFECTS OF INOTROPIC INTERVENTIONS

Different classes of inotropic interventions alter the isometric twitches of intact cardiac muscle in very different ways (Fig. 4), but all of the interventions altered the force–velocity curves in ways that were statistically indistinguishable from post–extrasystolic potentiation [5]. The differences in the shapes of the twitch can be explained either by changes in the time course of the myoplasmic calcium transient or by alterations in the calcium affinity of the thin filaments [6–8]. On the basis of this data, we believed that we had defined the range of possible mechanisms which alter the inotropic state of the myocardium. In terms of the "valve" concept of amplification, the effect of all the inotropic agents could be explained by their allowing more bridges to pass from inactive to active states.

As we were publishing this work, two other groups concluded that adrenergic stimulation acts directly on the contractile elements, independently of its effects on the activating system [9, 10]. They further noted that these effects were most prominent in muscles having a predominance of the fast, V1, myosin isoform. There are at least three possible explanations of the disparity between their conclusions and ours: 1) Since our experiments were done in adult rabbits that have a predominance of the slow, V3, isoform, the effects described by the other workers would have been less prominent. 2) Adrenergic stimulation of the mixed isoform muscles by the other workers might have selectively increased the activation of the V1 isoform by a mechanism of selective activation proposed t Winegrad and his colleagues [6]. 3) The effects described by the other workers might have been due to variations in the hypoxic core of their muscles; they activated their muscles continuously with barium contractures and the oxygen utilization could have varied both with the isoform composition and with the adrenergic tone of the preparation.

These considerations indicate that we have not yet answered the question of whether the usual inotropic interventions directly alter the contractility of the contractile elements in addition to their effect on the activating system. In addition, there are physiologically occurring negative inotropic interventions that probably do have such direct effects. We are now in the process of determining the extent to which these various inotropic interventions directly alter the contractile apparatus, once it becomes activated. As with our other work, our initial experiments are in skinned skeletal muscle, and much of the remainder of this presentation is a discussion of the theoretical implications of our present experiments.

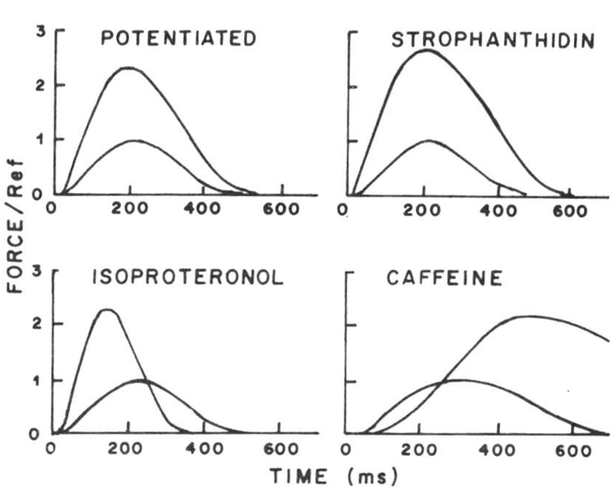

Figure 4. Effect of four interventions on twitches of rabbit papillary muscle at 23°C.

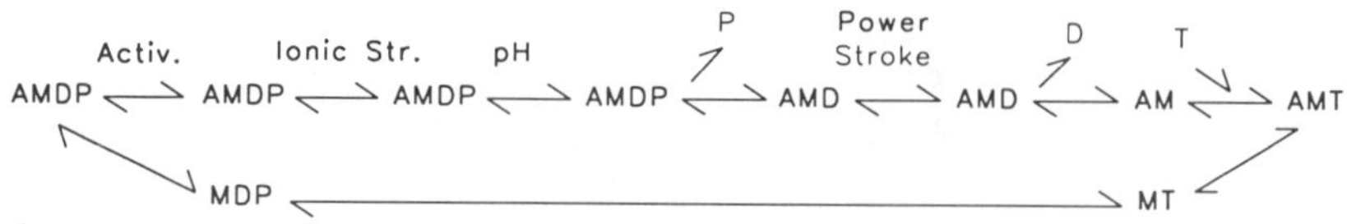

Figure 5. The crossbridge cycle. After the power stroke the myosin crossbridge (M) releases ADP (D), binds ATP (T), and detach from actin (A). The ATP is hydrolyzed before the bridge reattaches to the actin. The low–force attached bridge undergoes at least three transitions before the force–producing power stroke, as indicated.

The Crossbridge Cycle

It is generally believed that muscle contraction is produced by the cyclical attachment and detachment of myosin crossbridges to the actin filaments, with a force–producing power stroke occurring during the attached phase of the cycle. In addition, it is now known that multiple chemical transitions (ATP binding, hydrolysis, product release) and physical transitions (crossbridge attachment, power stroke, detachment) occur during the cycle (Fig. 5). The issue to be considered here is how alterations in these transitions affect shortening velocity, power output, and efficiency of the muscle.

Changes in Activation

Brenner et al. [11] have shown that bridges can attach to thin filaments even in the relaxed state, and that activation allows these initially attached bridges to move to other parts of the cycle (Fig. 5). The effect of activation is not to allow attachment, as implied by the simple scheme in Fig. 1C, but to allow initially attached bridges to move to states where they are less likely to detach. In the inactive state bridges accumulate either in the initially attached state or in the detached state, both states being in a rapid equilibrium. A very effective way of regulating the energy output of the muscle, therefore, is to regulate

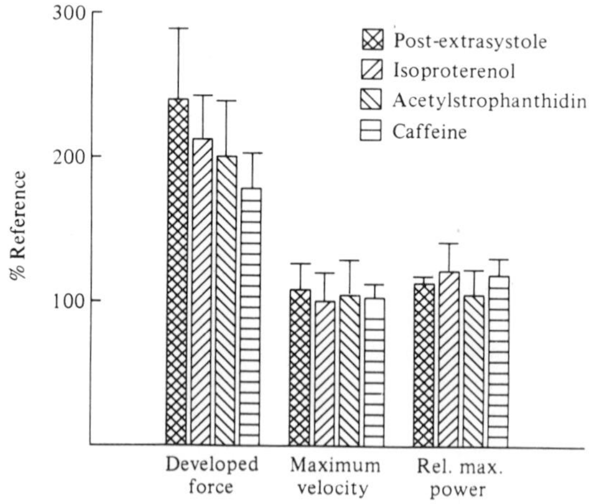

Figure 6. Effect of four interventions on the force–velocity parameters measured at the peak of the contraction. None of the parameters are significantly different from those measured during post–extrasystolic potentiation.

the rate at which bridges pass through the transition that is blocked by the troponin–tropomyosin system. The pioneering work of Allen and Blinks [12] showing that positive inotropic agents increase the amount of calcium released into the myofilament space supports the interpretation of the data in Fig. 6 that these agents mainly increase the degree of activation. The question to be considered here, therefore, is not whether these interventions increase activation, but to what extent, if any, they directly alter the cycling of crossbridges once they become activated. An additional issue is the expectations of physiological interventions with negative inotropic effects.

Effects on Velocity

The crossbridge theory predicts that velocity is determined by the rate at which attached bridges move through their several transitions and detach. At high loads the cycling rate is limited mainly by the rate at which bridges can pass through the power stoke while performing the work imposed by the external load. At velocities approaching the maximum, the low external load on the bridges does not greatly impede their movements, and velocity is instead limited by other transitions in the attached phase of the cycle. This consideration suggested that an inotropic intervention which altered a transition other than activation would also change velocity. An intervention that changes a transition during the attached phase would be likely to alter maximum velocity, since the attached phase transitions are the only impediments to shortening when there is no external load. An intervention that affects a transition during the detached phase would alter the fraction of bridges attached and thereby alter velocities in the middle of the curve. Thus far we have found that some interventions produce alternative transitions that have effects on velocity which we had not expected. These unexpected results have made us realize that more extensive experiments will be required to be certain that an intervention affects only activation. They also have led to the consideration that the muscle may have evolved some effective ways of shutting down contraction during fatigue and hypoxia.

An alternative pathway is illustrated by the effects of high ionic strength on contractile parameters [13]. Both low pH and high ionic strength diminish isometric force. The conditions to be illustrated (pH 6.35 vs. 7.35 and ionic strength 360 mM vs. 125 mM) both reduce isometric force by half. The low pH also reduces maximum velocity by 43% whereas the high ionic strength did not have a significant effect on velocity. Our earlier thinking would have suggested that low pH has a direct effect on the crossbridge cycle and that high ionic strength has an effect on the activating system. Tension transients show something else.

Tension Transients

When a length change is suddenly imposed on otherwise isometric sarcomeres the force undergoes a sequence of changes known collectively as tension transients [14]. During the length step, force changes in the direction of the step, and recovers in several characteristic stages following the step. The extent of the initial force change depends on the number of bridges that are attached and therefore in a position to resist the change. The ratio of the force change to the length change (i.e. the stiffness) is thus a measure of the number of attached bridges [15]. Figure 7 shows force records that have been scaled so that the isometric forces all have the same amplitude. Both low pH (Fig. 7A) and high ionic strength (Fig. 7B) decrease stiffness to a lesser extent than force, so that the initial force change associated with the length step is relatively larger. In absolute terms, both low pH and high ionic strength decrease force by about half and stiffness by about one–quarter, so that the relative stiffness is increased by about half. The lower absolute stiffness indicates that both interventions decrease the number of attached bridges, but the increased relative stiffness indicates that a larger fraction of the attached bridges are in low force states that precede the power stroke. This accumulation of bridges in low force states suggests that both interventions inhibit transitions that precede the power stroke. The force responses following the length change further indicate that the two interventions detain bridges in very different states which account for the differences in the effects of the two interventions on shortening velocity.

Figure 7A shows that the relatively greater force response seen at low pH is long–lived following release and short–lived following stretch. Fig. 7B show that high ionic strength produces the opposite directionality, the force differences are long–lived following stretch but decay rapidly following release. We interpret this as indicating that the bridges are detained in two different low force states by the two interventions, and that these states are differentiated by the strain dependence of the rates of detachment. A more extensive analysis showed an excellent correlation between the decreased maximum velocity and the internal load imposed by the bridges detained at low pH [13]. By contrast, high ionic strength does not effect velocity because the detained bridges detach following release and offer no resistance to shortening.

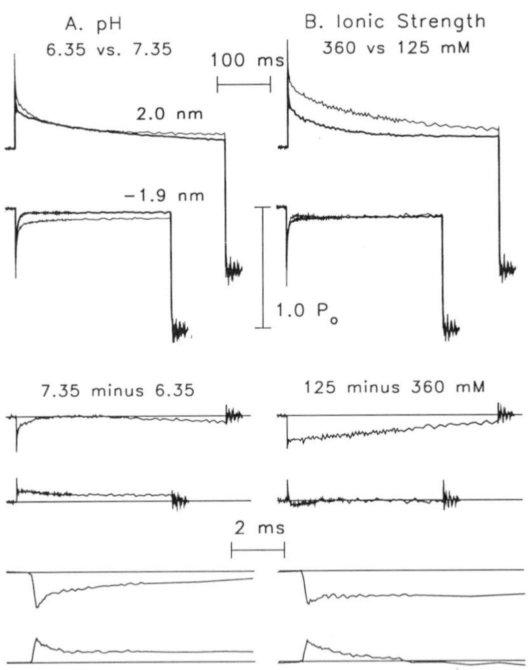

Figure 7. Effect of low pH (**A**) and high ionic strength (**B**) on the tension transients following a small stretch or release. A large step at the end of the record zeroes the transducer. The stretch was applied for a longer period because the responses were slower. Upper records: superimposed traces. Reference (thick – pH 7.35 in **A**, ionic strength 125 mM in **B**) and test (thin – pH 6.35 in **A**, ionic strength 360 mM in **B**) traces. Records have been scaled so that their isometric forces are the same. Sizes of the length steps are printed next to the records. The difference records (test minus reference) are plotted below. The lower pair of difference records are plotted at a 50 times greater speed to resolve the events associated with the step.

Effects on Energetics

Figure 7A shows that some interventions slow the crossbridge cycling rate by detaining bridges in states which resist shortening. The load imposed by these bridges decreases muscle efficiency since some of the energy of ATP hydrolysis must be expended in overcoming the internal load imposed by the detained bridges. This consideration has major implications for our expectations of inotropic interventions. In terms of the "valve" concept of amplification, an inotropic intervention that increases ATP hydrolysis rate by increasing the rate of only one transition might increase internal work and decrease muscle efficiency by causing bridges to accumulate behind other transitions. If large changes in efficiency are to be avoided, it might be necessary to make complementary changes in several transitions. This requirement for complementary changes could be especially important in the evolutionary differences in myosins of different species, which produce large changes in velocity [16], probably with only small changes in efficiency. The effects on energetic may be especially important for the negative inotropic consequences of fatigue and hypoxia.

Contraction during hypoxia causes a decrease of ATP and an accumulation of ADP, phosphate, and H^+. A speculation from my own institution [17] may have given rise to the common assumption that the depressed myocardial contractility during hypoxia results from low pH causing inactivation. The decreased activation would not, by itself, alter efficiency because crossbridge cycling rate, ATPase rate, and external work would all be lowered in the same proportion. The decreased pH would, however, decrease efficiency by detaining bridges in a state where they resist shortening, and this diminished efficiency would have deleterious effects when a muscle's substrate is already limited. It therefore seems likely that muscles have evolved strategies for avoiding this inefficiency. A possibility suggested by the finding of Allen et al. (1985) is that hearts do not become very acidotic during hypoxia, but that the decrease in contractility is produced by other metabolic derangements. This consideration raises the question of which metabolic alteration is responsible. It seems unlikely that either raised ADP and lowered ATP cause the contractile failure in hypoxia because both alterations increase force. This suspicion is strengthened by the consideration that both metabolic derangements detain bridges in a high force state [19], where they facilitate activation through a "cooperative" interaction between crossbridge and calcium binding [20]. Such facilitation of activation is likely to worsen the metabolic imbalance, with potentially catastrophic effects. The remaining metabolic consequence of hypoxia, increased phosphate, is likely to inhibit contraction in a manner that would not decrease muscle efficiency. Our work indicates that phosphate decreases force and has pH dependent effects on velocity [21]. At low pH phosphate decreases velocity but at high pH it increases velocity, apparently by increasing crossbridge detachment. If cardiac muscle behaves as our skeletal muscle, it might find it advantageous to avoid a low intracellular pH during hypoxia and allow an accumulation of phosphate to inhibit contraction. Such an accumulation would have a protective effect because the resulting inhibition of contraction would diminish further ATP hydrolysis with its attendant metabolic consequences.

DISCUSSION

Dr. Y. Kresh: What do you think happens in the state that has been termed "hibernating myocardium"? When the perfusion pressure is diminished, does a commensurate decrease in muscle function or contractility take place? What would be the mechanism under these conditions? Apparently the heart is not ischemic because this state is completely reversible and there is little memory of the "ischemic" event.

Dr. L.E. Ford: It seems that contraction is simply shut off. The most obvious candidate for a mechanism would be a reduction in the activation of the of the muscle, either because of a reduced calcium sensitivity of the activating system due to acidosis or because of a decreased calcium release.

Dr. Y. Kresh: It seems that the calcium transient has a lower amplitude.

Dr. L.E. Ford: To the extent that you lower the transient, you would then be likely to have a depressed contraction and less energy utilization.

Dr. Y. Kresh: How does the calcium flux get lowered? What is the stimulus?

Dr. L.E. Ford: I do not really know the answer to that. One would expect the calcium to increase in the muscle with ischemia according to the mechanism that Dr. Allen described here. This would eventually overload the SR. As we all know, when the SR becomes overloaded with calcium it starts releasing it spontaneously and this of course increases the metabolic deficit in an ischemic muscle and makes the situation worse. I do not really know the answer to your question of how the ischemic muscle would exclude calcium, or how it would reduce the transient.

Dr. E. Marban: The calcium transients do go down in some models of low flow ischemia which are rapidly reversible; I do not know whether it is appropriate to use the term "ischemia" because you can do it without any metabolic changes and we do not know what the transduction mechanism is. It is really a very interesting observation.

Dr. S. Sideman: Your review on calcium activation with Richard Podolin in 1983 [1] is quite impressive. Could you tell us how you got around to writing it?

Dr. L.E. Ford: This was written in response to an invitation from Chris Ashley, the editor of the Journal of Muscle Research and Cell Motility. I accepted his invitation because Richard Podolin was planning to join me for a year of research experience in the middle of his clinical training and the experience would give him a good background in the area we were about to investigate. The experience turned out to be especially rewarding, because Richard had a flair for writing, and the outcome is a thorough review which is often cited, although it did make me more than a little unpopular in some quarters.

REFERENCES

1. Podolin RA, Ford LE. The influence of calcium on shortening velocity of skinned frog muscle fibres. *J Muscle Res Cell Motility* 1983; 4: 263–282.
2. Podolin RA, Ford LE. Influence of partial activation on the force velocity properties of frog skinned muscle fibres in millimolar magnesium ion. *J Gen Physiol* 1986; 87: 607–631.
3. Moss RL. Effects on shortening velocity of rabbit skeletal muscle due to variations in the level of thin-filament activation. *J Physiol* 1986; 377: 487–505.
4. Chiu CY, Ballou EW, Ford LE. Force, velocity, and power changes during normal and potentiated contractions of cat papillary muscle. *Circ Res* 1987; 60: 446–458.
5. Chiu CY, Walley KR, Ford LE. Comparison of the effects of different inotropic interventions on force, velocity, and power in rabbit myocardium. *Circ Res* 1989; 65: 1161–1171.
6. Winegrad S. Regulation of cardiac contractile proteins: correlations between physiology and biochemistry. *Circ Res* 1984; 55: 564–574.
7. Blinks JR, Endoh M. Modification of myofibrillar responsiveness to Ca^{++} as an inotropic mechanism. *Circulation* 1986; 60 (Suppl. III): III–85–III–97.
8. Allen DG, Orchard CH. Measurement of intracellular calcium concentration in heart muscle; The effects of inotropic interventions and hypoxia. *J Mol Cell Cardiol* 1987; 16: 117–128.

9. Berman MR, Peterson JN, Yue DT, Hunter WC. Effect of isoproterenol on force transient time course and on stiffness spectra in rabbit papillary muscle in barium contracture. *J Mol Cell Cardiol* 1988; 20: 415–426.
10. Hoh JFY, Rossmanith GH, Lee JK, Hamilton AM. Adrenaline increases the rate of cycling of crossbridges in rat cardiac muscle as measured by pseudo–random binary noise perturbation analysis. *Circ Res* 1988; 62: 452–461.
11. Brenner B, Schoenberg M, Chalovich JM, Greene LE, Eisenberg E. Evidence for cross–bridge attachment in relaxed muscle at low ionic strength. *Proc Nat Acad Sci USA* 1982; 79: 7288–7291.
12. Allen DG, Blinks JR. Calcium transients in aequorin–injected frog cardiac muscle. *Nature* 1978; 273: 509–513.
13. Seow CY, Ford LE. High ionic strength and low pH detain skinned rabbit skeletal muscle crossbridges in a low force state. 1993, (sumbitted).
14. Huxley AF, Simmons RM. Proposed mechanism of force generation in striated muscle. *Nature* 1971; 233: 533–538.
15. Ford LE, Huxley AF, Simmons RM. The relation between stiffness and filament overlap in stimulated frog muscle fibres. *J Physiol* 1981; 311: 219–249.
16. Seow CY, Ford LE. Shortening velocity and power output of skinned muscle fibers from mammals having a 25,000–fold range of body mass. *J Gen Physiol* 1991; 97:541–560.
17. Katz AM, Hecht HA. The early pump failure of the ischemic heart. *Am J Med* 1969; 47: 497–502.
18. Allen DG, Morris PG, Orchard CH, Pirolo JS. A nuclear magnetic resonance study of metabolism in the ferret heart during hypoxia and glycolysis. *J Physiol* 1985; 361: 185–204.
19. Seow CY, Ford LE. ADP detains muscle cross–bridges near the end of their force producing power stroke (abstract). *Biophys J* 1992; 61: A294
20. Bremel RD, Weber A. A cooperation within actin thin filament in vertebrate skeletal muscle. *Nature New Biol* 1972; 238: 97–101.
21. Seow CY, Ford LE. Dual effect of phosphate on the crossbridge cycle of muscle (abstract). *Biophys J* 1993; 63: (in press).

CHAPTER 6

MECHANISMS OF ENDOCARDIAL ENDOTHELIUM MODULATION OF MYOCARDIAL PERFORMANCE

Stanislas U. Sys, Luc J. Andries, Thierry C. Gillebert, and Dirk L. Brutsaert[1]

ABSTRACT

The nature of modulation of myocardial performance by the endocardial endothelium (EE) is briefly described. Possible mechanisms of this modulation include a physical barrier effect, the release of various chemical messengers and a transendothelial physicochemical barrier.

INTRODUCTION

Ventricular function of the heart relies largely on autoregulatory mechanisms. Autoregulation is accomplished (i) through feedback of each cardiomyocyte by changes in length of the cardiac muscle or in volume of the cardiac chambers (heterometric autoregulation, Law of Starling), and (ii) through feedback mediated by neurohumoral control or by the coronary circulation (homeometric autoregulation). The endocardium may constitute yet another modulator of cardiac performance. The endocardium is the innermost structure of the heart, lined by a monolayer of endothelial cells. It occupies a unique position in the cardiovascular system. All circulating blood passes through the cavity of the heart at least once every 2 minutes; during exercise, this process may increase by a factor of 4 to 5. This intense pass–through flow allows for intimate contacts between the circulating blood and the inner surface of the heart; the endothelial cells of the endocardium are continuously exposed to the blood. In addition to the above autoregulatory mechanisms, recent evidence allowed to postulate that endocardial endothelial cells [1–4] as well as coronary vascular endothelial cells [5–8] directly control the cardiomyocytes and that the endothelial cells mediate feedback through interaction with the superfusing blood. Although the coronary endothelium may be considered by some as a more likely candidate for modulation of the

[1]Department of Physiology and Medicine, University of Antwerp, Antwerp, Belgium.

Interactive Phenomena in the Cardiac System, Edited by
S. Sideman and R. Beyar, Plenum Press, New York, 1993

myocardium than the endocardial endothelium (EE), the functional roles of EE and coronary endothelium may be complementary. In the coronary system, endothelial cells might be more specialized in responding to changes in blood flow, shear stress or other changes in the local environment. By contrast, the sensory function of the EE might perhaps be attributed a more global role, whereby substances in the blood entering the ventricles can induce immediate responses in cardiac output. This unique feature of the endocardium has been largely ignored. We will discuss some morphological and functional properties which led to the hypothesis that endocardial endothelial cells directly modulate the underlying cardiomyocytes. At this point, two questions will be treated. Firstly, what is the nature of EE modulation of myocardial performance? And secondly, which morphological and functional features of EE do provide a basis for its modulatory role, or what are the actual arguments supporting the hypothesis that EE cells do modulate myocardial performance?

NATURE OF EE MODULATION OF MYOCARDIAL PERFORMANCE

We have recently examined the possible functional role of EE in the control of subjacent myocardial function. We have developed various chemical, mechanical and pharmacological methods to destroy EE *in vitro* with no damage to subjacent myocardium [2, 9]. Regardless of the method, selective destruction of EE induced abbreviation of isometric twitch duration; isometric force decline occurred earlier during the twitch, with — except at high $[Ca^{++}]_o$ — a concomitant decrease in peak twitch force and some decline in late rate of rise of force. This was not accompanied by significant changes in maximal unloaded velocity of shortening. Conversely, the presence of an intact EE increased the contractile state of subjacent myocardium by prolonging the isometric twitch with concomitant increase in peak twitch. This response amounted up to about 15% for twitch duration and between 10 and 20% for peak twitch performance. This pattern differs from many positive inotropic conditions (beta-agonists, oubain, increased $[Ca^{++}]_o$, frequency and post-extrasystolic potentiation), and shows similarities with increased isometric twitch performance induced by increasing initial muscle length [10, 11]. These observations have been confirmed by various other laboratories [7, 12–14].

Similarly, transient suppression of EE function *in vivo* in the intact dog heart by intracavitary irradiation with high power, high frequency, continuous wave ultrasound induced premature pressure fall during relaxation accompanied by substantial alterations in segment length behavior of the ventricular wall during rapid reextension of the myocardial fibers [16]. These alterations in ventricular performance in the intact dog heart, as in isolated muscle, likewise amounted up to about 15% abbreviation in the timing of pressure fall. EE modulation of left ventricular systole interacts with heterometric and homeometric autoregulation: it appeared more pronounced at low filling pressures and low inotropic state [17].

MECHANISMS OF EE MODULATION OF MYOCARDIAL PERFORMANCE

In cat papillary muscles the EE is separated from the myocardium by a thick layer of connective tissue. This allowed destruction of the EE, without damage to the myocardium, by various techniques, such as scraping, Triton X-100 treatment, ultrasound treatment or blowing with dry air. Damage to EE was evaluated with scanning electron microscopy

[2, 9] and more recently by confocal scanning laser microscopy (CSLM) of EE stained with vital dyes [18]. Morphological integrity of the subjacent myocardium was demonstrated by 1) transmission electron microscopy; 2) CSLM of the actin striation pattern; 3) exclusion of fluorochromes such as lucifer yellow and propidium iodide. The latter technique also permitted detection of damage to fibroblast-like cells in endocardial connective tissue. Damage to interstitial cells could be prominent after Triton X–100 treatment, but was small after ultrasound treatment. In other animal species such as ferret and rat, which have a thin to very thin layer of endocardial interstitial tissue, transmission electron microscopy showed that the myocardium was also intact after Triton X–100 [19, 20].

Functional integrity of the myocardium was confirmed because 1) maximal peak isometric force of the muscles, at high $[Ca^{++}]_o$, and maximal unloaded velocity of shortening were unaltered by EE impairment; 2) there was no correlation to muscle thickness and the decrease in twitch duration induced by EE impairment; 3) once fully established, twitch duration never recovered to baseline levels for the entire duration of the experiment. When, by contrast, true myocardial depression is induced, twitches are affected differently; true myocardial depression is in general characterized by a fall in peak isometric force with a concomitant decrease in rate of both rise and decline of force. The latter changes are strongly correlated to muscle thickness, are often progressive, and may in some conditions recover. True myocardial depression is also manifested by a decreased peak twitch force at high $[Ca^{++}]_o$. Impairment of the endocardial surface thus influences mechanical performance of the underlying undamaged myocardium, particularly at a physiological $[Ca^{++}]_o$ and temperature. Because of the similarity in the pattern of changes induced by the presence or absence of a functional EE and those induced by increasing initial muscle length *in vitro* or by increasing end–diastolic volume *in vivo*, EE–dependent events may similarly be mediated through increased sensitivity of the myofilaments to $[Ca^{++}]_i$. Findings by other investigators seem to support this idea. For example, simultaneous measurements of aequorin induced light signals and isometric twitch force in isolated cardiac muscle from ferret hearts have demonstrated that intact EE does indeed enhance myocardial performance by increasing myofibrillar Ca^{++} sensitivity [15]. It would also seem that the main mechanical manifestation of such changes is a delayed onset of twitch tension decline during relaxation.

The ultrastructure of the intercellular junctional region and the paracellular permeability of ventricular EE are suggestive for its possible modulatory role. The surface area of EE cells was larger than in microvascular endothelial cells. In addition, intercellular clefts in EE were deeper than in myocardial capillary endothelium, whereas tight junctions had a similar structure in both endothelia. Accordingly, EE might be expected to have a lower permeability than capillary endothelium. However, CSLM showed that negatively charged dextran with MW 10000 (coupled to lucifer yellow), when intravenously injected, penetrated first through EE and only later through subendocardial capillary endothelium [21]. Penetration of tracer through EE probably results from differences in hydrostatic pressure. The observed ultrastructure of EE possibly represents an adaptation which limits diffusion driven by high hydrostatic pressure in the heart. Differences in paracellular diffusion of fluid and small solutes, between EE and myocardial vessels, illustrate the characteristic permeability properties in endocardium and subjacent myocardium. To what extent the negatively charged fibrous matrix of the intercellular clefts and the organization of the zonula adherens–like junction in EE influence paracellular permeability remains to be investigated. Paracellular diffusion of fluid and small solutes through EE precludes the possibility that substances produced by the EE can rapidly reach the underlying myocardial tissue.

Next, there is recent experimental evidence that EE cells release substances with inotropic properties. Effluent from superfused porcine cultured right ventricular EE cells was bio–assayed with endothelium–denuded pig coronary artery rings or with EE–denuded ferret papillary muscles [22]. The cultured EE cells tonically released (i) an unstable EDRF–like substance, and (ii) an unidentified stable substance which in EE–denuded papillary muscles reversed the changes in mechanical performance seen after EE removal. Moreover, in isolated ferret papillary muscles, EE could be stimulated by substance–P to release an EDRF–like agent which elevated myocardial c–GMP, whereas removal of EE was mimicked by but not itself associated with elevation of myocardial c–GMP [22]. The recent demonstration of NO–synthase in EE cells [23] would further suggest a contribution of NO in EE modulation. Tonic EDRF activity appears to be low, as inhibition of EDRF synthesis by L–NMMA does not prolong twitch duration in isolated cardiac muscle [14]; its release may be stimulated, however, by various stimulants such as bradykinin and substance P. Moreover, EE cells in culture produce significant amounts of prostacyclin [24, 25].

We previously hypothesized the existence of an endocardially released positive inotropic factor which prolongs contraction possibly by increasing the sensitivity of the myofilaments to $[Ca^{++}]_i$ (myocardium contracting factor, MCF) as well as of an endocardially released agent which induces premature relaxation of the myocardium (myocardium relaxing factor, MRF). Normally, as the presence of a functional EE delays the onset of isometric tension decline and the removal of EE abolishes this effect, one may expect MRF activity to be overridden by MCF. Whether the myocardial inotropic action of endothelin and the presence of endothelin–receptors on the cardiomyocytes can be invoked to postulate release of endothelin by neighboring (endocardial) endothelial cells [6] needs further attention. Interestingly, and similarly as in vascular endothelium, release of prostacyclin by the EE may contribute to MRF activity. Indomethacin, a known inhibitor of cyclo–oxygenase was indeed suggested to elicit an EE mediated activation of myocardial function with increased contraction duration, both *in vivo* and *in vitro*. In other studies, tissue cyclo–oxygenase was found to be about twice as high in the endocardium as in the myocardium, and located specifically in the endothelial cell fraction [26]. The physiological roles of MCF and MRF are speculative at present. The half–life of EDRF, and to a lesser extent that of prostacyclin, is too short for it to penetrate a substantial portion of subjacent myocardium, unless these substances would control myocardial performance indirectly through physicochemical linkage. In addition, both substances may help to inhibit platelet adhesion and intraventricular thrombus formation. By contrast, MCF with its greater stability could control myocardial contraction both directly through diffusion and indirectly by transport from the cardiac cavities into the coronary circulation.

The participation of the EE in the inotropic response to various agents further supports the involvement of EE in modulation of myocardial performance. Both the activity of the $\alpha 1$–agonist phenylephrine and atrial natriuretic peptide (ANP) on the myocardium required an intact EE. Low concentrations of the $\alpha 1$–agonist induced a positive inotropic response with twitch prolongation [27], whereas ANP induced an opposite effect with an early tension decline [28]. These inotropic response to the alpha1–agonist and to ANP were proposed to result from the EE release of myocardium contracting and relaxing factor respectively. The involvement of ANP in the modulation of myocardial performance is not surprising, since immunohistochemical and in–situ hybridization studies have demonstrated the presence of specific ANP receptors on EE cells in left and right ventricle [29, 30]. Few receptors were detected in ventricular myocardium. Other substances as serotonin, vasopressin, angiotensin, and endothelin also might induce a change in the release of MCF or MRF in EE, thereby modifying the direct response of these substances on the myocardium. The presence of several types of receptors in EE suggests that EE might have a sensory function for various substances circulating in the superfusing blood.

Morphologically, the prominent trabecular structure of the cavitary side of the ventricular wall and the surface characteristics of EE cells with numerous microvilli and invaginations offer a high ratio of cavitary surface area to ventricular volume. At peak systole, trabecular muscles are squeezed together, and intertrabecular spaces are reduced in volume displacing blood from the valleys and facilitating exchange of the EE with the superfusing blood. From recent functional morphological investigations, EE cells appear to highly active with well developed Golgi complex and with gap junctions. Moreover, EE cells demonstrate structured contractile proteins, allowing for shape changes, regulation of permeability and some degree of motility. In addition to shear stress, mechanical stress by dimensional changes of the heart will during the cardiac cycle might influence EE cell shape, organization of the cytoskeleton and distribution of von Willebrand factor. These features and the aforementioned presence of receptors suggest the possibility that EE may be subject to direct physiological regulation acting as a finely tuned dynamic interface between the superfusing blood and the myocardium.

Finally, the epithelial-like organization of EE as well as many of the above functional morphological features, in particular the long intercellular contacts with complex interdigitations and the presence of numerous gap and tight junctions, would support the existence of a transcellular or transendothelial physicochemical control. A transcellular potential difference would require a strong electrochemical gradient for certain ions as well as a selective boundary barrier. The basement membrane below the EE has also been suggested to be important in limiting permeability to certain ions, by the presence of anionic sites. Even the permeability for small substances, like potassium ions, varies significantly within different vascular beds [31]. How a transendothelial electrochemical potential would then participate in a cascade of EE-derived events leading to changes in the sensitivity of the myofilaments to $[Ca^{++}]_i$ is unclear. There has been recent evidence that EE damaged-induced abbreviation of twitch contraction in isolated muscle is not accompanied by significant changes in action potential duration of subjacent myocardium [32]. These observations do not preclude, however, the existence of functional electrical coupling between the EE and subjacent cells, despite the ultrastructural absence of heterocellular contacts [33]. On theoretical grounds, coupling of a transendocardial electrical potential to the electrochemical properties of the myocardial sarcolemma could create a variable, EE-mediated electrotonic control of a substantial portion of subjacent myocardium in the ventricular wall. It remains to be resolved whether and to what extent such electrophysiological properties of individual EE cells would participate in the establishment of a transcellular electrical potential difference across the entire EE.

CONCLUSION

Different steps in the EE-mediated events which link function of the EE cells to the myofilaments, were described and are still partly speculative. Could EE act as a physical barrier inhibiting penetration of some agents to the myocardium ? A simple barrier effect, however, cannot explain modulation by the EE of the inotropic response to the great variety of substances which have been described. EE could, in a manner analogous to endothelial regulation of vascular smooth muscle tone, affect myocardial performance either by releasing various chemical messengers, or by the establishment of a transendothelial physicochemical control, or by the combination of both mechanisms.

DISCUSSION

Dr. R. Beyar: How can you prove that you damage only the endothelium and not, at least partially, the muscle? This may affect some of your results.

Dr. S. Sys: There are several arguments to prove that the myocardium is not damaged. At the high calcium concentration there is no decrease in the maximally developed force of the muscles. If there would be damage, it would be all along the entire muscle and the functional cross–sectional area would be diminished, so the total force, even after normalization for the total cross–section, would be decreased. We also have functional morphological arguments. If you look at the underlying tissue you can see the basal lamina, which is in many cases still quite intact although the endocardial/endothelial cells on top of that basal lamina are damaged to a very large extent, and with extracted nuclei.

Dr. D. Allen: I always have great difficulty understanding how this monolayer of cells on the surface of the thick ventricular wall is going to affect the cells right in the middle. Now it is hard enough to understand in the papillary muscle, which is approx. 1 mm thick and has no flow through it. It is much harder in the LV wall which is perhaps a couple of centimeters thick and has millions of capillaries going through it, which would presumably carry away any diffusible activator.

Dr. S. Sys: This argument is mainly related to the fact that it would be due to diffusion of different substances. From the available evidence, EE cells certainly do release different substances with inotropic properties. If the effects of EE would be due only to diffusion of different substances, you might indeed expect in the isolated muscle an effect of cross–sectional area; in the larger muscles the effect would be less, in fact than in the smaller muscles. If it is consumed, you expect more of the diffusible substance at the place where it is made and it appears that the effect of damage in the EE is not dependent on the muscle cross–sectional area.

Another fact is that the effect is quite immediate. After the triton immersion, if you can return the muscle back into the same solution which has the same conditions as before the triton immersion, then you immediately see a shortening of the twitch duration with very little effect on the contraction phase. This is another argument for a mechanism, other than only diffusible substances. The other possibility then is that it might have something to do with an electrotonic potential. The EE may be quite similar to the epithelium in the renal tubuli, an endothelium or epithelium which can act in fact as a physicochemical barrier and which can support a potential difference across not the membrane but across the whole endothelium or epithelium, it depends on which case you are looking at. If it would be an electrotonic control, its effects could carry far away in a short time.

Dr. H. Strauss: A question pertaining to the treatment of the endothelium to remove function, by exposure to triton–x. It pertains to the depth of the muscle to which triton diffuses through and modifies the myocardium as well as the endocardium and the other is what happens to those membranes. Do those cells uncouple? Does this generate a passive current leak that leads to a shortening in repolarization and a reduction in Ca^{2+} available for contraction instead of some sort of chemical signal between the endothelium and the muscle?

Dr. S. Sys: Your first question is the depth of the damaging treatment with the triton. From the morphological and functional evidence, we are pretty sure that it is only the endocardial endothelial layer and not muscle tissue which has been damaged by the triton treatment. Regarding your question on a change in repolarization: We think that it is not a change in the repolarization because certainly at 12/min in normal conditions, damaging EE does not change the action potential duration. We have not seen any changes in action potential so probably it is not an early repolarization. This is consistent with the finding that it would be mainly calcium sensitivity.

REFERENCES

1. Brutsaert DL, Meulemans AL, Sipido KR, Sys SU. The endocardium modulates the performance of myocardium. *Arch Int Physiol Biochem* 1987; 95: 4.
2. Brutsaert DL, Meulemans AL, Sipido KR, Sys SU. Effects of damaging the endocardial surface on the mechanical performance of isolated cardiac muscle. *Circ Res* 1988; 62: 357–366.
3. Brutsaert DL. The endocardium. *Annu Rev Physiol* 1989; 51: 263–273.
4. Brutsaert DL, Andries LJ. The endocardial endothelium. *Am J Physiol* 1992; 263: H985–H1002.
5. Henderson Ah, Lewis MJ, Shah AM, Smith JA. Cutting edge of cardiovascular research. Endothelium, endocardium, and cardiac contraction. *Cardiovasc Res* 1992; 26: 305–308.
6. Krämer BK, Nishida M, Kelly RA, Smith TW. Endothelins. Myocardial actions of a new class of cytokines. *Circulation* 1992; 85: 305–356.
7. Li K, Stewart DJ, and Rouleau J–L. Myocardial contractile actions of endothelin–1 in rat and rabbit papillary muscles. Role of endocardial endothelium. *Circ Res* 1991; 69: 301–312.
8. Li K, Rouleau J–L, Andries LJ, Brutsaert DL. Effect of dysfunctional vascular endothelium on myocardial performance in isolated papillary muscles. *Circ Res* 1993; 72: in press.
9. Andries LJ, Meulemans AL, Brutsaert DL. Ultrasound as a novel method for selective damage of endocardial endothelium. *Am J Physiol* 1991; 261: H1636–H1642.
10. Allen DG, Kentish JC. The cellular basis of the length–tension relation in cardiac muscle. *J Mol Cell Cardiol* 1985; 17: 821–840.
11. Hibberd MG, Jewell BR. Calcium– and length–dependent force production in rat ventricular muscle. *J Physiol (Lond)* 1982; 329: 527–540.
12. Bourreau JP, Banijamali HS, Challice CE. Modulation of E–C coupling in cat myocardium by endocardial endothelium. *Biophys J* 1990; 57: 175a.
13. Housmans PR. Regulation of cardiac muscle relaxation. *Biophys J* 1990; 57: 11a.
14. Henderson AH, Lewis MJ, Shah AM, Smith JA. Endothelium, endocardium, and cardiac contraction. *Cardiovasc Res* 1992; 26: 305–308.
15. Wang J, Morgan JP. Endocardial endothelium modulates myofilament Ca^{++} responsiveness in aequorin–loaded ferret myocardium. *Circ Res* 1992; 70: 754–760.
16. Gillebert TC, De Hert SG, Andries LJ, Jageneau AH, Brutsaert DL. Intracavitary ultrasound impairs left ventricular performance: presumed role of endocardial endothelium. *Am J Physiol* 1992; 263: H857–H865.
17. De Hert SG, Gillebert TC, Brutsaert DL. Modulation of left ventricular performance by intracavitary ultrasound depends on volume, inotropic state and adrenergic control. *Circulation* 1993: in press.
18. Li K, Rouleau JL, Calderone A, Andries JL, Brutsaert DL. Endocardial function in pacing–induced heart failure in the dog. *J Mol Cell Cardiol* 1993: in press.
19. Finkel MS, Oddis CV, Jacob TD, Watkins SC, Hattler BG, Simmons RL. Negative inotropic effects of cytokines on the heart mediated by nitric oxide. *Science* 1982; 257: 387–389.
20. Shah AM, Smith JA, Lewis MJ. The role of endocardium in the modulation of contraction of isolated papillary muscles of the ferret. *J Cardiovasc Pharmacol* 1991; 17: S251–S257.
21. Andries LJ, Brutsaert DL. Endocardial endothelium: junctional organization and permeability. *Cell Tissue Res* 1993: submitted.
22. Smith JA, Shah AM, Lewis MJ. Factors released from endocardium of the ferret and pig modulate myocardial contraction. *J Physiol* 1991; 439: 1–14.
23. Schulz R, Smith JA, Lewis MJ, Moncada S. Nitric oxide synthase in cultured endocardial cells of the pig. *Br J Pharmacol* 1991; 104: 21–24.
24. Manduteanu I, Popov D, Radu A, Simionescu M. Calf cardiac valvular endothelial cells in culture: production of glycosaminoglycans, prostacyclin and fibronectin. *J Mol Cell Cardiol* 1988; 20: 103–118.
25. Mebazaa A, Martin LD, Robotham JL, Maeda K, Gabrielson EW, Wetzel RC. Right and left ventricular cultured endocardial endothelium produces prostacyclin and PGE_2. *J Mol Cell Cardiol* 1993: in revision.
26. Brandt R, Nowak J, Sonnenfeld T. Prostaglandin formation from exogenous precursor in homogenates of human cardiac tissue. *Basic Res Cardiol* 1984; 79: 135–141.
27. Meulemans AL, Andries LJ, Brutsaert DL. Endocardial endothelium mediates positive inotropic response to α1–adrenoceptor agonist in mammalian heart. *J Mol Cell Cardiol* 1990; 22: 667–685.

28. Meulemans AL, Sipido KR, Sys SU, Brutsaert DL. Atriopeptin III induces early relaxation of ventricular cardiac muscle. *Circ Res* 1988; 62: 1171–1174.
29. Rutherford RAD, Wharton J, Gordon L, Moscoso G, Yacoub MH, Polak JM. Endocardial localization and characterization of natriuretic peptide binding sites in human fetal and adult heart. *Eur J Pharmacol* 1992; 212: 1–7.
30. Wilcox JN, Augustine A, Goeddel DV, Lowe DG. Differential regional expression of three natriuretic peptide receptor genes within primate tissues. *Mol Cell Biol* 1991; 11: 3454–3462.
31. Jain RK. Transport of molecules across tumor vasculature. *Cancer Metastasis Rev* 1987; 6: 559–593.
32. Shah AM, Shattock MJ, Lewis MJ. Action potential duration and endocardial modulation of myocardial contraction. *Cardiovasc Res* 1992; 26: 376–378.
33. Andries LJ, Brutsaert DL. Differences in functional structure between endocardial endothelium and vascular endothelium. *J Cardiovasc Pharmacol* 1991; 17: S243–S246.

CHAPTER 7

CALCIUM KINETIC AND MECHANICAL REGULATION OF THE CARDIAC MUSCLE

Amir Landesberg and Samuel Sideman[1]

ABSTRACT

A comprehensive dynamic model of the excitation contraction coupling, developed for a single cardiac muscle, is extended to a multi–cell system (duplex). The model defines the mechanical activation level based on calcium kinetics and crossbridge cycling and emphasizes the central role of the troponin regulatory proteins in regulating muscle activity. The intracellular control mechanism includes two feedback loops that affect the affinity of troponin for calcium and the crossbridge cycling. The model is used to simulate the basic mechanical characteristics of the cardiac muscle, i. e. the force–length and the force–velocity relationships, and describes their dependence on the mechanical activation level. The two–cell duplex unit is used to study the influence of inter–cellular interactions and the effect of inhomogeneity on muscle performance, due to non–uniformity in the electrical stimulation or inhomogeneity in calcium kinetics. Better understanding of the performance of the inhomogeneous muscle is obtained due to our ability to describe the control of the activation level in each cell.

INTRODUCTION

Cardiac muscle models are based on the two fundamental mechanical characteristics: the force–length and force–velocity relationships [1–3]. However, these relationships depend on the mechanical activation level [4, 5], and the ability to simulate the mechanical activity depends on a reasonable description of the mechanical activation function. Different activation functions were used in modeling the cardiac activity, including a simple half sinus [1], an exponential [3] a combination of sinusoidal contraction and exponential

[1]Heart System Research Center, The Julius Silver Institute, Department of Biomedical Engineering, Technion–Israel Institute of Technology, Haifa, 32000 Israel.

relaxation [6], or a complicated time dependent function [2]. Clearly, each function yields a different description of the mechanical performance. Because all these definitions represent the activation function as a deterministic function of time, they can not be used to characterize the intracellular control mechanism that affect the activation level and the excitation–contraction coupling. Ford [4] proposed to define the activation level by the number of sites on the thin actin filaments which are *available* for attachment to myosin crossbridges. This definition is based on Huxley's model [7], and attempts to describe the mechanism of regulation of muscle contraction. This definition is particularly useful as it highlights the central role of the troponin in controlling force development.

Consistent with Ford's definition [4] of activation, the present model defines the activation level as the *ability* of the muscle to generate force. Based on a biochemical model of muscle contraction [8], the activation level can be described by the number of available crossbridges in the weak, non–force generating conformation that can convert to the strong force generating conformation.

The present study describes the performances of the contractile element (Fig. 1), and couples the free calcium transient with the mechanical activity. The model simulates the kinetics of calcium binding to troponin–c, and the regulation of crossbridge cycling by the troponin regulatory proteins. The model has two feedback mechanisms, a negative one and a positive one. The negative feedback loop is a mechanical one, wherein increasing the shortening velocity of the filaments increases the rate of crossbridge cycling from the strong to the weak conformation, thus reducing the generated force. The positive feedback loop, called "cooperativity," is a biochemical one wherein an increase in the number of crossbridge in the strong conformation increases the affinity of Troponin–C for calcium.

The cooperativity feedback mechanism is based on our earlier study which relates to data from skinned cardiac cells [9]. Measurement of the force and the bound calcium to troponin with and without vanadate by Hofmann and Fuchs [10, 11] and the measurements of the force–length–free calcium by Kentish et al. [12] and Hibberd and Jewell [13] were used to described the dependence of the affinity of Troponin for calcium on the amount of cycling crossbridges at the strong state and on the free calcium concentration.

The earlier study is extended here to simulate the behavior of the intact cell, with transient free calcium concentration, at various mechanical conditions. The performance of

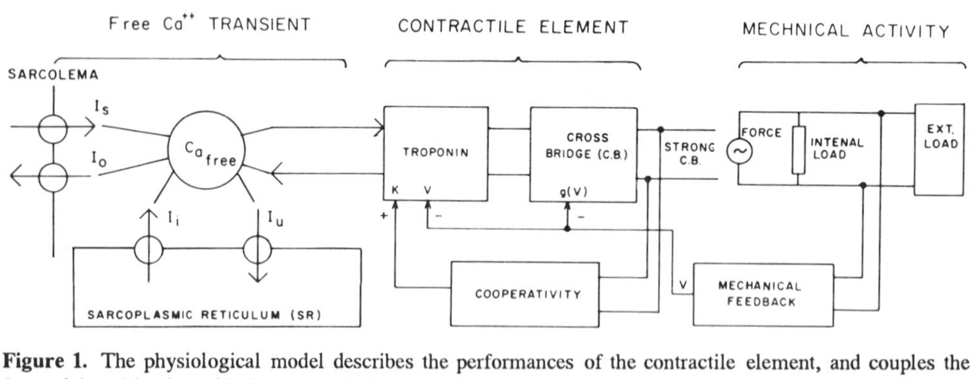

Figure 1. The physiological model describes the performances of the contractile element, and couples the free calcium kinetics with the mechanical activity. The model contains two main feedback mechanisms; a mechanical negative feedback and a positive feedback, termed cooperativity. I_i, I_s – calcium influx; I_o, I_u – calcium eflux currents are based on Lee and Allen [30]. K– calcium binding coefficient; V – sarcomere sliding velocity; g(V) – crossbridge turnover from strong to weak conformation.

a two–cell system (duplex), is studied in order to test the effect of non–uniformity in the electrical stimulation and inhomogeneity in calcium kinetics at the various cells.

THE PHYSIOLOGICAL MODEL

The Basic Assumptions

The main assumptions of the model are:

1. A single Troponin complex, with the adjacent seven actin molecules and the two heads of the myosin, is considered as one regulated unit.
2. The crossbridges exists in two main conformations [8, 14]: a strong force generating one and a weak non–force generating one.
3. Crossbridge cycling between these conformations is described by the rate limiting processes. The rate limiting step in the transition from the weak to the strong conformation is the hydrolysis of ATP and phosphor release [15]. The rate of transition from the strong to the weak conformation is affected by the motion of the crossbridges from the strained 45° to the 45° conformation [8]. Thus the filaments sliding velocity affects the rate of crossbridges turnover to the weak state.
4. Calcium binding to the low affinity sites regulates the activity of the ATPase [16] and the crossbridge cycling, since ATP hydrolysis is required for the transition of the crossbridges to the strong conformation [8].
5. There is a loose coupling between calcium kinetic and crossbridge cycling; Calcium can detach from the troponin before the crossbridge turn back to the weak conformation, leaving the crossbridge in the strong conformation without bound calcium on the neighbour troponin.
6. The kinetics of calcium binding to the low affinity sites on the troponin depends on crossbridge conformation [9, 17, 18] and on troponin–tropomyosin–actin interactions along the sarcomere [17, 19, 20] which is described by the cooperativity feedback.
7. There are regions of *non–overlap, single–overlap* and *double–overlap* between the thin and the thick filaments. Force is generated only by crossbridges in the strong conformation in the *single–overlap* region. No force is generated in the non–overlap and the double–overlap regions [21], henceforth referred to as the 'non force generating (NFG) regions."

The State Variables of the Regulatory Troponin Complex

The regulatory troponin units exist in different states which are grouped according to three criteria (Table 1):

1. The position of the units is either in the single overlap region, or in the non–force generating (NFG) regions.
2. The existence of bound calcium on the troponin, and
3. The conformation of the adjacent crossbridge: strong or weak?

Table 1. State Variables Used in the Model.

State of Troponin Complex	Overlap	Calcium	Crossbridge
R_n	Non	-	—
S_n	Non	BOUND	—
R	Single	-	Weak
S	Single	BOUND	Weak
T	Single	BOUND	STRONG
U	Single	-	STRONG

The transitions between the different states are defined by calcium binding to troponin, by crossbridge cycling and by filament sliding. Figure 2 shows the interactions between the states of the troponin regulatory units in the isometric regime.

Four states exist in the single–overlap, force generating, region. *State R* represents the rest state, wherein no calcium is bound to troponin, and the crossbridges are in the weak conformation. In *state S* calcium is bound to troponin but the crossbridges are still in the weak conformation. Crossbridge cycling leads to *state T* where calcium is still bound to the low affinity sites but the crossbridges are in the strong conformation. Calcium detachment from the troponin at state *T* lead to *state U*, representing a situation in which the crossbridges are in the strong conformation but calcium has already been released from the low affinity sites.

State S describes the level of the mechanical activation: it represents the number of available crossbridges in the weak conformation that can turn to the strong, force generating, conformation, i.e. the ability of the muscle to generate force. State U represents the loose coupling between calcium binding to Troponin and crossbridge cycling.

The present study relates only to the force generation and the total amount of bound calcium to the troponin. According to assumption No. 7 the force in the NFG regions is zero, thus only the total amount of bound calcium is calculated in the double–overlap and non–overlap regions. Consequently, only two states, R_n and S_n, are considered in the NFG regions, corresponding to R and S in the single–overlap region.

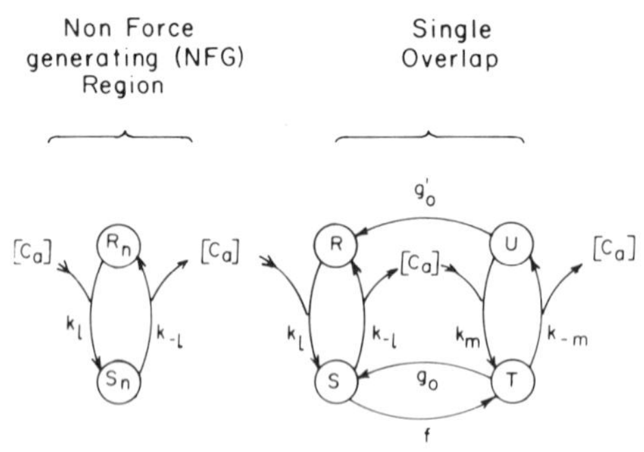

Figure 2. Schematic diagram showing the transitions between the various states of the troponin regulatory units in the isometric regime. The transitions are defined by calcium kinetics (k_ℓ, $k_{-\ell}$, k_m, k_{-m}) and by crossbridge cycling (f, g, g'). [Ca] is the free calcium concentration.

Filament Sliding and Crossbridge Distribution

Filaments sliding has two effects:

1. Filament sliding affects the transfer of troponin regulatory units from the single–overlap to the NFG region during muscle shortening–contraction (Fig. 3a) and the transfer of troponin units in the opposite direction as the muscle elongates during relaxation (Fig. 3b). The amount of troponin regulatory units that are transferred between these regions as a consequence of filament sliding is proportional to the sliding velocity of the filaments and to the instantaneous density of the troponin in each particular state of the troponin.
2. According to assumption No. 3 the filaments sliding velocity affects the rate of transition from the strong to the weak conformation [8]. A linear dependence of this transition rate on the velocity of the filaments sliding is assumed here.

THE MATHEMATICAL MODEL OF THE CONTRACTILE ELEMENT

The overlap ratio (α) is defined as the ratio of the single overlap region length (L_o) of the thick filament to the total lenght (L_m) of this filament.

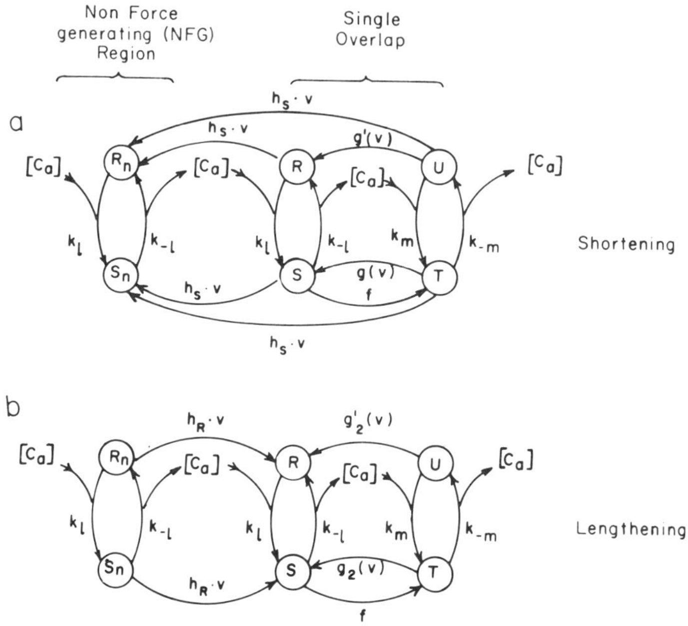

Figure 3. Schematic diagram of the transitions between the various states of the troponin regulatory units during sarcomere sliding. **a:** Sarcomere shortening–contraction. **b:** Sarcomere lengthening–relaxation. The transitions between the states are defined by calcium kinetics (k_ℓ, $k_{-\ell}$, k_m, k_{-m}), by crossbridge cycling (f, g(V), g'(V)), and by filament sliding (h_sV, h_RV). V is the rate of change of the single overlap ratio. [Ca] is the free calcium concentration ($h_s = 1/L_o$, $h_R = 1/(L_d + L_n)$).

$$\alpha \triangleq \frac{L_o}{L_m} \tag{1}$$

Note that $\alpha = 1$ for maximal single–overlap length. Under normal physiological conditions, sarcomere length is greater than the thick filament length ($SL > L_m$) and is given by $SL = 2 \cdot (L_n + L_o + L_d)$, where L_n and L_d are the non–overlap and double–overlap lengths. The sarcomere shortening velocity V_{SL} is given by:

$$V_{SL} = L_m V \tag{2}$$

where V is the rate of change of the overlap ratio, i. e. $V = -d\alpha/dt = \dot{\alpha}$.

As seen in Fig. 2, most of the transitions between the states are bi–directional, except those caused by: 1) The transfer between the states in the border between the single–overlap and the NFG regions i. e. between U and R_n and between T and S_n, (Fig. 3), and 2) the transitions from U to R, corresponding to assumption No. 4 above, which states that calcium is essential for triggering crossbridge cycling from the weak to the strong conformation.

We now define $\bar{R}$, $\bar{S}$, $\bar{T}$, $\bar{U}$, $\bar{R}_n$, $\bar{S}_n$ as the density of the troponin state in its corresponding region i.e. $\bar{R} = R/L_o$, $\bar{S} = S/L_o$, $\bar{T} = T/L_o$, $\bar{U} = U/L_o$, $\bar{R}_n = R_n/(L_n+L_d)$ and $\bar{S}_n = S_n/(L_n+L_d)$. The transitions between the density state variables within the single–overlap region are given by:

$$\begin{bmatrix} \dot{\bar{R}} \\ \dot{\bar{S}} \\ \dot{\bar{T}} \\ \dot{\bar{U}} \end{bmatrix} = \begin{bmatrix} -K_\ell & k_{-\ell} & 0 & g_0' + g_1'V \\ K_\ell & -f-k_{-\ell} & g_0 + g_1V & 0 \\ 0 & f & -g_0-g_1V-k_{-m} & K_m \\ 0 & 0 & k_{-m} & -K_m-g_0'-g_1'V \end{bmatrix} \cdot \begin{bmatrix} \bar{R} \\ \bar{S} \\ \bar{T} \\ \bar{U} \end{bmatrix} \tag{3}$$

where $K_\ell = k_\ell \cdot [Ca]$; $K_m = k_m[Ca]$; [Ca] denotes the free calcium concentration; f, g_o, g_o', g_1, g_1' represent the crossbridge turnover rate kinetics. The rate coefficients k_ℓ and $k_{-\ell}$ represent the rate constants of calcium binding to low affinity sites of troponin when the regulated crossbridges are in the weak conformation; k_m and k_{-m} represent the rate constants of calcium binding to the low affinity sites when the regulated crossbridges are in the strong conformation.

The transitions between the density state variables for the NFG region are described by:

$$\begin{bmatrix} \dot{\bar{R}}_n \\ \bar{S}_n \end{bmatrix} = \begin{bmatrix} -K_\ell & k_{-\ell} \\ K_\ell & -k_{-\ell} \end{bmatrix} \cdot \begin{bmatrix} \bar{R}_n \\ \bar{S}_n \end{bmatrix} \tag{4}$$

The rate coefficients k_ℓ, $k_{-\ell}$, k_m, k_{-m} depend on the number of cycling crossbridges at the strong conformation due to the cooperativity feedback.

The total amount of bound calcium (BCa) is given by:

$$BCa = (\bar{S} + \bar{T}) \cdot L_o + \bar{S}_n \cdot (L_n + L_d) \tag{5}$$

The present model describes the rate limiting processes, which are related to crossbridge cycling between the weak and the strong conformation. The rate of crossbridge attachment and detachment is at least an order of magnitude faster than the rate of cross-bridge cycling between the weak and the strong conformation [22]. The slow rate constants f and g of Huxley [7] actually characterize the crossbridge cycling between the weak and the strong conformations, rather than the rate of attachment and detachment [22], and the crossbridges reach equilibrium between attachment and detachment quite rapidly, relative to the rates of transition between the weak and strong conformation. Denoting the proportionality constant ($\bar{F}$) as the average force developed by each crossbridge we obtain (by assumption No. 7), that the force F per unit filament cross-section:

$$F = \bar{F}\,(\bar{T} + \bar{U})\cdot L_o \tag{6}$$

The internal load is simulated here by the following passive element [1]:

$$F_{PE} = \begin{cases} E\left(e^{D(SL/Sp_o)-1} - 1\right) & SL \geq Sp_o \\ -B\left(1 - \dfrac{SL}{Sp_o}\right) & SL < Sp_o \end{cases} \tag{7}$$

where SL is the sarcomere length, Sp_o is the length of the unstressed sarcomere, and E, D and B are empirical constants [1].

The description of the sarcolemmal and the sarcoplasmic reticulum (SR) calcium flow (Fig. 1) is based on the model of Lee and Allen [23], wherein the calcium currents through the sarcolemma and the SR are described by a deterministic functions of the time, extra cellular calcium and the intra SR calcium concentration.

RESULTS

Analysis of the Intact Muscle

The Force–Length Relationship (FLR): Figure 4a depicts isometric contractions at different sarcomere lengths leading to the force–length relationship. Isometric contractions exhibit three phenomena which are related to the cooperativity mechanism: 1. An increase in the first free calcium transient after muscle length shortening (Fig. 4b), corresponding to the data of Allen and Smith [24] (inset in Fig. 4b). 2) The time to peak force increases with the increase in the sarcomere length (Fig. 4c), corresponding to the data of Allen and Kurihara [25]. 3) As shown by Allen and Kentish [26], the force–length relationship of the intact cell is steeper then in the skeletal muscle (Fig. 5).

Simulations of the effect of different extra cellular calcium concentration on the FLR are shown in Fig. 5. An increase in the extra cellular calcium concentrations reduces the steepness of the FLR and shift the curve to the left, consistent with the measurements Allen and Kentish [26]. The steepness of the FLR is determined by the cooperativity feedback; interventions that raise the free calcium, or increase calcium binding to troponin, elevate the activation level (state S) and shift the FLR curve to the left. The length dependent sensitivity to calcium [26] is explained by the cooperativity feedback: an increase in the sarcomere length increases the number of available cycling crossbridges in

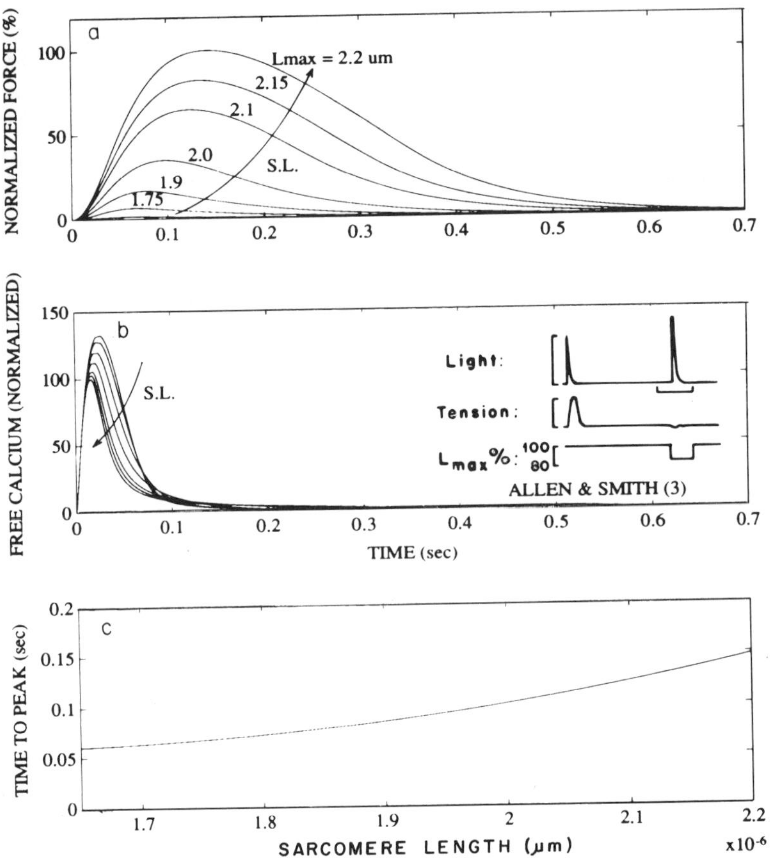

Figure 4. Simulation of isometric contraction for different muscle lengths. **a:** normalized force; **b:** the first free calcium transient obtained after muscle length shortening; {inset in 4b – measurements of Allen and Smith [24]}; **c:** time to peak force, at different sarcomere lengths. [Ca] is normalized by peak [Ca] at SL_{max}. Force is normalized by peak force at SL_{max}. SL – sarcomere length.

the single–overlap region that increases the activation level, state S. Elevation the activation level increases the number of crossbridges in the strong conformation and, through the cooperativity feedback, elevates the affinity of troponin for calcium.

The Force–Velocity Relationship (FVR): Figure 6 shows the FVR at different initial muscle lengths, calculated from the isometric – isotonic change–over contractions measured by Braunwald [27]. Using Eqs. (1) to (5), the velocity of sarcomere shortening at any level of activation in the isotonic regime is given by:

$$V_{isotonic} = \frac{\overline{F}f \cdot S - g_0 \cdot F}{(g_1 + \frac{2}{\alpha})F + K_{PE}} \cdot L_m \qquad (8)$$

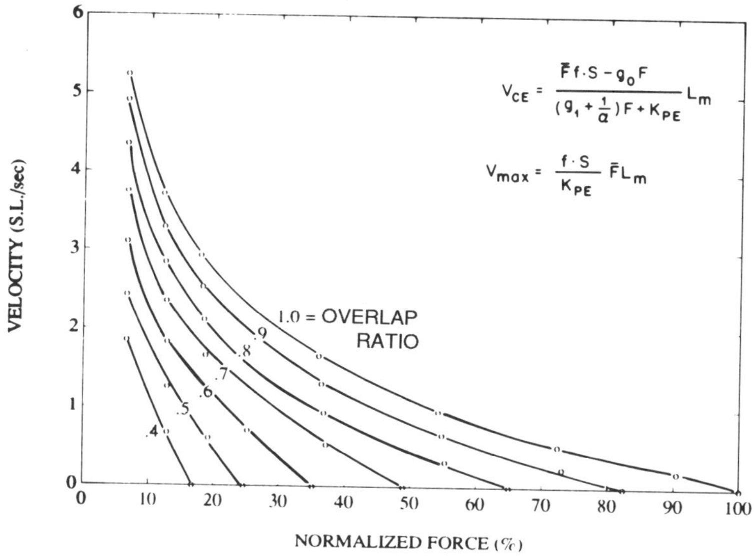

Figure 5. Force–length relationship at different extra-cellular calcium concentration $[Ca]_{out}$. Measurements of Allen and Kentish [26] are shown in the inset. Circles represent the points of model simulation. Note that increasing $[Ca]_{out}$ shifts the force–length relationship to the left and reduces its steepness.

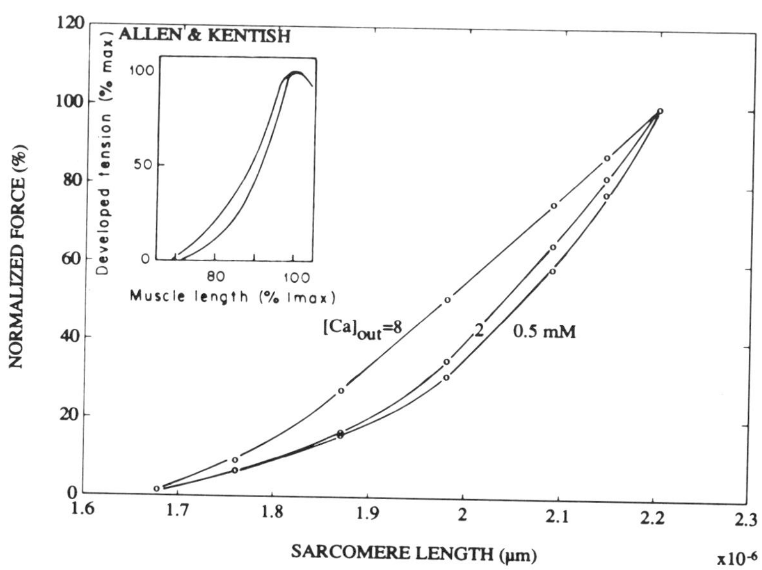

Figure 6. Force–velocity relationships for different sarcomere lengths. Simulation of the measurements of Braunwald [27]. Circles represent calculated points by model simulation. The simulation demonstrates the importance of the activation and the internal load.

where $K_{PE} = dF_{PE}/d\alpha$ relates to the parallel element (internal load) stiffness, and is calculated from Eq. (7). Note that the velocity of shortening relates directly to the activation level and is inversely related to the internal load stiffness K_{PE} and to the force

F, since $f \cdot S >> g_0 \cdot F$ at contraction. The maximal unloaded velocity, V_{max} is obtained from Eq. (8) and is given by:

$$V_{max} = \bar{F} L_m \frac{fS_o}{K_{PE}} \tag{9}$$

Equation (9) is supported by experimental evidence showing that the maximal unloaded velocity depends on:

1. The level of activation, as stipulated by Ter Keurs [28] and Zahalak [5].
2. The rate of crossbridge cycling from the weak to strong conformation, f, i.e. the rate of ATP hydrolysis and P release, as suggested by Eisenberg [8, 15], and
3. The relation between the level of activation, and the stiffness of the internal load, K_{PE}, as shown by Ford [4].

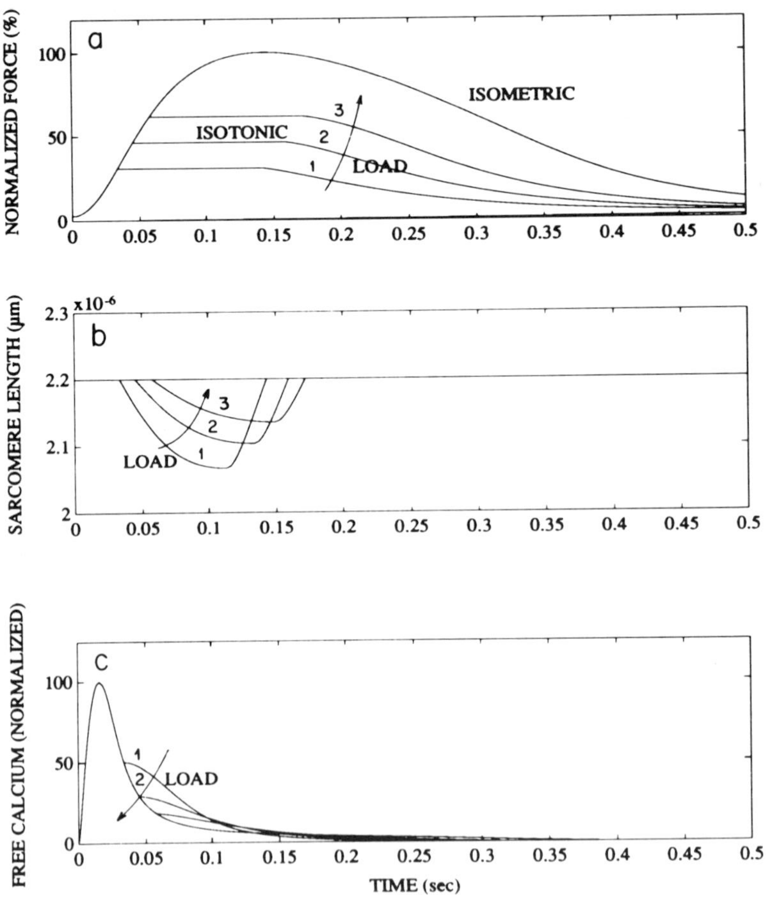

Figure 7. Load dependence of relaxation. **a:** Normalized force for different levels of isotonic loading. **b:** Sarcomere lengths; note the reduction in contraction duration when the load is reduced, corresponding to the measurements of Brutsaert and Sys [29]. **c:** The free calcium transient is reduced as the load is increased, corresponding to the data of Lab et al. [30].

The internal load is especially significant at low levels of activation and short sarcomere lengths [4], when the magnitude of the internal load is of the order of the developed force.

Load Dependent Relaxation: Simulations of muscle contraction at various afterloads (Fig. 7) demonstrate the load dependence of relaxation, in agreement with the data of Brutsaert and Sys [29]. Increasing the load elongatates the duration of contraction; decreasing the load shortens the duration of contraction. The model explains this phenomena by the negative feedback of the filament velocity of crossbridge cycling; load reduction increases the velocity of shortening (Fig. 7b), which in turn increases the rate of crossbridge turnover to the weak conformation. Therefore, the higher the velocity of filament sliding, the faster is the onset of relaxation. The simulation also demonstrates the influence of the mechanical loading condition on the free calcium transient (Fig. 7c) shown by Lab et al. [30]. The calculated calcium transient in the isotonic contraction is wider than in the isometric contraction. Due to the mechanical feedback and the cooperativity the free calcium transient is wider when the load is reduced in isotonic contractions.

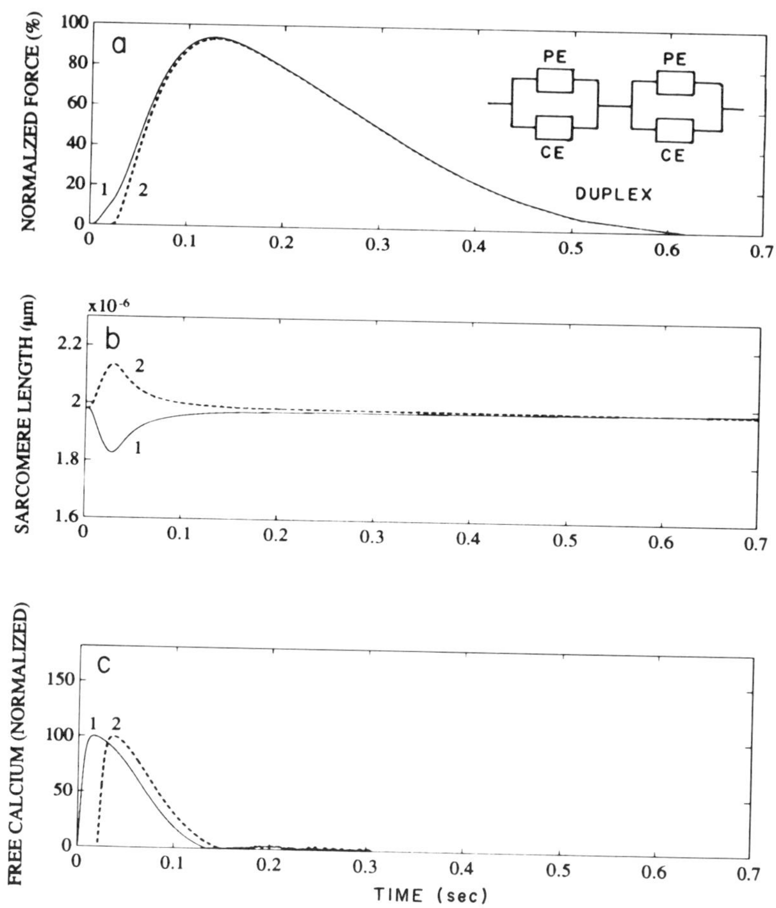

Figure 8. Effect of delay in electrical stimulation on duplex performance. The two cardiac cells are connected serially **(inset)**. Only the contractile element (CE) and the parallel element (PE) are considered. **a:** The force generated by each contractile element, normalized to the maximal force (without delay between the cells). **b:** The sarcomere length of each cell in the duplex. **c:** The free calcium transient of each cell. Note the effect of the control mechanism of the mechanical activity in ameliorating the homogeneity of muscle contraction.

Analysis of a Duplex

So far we have demonstrated the ability of the *dynamic loose coupling model* to describe the basic mechanical property of the intact cardiac muscle: the FLR, the FVR, the control of relaxation, and the influence of mechanical perturbations on the free calcium transient (Figs. 4b and 7c). We now extend the model to describe the interaction between two cells, a duplex, in the cardiac muscle under different conditions. The two cells, or segments of cardiac muscle, are connected serially.

Delay in electrical stimulation: Figure 8 demonstrates the effect of delay in the electrical excitation on the mechanical performance. Delay in the stimulation of the second cell causes a delay in the uprise of calcium transient (Fig. 8c), and in the force development (Fig. 8a). This non–uniformity in the rate of force generation leads to the difference in the cells contraction: the first cell shortens while the delayed cell is stretched (Fig. 8b). However, due to the control mechanism of the mechanical activity, this difference in the cells contractions is attenuated during the contraction, and the relaxation is almost uniform (Figs. 8a and 8b).

Figure 9 shows the effects of different delay intervals in the stimulation of the second segment, on the contraction of the *first* segment. Increasing the delay interval increases the non–uniformity in segments contractions (Fig. 9b) and reduces the maximal force and the rate of force development (Fig. 9a). However, the mechanical feedback tends to attenuate the differences in the contraction of the segments: delay of 50 msec causes only 20 per cent reduction in the force. Thus reasonable delay in electrical stimulation of normal cells (less then 20 msec) can not lead to a polyphasic muscle contraction, if calcium kinetics and the affinity of troponin for calcium is identical in the two segments.

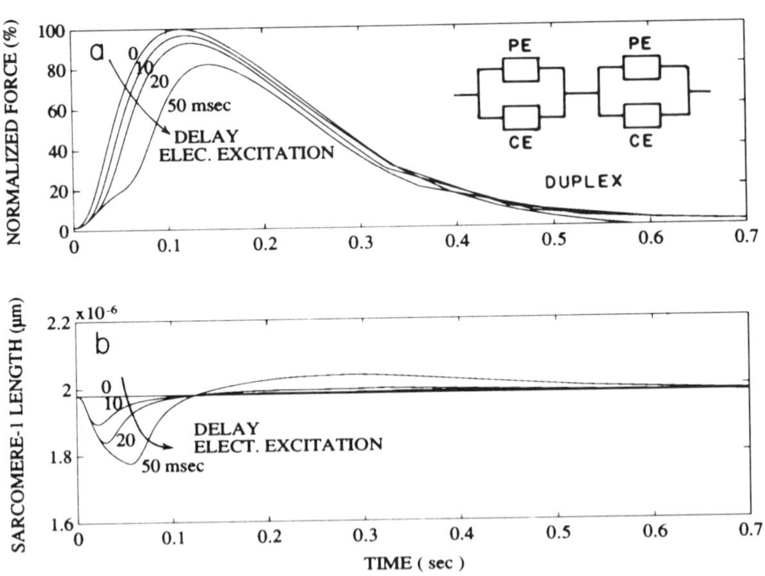

Figure 9. Effect of different delay intervals in the activation of the second cell, on the performances of the first cell, in the duplex. **a:** The force developed by the contractile element, normalized to the no–delay maximal force. **b:** The sarcomere length. Note that for a reasonable delay in the electrical excitation – no significant polyphasic contraction is detectable, except for the non–uniformity at the beginning of the contraction.

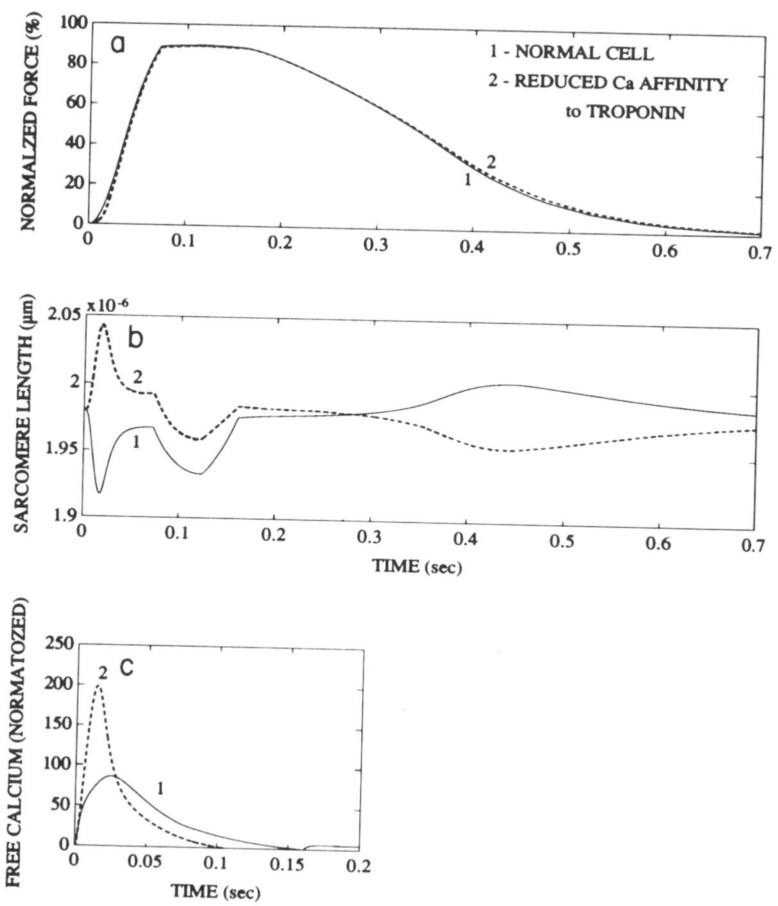

Figure 10. Effect of inhomogeneity in calcium kinetics. The first cell is normal while the second cell has a decrease in the affinity of troponin for calcium, which is a one of the main consequence of ischemia and intracellular acidosis [31, 32]. **a:** The force developed by each contractile element, normalized to the no-delay normal force. **b:** The sarcomere length. **c:** Free calcium concentration. Note the significant polyphasic contraction with early and late elongation of the weak segment, as was reported by Wiegner et al. [33].

Non-uniformity in calcium kinetics: Blink and Endo [31] have demonstrated that the sensitivity of the myofilaments to calcium is decreased when the PH is reduced. Blanchard and Solaro [32] have shown that the effect of acid pH on the activity of the myosin ATPase is related to the changes in calcium binding to Troponin. The activity of the ATPase remains the same function of the *bound calcium* at the different pH. Thus, the acid pH causes reduction in force generation mainly due to reduction in the amount of bound calcium to the Troponin, as a result of decrease in the affinity of troponin for calcium. Here we can study the influence of non-uniformity between "normal" and "ischemic" cell by reducing the affinity of troponin for calcium in one, while the other cell remains "normal". This disparity leads to non-uniformity in the muscle length contraction (Fig. 10b). with polyphasic contraction: the weak cell demonstrates early and late elongation while the "normal" cell shorten. The results are in good agreement with the results of Wiegner [33] and may relate to the early and late systolic bulging of the ischemic myocardium. The rise in the free calcium in the ischemic cell (Fig. 10c) is due to the reduced affinity of troponin for calcium. Thus, non–uniformity in calcium kinetics may leads to polyphasic contraction.

DISCUSSION

The study defines the role of the troponin regulatory proteins in regulating muscle activity, and characterizes the function of activation, based on a biochemical model of crossbridge cycling and calcium kinetics.

The application of only one type of cooperativity in the model is based on our previous analysis [9] of the force–length–free calcium relationships in the skinned cell and on the measured data of bound calcium to troponin. This cooperativity which links the apparent calcium binding coefficient with the number of crossbridges in the strong conformation, is the dominant feedback mechanism that regulates calcium binding to troponin. Other types of cooperativity which may exist have but a negligible effect on the mechanical performance.

The most important advantage of the model is its ability to describe the force–length and the force–velocity relationships as functions of the activation level, and the ability to describe the effect of mechanical conditions and interventions on the activation level.

The model describe the instantaneous relationships between the force, velocity of shortening, crossbridge cycling, calcium binding to troponin and the activation level. The ability to describe these relationship is essential for the description of the intracellular excitation–contraction coupling and is important for the simulation of intercellular interaction in a multi–cell system.

Pietrabissa et al. [2] described a "multicomponent cardiac fiber model" where each unit is represented by Hill's three–element model [2]. The contractile element of each unit is considered as a time dependent shortening generator. Using their phenomenological model Pietrabissa et al. try to simulate the effect of delay in electrical stimulation on the mechanical performance of the cardiac fiber. They assume that both the tension and the shortening of the contractile element depend only on the time and the preload (which is defined as the extension of the units *before* the activation). However, Zahalak [34] has demonstrated, based on Huxley's model of crossbridge kinetics of attachment and detachment, that consistent with experimental data, length perturbation during contraction has a significant effect on muscle mechanical activity. Moreover, given different lengths and times the muscle contracts at different shortening velocities [35], depending on the history of contraction till the given point of time and length. Thus, the mechanical activation function is not only a function of the time and preload but also has a "memory" which determines the muscle performance dependence on the history of contraction. The model of Pietrabissa et al. can not simulate, for example, the effect of different loading during the contraction on the duration of contraction shown by Brutsaert and Sys [29]. Rather, the duration of isotonic contraction in their model is determined (Fig. 10 in [2]) by the shape of shortening of the "ideal shortening generator". Pietrabissa et al. conclude that the inhomogeneity in the mechanical performance of a serial multicomponent fiber is due to inhomogeneity in the preload of each unit: each unit "feels" a different preload, depending on its position inside the fiber or its distance from the point of initial electrical stimulation. The first unit that is activated contracts and stretches the other units. The later the unit is activated, the more it is stretched before activation, and the preload is increased. However, a more realistic description of the control of contraction within the cell and the mechanical interaction between the cells is needed in order to study the interaction between the cardiac cells due to inhomogeneity of the electrical stimulation.

The present study, unlike the above phenomenological model [2], simulates the effect of the instantaneous loading and geometrical constrain during the contraction on the crossbridge cycling and calcium kinetics and thus on the mechanical activation function, it is not limited to the effect of the preload.

The duplex simulation demonstrates that the control mechanism within the cardiac cell tends to attenuate the inhomogeneity in the mechanical activity that is caused by the non–uniformity in the electrical activation and the inhomogeneity in the preload. Thus, a reasonable delay in the onset of calcium transient at the beginning of contraction in the different cells, leads to inhomogeneity in the early contraction, but this inhomogeneity is attenuated during the contraction and practically disappears at the time of peak force. The control mechanism ameliorates the uniformity of muscle contraction, and attenuates polyphasic contraction due to delay in the electrical stimulation.

It is of course important to investigate what happens when the control mechanism within the cell is affected by pathological processes, such as acidosis, and if the cells are not identical in their control mechanism and their calcium kinetics.

The present duplex simulation also demonstrates that inhomogeneity in the control mechanism due to changes in calcium kinetic can easily produce polyphasic contraction. Wiegner et al. [33] have studied the interaction between inhomogeneous cardiac muscle segment in series at isotonic loading, when one segment was normal while the other was hypoxic. They have demonstrated polyphasic contraction of the muscle, and define three phase of motion of the weak segment, similar to the simulation shown in Fig. 10. The first phase is an early stretch of the weak segment, which is due to a slower rate of force development in the weak segment in comparison to the normal segment (in the presented simulation). The second phase is a late systolic lengthening of the weak segment which result, in the simulation, from earlier termination of shortening "early relaxation". The third phase is late shortening of the weak segment, due to slower rate of force decline in the weak segment relatively to that of the normal segment. Thus the polyphasic contraction is obtained due to slower rate of contraction and relaxation of the weak segment.

Inhomogeneity in cells contraction and polyphasic contraction reduce the rate of force development, reduce the maximal force and lead to earlier relaxation of the duplex. Thus the intracellular control mechanism is important in regulating the mechanical activity of each cell.

The present simulation included no changes in the stiffness and passive properties. The serial passive element was disregarded here because the cells in the duplex are connected serially and thus their serial element have the same force and the same length. Note that introducing changes in the passive property, which appear after the rapid change in active property of the sarcomere, will further aggravate the demonstrated inhomogeneity.

CONCLUSIONS

1. The dynamic loose coupling model proposed here, based on calcium kinetics and crossbridge cycling, describes the basic mechanical property of the cardiac muscle: the FLR, the FVR, and the control of relaxation.
2. The model describes the influence of mechanical perturbations on the free calcium transient, through mechanical feedback and cooperativity.
3. The mechanical activation level is defined by state S, which accounts for the ability of the muscle to generate force. State S describes the amount of the troponin

complex with bound calcium, but with crossbridges in the weak conformation that can turn to the strong, force generating, conformation.

4. The mechanical activation function is affected by intercellular mechanical interaction and can be used in multi–cell systems. The intracellular control mechanism is important in regulating intercellular interaction and vice versa.
5. Non–uniformity in calcium kinetics and affinity to troponin leads to polyphasic contractions, and is important in the description of the mechanical performance of ischemic muscle.
6. The duplex can serve to study the influence of intercellular interaction on mechanical activation function.

Acknowledgment

This study is sponsored by the Women's Division, American Technion Society, N.Y. and supported in part by the Fund for the Promotion of Research at the Technion (SS), the Henri Gutwirth Fund for the Promotion of Research (SS), the Miriam and Aaron Gutwirth Memorial Fellowship, and the Al and Phyllis Newman Endowment fund.

DISCUSSION

Dr. L.E. Ford: This is very nice indeed. Inevitably, the muscle shortens. The sarcomeres shorten by about 5% of the muscle length as force develops. Have you looked at the influence of serial elasticity on the time course of the twitch?

Dr. A Landesberg: We have modeled the contractile element and the parallel element but did not include the serial element. We tried to emphasize the importance of calcium kinetics in the regulation of the mechanical activity and the importance of inhomogeneity in calcium kinetics between the cells. The cells are identical in their passive property in the simulation, and are connected serially. The force in the serial element is the same in both cells, and therefore introducing a serial element will not attenuate the inhomogeneity of the segment contraction in the duplex presented here. Moreover, there is a disagreement about the nature of the serial element. Some say that it is mainly an artifact due to the damage to the end of the muscle strip.

Dr. L.E. Ford: Several very simplified models have been published that relate calcium release to the developed force without accounting for the real behavior or the contractile elements. It is very important to look at the dynamics in the way you have, both in the dynamics of the crossbridges cycling and the dynamics of muscle shortening. Inevitably the muscles will shorten internally and a computer model must account for this if it is to be realistic.

Dr. A. Landesberg: I want to emphasize that the mechanical activation is a dynamic function which also depends on the mechanical constrains. To describe the interaction between the cells we need, for each cell, a more realistic activation function which can describe how the contraction of one cell affects the performance of the other cell; how the normal cell influences the performance of the ischemic cell, and vice versa.

Dr. T. Arts: When you have two muscles in series and one is activated earlier than the other, I thought the relaxation was nearly parallel. We had an idea that early activated muscles are deactivated earlier. How is it in your model?

Dr. A. Landesberg: The contraction of the two cells (duplex) in series is shown in Fig. 8. The duplex is at isometric regime, with a relatively small delay in the electrical stimulations. Due to the control mechanism the relaxation is almost parallel. In general you are right; the earlier activated cell is deactivated earlier. This is not because the duration of activation is constant in the two segments. The early activated cell deactivates earlier but the duration of the contraction is longer than the duration of contraction of the delayed cell at the described mechanical constrain (the cells are connected serially at the isometric regime). Your observations are better noted when the delay in the electrical stimulation is increased or when the duplex is allowed to contract un-isometrically; when the effect of "shortening deactivation" is increased.

Dr. T. Arts: In our laboratory, Dr. Prinzen was looking in the same heart at early and late activated muscle. There was less shortening in the early activated areas and it appeared that the early activated parts had to do less work than the late activated parts. Here I can not find that. So I am still puzzled.

Dr. A. Landesberg: You can find it in an isotonic or physiological contraction, where the duplex is allowed to shorten. In general, it is true for cells connected serially, as shown by the simple model of Pietrabissa [2]: contraction of the early activated area increases the preload of the late activated area and thus can increase the work that is performed in this area. However, the description of the interaction between cells merely by the effect of the preload is an over simplification. The ability of the cells to control their level of activation ameliorate the uniformity in the contraction and the work performed by the cells.

Dr. F. Prinzen: If I remember the H. Wiegner paper correctly, their signals were not the same as your's, so there is a difference that may depend on the loading conditions you are modeling. As to the difference in activation states between early and late activated cells or the synchronous activation, compared with an isometric contraction. You suggest that the late activated fiber has a lower state of activation. Our results indicate the opposite. But we have found it in the whole heart, and it is a very complex mechanical situation, so this should be easier to check on in your model.

Dr. A. Landesberg: The loading condition is the same: an isotonic contraction. However, Wiegner did not measure the free calcium transient in the two segments. I want to show, qualitatively, that the mechanical performance is sensitive to a change in calcium kinetics, which control the mechanical activity. Therefore, the interaction between cells is influenced by the inhomogeneity in calcium kinetics of the cells. As to the delay in the activation: The late activated cell has a higher activation level. The activation level is also a function of the single overlap length, therefore stretching the cell in the ascending limb will increase the activation level.

Dr. F. Prinzen: Have you decreased the activation of the first cell only?

Dr. A. Landesberg: You can interpret it in this way, even as "shortening deactivation." Shortening of the first cell, through the mechanical feedback and the cooperativity, reduces the level of activation of the cell, as is demonstrated in Fig. 9c for a different delay in the excitation of the second cell. This is also the reason the relaxation will begin earlier at isotonic contraction.

Dr. D. Allen: One of the traditional problems in cardiac physiology has been the steepness of the steady-state pCa-tension curve. There is only one binding site on troponin. Clearly the various feedbacks that you have put into your model will make it steeper. I wonder if you could tell us how steep the pCa-tension curve is in your model compared with reality?

Dr. A. Landesberg: The model simulates the performances of the contractile element in the intact cell, where we have transient rise and fall of the free calcium concentration. The amount of the total free calcium has a significant effect on the steepness of the force-length. This is shown in Fig. 5. The pCa-tension in the model is not affected only by the peak free calcium transient, but also by the shape of the curve, by the magnitude and the rise and fall time of the various currents. These currents are taken, as mentioned, from the Lee and Allen model [23].

Dr. D. Allen: I am suggesting to set the calcium constant and measure the tension your model produces and then do that at a range of calcium. Then you could plot a relationship between steady state free calcium and tension.

Dr. A. Landesberg: We did that for the data of the skinned cell [9], based on the measurements of Kentish et al. [12] and Hibberd and Jewell [13]. In skinned cells you have constant free calcium and you can measure the force at different free calcium levels. We used this data to characterize the cooperativity feedback [9].

Dr. J. Bassingthwaighte: What is the Hill coefficient for that relationship?

Dr. A. Landesberg: We did not calculate the Hill coefficient for the intact cell. The apparent calcium binding coefficient in the model is not a direct function of the free calcium concentration but a function of the amount of crossbridges in the strong conformation—the force level. For the skinned cell, where the force and the free calcium are constant, the Hill coefficient, according to Hibberd and Jewell, is between 2.48 and 2.94 [13].

REFERENCES

1. Beyar R, Sideman S. A computer study of the left ventricular performance based on fiber structure, sarcomere dynamics, and transmural electrical propagation velocity. *Circ Res* 1984; 55: 358–375.
2. Pietrabissa R, Montevecchi FM, Fumero R. Mechanical characterization of a model of a multicomponent cardiac fiber. *J Biomed Eng* 1991; 13: 407–414.
3. Wong ALK. Mechanics of cardiac muscle, based on Huxley's model: mathematical simulation of isometric contraction. *J Biomechanics* 1971; 4: 529–540.
4. Ford EL. Mechanical manifestations of activation in cardiac muscle. *Circ Res* 1991; 68: 621–637.
5. Zahalak IG, Shi-ping MA. Muscle activation and contraction: constitutive relations based directly on crossbridge kinetics. *J Biomechan Eng* 1990; 112: 52–62.
6. Beyar R, Sideman S. Atrioventricular interaction: a computer study. *Am J Physiol* 1987; 252: H653–H665.
7. Huxley AF. Muscle structure and theories of contraction. *Prog Biophys Biophys Chem* 1957; 7: 255–318.
8. Eisenberg E, Hill TL. Muscle contraction and free energy transduction in biological system. *Science* 1985; 227: 999–1006.
9. Landesberg A, Sideman S. Coupling calcium binding to Troponin–C and crossbridge cycling kinetics in skinned cardiac cells. *Am J Physiol* 1992; submitted.
10. Hofmann PA, Fuchs F. Effect of length and crossbridge attachment on Ca2+ binding to cardiac troponin–C. *Am J Physiol* 1987; 253: C90–C96.
11. Hofmann PA, Fuchs F. Evidence for force-dependent component of calcium binding to cardiac troponin–C. *Am J Physiol* 1987; 253: C541–C546.
12. Kentish JC, ter Keurs HED, Noble MIM, Ricciardi L. The relationship between force, calcium and sarcomere length in skinned trabeculae from rat ventricle. *J Physiol* 1983; 345: 24P.
13. Hibberd MG, Jewell BR. Calcium and length-dependent force production in rat ventricular muscle. *J Physiol* 1982; 329: 527–540.
14. Brenner B, Eisenberg E. The mechanism of muscle contraction. Biochemical, mechanical, and structural approaches to elucidate crossbridge action in muscle. *Basic Res Cardiol* 1987; 82(Suppl. 2): 2–16.
15. Brenner B, Eisenberg E. Rate of force generation in muscle: correlation with actomyosin Atpase activity in solution. *Proc Natl Acad Sci* 1986; 83: 3542–3546.
16. Chalovich JM, Eisenberg E. The effect of troponin – tropomyosin on the binding of heavy meromyosin to actin in the presence of ATP. *J Biol Chem* 1986; 261: 5088–5093.
17. Grabarek Z, Grabarek J, Leavis PJ, Gergely J. Cooperative binding to Ca – specific sites of troponin C in regulated actin and actomyosin. *J Biol Chem* 1983; 258: 14098–14102.
18. Greene LE, Eisenberg E. Relationship between regulated actomyosin ATPase activity and cooperative binding of myosin to regulated actin. *Cell Biophys* 1988; 12: 59–71.
19. Guth K, Potter JD. Effect of rigor and cycling crossbridges on the structure of troponin–C and on the Ca2+ affinity of the Ca2+–specific regulatory sites in skinned rabbit spoas fibers. *J Biol Chem* 1987; 262: 15883–15890.

20. Williams DL, Greene LE, Eisenberg E. Cooperative turning on of myosin subfragment-1 ATPase activity by the troponin-tropomyosin-actin complex. *Biochemistry* 1988; 27: 6987–6993.
21. Stephenson DG, Stewart AW, Wilson GJ. Dissociation of force from myofibrillar MgATPase and stiffness at short sarcomere length in rat and toad skeletal muscle. *J Physiol* 1989; 410: 351–366.
22. Brenner B. Rapid dissociation and reassociation of actomyosin crossbridge during force generation: A newly observed facet of crossbridges action in muscle. *Proc Natl Acad Sci* 1991; 88: 10490–10494.
23. Lee JA, Allen DG. EMD 53998 Sensitizes the contractile proteins to calcium in intact ferret ventricular muscle. *Circ Res* 1991; 69: 927–936.
24. Allen DG, Smith GL. The first calcium transient following shortening in isolated ferret ventricular muscle. *J Physiol* 1985; 366: 83P.
25. Allen DG, Kurihara S. The effect of muscle length on intracellular calcium transient in mammalian cardiac muscle. *J Physiol* 1981; 327: 79–94.
26. Allen DG, Kentish JC. The cellular basis of the length-tension regulation in cardiac muscle. *J Mol and Cellular Biol* 1985; 17: 821–840.
27. Braunwald E. *Heart Disease, A Textbook of Cardiovascular Medicine*, third, edition. 1988; pp 394–401.
28. ter Keurs HEDJ, de Tombe PP. The velocity of sarcomere shortening in mammalian myocardium (abstract). *The 10th Int Conf Cardiovasc System Dynamics Soc*, Japan, September 1992.
29. Brutsaert DL, Sys SU, Rademakers FE. Triple control of relaxation: implications in cardiac disease. *Circulation* 1984; 69: 190–196.
30. Lab MJ, Allen DG, Orchard CH. The effect of shortening on myoplasmic calcium concentration and on action potential in mammalian ventricular muscle. *Circ Res* 1984; 55: 825–829.
31. Blink JR, Endo M. Modification of myofibrillar responsiveness to Ca^{++} as an inotropic mechanism. *Circulation* 1986; 73: suppl-III, 85–98.
32. Blanchard EM, Solaro J. Inhibition of the activation and troponin calcium binding of dog cardiac myofibrils by acid pH. *Circ Res* 1984; 55: 382–391.
33. Wiegner AW, Allen GJ, Bing OHL. Weak and strong myocardium in series: implications for segmental dysfunction. *Am J Physiol* 1978; 4(6): H776–H783.
34. Zahalak IG. Modeling muscle mechanics (and energetics). In: *Multiple Muscle System: Biomechanics and Movement Organization*, Winters JM and Woo SLY (eds). Springer-Verlag: NY. 1990, pp 1–23.
35. Zahalak IG. A distribution-moment approximation for kinetic theories of muscle contraction. Mathematical Biosience, kinetics. *Mathematical Biosience* 1981; 55: 89–114.

CHAPTER 8

CELLULAR RESPONSES TO ELECTRICAL STIMULATION: A STUDY USING A MODEL OF THE VENTRICULAR CARDIAC ACTION POTENTIAL

Yoram Rudy and Ching-hsing Luo[1]

ABSTRACT

A mathematical model of the membrane action potential of a ventricular cardiac cell is used to examine the cellular responses to premature stimulation. Results demonstrate the importance of the slow recovery of I_{Na} in determining the response of the cell. Simulated responses to periodic stimulation include monotonic Wenckebach patterns and alternans in APD at normal $[K]_o$. At low $[K]_o$, nonmonotonic Wenckebach periodicities, aperiodic patterns, and enhanced supernormal excitability that results in unstable responses ("chaotic activity") are observed. These observations are consistent with recent experimental results, and the simulations provide insights into the underlying mechanisms at the level of membrane ionic channel kinetics.

INTRODUCTION

The response of cardiac cells to premature stimulation that occurs prior to complete recovery of membrane excitability is an important factor in the generation, maintenance, and termination of cardiac arrhythmias. Premature stimulation frequently occurs during cardiac pacing and defibrillation. Premature stimuli may be generated intrinsically by abnormal cellular activity (e.g., early and delayed afterdepolarizations [1]) or by depolarizing pulses that emerge from local reentrant activity. In addition, premature stimulation is a phenomenon that is associated with the reentrant action potential itself since interaction between depolarization and repolarization (i.e. "head" and "tail" of the reentrant action potential) usually occurs on the reentry pathway (a similar interaction occurs during fibrillation as well). Our model simulations of reentry [2] demonstrated the

---

[1]Department of Biomedical Engineering, Case Western Reserve University, Cleveland, OH 44106, USA.

Interactive Phenomena in the Cardiac System, Edited by
S. Sideman and R. Beyar, Plenum Press, New York, 1993

importance of the interaction between depolarization and repolarization in the induction and sustenance of reentrant activity. More recently, we have investigated the role of a single premature stimulus in the termination of reentry [3]. In this chapter we examine the response of a single ventricular cell to premature stimulation under a variety of conditions and stimulation protocols. Various phenomena that involve interaction between depolarization and repolarization are investigated. These include slow recovery from inactivation of the fast sodium current, supernormal excitability, Wenckebach periodicity, and aperiodic response of the cell to periodic stimulation. These phenomena are explained in terms of the kinetics of membrane ionic currents. Details can be found in a recent publication [4].

METHODS

A mathematical model of the ventricular cardiac action potential (Fig. 1) was developed (the L–R model, [4]) and was used in the simulations presented here. The model is based, whenever possible, on recent single–cell and single–channel data. It incorporates the possibility of changing extracellular potassium concentration, $[K]_o$, and accounts for the dependence of the conductances of the potassium currents, I_K and I_{K1}, on $[K]_o$. The fast sodium current, I_{Na}, is characterized by fast upstroke velocity ($\dot{V}_{max}$ = 400 V/sec) and slow recovery from inactivation (the Hodgkin–Huxley–type formulation of I_{Na} incorporates both a fast inactivation gate, h, and a slow inactivation gate, j). The current–voltage (I–V) curves of the time–independent potassium current, I_{K1}, include a negative–slope phase and display significant crossover as $[K]_o$ is varied [5]. The time–dependent potassium current, I_K, shows only minimal degree of crossover [6]. A novel potassium current, I_{KP}, that activates only at plateau potentials is included in the model [7]. The simulated action potential duplicates the experimentally observed effects of changes in $[K]_o$ on action potential duration (APD) and rest potential. It should be emphasized that the L–R model as used in the simulations presented here, retains the Beeler–Reuter (B–R, [8]) formulation of the slow inward current. However, we use the model to investigate phenomena that are dominated by the sodium and potassium currents and are only minimally influenced by the

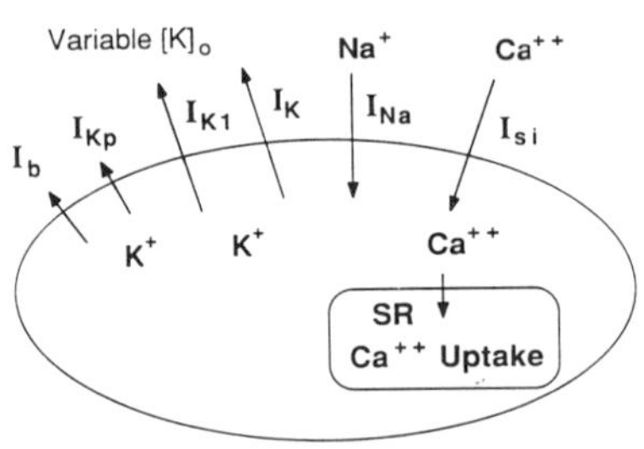

$$I_{Na} = \overline{G}_{Na} \cdot m^3 \cdot h \cdot j \cdot (V - E_{Na}) \qquad \tau_m = 0.03;\ \tau_h = 9.7;\ \tau_j = 79\ \text{(msec)}$$

$$I_{si} = \overline{G}_{si} \cdot d \cdot f \cdot (V - E_{si}) \qquad d[Ca]_i/dt = -10^{-4} \cdot I_{si} + 0.07(10^{-4} - [Ca]_i)$$

$$I_K = \overline{G}_K \cdot X \cdot X_i \cdot (V - E_K) \qquad \overline{G}_K = 0.282 \cdot \sqrt{[K]_o/5.4}$$

$$I_{K1} = \overline{G}_{K1} \cdot K1_\infty \cdot (V - E_{K1}) \qquad \overline{G}_{K1} = 0.647 \cdot \sqrt{[K]_o/5.4}$$

$$I_{Kp} = \overline{G}_{Kp} \cdot Kp \cdot (V - E_{Kp})$$

Figure 1. Schematic representation of the ventricular cell model and related equations.

slow inward current. A more complete model (the phase 2 L–R model) that includes ionic pumps and exchange mechanisms, a correct representation of the membrane calcium currents, calcium release and uptake by the sarcoplasmic reticulum (SR) and calcium buffering in the myoplasm and in the SR has been recently developed in our laboratory [9]. This model is capable of simulating dynamic changes in ionic concentrations such as the calcium transient during the action potential.

SIMULATIONS AND RESULTS

Recovery of Membrane Excitability

The simulations in this section demonstrate the importance of the slow inactivation property of I_{Na} in determining the time course of membrane reactivation and of the cellular response to stimulation during the recovery phase. The experimental reactivation data of Ebihara et al. (Fig. 3 of Reference [10]) are duplicated in Fig. 2A. Figure 2B shows the

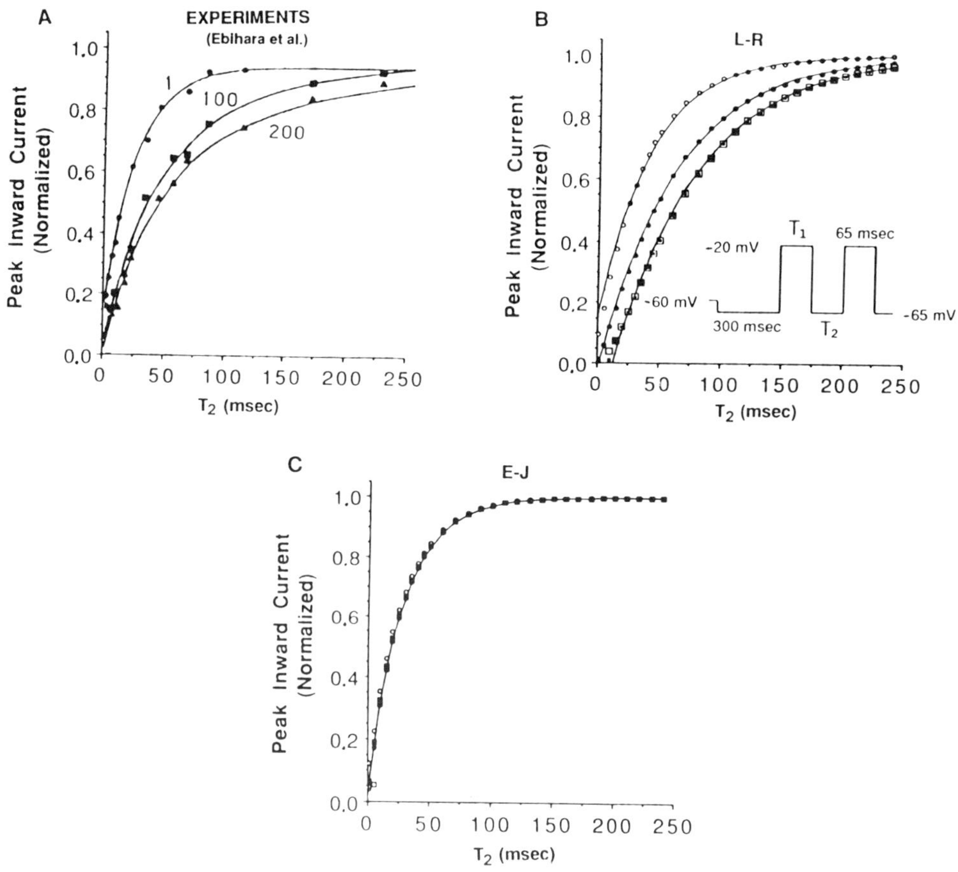

Figure 2. Reactivation of the sodium channel. The protocol is illustrated in panel B. **A:** Experimental results of Ebihara et al. [10] for T1 = 1, 100, and 200 msec. **B:** Simulations using the L–R model for T1 = 1,5,20, and 50 msec. **C:** Simulations using the Ebihara–Johnsonn (E–J) model for same T1 values as in panel B (from [4], by permission of the American Heart Association, Inc.).

results of a simulation using the L–R model. The protocol used both in the experiment and in the model simulations is also illustrated in this figure. Figure 2C is a simulation using the Ebihara–Johnson (E–J, [11]) model of I_{Na}. Note that the L–R model includes the property of slow recovery of I_{Na} while the E–J model does not. In the L–R model this property is introduced by a slow inactivation gate, j, with a voltage–dependent time constant, τ_j, that has a value close to 80 msec at a membrane potential V = −65 mV. The protocol is as follows: two depolarizing voltage pulses with 45 mV amplitude are applied after preclamping the membrane at −65 mV for 300 msec. The first pulse of duration T_1 inactivates the sodium channel. T_2, the interval between the depolarizing pulses, is varied to provide different reactivation times before the second test pulse of a constant duration (65 msec) is applied. The membrane response to the second pulse in terms of the peak inward current is plotted as a function of T_2.

The experimental behavior (panel A) is well duplicated by the L–R model (panel B). The individual curves in panel A are obtained for T1 in the range 1–200 msec, while in panel B the range is 1–50 msec. This quantitative difference probably reflects the different species (chicken embryo and guinea pig). The E–J model (panel C) completely fails to duplicate the dependence on T_1, and the curves obtained for different T1 values overlap.

The E–J model (panel C) fails to separate the curves for different T1 values because slow recovery (j gate) is not part of this model, so that inactivation and reactivation of the sodium channel are controlled by the fast inactivation h gate. Because in this model h is almost completely inactivated in 1 msec when the membrane potential is depolarized to −20 mV (τ_h = 0.33 msec at −20 mV), all curves for $T_1 \geq 1$ msec overlap. In contrast, the L–R model (panel B) generates different reactivation curves for different values of T_1, as observed experimentally. This is because the model incorporates a slow inactivation j gate (τ_j = 4.34 msec at −20 mV). This implies that for T_1 = 1 and 5 msec the j gate at the end of T_1 is inactivated to a different degree, resulting in different reactivation curves. For $T_1 \geq 20$ msec, the j gate is completely inactivated at a membrane potential of −20 mV, and all the curves overlap. In addition, since for $T_1>1$ msec the recovery process is controlled by the j gate, all reactivation curves can be fit by a single exponential. In particular, for $T_1 \geq 20$ msec all curves are represented by the same time constant (τ = 70 msec), which is very close to the τ_j value at V = −65 mV (τ_j = 77.4 msec), as expected. These results demonstrate the importance of the process of slow inactivation I_{Na} in determining the time course of recovery of membrane excitability.

Supernormal Excitability

Supernormality, which can be defined as greater than normal excitability during or immediately following the action potential repolarization phase, is a known property of cardiac preparations at low extracellular potassium concentrations [12–15]. The strength–interval curve, used to investigate supernormality, is obtained by applying a test pulse, S_2, following an action potential generated by a stimulus, S_1. By varying the S_1S_2 interval and the current amplitude of S_2, the threshold current (I_{th}) for exciting a second action potential by S_2 is obtained as a function of the S_1S_2 interval. Based on such excitability measure–ments, Spear and Moore found that 1) supernormality disappears when $[K]_o$ is elevated above 5 mM and 2) the supernormal period at fixed $[K]_o$ is independent of the APD and is determined by the characteristics of the membrane potential during repolarization. I_{K1} and I_K of the L–R model can change their reversal potentials and conductances in response to variations in $[K]_o$. We used the L–R model to simulate and investigate supernormality.

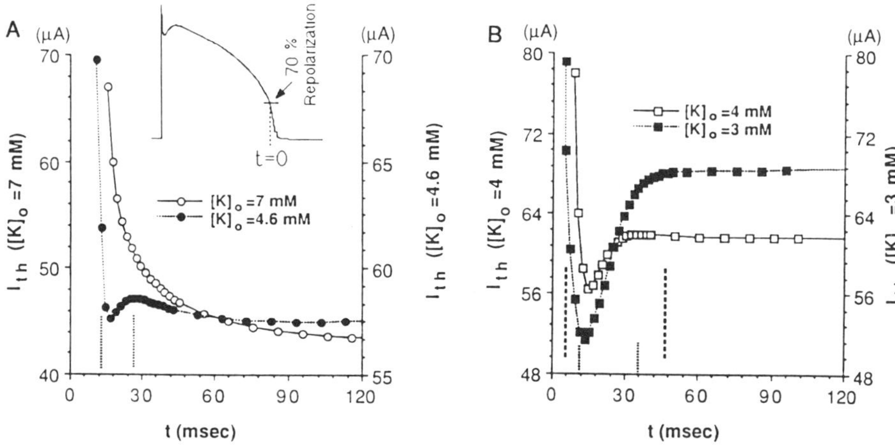

Figure 3. Strength–interval curves for different concentrations $[K]_o$. Ith is plotted as a function of recovery time t (t = 0 is set at 70% repolarization). **A:** $[K]_o$ = 7 and 4.6 mM. **B:** $[K]_o$ = 4 and 3 mM. The two vertical broken lines define the supernormal window for each curve (from [4], by permission of the American Heart Association, Inc.).

Figure 3 shows the simulated strength–interval curves for $[K]_o$ = 7, 4.6, 4, and 3 mM, covering late phase 3 and early phase 4 of the action potential. The simulated protocol followed the experimental protocol described above. I_{th} is defined as the critical current amplitude for which the peak sodium current is greater than 4 μA (1% of the maximum current for a fully recovered membrane and suprathreshold stimulus). Note that test stimuli of very short duration (T = 0.5 msec) were used to investigate the instantaneous membrane excitability at that S_1S_2 interval. The abscissa is normalized by setting the 70% repolarization of the action potential as time zero. Clearly, supernormality is observed for $[K]_o \leq 4.6$ mM (but not for $[K]_o$ = 7 or 5.4 mM) as a notch (local minimum followed by a local maximum) in the strength–interval curve. With decreasing $[K]_o$, the peak–to–peak amplitude of the notch increases and so does the width of the "super–normal window". This time window is defined as the interval during which the threshold is lower than the local maximum that follows the notch. The supernormal window is indicated in the figures by two broken vertical lines.

To explain the underlying mechanism of supernormality in terms of membrane channel kinetics, the following simulation was carried out for $[K]_o$ = 7 mM. The j gate of the sodium channel was clamped at the value of 1 for all times and the strength–interval curve was computed (Fig. 4). The unclamped strength–interval curve is also plotted for comparison. With j = 1, sodium channel recovery from inactivation is controlled by the h gate and its much faster kinetics ($\tau_h \ll \tau_j$). Under these conditions, supernormality is observed in Fig. 4 even for $[K]_o$ = 7 mM. In contrast, when j is free to vary according to its normal kinetics, no supernormality is observed for this concentration of K_o, in agreement with the experimental behavior [12, 15]. This simulation clearly suggests that the nonmonotonic, supernormal behavior is determined by the time course of recovery of the sodium channel. The sodium channel recovers faster at low $[K]_o$, creating a super–normal phase when $[K]_o \leq 4.6$ mM. Specifically, as $[K]_o$ decreases from 7 to 3 mM, the resting membrane potential changes from −78.2 to −95.5 mV, resulting in a decrease of (the voltage dependent) τ_j from 33 to 7 msec during late phase 3 and phase 4 of the action

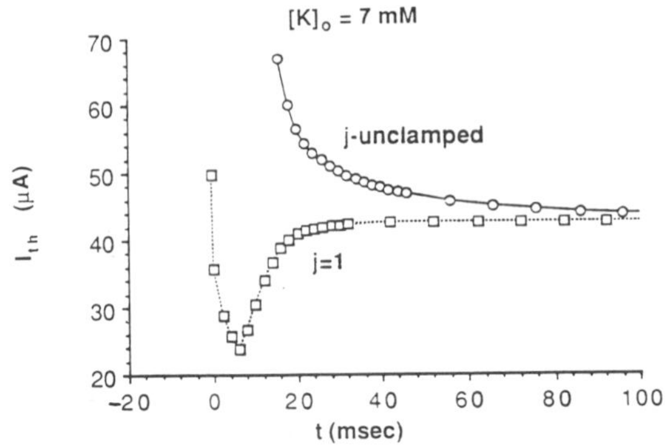

Figure 4. Strength–interval curve for $[K]_o$ = 7mM under two conditions: j clamped at the value of 1 (j = 1, lower curve) and j free to vary (j – unclamped, upper curve) (from [4], by permission of the American Heart Association, Inc.).

potential. Therefore, the sodium channel recovers earlier at lower $[K]_o$, creating the conditions for supernormal excitability. It should be emphasized that the slow inactivation and recovery process of I_{Na} (the j–gate) determine this behavior. Models that do not include these processes (e.g. the E–J model, the Drouhard and Roberge model [16]) generate strength–interval curves that are similar to the strength–interval curves obtained by the L–R model with j = 1. As shown (Fig. 4), under these conditions, supernormality is a property of the model even for high extracellular concentrations ($[K]_o$ = 7 mM) in contradiction to experimental observations [12], [15]. This, of course, is a nonphysiological behavior that results from a nonphysiological fast recovery of the sodium channel.

Response to Periodic Stimulation at Normal $[K]_o$

In the following simulation the L–R cell model was stimulated periodically at a basic cycle length (BCL) ranging from 160 to 2,000 msec (stimuli of strength 3.06 µA and duration 20 msec were used, which corresponds to threshold stimulation at S_1S_2 = 882 msec). Simulated activation patterns for different BCLs are shown in Fig. 5A. A staircase plot of response–to–stimulus (R:S) ratios versus BCL is shown in Fig. 5B (numbers in the figure indicate stimulus to response [S:R] ratios). The staircase pattern demonstrates phase–locking at S:R of integer values (1:1, 2:1, 3:1, etc.) and sharp transitions between these values through many noninteger S:R ratios ("Wenckebach periodicities"). This pattern is in good agreement with the experimental behavior observed by Chialvo et al. [12]. Additional simulations [4] demonstrated that this response is dominated by the activation kinetics of the time–dependent potassium current, I_K. It should be added that when the staircase of Fig. 5B is shifted toward shorter BCLs (by increasing the stimulus strength), the transition from a 1:1 pattern to a 2:1 pattern is preceded by alternans in the action potential duration (APD) as BCL is decreased in the range of 1:1 response, approaching the transition to 2:1. These alternans result mostly from alternating kinetics of I_K at the range of shorter BCLs.

Response to Periodic Stimulation at Low $[K]_o$

The response patterns discussed above (Fig. 5) were obtained in the setting of normal extracellular potassium concentration ($[K]_o$ > 4.6 mM). Under these conditions, the

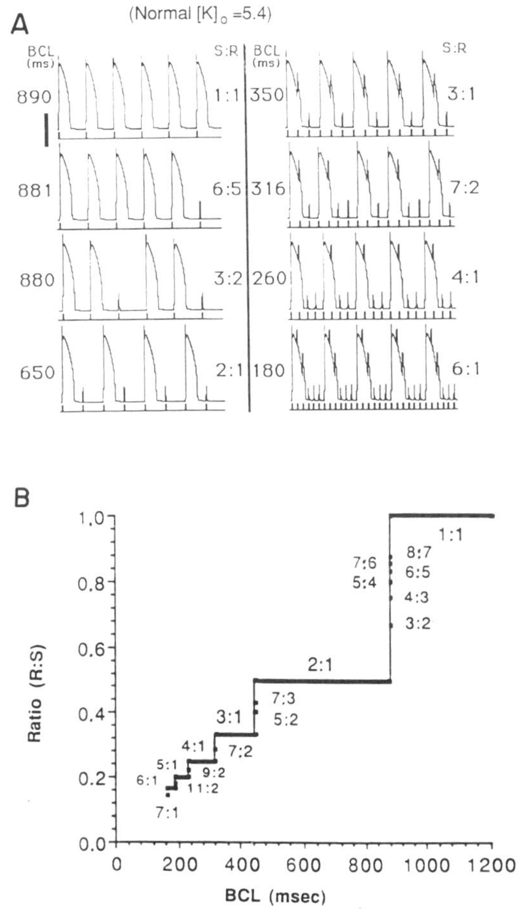

Figure 5. Periodic rate-dependent patterns for normal $[K]_o$ = 5.4 mM. **A:** Examples of activation patterns (calibration bar, 52.5 mV). Numbers on the left indicate basic cycle length (BCL), whereas ratios on the right are the resulting stimulus-to-response (S:R) ratios. The train of stimuli is indicated below each pattern. **B:** The staircase plot of response-to-stimulus (R:S) ratios as a function of BCL. The numbers inside the panel indicate the S:R ratios (from [4], by permission of the American Heart Association, Inc.).

strength interval curve is decreasing monotonically (see Fig. 3A, trace for $[K]_o$ = 7 mM). This monotonic behavior is reflected in the monotonic staircase of Fig. 5B. A different pattern is observed for low extracellular potassium concentrations as a result of the nonmonotonic recovery of excitability that is introduced by the supernormal phase (see Fig. 3B). In Fig. 6, the results of a simulated repetitive stimulation experiment at low $[K]_o$ ($[K]_o$ = 4 mM) are shown as the staircase plot of the R:S ratio versus BCL of stimulation. A comparison of Fig. 6 ($[K]_o$ = 4 mM) and Fig. 5B ($[K]_o$ = 5.4 mM) clearly demonstrates that the activation patterns are different under these two different conditions. For normal $[K]_o$ (no supernormality) a monotonic progression of the activation ratio (a monotonic staircase) is observed (Fig. 5B). In contrast, a nonmonotonic staircase of the activation ratio is observed for low $[K]_o$, in the presence of supernormality (Fig. 6). A stable 1:1 pattern is followed by a region of nonmonotonic behavior as BCL is decreased below 458 msec (right arrow). This nonmonotonic region covers a range of BCLs from 458 to 415 msec.

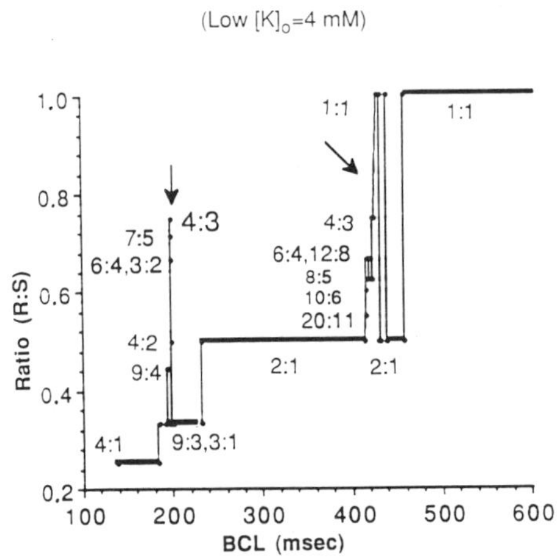

Figure 6. Periodic rate-dependent patterns for low $[K]_o$ = 4 mM. Note the nonmonotonc behavior of the R:S staircase plot (arrows) caused by the phase of supernormal excitability. Format is the same as in Fig. 5B (from [4], by permission of the American Heart Association, Inc.).

Below 415 msec another regular region of a 2:1 pattern is obtained, followed by another region of nonmonotonic behavior. (BCLs from 205 to 190 msec, left arrow). Note that the same patterns are repeated for different regions of BCL. For example, a 1:1 pattern is observed for a BCL of 500, 438 and 428 msec. These regions are separated by regions of 2:1 patterns. This nonmonotonic behavior was observed experimentally as well [12] and, as stated above, reflects the nonmonotonic strength–interval curve when supernormality is present at low $[K]_o$.

In Fig. 6 as the BCL is reduced below 205 msec, irregular activation patterns are observed (BCL = 200.4 msec, left arrow). For this particular BCL, unstable patterns are observed and no regular periodicity is established for more than 250 consecutive stimuli. This behavior is consistent with the experimental findings of Chialvo et al. [12], who observed highly aperiodic activity (termed "chaotic activity") at a BCL of 200 msec with no repeated patterns for recording periods that encompassed 100 or more stimuli.

The highly aperiodic response can be explained by the strength–interval curve and the action potential duration (APD) restitution curve that are obtained under the conditions of the simulated experiment of Fig. 6 (i.e., $[K]_o$ = 4 mM). These curves are shown in Fig. 7A and 7B, respectively, In Fig. 7A, the horizontal dotted line indicates the current amplitude of the stimuli during the repetitive stimulation of Fig. 6 (3.13 μA). For this level of stimulation, four different regions exist on the strength–interval curve, as characterized by their responses. Regions 1 and 3 are excitable, whereas regions 2 and 4 are inexcitable. Note that excitable and inexcitable regions alternate, resulting in the nonmonotonic behavior of Fig. 6. The corresponding four regions are identified on the APD restitution curve (Fig. 7B). Note the discontinuity of this curve in region 2, corresponding to the inexcitable region in Fig. 7A. Also, APD is almost constant in region 1, while in region 3 a fast rate of change (very steep slope) is observed. (This fast change of APD is caused by the fast decrease of the I_K X–gate during this phase). The highly aperiodic activity occurs at a BCL below 205 msec. For this range, the stimuli are frequently applied during region 3 of the strength–interval curve (supernormal phase). In this region, the APD

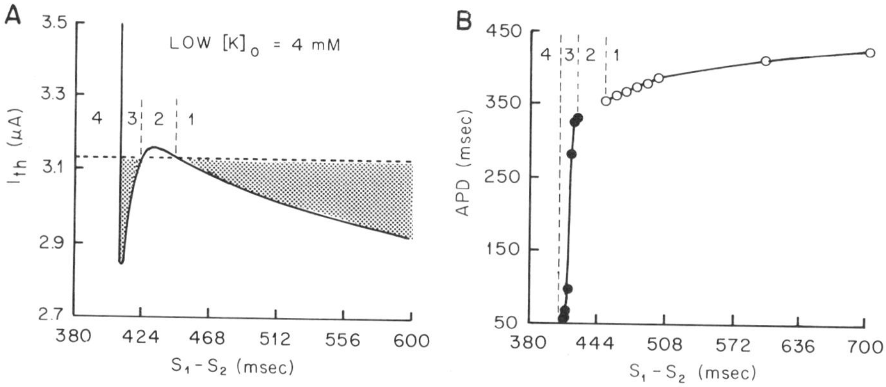

Figure 7. A: Strength–interval curve and **B:** APD restitution curve, for low $[K]_o$ = 4 mM. The horizontal dotted line in **A** indicates the stimulus strength used in the simulation of Fig. 6. Excitable regions (1 and 3) are shaded to distinguish them from inexcitable regions (2 and 4). The restitution curve in **B** is discontinuous because of the inexcitable region 2. Note the steep slope of the restitution curve in **B** in the supernormal region 3 (from [4], by permission of the American Heart Association, Inc.).

depends very strongly on the time of stimulation. In fact, APD changes by 281 msec over an interval of only 15 msec (Fig. 7B). As a result, a small change in the time of stimulation during the supernormal phase can cause a very large change in the duration of the elicited action potential and in the timing, relative to the elicited action potential, of the next stimulus. Consequently, small variations in the time of stimulation in region 3 shift the timing of the next stimulus between different regions of the strength–interval curve, eliciting a very different response. This high sensitivity to the timing of stimulation ("initial conditions") is the basis for the unstable patterns ("chaotic activity"). It should be mentioned that in addition to the slow recovery of I_{Na} and the kinetics of the I_K activation process, the negative slope characteristic of I_{K1} plays an important role in this behavior. When we eliminate the negative slope, unstable patterns do not develop.

DISCUSSION AND CONCLUSIONS

This chapter addresses various cellular phenomena that result from the interaction of excitation and repolarization. These phenomena are important in the context of cardiac arrhythmias since arrhythmogenic activity usually involves interactions between excitation processes and repolarization processes. An important conclusion of the simulations is that the process of slow recovery from inactivation of I_{Na} plays a very important role in determining the membrane response to premature stimulation. This process controls the membrane responsiveness since, during repolarization, the slow inactivation gate, j, is almost completely inactivated and since its time constant is much greater than the time constant of the fast inactivation gate, h, (i.e. $\tau_j >> \tau_h$). In addition, the slow recovery process determines the degree of supernormal excitability at different extracellular potassium concentrations, $[K]_o$.

The simulations of membrane response to premature stimulation predict a variety of rate–dependent phenomena. These include Wenckebach periodicities, beat–to–beat alternans of APD, and (because of super–normality at low $[K]_o$) unstable aperiodic response patterns that display high sensitivity to initial conditions. The occurrence of Wenckebach periodicities in our simulations support other observations [12, 17] that this phenomenon is an intrinsic property of single cardiac cells. This observation suggests that the single–cell response under a variety of conditions might play an important role in arrhythmogenesis. The occurrence of beat–to–beat alternans in the simulations is intriguing. Beat–to–beat alternans in APD are a property of reentrant action potentials [2, 18]. In a broader sense, electrical alternans are detected in many circumstances that are associated with ventricular fibrillation and, as suggested by Guevara et al. [19], may reflect the first in a cascade of period–doubling bifurcations that eventually result in chaos, that is, fibrillation [20]. As with Wenckebach periodicity, the observation that alternans can be generated at the level of the single cell points to the possible important role of the single–cell response in arrhythmogenesis. Finally, the appearance of highly aperiodic patterns that are extremely sensitive to initial conditions might also be related to arrhythmogenesis since it implies that short propagation delays (˜1 msec) can initiate very different responses in neighboring cells (or multicellular fiber bundles). Note that propagation delays of this magnitude can occur across gap junctions under a very moderate degree of cell–to–cell uncoupling [21, 22].

Acknowledgements

Supported by grant HL–33343 from the National Heart, Lung, and Blood Institute, National Institutes of Health, and by a fellowship from the Ministry of Education, Republic of China.

DISCUSSION

Dr. R. Beyar: Can you relate to your model as an electromechanical coupler between electro–physiology and mechanics?

Dr. Y. Rudy: This model can be used in many different ways, but for the sake of people who are interested in calcium and excitation–contraction coupling, this model provides one important component of excitation–contraction coupling, namely the correct dynamic calcium transient during normal and abnormal conditions. In fact, we have already used this model to simulate mechanically related phenomena. For example, post extrasystolic potentiation was simulated with this model and we obtained the correct behavior and also were able to show that the mechanism of this phenomenon has to do with the time delay or the time constant of translocation of calcium from the network to the junctional SR. This is one example that illustrates that, in addition to purely electrical phenomena, this model can provide the basis for simulations of excitation–contraction coupling processes and can be used to bridge the gap between purely electrical and purely mechanical models at the cellular level.

Dr. E. Marban: How did you model the sodium–calcium exchange and what effect does inhibition of the sodium–calcium exchange have on action potential repolarization?

Dr. Y. Rudy: The sodium calcium exchange current in our model is based on the formulation proposed by Mullins and later simplified by DiFrancesco and Noble. However, we have modified this formulation substantially so that the dependence of the exchange current on extracellular concentrations of sodium and calcium, and its saturation oat very negative potentials are represented correctly in the model.

Regarding the second question, the sodium–calcium exchange current does not contribute significantly to the action potential during the plateau. However, it influences the rate of membrane repolarization during the repolarization phase. Since it is a depolarizing current during this phase, it slows the rate of repolarization and prolongs the action potential duration. This simulated effect is in agreement with the action potential clamp results of Doerr et al. from Trautwein's laboratory.

Dr. J. Bassingthwaighte: Is your model available for other people to use?

Dr. Y. Rudy: The first phase of the model that I have described was published in *Circ Res* [4]. The paper includes a table that contains all the equations and parameter values needed for implementation on a personal computer. Many people are already using the first phase model, based on this published information, for propagation studies, for single cell studies, and even as an instructional tool in physiology.

The second phase model is currently in the process of being reviewed. Again, our attitude is that we want to share it with everyone and see it used for simulation studies of arrhythmias, calcium dynamics, excitation contraction coupling, as well as studies of propagation of excitation in cardiac tissue. The submitted manuscript includes a detailed discussion of the experimental basis for the model formulation. All equations and parameter values are provided in tables and can be implemented on a personal computer.

REFERENCES

1. Cranefield PF, Aronson RS. Cardiac Arrhythmias: *The Role of Triggered Activity and Other Mechanisms.* Futura Publishing Company Inc.: New York, 1988.
2. Quan W, Rudy Y. Unidirectional block and reentry of cardiac excitation: A model study. *Circ Res* 1990; 66: 367–382.
3. Quan W, Rudy Y. Termination of reentrant propagation by a single stimulus: A model study. *PACE* 1991; 14: 1700–1706.
4. Luo C, Rudy Y. A model of the ventricular cardiac action potential: Depolarization, repolarization, and their interaction. *Circ Res* 1991; 68: 1501–1526.
5. Sakmann B, Trube G. Conductance properties of single inwardly rectifying potassium channels in ventricular cells from guinea-pig heart. *J Physio (Lond)* 1984; 347: 641–657.
6. Matsuura H, Ehara T, Imoto Y. An analysis of the delayed outward current in single ventricular cells of the guinea pig. *Pflugers Arch* 1987; 410: 596–603.
7. Yue DT, Marban E. A novel cardiac potassium channel that is active and conductive at depolarized potentials. *Pflugers Arch* 1988; 413: 127–133.
8. Beeler GW, Reuter H. Reconstruction of the action potential of ventricular myocardial fibers. *J Physiol (Lond)* 1977; 268: 177–210.
9. Luo C, Rudy Y. A dynamic model of the cardiac ventricular action potential: Ionic currents and concentration changes. AHA 65th Scientific Sessions, New Orleans, November 16–19, 1992. *Circulation*, 1992; 86, No 4: I–563 (Abst).
10. Ebihara L, Shigeto N, Lieberman M, Johnson EA. A note on the reactivation of the fast sodium current in spherical clusters of embryonic chick heart cells. *Biophys J* 1983; 42: 191–194.
11. Ebihara L, Johnson EA. Fast sodium current in cardiac muscle: A quantitative description. *Biophys J* 1980; 32: 779–790.
12. Chialvo DR, Michaels DC, Jalife J. Supernormal excitability as a mechanism of chaotic dynamics of activation in cardiac Purkinje fibers. *Circ Res* 1990; 66: 525–545.
13. Hoff HE, Nahum LH. The supernormal period in the mammalian ventricle. *Am J Physiol* 1938; 124: 591–595.
14. Weidmann S. Effects of calcium ions and local anaesthetics on electrical properties of Purkinje fibers. *J Physiol (Lond)* 1955; 129: 568–582.
15. Spear JF, Moore EL. The effect of changes in rate and rhythm on supernormal excitability in the isolated Purkinje system of the dog. *Circulation* 1974; 50: 1144–1149.
16. Drouhard JP, Roberge FA. Revised formulation of the Hodgkin–Huxley representation of the sodium current in cardiac cells. *Comput Biomed Res* 1987; 20: 333–350.
17. Delmar M, Michaels DC, Jalife J. Slow recovery of excitability and the Wenckebach phenomenon in the single guinea pig ventricular myocyte. *Circ Res* 1989; 65: 761–774.

18. Frame L, Simson M. Oscillations of conduction, action potential duration, and refractoriness. *Circulation* 1988; 78: 1277–1287.
19. Guevara MR, Alonso F, Jeandupeux D, Van Ginneken ACG. Alternans in a periodically stimulated isolated ventricular myocytes: Experiment and model. In: Goldbeter A (ed), *Cell to Cell Signalling: From Experiments to Theoretical Models*. Academic Press, Inc: New York, 1989: 551–563.
20. Adam DR, Smith JM, Akselrod S, Nyberg S, Powell AO, Cohen RJ. Fluctuations in T-wave morphology and susceptibility to ventricular fibrillation. *J Electrocardiol* 1984; 17: 209–218.
21. Rudy Y, Quan W. A model study of the effects of the discrete cellular structure on electrical propagation in cardiac tissue. *Circ Res* 1987; 61: 815–823.
22. Rudy Y, Quan W. Propagation delays across cardiac gap junctions and their reflection in extracellular potentials: A simulation study. *J Cardiovasc Electrophysiol* 1991; 2: 299–315.

CHAPTER 9

Excitation–Contraction Coupling and Contractile Protein Function in Failing and Nonfailing Human Myocardium

Gerd Hasenfuss[1], Burkert Pieske[1], Christian Holubarsch[1], Norman R. Alpert[2] and Hanjörg Just[1]

ABSTRACT

Isometric force, heat output, and aequorin light emission were measured in isolated muscle strips from nonfailing human hearts and from hearts with endstage failing dilated cardiomyopathy (37°C; 30–180 beats per minute (bpm)). In nonfailing myocardium, peak twitch tension increased with higher rates of stimulation, whereas the force–frequency relation was inverse in the failing myocardium. At 60 bpm and at higher rates of stimulation, peak twitch tension was reduced significantly in the failing myocardium. Myothermal measurements, performed at 60 bpm, indicated that the number of crossbridge interactions and the amount of calcium cycling are reduced significantly in the failing myocardium. Furthermore, aequorin light transients indicated that the inverse force–frequency relation in failing myocardium results from altered calcium cycling; with increasing rates of stimulation aequorin light emission increased continuously in the nonfailing and decreased continuously in the failing myocardium. The data suggest that impaired myocardial performance in failing human myocardium may result primarily from disturbed excitation–contraction coupling processes with a reduced amount of calcium cycling and, thus, a decreased activation of contractile proteins.

INTRODUCTION

During the last years important experimental studies have been performed in isolated human myocardium. Although different abnormalities have been described in sarcolemmal

---

[1]Medizinische Klinik III, Universität Freiburg, FRG and [2]Department of Physiology and Biophysics, University of Vermont, Burlington, VT 05401, USA.

Interactive Phenomena in the Cardiac System, Edited by
S. Sideman and R. Beyar, Plenum Press, New York, 1993

receptor systems [1, 2], in contractile proteins [3, 4] or in mitochondria [5], there is accumulating evidence that altered excitation–contraction coupling may be the major disturbance underlying reduced systolic and diastolic function of the failing human heart [3, 6, 7].

Excitation–contraction coupling comprises of 1) entry of calcium into the cell through L–type voltage gated calcium channels; 2) calcium triggered calcium release from sarcoplasmic reticulum (SR) through ryanodine–sensitive calcium–release channels; 3) activation of contractile proteins, following calcium binding to troponin–C; and 4) removal of calcium predominantly by SR–Ca^{2+}–ATPases, and, to a lesser extent, by sarcolemmal Na^{+}–Ca^{2+}–exchanger and sarcolemmal Ca^{2+}–ATPase.

In the present paper we report on our mechanical and biophysical measurements performed in isolated nonfailing and failing human myocardium which suggest that reduced systolic performance of failing human myocardium results from reduced activation of contractile proteins due to disturbed excitation–contraction coupling processes with a reduced amount of calcium released and cycling [3, 8–10].

METHODS

Muscle Preparation

Failing myocardium: Experiments were performed in 31 left ventricular muscle strip preparations dissected from hearts obtained from 21 patients with end–stage failing dilated cardiomyopathy (New York Heart Association class IV) undergoing cardiac transplantation surgery.

Nonfailing myocardium: Nonfailing myocardium (23 muscle strip preparations) was prepared from left ventricular biopsies obtained during coronary artery bypass surgery from seven patients with coronary artery disease and normal left ventricular function and from left ventricles of five donor hearts, which could not be transplanted for technical reasons. The myocardial biopsies (1.5 x 1.5 x 12 mm) were dissected from the epicardial surface of the anterior wall of the left ventricle immediately after complete cardioplegia as described [11].

The excised myocardium was immediately submerged in a protective solution at room temperature and oxygenated by bubbling with 95% O_2, 5% CO_2. The protective solution consists of Krebs–Ringer solution to which 2,3–butanedione monoxime is added [12]. To prepare the experimental intact muscle strip, the excised myocardium was clamped between the ends of plastic rods, submerged in protective solution in a dissection chamber and dissected as described [11, 12]. Cross–sectional areas of the final strip preparations have been shown to be below the critical cross–sectional area for adequate oxygenation on the basis of the Paradise protocol performed in studies from tissue of the same hearts in our laboratory [3, 8, 11, 12].

Experimental Procedure

To perform the measurements, the muscle was mounted to the apparatus and connected to the force gauge. The muscle was then submerged in normal oxygenated Krebs–Ringer solution to wash out the 2,3–butanedione monoxime. After an equilibration period of 30 to 90 minutes, the muscle was stretched gradually (0.05 – 0.1 mm steps) to the length at which maximum steady–state twitch force was reached (l_{max}). When steady state conditions were reached at l_{max}, measurements were performed.

Myothermal measurements: Heat measurements were performed as described recently [3, 13–15]. Heat measurements in conjunction with the mechanical performance were used to quantify the extent and rate of the reactions involved in crossbridge interactions and excitation–contraction coupling. Under steady state isometric conditions all of the energy turned over by the muscle is liberated as heat by the end of the twitch. The total activity related heat is divisible into initial and recovery components. Initial heat is composed of the tension–dependent heat and tension–independent heat. Tension–dependent heat results from high–energy phosphate hydrolysis by cycling crossbridges. Assuming one high energy bond is hydrolyzed during each crossbridge cycle, tension–dependent heat reflects the number of crossbridge interactions during the twitch. Tension–independent heat is associated with high– energy phosphate hydrolysis by sarcoplasmic reticulum calcium pumps, predominantly, and, to a lesser extent, with high energy phosphate hydrolysis by sarcolemmal calcium pumps, sarcolemmal sodium–potassium ATPases and other ATP utilizing pumps [15]. During steady–state conditions, tension–independent heat mainly reflects the amount of calcium removed and, therefore, the amount released and cycled during the twitch [3, 14, 15].

Force–frequency relationship: The force–frequency relationship was investigated by recording isometric twitches under steady state conditions at frequencies of 30, 60, 90, 120, 150, and 180 bpm.

Aequorin measurements: Intracellular calcium was evaluated using the photoprotein aequorin. Aequorin was introduced intracellularly by a macro–injection technique [16, 17].

Statistical analysis: Data are expressed as mean ± standard error of the mean (SEM). Differences between failing and nonfailing myocardium were determined by the nonpaired t–test. A p value <0.05 was accepted as statistically significant.

RESULTS

Figure 1 illustrates the altered force–frequency relationship of failing human myocardium. At a stimulation rate of 30 bpm, peak twitch tension was similar in failing and nonfailing human myocardium. However, at higher stimulation rates peak twitch tension increased in the nonfailing and decreased in the failing human myocardium. Thus, at 60 bpm and at higher frequencies, peak twitch tension was significantly reduced in failing compared to nonfailing human myocardium.

To elucidate the subcellular alterations underlying the contractile deficit of failing myocardium, simultaneous heat and force measurements were performed at a stimulation rate of 60 bpm. Under those conditions, in failing compared to nonfailing myocardium, peak twitch tension was reduced by 46% ($p<0.05$), maximum rate of tension rise by 51% ($p<0.01$) and maximum rate of tension fall by 46% ($p<0.05$). Initial heat, which results from high–energy phosphate hydrolysis of excitation–contraction coupling processes and crossbridge interactions, was reduced by 61% ($p<0.01$) in the failing compared to nonfailing human myocardium (Fig. 2). The reduction of initial heat in the failing human myocardium resulted from both decreased tension–dependent heat by 61% ($p<0.01$) and decreased tension–independent heat by 69% ($p<0.05$) (Fig. 2). Decreased tension–dependent heat indicates that fewer high–energy phosphate bonds are hydrolyzed by contractile proteins and reflects a reduced number of crossbridge interactions during the contraction–relaxation cycle in the failing human myocardium. As shown in Fig. 3, there was a close correlation between peak twitch tension and tension–dependent heat. This indicates that low force production in failing myocardium is associated with a decreased number of crossbridge interactions, whereas both number of crossbridge interactions and force production are higher in nonfailing human myocardium. Reduced tension–independent heat reflects decreased high–energy phosphate hydrolysis by excitation–contraction coupling processes and indicates a considerable reduction in the amount of calcium ions cycling during the isometric twitch in the failing human myocardium.

Tension–independent heat rate, reflecting the average rate of calcium removal, predominantly, was also reduced by 71% in failing compared to nonfailing human myocardium.

Isometric tension and light emission were measured simultaneously at different rates of stimulation. There was a parallel increase in peak twitch tension and aequorin light emission in nonfailing myocardium, whereas both tension and light decreased with

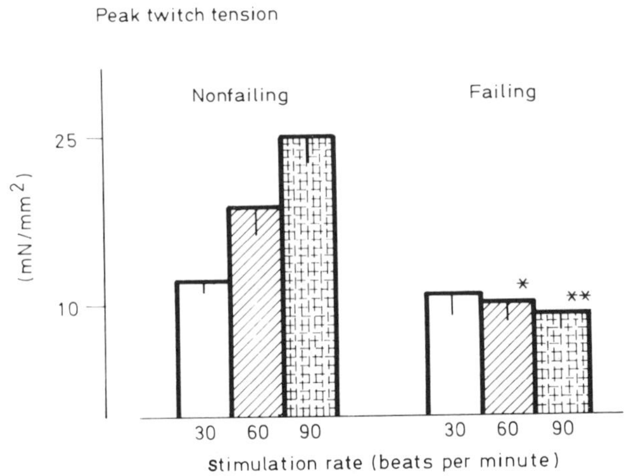

Figure 1. Relationship between peak twitch tension and stimulation frequency in nonfailing and failing human myocardium. * = p<0.05 and ** = p<0.01 versus nonfailing myocardium. Reproduced with permission from [29].

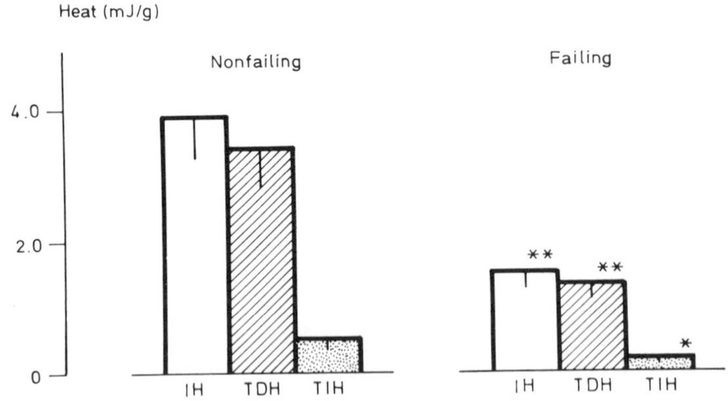

Figure 2. Initial heat liberation (IH) and partitioning of initial heat into tension–dependent heat (TDH) and tension–independent heat (TIH) in nonfailing and failing human myocardium. TDH and TIH result from high–energy phosphate hydrolysis of crossbridge cycling and excitation–contraction coupling processes (calcium cycling), respectively. * = p<0.05 and ** = p<0.01 compared to nonfailing myocardium. Reproduced with permission from [29].

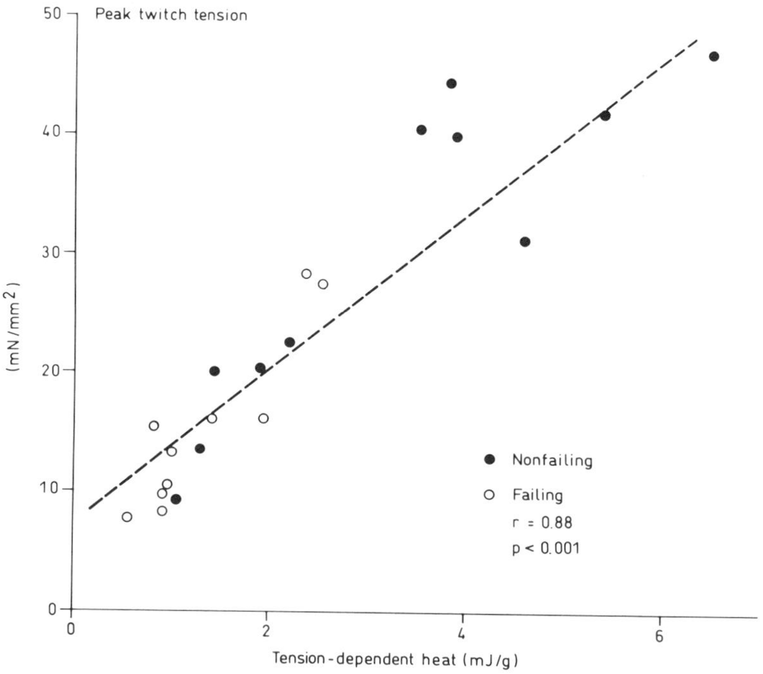

Figure 3. Relationship between peak twitch tension and tension–dependent heat in failing (○) and nonfailing (●) human myocardium. Tension–dependent heat reflects the number of crossbridge interactions during the contraction–relaxation cycle.

increasing rate of stimulation in the failing myocardium. At 180 compared to 30 bpm, peak aequorin light signal was increased by 88% ($p<0.05$) in nonfailing and decreased by 23% ($p<0.01$) in the failing human myocardium.

DISCUSSION AND CONCLUSION

The present data suggest that disturbed excitation–contraction coupling with a reduced amount of calcium ions cycling may be the major cause of myocardial failure in dilated cardiomyopathy. Furthermore, there is considerable evidence that the disturbance of excitation–contraction coupling increases at higher rates of stimulation.

Altered excitation–contraction coupling as the primary cause of the contractile deficit observed at 60 bpm in failing human myocardium is obvious from the parallel reduction of peak twitch tension, tension–dependent heat and tension–independent heat. Tension–independent heat results from high–energy phosphate hydrolysis by excitation–contraction coupling processes. This includes sarcoplasmic reticulum (SR) Ca^{2+}–ATPases, predominantly, and to a lesser extent sarcolemmal Ca^{2+}–ATPases, sarcolemmal Na^{+}–K^{+}–ATPases and other ATP hydrolyzing pumps; the sarcolemmal Na^{+}–Ca^{2+}–exchanger is energetically linked to the Na^{+}–K^{+}–ATPase [3, 14, 15]. Accordingly, since tension–independent heat results from high–energy phosphate hydrolysis associated with calcium removal, predominantly, the reduction of tension–independent heat by 69% indicates decreased calcium cycling during the isometric twitch in the failing human myocardium.

Tension–dependent heat reflects high–energy phosphate hydrolysis by crossbridges. Assuming that one high–energy bond is hydrolyzed during each crossbridge cycle in failing and nonfailing human myocardium, the reduced tension–dependent heat indicates that the total number of crossbridge interactions during the isometric twitch is reduced by 61% in the failing myocardium. Furthermore, the close correlation between peak twitch tension and tension–dependent heat indicates that the contractile deficit in failing human myocardium results from a reduced number of crossbridges activated. Taken together, the myothermal data suggest that reduced tension development in the myocardium from end–stage failing dilated cardiomyopathic hearts results from reduced calcium activation of contractile proteins. In addition, mechanical and aequorin measurements performed at different rates of stimulation indicate that the contractile deficit and the disturbance of calcium cycling increase with higher rates of stimulation in the failing human myocardium.

Differences in peak Ca^{2+}–concentration between failing and nonfailing human myocardium have not been seen in earlier studies using the aequorin technique although in those experiments prolonged aequorin transients, indicative for disturbed calcium removal, have been observed [6, 18, 19]. However, this apparent discrepancy can be explained by different experimental conditions, since most previous aequorin studies in human myocardium were performed at 30°C with stimulation rates of 20 bpm [6, 18, 19]. Because of the different force–frequency relation in failing and nonfailing human myocardium, force and intracellular calcium are similar in both types of human myocardium at low stimulation rates but reduced significantly in the failing compared to nonfailing myocardium at physiologic rates of stimulation (Fig. 1). Our finding of a reduced amount of calcium cycling in muscle strips from failing human myocardium is in accord with recent measurements in single ventricular myocytes using the Ca^{2+}–indicator fura–2 [7]. In those experiments, it was shown that peak Ca^{2+}–transients were significantly smaller in myocytes isolated from failing compared to nonfailing human hearts.

The question arises by what mechanisms calcium cycling may be reduced in the failing human myocardium. The following possibilities should be discussed: 1) Fewer calcium ions may enter the cell through the L–type calcium channels, and, therefore calcium triggered calcium release from the SR may be reduced. 2) Calcium release from the SR may be impaired by alterations of the ryanodine–sensitive SR calcium release channel. 3) Calcium release may be reduced due to decreased SR calcium re–uptake and thus, SR calcium depletion.

Regarding the L–type sarcolemmal calcium channels, it is unclear yet, whether or not altered density or function may be of relevance in the failing human heart. Dihydropyridine binding studies and functional measurements by voltage–clamp techniques indicated unaltered density and properties of this protein [20, 21]. However, molecular biology measurements recently showed that mRNA expression of the dihydropyridine receptor is reduced significantly in hearts with dilated or ischemic cardiomyopathy [22].

Regarding the ryanodine receptor, reduced mRNA expression of this protein has been observed in ischemic cardiomyopathy, whereas no significant changes in expression have been described in dilated cardiomyopathy [22]. Functional measurements of isolated SR calcium–release channels using a modified voltage–clamp technique suggested normal function in failing human myocardium from both ischemic and dilated cardiomyopathic hearts [23]. However, another study using caffeine stimulation indicated altered gating properties of this channel in dilated cardiomyopathy [24].

Regarding calcium re–uptake from the cytosol, there are several reports demonstrating that expression of SR–Ca^{2+}–ATPase is reduced at the levels of mRNA and protein in failing human myocardium from hearts with ischemic and dilated cardiomyopathy [25–27]. Accordingly, reduced SR calcium re–uptake in the failing human heart was suggested from $^{45}Ca^{2+}$–uptake measurements in homogenates from human myocardium [28]. In addition, aequorin measurements and heat measurements in muscle strips or Fura–2 measurements in isolated myocytes form human hearts indicated that calcium removal may be altered in the failing heart [3, 6, 7]. Taken together, there is good evidence that SR calcium re–uptake is impaired in the failing human myocardium due to a reduced number of the SR–Ca^{2+}–ATPases.

It should be pointed out here that calcium re–uptake may also be impaired due to energy lack in the failing myocardium, which may result from disturbed mitochondrial function [5]. The latter, however, was not obvious from myothermal measurements which indicated unaltered efficiency of metabolic recovery processes in the failing human myocardium [3].

Assuming that reduced calcium cycling in the failing human myocardium may result from decreased SR calcium re–uptake with SR calcium depletion and, therefore, reduced SR calcium release, this hypothesis may also explain the altered force–frequency relationship in the failing human myocardium. An increase in the stimulation frequency reduces the time available for SR calcium transport and thus, in presence of depressed SR calcium transport capacity, may further reduce calcium re–uptake and the availability of calcium to be released during the following twitch.

In conclusion, disturbed excitation–contraction coupling with a reduction in the amount of calcium cycling provides a potential subcellular explanation for disturbed myocardial function in failing human hearts.

DISCUSSION

Dr. D. Allen: Has anybody measured metabolite levels in these samples from the failing hearts?

Dr. G. Hasenfuss: That is a good question. It has not been done yet. Our plan is to measure metabolites at the highest rate of stimulation in failing and nonfailing human myocardium.

Dr. G. Allen: Obviously, another interpretation would be that the SR is failing because the metabolite levels fall more rapidly in the failing hearts.

Dr. G. Hasenfuss: Yes, that would be the alternative explanation. However, we have found a close correlation between force–frequency relation and expression of SR–Ca^{2+}–ATPase. Therefore, there is considerable evidence that the altered force–frequency relation results from decreased expression of the SR–Ca^{2+} pumps.

Dr. G. Allen: Your results look remarkably like what would happen if you take a papillary muscle and put it in an anoxic solution. Then you see exactly the same phenomenon that the increase in force at high frequencies disappears. I am not suggesting that yours are anoxic, merely that the energy producing pathways inside them might be depressed, much as in an anoxic preparation.

Dr. G. Hasenfuss: While this is not a definite proof, we did an oxygen tension reduction test. That means in normal Krebs–Ringer solution the concentration of oxygen is 95% and 5% CO_2. In the tests we reduce the oxygen tension to 80% and the assumption is that if there was already a hypoxic core with 95% oxygen, then you immediately should see a further decrease in force when you go to 80% oxygen and those muscles which show a decrease in force by more than 10% were not included in the analysis. The other possibility would be to measure metabolites and it is the plan to do that. On the other hand, you showed us that during hypoxia you would see an increase in the calcium cycling and this is what we do not see. We see a decrease in calcium cycling and a parallel decrease in force.

Dr. G. Allen: Actually whether you get an increase in calcium on hypoxia depends on the glycogen level in the muscle *[Lee and Allen, Pflugers Archiv, 1988; 413: 83–89]*.

Dr. E. Marban: Under what stimulation conditions did you measure the tension independent heat?

Dr. G. Hasenfuss: That was 60 bpm.

Dr. E. Marban: Would there still be a difference if you had done it at 30 bpm?

Dr. G. Hasenfuss: Well, we did not do that but I would expect that there would be no difference at a low rate of stimulation. This can be seen from the aequorin signal: the higher you go with the rate of stimulation the bigger the difference in force and intracellular calcium between the failing and the nonfailing myocardium.

Dr. E. Marban: I did not catch the methodology. Did you use BDM for that?

Dr. G. Hasenfuss: We used BDM to partition the initial heat into tension–dependent and tension–independent heat. We showed that at concentrations of BDM up to 4 millimolar you get only a small depression in the intercellular calcium signal. These experiments were performed in Jim Morgan's lab.

Dr. E. Marban: So even though it is Jim Morgan's lab, you contradict Gwathmey's data.

Dr. G. Hasenfuss: The difference can be explained by differences in experimental conditions. They used a low rate of stimulation and a low temperature and do not see differences in terms of isometric tension development. And if we use a low rate of stimulation we also do not see a difference in tension development. But when we use a physiological stimulation frequency, twitch tension is reduced significantly in the failing compared to nonfailing human myocardium.

Dr. H. Halperin: Have you looked at any of these kinds of situations with more intact models where substrate delivery would not be a problem, such as more intact hearts where you could pace them faster and see if in fact these tensions do drop at higher rates?

Dr. G. Hasenfuss: We did clinical studies in patients. We used RV stimulation in patients with normal LV function and patients with dilated cardiomyopathy. There is an increase in maximum rate of tension rise when you increase the rate of stimulation in the non failing hearts. When you do the same in failing hearts you do not see an increase in maximum rate of tension rise.

Dr. L.E. Ford: If you are working with human myocardium you must be studying hearts that were diseased for a variety of reasons yet they all seemed to have the same outcome. This leads to the questions of whether some of the hearts have failed because of coronary artery disease and you have taken pieces of muscle that have normal concentrations of myosin. Could you have obtained a normal piece of muscle from a heart that was simply loaded abnormally?

Dr. G. Hasenfuss: This is an important issue. The data I presented was obtained in dilated cardiomyopathy and there may be a big difference between dilated cardiomyopathy and ischemic cardiomyopathy. In ischemic cardiomyopathy you might have a kind of normal functioning myocardium and failure might result from an increase in scar tissue. In dilated cardiomyopathy the problem is located at the level of the myocyte. We did some heat measurements in myocardium from ischemic cardiomyopathy and the myocardium was taken from non–infarcted areas. In those hearts we found that force production was quite normal. Also, the number of crossbridge interactions per twitch, was no different compared to the non–failing myocardium, but there was a significant difference between failing myocardium from ischemic and dilated cardiomyopathy.

REFERENCES

1. Bristow MR, Ginsburg R, Minobe W, Cubicciotti RS, Sagman WS, Kurie K, Billingham ME, Harrison DC, Stinson EB. Decreased catecholamine sensitivity and ß–adrenergic–receptor density in failing human hearts. *N Engl J Med* 1982; 307: 205–211.
2. Böhm M, Gierschik P, Erdmann E. Quantification of G_{ia}–proteins in the failing and nonfailing human myocardium. *Basic Res Cardiol* 1992; 87(1): 37–50.
3. Hasenfuss G, Mulieri LA, Leavitt BJ, Allen PD, Haeberle JR, Alpert NR. Alteration of contractile function and excitation–contraction coupling in dilated cardiomyopathy. *Circ Res* 1992; 70: 1225–1232.
4. Margossian SS, White HD, Calfield JB, Norton P, Taylor S, Slayter HS. Light chain 2 profile and activity of human ventricular myosin during dilated cardiomyopathy. Identification of a causal agent for impaired myocardial function. *Circulation* 1992; 85: 1720–1733.
5. Schultheiss H–P. Dysfunction of the ADP/ATP carrier as a causative factor for the disturbance of the myocardial energy metabolism in dilated cardiomyopathy. *Basic Res Cardiol* 1992; 87(1). 311–320.
6. Morgan JP. Abnormal intracellular modulation of calcium as a major cause of cardiac contractile dysfunction. *N Engl J Med* 1991; 325: 625–632.
7. Beuckelmann DJ, Näbauer M, Erdmann E. Intracellular calcium handling in isolated ventricular myocytes from patients with terminal heart failure. *Circulation* 1992; 85: 1046–1055.
8. Mulieri LA, Hasenfuss G, Leavitt BJ, Allen PD, Alpert NR. Altered myocardial force–frequency relation in human heart failure. *Circulation* 1992; 85: 1743–1750.
9. Pieske B, Hasenfuss G, Holubarsch Ch, Schwinger R, Böhm M, Just H. Alterations of the force–frequency relationship in the failing human heart depend on the underlying cardiac disease. *Basic Res Cardiol* 1992; 87(1): 213–221.
10. Pieske B, Kretschmann B, Holubarsch CH, Posival H, Just H, Hasenfuss G. Alteration of intracellular calcium handling causes inverse force–frequency relation in the failing human myocardium. 1993; (in preparation).
11. Mulieri LA, Leavitt BJ, Hasenfuss G, Allen PD, Alpert NR. Contractile frequency dependence of twitch and diastolic tension in dilated cardiomyopathy. *Basic Res Cardiol* 1992; 87(1): 199–212.
12. Mulieri LA, Hasenfuss G, Ittleman F, Blanchard EM, Alpert NR. Protection of human left ventricular myocardium from cutting injury with 2,3–butanedione monoxime. *Circ Res* 1992; 65: 1441–1444.
13. Mulieri LA, Luhr G, Trefry J, Alpert NR. Metal–film thermopiles for use with rabbit right ventricular papillary muscle. *Am J Physiol* 1977; 233: C146–C156.
14. Hasenfuss G, Mulieri LA, Blanchard EM, Holubarsch Ch, Leavitt BJ, Ittleman F, Alpert NR. Energetics of isometric force development in control and volume overload human myocardium. Comparison with animal species. *Circ Res* 1991; 68: 836–846.
15. Alpert NR, Blanchard EM, Mulieri LA. Tension independent heat in rabbit papillary muscle. *J Physiol (Lond)* 1989; 414: 433–453.
16. Kuihara Y, Morgan J. A comparative study of three methods for intracellular loading of the calcium indicator aequorin in ferret papillary muscles. *Biochem Biophys Res Com* 1989; 162: 402–407.
17. Wang J, Morgan JP. Endocardial endothelium modulates myofilament Ca^{2+} responsiveness in aequorin–loaded ferret myocardium. *Circ Res* 1992; 70: 754–760.
18. Gwathmey JK, Copelas L, Mackinnon R, Schoen FJ, Feldman MD, Grossman W, Morgan JP. Abnormal intracellular calcium handling in myocardium from patients with end–stage heart failure. *Circ Res* 1987; 61: 70–76.
19. Gwathmey JK, Slawsky MT, Hajjar RJ, Briggs GM, Morgan JP. Role of intracellular calcium handling in force interval relationship of human ventricular myocardium. *J Clin Invest* 1990; 85: 1599–1613.
20. Rasmussen PR, Minobe W, Bristow MR. Calcium antagonist binding sites in failing and nonfailing human ventricular myocardium. *Biochemical Pharmacol* 1990; 39: 691–696.
21. Beuckelmann DJ, Näbauer M, Erdmann E. Characteristics of calcium–current in isolated human ventricular myocytes from patients with terminal heart failure. *J Mol Cell Cardiol* 1991; 23: 929–937.
22. Brillantes AM, Allen PD, Takahashi T, Izumo S, Marks AR. Differences in cardiac calcium release channel (ryanodine receptor) expression in myocardium from patients with end–stage heart failure caused by ischemic versus dilated cardiomyopathy. *Circ Res* 1992; 71: 18–26.
23. Holmberg S, Williams AJ. Single channel recordings from human cardiac sarcoplasmic reticulum. *Circ Res* 1989; 65: 1445–1449.

24. D'Agnolo A, Luciani GB, Mazzucco A, Gallucci V, Salviati G. Contractile properties and Ca^{2+} release activity of the sarcoplasmic reticulum in dilated cardiomyopathy. *Circulation* 1992; 85: 518–525.
25. Mercadier JJ, Lompre AM, Duc P, Boheler KR, Fraysse JB, Wisnewsky C, Allen PD, Komajda M, Schwartz K. Altered sarcoplasmic reticulum Ca^{2+}–ATPase gene expression in the human ventricle during end–stage heart failure. *J Clin Invest* 1990; 85: 305–309.
26. Studer R, Reinecke H, Bilger J, Eschenhagen Th, Böhm M, Hasenfuss G, Just H, Holtz J, Drexler H. Gene expression of the cardiac sodium–calcium exchanger in end–stage human heart failure. J Clin Invest (submitted).
27. Takahashi T, Allen PD, Izumo S. Expression of A–, B–, and C–type natriuretic peptide genes in failing and developing human ventricles. correlation with expression of the Ca^{2+}–ATPase gene. *Circ Res* 1992; 71: 9–17.
28. Limas CJ, Olivari M, Goldenberg JF, Levine TB, Bendit DG, Simon A. Calcium uptake by cardiac sarcoplasmic reticulum in human dilated cardiomyopathy. *Cardiovasc Res* 1987; 21: 601–605.
29. Hasenfuss G, Mulieri LA, Holubarsch C, Pieske B, Just H, Alpert NR. Energetics of calcium in nonfailing and failing human myocardium. *Basic Res Cardiol* 1992; 87(2): 81–92.

Mechanics and Microcirculation

CHAPTER 10

ESTIMATION OF MYOCARDIAL MECHANICAL PROPERTIES WITH DYNAMIC TRANSVERSE STIFFNESS

Henry R. Halperin, Joshua E. Tsitlik, Barry K. Rayburn, Jon R. Resar, Julie Z. Livingston, and Frank C.P. Yin[1]

ABSTRACT

There are currently no validated methods for accurately estimating regional ventricular mechanical properties. We recently developed a dynamic indentation system that can determine dynamic transverse stiffness (the slope of the relation between the indentation stress and indentation strain during high frequency indentations) in as little as 10 msec. The apparatus consists of an indentation probe coupled to a linear–motor and a computerized control system. This indentation system was tested on beating, canine ventricular septa that were mounted in a biaxial system that could apply strains in the plane of the septum and measure the resulting in–plane stresses. The probe indented the septa with peak displacements of 0.1–0.5 mm at frequencies of 20 and 50 Hz. The transverse stiffness was shown to be related to the in–plane stress and stiffness in the isolated septa. Dynamic transverse stiffness was then used to study the effects of myocardial perfusion on passive tissue stiffness and on contractility. In addition, the transverse stiffness was studied in intact canine hearts during diastole, where it was related to the chamber stiffness. Thus, dynamic transverse stiffness appears to allow estimation of myocardial mechanical properties.

INTRODUCTION

Multiple factors can influence regional function in diseased hearts, including regional variations in loading, contractility, vascular supply, external restraints, neural supply, wall thickness, and wall curvature [1–7]. With currently available methods, it is difficult to separate these factors [5, 8, 9]. In order to distinguish regional loading

---

[1]Peter Bolfer Cardiac Mechanics Laboratory, Department of Medicine, The Johns Hopkins Medical Institutions, Baltimore, MD 21205, USA.

Interactive Phenomena in the Cardiac System, Edited by
S. Sideman and R. Beyar, Plenum Press, New York, 1993

differences from regional mechanical property changes, and to validate model predictions of wall stress [10–12], we must be able to quantify the regional muscle mechanical properties, which are embodied in the regional stress–strain relationships.

Regional wall strain can be measured reasonably accurately *in vivo* by optical techniques [13, 14], by ultrasonic techniques [7, 15], and by multiple markers visualized with radiographic techniques [16, 17]. Regional wall stress, however, is much more difficult to accurately quantify. The various strain gauge devices [18, 19] used give uncertain results because of the unknown degree of coupling between the transducer and ventricular wall [5, 20], and the mathematical predictions [10–12] remain unvalidated [5].

We showed in isolated ventricular septa that, during steady–state indentations, the transverse stiffness (TS – the ratio of indentation stress to indentation strain) was proportional to, and could be used as an estimate of, the in–plane wall stress [21]. While the slopes of the relationships between the transverse stiffness and in–plane wall stress were similar for actively generated and passively applied stress, the intercepts (transverse stiffness axis) for active contractions were significantly greater ($p<.015$). Moreover, the intercepts could be estimated from the slopes and intercepts of the relations between the transverse stiffness and the in–plane wall *strain* ($p<.002$). Since both the transverse stiffness and the in–plane wall strain could be measured, the in–plane wall stress could be estimated from measured quantities. With these steady–state indentations, however, the transverse stiffness could be determined only every 20–40 seconds because the indenting probe had to be accurately positioned at 6–10 different depths in the muscle, with each maintained constant for 2–3 cycles. These steady–state transverse stiffness determinations preclude measurement of changes in wall stress throughout the cardiac cycle, and cannot easily be performed on intact hearts.

Recently, we modified the transverse indentation apparatus to eliminate the requirement for prolonged indentations. A servo–controlled linear–motor system was developed to allow dynamic indentations throughout the course of a single contraction. Validation studies were performed on isolated perfused canine ventricular septa and isolated, perfused canine intact hearts. In addition, the effects of coronary perfusion on diastolic stiffness and contractility were studied using TS.

METHODS

Dynamic Indentation Apparatus

The dynamic indentation apparatus (Fig. 1) consists of an indentation probe coupled to a linear–motor (Model 203, Ling Dynamic Systems) by a cable assembly. A spring maintains tension on the cable and moves the probe toward the specimen. The position of the probe is measured by an LVDT (linear variable differential transformer, Model 241, Transtech Inc.). The probe consists of a circular, fluid–filled chamber, with a membrane covering the open end. The end of the chamber covered by the membrane indents the specimen, and the pressure in the chamber is equal to the average magnitude of the normal–stress acting on the membrane during the indentations (indentation stress), since the membrane is flat and the fluid is incompressible. The pressure is measured by a high–fidelity micromanometer (Model PC–450, Millar Instruments Inc). A microcomputer (IBM–AT) is used to produce displacement oscillations of the probe about a specified position. These linear displacement oscillations produce the cyclic indentations of the test specimen. During these indentations, as the probe cyclically indents the test specimen more and then less deeply, the indentation stress obviously increases to a maximum and then decreases

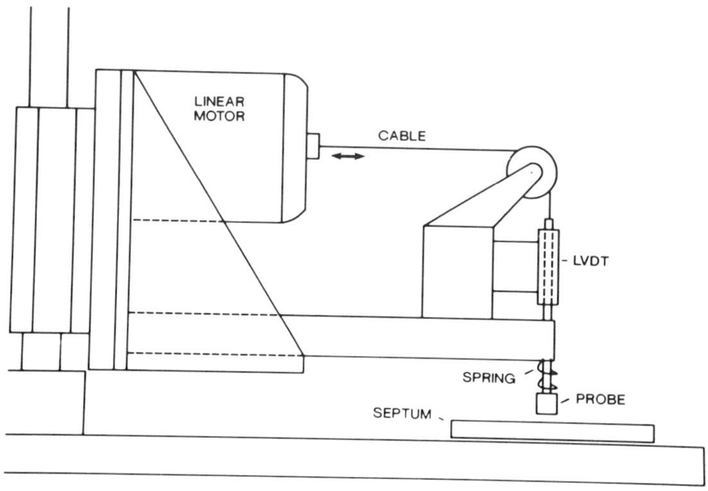

Figure 1. Dynamic indentation system. The arrow indicates the direction of motion of the linear motor shaft. Reprinted with permission from ref. [23] (©1991 IEEE).

to a minimum. If the probe loses contact with the specimen during part of the indentation cycle, the indentation stress would be zero during that part of the cycle. It is desired, however, for the probe to maintain contact with the test specimen throughout the indentation cycle, while maintaining the minimum indentation stress at a specified level (Fig. 2). The minimum value of indentation stress is determined for each indentation cycle. If the minimum value is above the specified level, the mean position of the probe is moved away from the test specimen, and likewise, if the minimum value is below the specified level, the mean position of the probe is moved toward the test specimen (Fig. 2).

Once the indentation stress and indenter position are measured, the transverse stiffness is calculated as the slope of the relation between the indentation stress and indentation strain for each indentation cycle. The indentation stress is measured directly. The indentation strain is defined as the non–indented thickness of the specimen, minus the indented thickness, all divided by the non–indented thickness.

Experimental Studies

The relationship between the dynamic transverse stiffness and the in–plane wall stress was studied in 10 isolated, perfused canine ventricular septa. The septal preparation has been previously described [21]. Briefly, canine hearts were arrested with cold potassium cardioplegia. The left and right ventricular free walls were removed, leaving the interventricular septum. The septal artery was cannulated, and the septum was perfused with oxygenated fluorocarbon (Oxypherol–ET, Alpha Therapeutics). The septum was then mounted in an apparatus that could apply biaxial in–plane strains, while measuring the resulting in–plane stresses [21]; e.g. The septum was attached like a trampoline to two, orthogonal sets of carriages by loops of 3–0 silk thread. In–plane force was measured by transducers coupled to the carriages, and in–plane length was measured between pairs of centrally placed carbon markers by two video analyzers [22]. Active contractions were produced as in previous studies [21], and the in–plane stress at peak contraction was increased by stretching (preloading) the specimen in steps under computer control (stretching protocol).

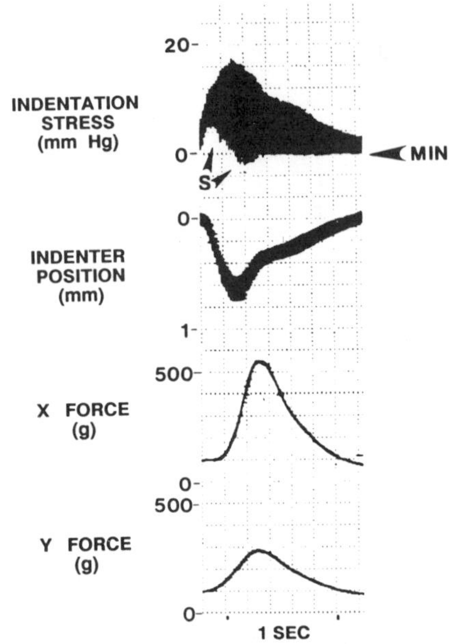

Figure 2. Dynamic indentations during an active contraction in a septum. A servo system moves the indenter to maintain the minimum indentation stress (MIN), but there is some servo error (S). The X and Y forces are in-plane. Reprinted with permission from ref [23] (©1991 IEEE).

Each level of preload was maintained for two contractions. Eight increments of preload were studied. Transverse indentations were performed on the central area of the specimen with peak displacements of 0.1–0.5 mm at frequencies of 20 Hz and 50 Hz.

To determine comparable relationships in intact hearts, the transverse stiffness was studied in four isolated, perfused canine intact hearts. The hearts were subjected to 12–15 minutes of warm ischemia followed by reperfusion with oxygenated fluorocarbon to prompt edema formation and allow for measurements in different mechanical states (less and more stiff). Transverse indentations were performed as with the septa.

Effects of Coronary Perfusion

Although left ventricular chamber compliance is affected by coronary perfusion, the relationship between myocardial tissue stiffness and coronary perfusion has never been directly measured. Seven isolated, perfused canine interventricular septa were studied during prolonged diastoles. The septa were maximally vasodilated with adenosine and perfused with Fluosol. The role of small vessels on TS was assessed by embolizing the septal bed with 15μ polystyrene microspheres. TS before and after embolization was linearly related to perfusion.

Evidence for the Gregg phenomenon (higher contractility with increased perfusion pressure) is conflicting due, in part, to difficulties in measuring small contractility differences and to the dynamic nature of contraction in the beating heart. Since TS is closely related to stiffness, it was used to index changes in systolic stiffness or contractility. TS was, therefore, used as an index of contractility at multiple perfusion pressures (PP) in six, isolated tetanized canine septa. Ryanodine 5μM allowed repeated tetanization and 5mM

2, 3–butane dione monoxime (BDM) produced a second, lower inotropic level. TS and PP were averaged over one second during a steady–state tetanus at multiple PP.

RESULTS

Validation Studies

Representative indentations (0.2 mm, 50 Hz) of an actively contracting septum are shown in Fig. 2. At a relatively constant oscillation amplitude, the amplitude of the indentation stress increased as the force of contraction increased, and decreased as the force of contraction decreased. The indentation stress was linearly related to the indentation strain (Fig. 3), with a high degree of correlation. The slope of the relation between the indentation stress and indentation strain (transverse stiffness) was, therefore, independent of the depth

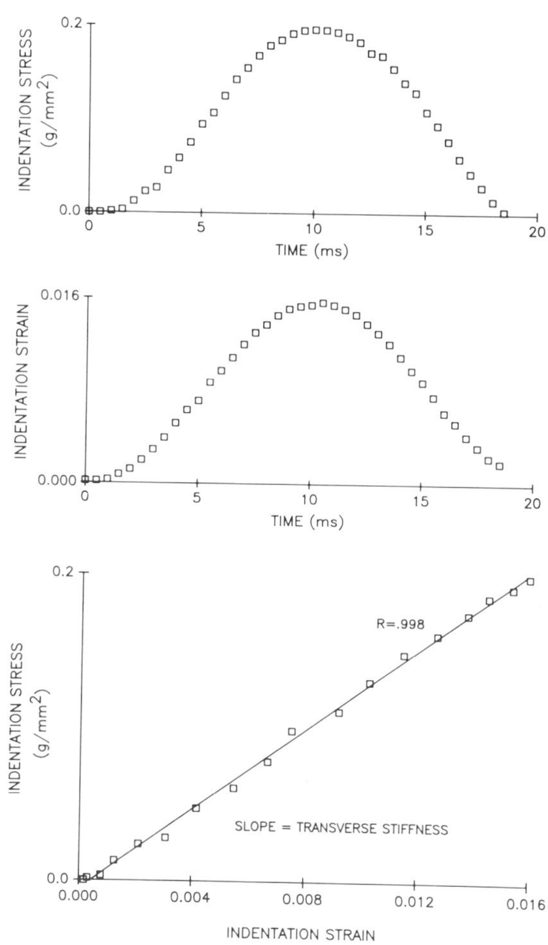

Figure 3. Indentation stress (top panel) and indentation strain (middle panel) for one 50 Hz indentation cycle (2 KHz digitizing). The transverse stiffness (lower panel) is the slope of the relation between the indentation stress and strain. Reprinted with permission from ref [23] (©1991 IEEE).

of penetration for these small indentation strains. Repeat determinations of transverse stiffness performed under identical loading conditions were within 5% of each other. In addition, there was no significant differences between transverse stiffness determinations done at 50 Hz and those at 20 Hz.

The relationships between the in–plane stress index, the in–plane strain index, and the transverse stiffness for one of the stretching protocols is shown in Fig. 4. Each panel of Fig. 4 shows the relations at peak–contraction, as well as at end–diastole. The in–plane stress–strain relation at peak contraction is nearly linear as contrasted with the exponential stress–strain relation at end–diastole (upper panel). The relations between the transverse stiffness and the in–plane strain (center panel) are similar; i.e. the relation at peak contraction is essentially linear, while the relation at end–diastole is exponential. However, despite the different behaviors of the relations between the transverse stiffness and the in–plane strain, the relations between the transverse stiffness and in–plane stress (lower panel) are nearly–linear.

For the intact hearts, the slopes (SL) of the passive (diastolic) pressure volume (PV) relationships for each heart (range: 1.8–6.4) mmHg/ml) were compared to the TS (range: 1.3–102 g/mm^2). The TS was obtained at low intracavitary pressures to minimize the effect of LV pressure. The TS and SL were strongly correlated and were related nonlinearly by:

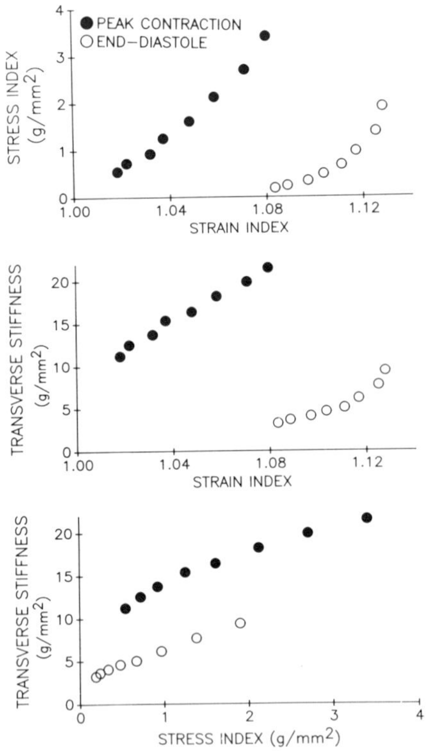

Figure 4. Measured relations between the in–plane stress and strain (upper panel), transverse stiffness and in–plane strain (center panel), and transverse stiffness and in–plane stress (lower panel). Each point is data from one contraction (peak contraction – filled circles, end diastole – open circles). The strain index is the root mean square of the in–plane stretch ratios (deformed length ÷ reference length). The stress index is the root mean square of the two in–plane stresses.

TS = 2.5 x SL^2 – 5.3 (n = 7, r = 0.99, $p<0.001$). Since the slope of the PV relation represents overall cavitary stiffness with contributions from both the muscle properties and the complex geometry of the intact ventricle, these data are consistent with the TS estimating muscle properties as in the septa, and the TS–SL relationship being nonlinear because of geometric factors.

Effects of Coronary Perfusion

TS before and after embolization was linearly related to perfusion pressure (PP) from zero–flow pressure to the physiologic range (80–100 mmHg). For all specimens, the slopes before and after embolization were significantly different (0.021 vs 0.006, $p<0.05$) indicating that embolization decreased stiffness at each PP. These results are the first direct demonstration of the effect of coronary perfusion on passive myocardial tissue stiffness. Furthermore, this effect is primarily dependent upon perfusion of post–arteriolar vessels.

For hearts treated with BDM, random effects ANOVA revealed a direct relationship between TS and PP at both inotropic levels, with no differences in slopes (0.025 vs 0.025, p = NS) but a lower intercept after BDM (3.24 vs 5.78, $p<0.001$). Thus, these data confirm the presence of the Gregg phenomenon in this vasodilated preparation.

DISCUSSION

The new indentation system allows dynamic determination of transverse stiffness throughout a single cardiac contraction, rather than requiring the multiple beats of the previous system [21]. The stresses in the plane of the ventricular septum must be equivalent at each depth that the indentation stress and indentation strain are measured. In the previous apparatus, the transverse indentations were done slowly and in steps, with each step lasting for a number of seconds. The relation between the indentation stress and indentation strain was determined by using indentation data measured at equivalent in–plane stresses during each step. Each contraction of the septum would, therefore, yield only one value of indentation stress and indentation strain. In the revised apparatus, the transverse indentations are done rapidly enough that the stresses in the plane of the septum do not change significantly during one indentation cycle; e.g. the new system can move the indenting probe at over 100 mm/sec, so that the 0.1–0.5 mm of indentation required for determination of transverse stiffness can readily be done in 10–20 msec. Since the in–plane wall stress does not change significantly over 10–20 msec, transverse stiffness can be determined many times during each contraction.

Previous studies [21], using steady–state indentations, have shown that the in–plane wall stress can be estimated from the transverse stiffness, and the transverse stiffness -- in–plane stress relation (determined from the transverse stiffness -- in–plane strain relation). The apparatus used in the previous studies had severe limitations, since it took as long as 40 sec for one transverse stiffness determination; i.e. the specimen had to be extremely stable to yield any useful data, and even if the specimen was quite stable, only a limited amount of data could be obtained from it. The current apparatus, with its dynamic determination of transverse stiffness, eliminates those limitations. The relations between the dynamic transverse stiffness and in–plane stress (Fig. 4) are consistent with our earlier studies using steady–state indentations [21], implying that both steady–state and dynamically determined transverse stiffness are related to the in–plane stress. The values of the dynamically determined transverse stiffnesses are higher, indicating that viscous properties may be important. The exact details of these relations remain to be determined.

Both the transverse stiffness and the in–plane stretch are easily measurable in the isolated septum, and are likely measurable in the intact heart. Since the relationships between the transverse stiffness and the in–plane stretch are similar to the material's stress–stretch behavior (near–linear versus exponential for activated versus diastolic muscle), it follows that it is probably possible to distinguish between these materials simply by measuring the transverse stiffness and the in–plane stretch.

The transverse stiffness appears to be a useful way of studying the effects of coronary perfusion on myocardial mechanical properties. Studies using the transverse stiffness are the first direct demonstration of the effect of coronary perfusion on passive myocardial tissue stiffness, and show that this effect is primarily dependent upon perfusion of post–arteriolar vessels. Studies using the transverse stiffness have also confirmed the presence of the Gregg phenomenon during steady–state contractions in a vasodilated preparation.

CONCLUSION

A new apparatus was developed that can perform dynamic indentations of muscle. This apparatus makes it practical to determine the transverse stiffness at various times in a contraction cycle, and if further validated, may form a basis for estimating in–plane mechanical properties. Since no validated methods have heretofore been available that can reliably quantify regional myocardial mechanical properties, this method may help to improve our understanding of regional ventricular function, and the role that altered wall stress and mechanical properties have in various disease states.

Acknowledgement

Supported by NHLBI R01 HL44092; an Established Investigatorship Award (H.H.) from the American Heart Association with funds contributed in part by the AHA Maryland Affiliate, Inc; and a grant from the W.W. Smith Foundation.

DISCUSSION

Dr. T. Arts: You are measuring force and displacement when you indent your muscle surface, so you are in fact measuring stress perpendicular to the fibers. You claim that you are measuring strain in the plane of the fiber, different from what other people do. But, in fact you are doing the same. You are using a mathematical model to relate transverse stiffness to in–plane stiffness. In the real ventricle you measure LV pressure which is perpendicular, and then you are using a mathematical model, like many people do, and calculate the stress in the plane of the wall. I do not see very much difference in the way you are handling in–plane stress. You are using a mathematical model too, and it is also dependent on material properties. What is the real gain of this technique over the current techniques on pressure–volume relation? Wall stress calculations are presented in many models, using the radius or curvature and so on.

Dr. H. Halperin: There is actually a fundamental benefit from our technique. We are trying to do a stepwise estimation. We are not just doing a Mirsky type ellipsoidal or spherical model where you assume certain materials, or assume that the materials are not important. First, we go through validation processes where we measure the transverse stiffness and the in–plane stresses directly. The mathematical model we use is not a model of stress from geometry. It gives the relationship between the transverse stiffness and the in–plane properties. That is a mathematical model, but the difference here is that we can validate it because we are measuring the transverse stiffness and the stresses. In many kinds of situations we included BDM, differences in perfusion pressure and ischemia reperfusion. If we can get a nice relationship between the transverse stiffness and the in-plane stress in all those circumstances, then we are a big step ahead of just simply using a mathematical model to calculate stress. In fact, it looks like the transverse stiffness is related to material properties. We do not know in the other mathematical models what the material properties are. The issue is to do enough validation studies with the transverse stiffness so as to know the relationship between it and the in-plane material properties and the stress. There are a few tricks you can use too. In the relatively unloaded state, where wall stress is very low, the transverse stiffness is a direct estimate of the in-plane stiffness. Under those circumstances, at least, you have one particular calibration point because the transverse stiffness gives you the in-plane stiffness there directly without any assumptions at all. You can use a few tricks like that in addition to these validation studies to get a better handle on material properties than by simply using a mathematical model.

Dr. T. Arts: Did you measure pressure in the intact heart.

Dr. H. Halperin: We have not used the pressure in this model because the transverse stiffness and the strain seem to be sufficient to determine what the stresses are, independent of what the pressure is. Obviously we want to do that. In fact, in the intact hearts, with the symmetrical ventricles, there is no big argument. It is in the asymmetrical ventricles what we are interested in.

Dr. R. Chadwick: Why do you vibrate the indentation probe?

Dr. H. Halperin: We vibrate the indentation probe because we want to have a value of transverse stiffness over a very short period of time. If you do a slow indentation, the heart will move away during the course of the indentation and you do not know what the relationship between the indentation stress and indentation strain is. During that quick indentation the properties of the heart muscle are not changed; the heart muscle properties are the same in the 20–30 points that we get in 10–20 ms indentations. That way the slope of that relationship between the indentation stress and indentation strain in that determination is done with the heart muscle properties unchanged.

Dr. Y. Lanir: One advantage of this technique is the potential ability to measure local stress. That is very important in case of a local damage to the heart. In the models, one has usually to assume some kind of global geometry and global properties. Local inhomogeneities are difficult to model.

Dr. H. Halperin: That the transverse stiffness does track the pressure, as you would expect it to. We started at different points on the same heart to see if the stresses were the same, and they were not. Yet, your mathematical model would say they are. So we though that this technique has a problem. Using 2D echocardiography to look at the detailed geometry of the heart showed it was not very symmetrical. That is fascinating because it leads us to believe that the mathematical models have real flaws.

Dr. T. Arts: I don't agree.

Dr. R. Mates: Did you vary the frequency of the stimulator to see whether there were any appreciable viscoelastic affects?

Dr. H. Halperin: We used a few different frequencies. We used 20 Hz and 50 Hz. We can not go below that because it is difficult to separate the data from the intrinsic contraction. There are clearly some viscoelastic properties. The relations at 20 Hz are not exactly the same as at 50 Hz. We have not done enough analysis to look at those differences. All these relationships have a similar form at the different frequencies, but they are not identical.

Dr. J. Bassingthwaighte: My experience with using isolated heart preparations is that if you have any catheter or other material object that is in the cavity close to the ventricular wall, it creates damage, hematomas and what not. It is almost impossible to avoid. What kind of damage does your probe produce?

Dr. H. Halperin: There was no noticeable damage on the epicardial surface. We have only done isolate flurosol perfused intact hearts, and you can not notice an indentation when you take it away. Certainly that is an issue. We have not noticed any real local damage; it is not a spear, like in a catheter, but a flat probe that is from 4–7 mm in diameter, which sits nicely on the surface.

REFERENCES

1. Tennant R, Wiggers CJ. The effect of coronary occlusion on myocardial contraction. *Am J Physiol* 1935; 112: 351–361.
2. Ross J Jr, Sonnenblick EH, Covell JW, Kaiser GA, Spiro D. The architecture or the heart in systole and diastole. *Circ Res* 1967; 21: 409–421.
3. Tyberg JV, Forrester JS, Parmley WW. Altered segmental function and compliance in acute myocardial ischemia. *Eur J Cardiol* 1974; 14: 307–317.
4. Hutchins GM, Bulkley BH, Moore GW, Piasio MA, Lohr FT. Shape of the human cardiac ventricles. *Am J Cardiol* 1978; 41: 646–654.
5. Yin FCP. Ventricular Wall Stress. *Circ Res* 1981; 49: 829–842.
6. Janicki JS, Weber KT, Gochman RF, Shroff S, Geheb FJ. Three-dimensional myocardial and ventricular shape: a surface representation. *Am J Physiol (Heart Circ Physiol)* 1981; 10: H1–H11.
7. Gallagher KP, Osakada G, Hess OM, Koziol JA, Kemper WS, Ross J Jr. Subepicardial segmental function during coronary stenosis and the role of myocardial fiber orientation. *Circ Res* 1982; 50: 352–359.
8. Ross J Jr. Assessment of cardiac function and myocardial contractility. In: Hurst JW, ed. *The Heart.* New York: McGraw–Hill, 1982; pp 310–33.
9. Ross J Jr. Cardiac function and myocardial contractility: A perspective. *J Am Coll Cardiol* 1983; 1: 52–62.
10. Sandler H, Dodge HT. Left ventricular tension and stress in man. *Circ Res* 1963; 13: 91–104.
11. Mirsky I. Effects of anisotropy and nonhomogeneity on left ventricular stresses in the intact heart. *Bull Math Biophys* 1973; 32: 197–213.
12. Janz RF, Grimm AF. Finite–element model for the mechanical behavior of the left ventricle. *Circ Res* 1972; 30: 244–252.
13. Peters WH, Ranson WF. Digital imaging techniques in experimental stress analysis. *Optical Eng* 1982; 21(3): 427–431.
14. Prinzen TT, Arts T, Prinzen FW, Reneman RS. Mapping of epicardial deformation using a video processing technique. *J Biomech* 1986; 19: 264–263.
15. Theroux P, Franklin, Ross J Jr, Kemper WS. Regional myocardial function during acute coronary occlusion and its modification by pharmacological agents in the dog. *Circ Res* 1974; 35: 896–908.
16. Hinds JE, Hawthorne EH, Mullins CB, Mitchell JH. Instantaneous changes in the left ventricular lengths occurring in dogs during the cardiac cycle. *Fedn Proc Fedn Am Soc Exp Biol* 1969; 28: 1351–1357.
17. Walley KR, Grover M, Raff GL, Benge JW, Hannaford B, Glantz SA. Left ventricular dynamic geometry in the intact and open chest dog. *Circ Res* 1982; 50: 573–589.
18. Feigl EO, Simon GA, Fry DL. Auxotonic and isometric cardiac force transducers. *J Appl Physiol* 1967; 23: 597–600.
19. Burns JW, Covell JW, Myers R, Ross J Jr. Comparison of directly measured left ventricular wall stress calculated from geometric reference figures. *Circ Res* 1971; 28:611–621.
20. Huisman RM, Elzinga G, Westerhoff N, Sipkema P. Measurement of left ventricular wall stress. *Cardiovasc Res* 1980; 14: 142–153.
21. Halperin H, Chew PH, Weisfeldt ML, Sagawa K, Humphrey JD, Yin FCP. Transverse stiffness: A method for estimation of myocardial wall stress. *Circ Res* 1987; 61(5): 695–703.
22. Yin FCP, Tompkins WR, Peterson KL, Intaglietta M. A video dimension analyzer. *IEEE Trans Biomed Eng* 1972; BME–19: 376–381.
23. Halperin HR, Tskitlik JE, Gelfand M, Downs J, Yin FCP. Servo–controlled indenter for determining the transverse stiffness of ventricular muscle. *IEEE Trans Biomed Eng* 1991; 38(6): 605.

CHAPTER 11

INTRAMYOCARDIAL MECHANICAL STATES: VESSEL–INTERSTITIUM–MUSCLE INTERFACE

J. Yasha Kresh[1]

ABSTRACT

The intramural blood vessels and fluid–filled interstitial space form a hydraulic continuum enmeshed by myocardial muscle layers and collagen matrix. Coronary circulation was found to be strongly influenced by passive and active properties of the muscle surrounding the coronary microvasculature. Selective remodeling of the extracellular collagen–matrix and partial uncoupling of the intramyocardial structure(s) cause profound functional alterations in the coronary circulation and interstitial compartment fluid–dynamics. Mechanical impediment to coronary inflow resides in the muscle fiber–interstitium–microvessel interface, functioning independently of the generated chamber pressure conditions.

INTRODUCTION

The interaction of the cardiac muscle with intramural vascular structures during active contraction and relaxation is without a unified hypothesis [1–4]. The understanding of coronary circulation and myocardial perfusion dynamics has been limited in–part by an erroneous characterization of the extravascular tissue pressure and intramyocardial wall stress distribution [5–8]. The morphological microscopic evidence [9] revealed that myocardial muscle cells are tightly bound to each other and to adjoining blood vessels by a dense collagen matrix. The interaction (hydraulic) of intramyocardial compartments (intravascular–interstitial–intracellular) and traction of the microcirculation will alter dynamically (non–linear/time–varying) capacitance–resistance components [10]. The active contraction process and force generation is in the myocardium. The ventricular chamber

[1]Likoff Cardiovascular Institute, Departments of Cardiothoracic Surgery and Medicine, Philadelphia, PA 19102, USA.

Interactive Phenomena in the Cardiac System, Edited by S. Sideman and R. Beyar, Plenum Press, New York, 1993

pressure is generated by myocardial cells whose deformation is influenced by both intrinsic and extrinsic loads. Furthermore, when the "afterload" is removed (LVP = 0), intramyocardial tissue stress, intramyocardial fluid pressure and phasic near "normal" inflow–outflow features are retained [10]. In contrast, flow measured in a saphenous–vein bypass–graft (in patients), supplying a dyskinetic region, displays a dominant systolic flow component (unpublished data). In effect the ventricular chamber dynamics are causally uncoupled from being the primary control of myocardial perfusion [11]. The intramyocardial stress fields and resultant muscle "traction" surrounding the coronary vasculature modulate the inflow–outflow pattern and perfusion distribution in the myocardium [10, 12]. This line of thinking is in part motivated by observations we made on isolated collapsible vessels fixed in a pressurized chamber and subjected to periodic extramural modulation. In such a system the modulating waveform is partially transduced through the vessel wall, augmenting the effective intraluminal pressure. A transiently greater local pressure will oppose the upstream perfusion pressure (head pressure), without necessitating large displacement of vascular volume and/or sizable intramyocardial vessel collapse. Under *in vivo* conditions, changes in vessel geometry (cross–section and length) are in part dependent upon traction forces imposed on intramural vessels by the surrounding environment (e.g. collagen struts, interstitial fluid pressure).

The work reported here was motivated by a series of experiments using an *in vivo* canine preparation, in which local myocardial contractility and vascular tone were controlled independently of global hemodynamic variables. In these experiments a separate perfusion system was used to supply blood to the cannulated left anterior descending coronary artery, from a canula in the femoral artery, maintaining constant perfusion pressure and normothermia.

Local myocardial contractile performance in both the normal and maximally dilated (adenosine) coronary bed was modified by infusing the beta agonist isoproterenol and beta blocker Esmolol. Coronary blood flow (CBF) and intramyocardial pressure (IMP) were the variables monitored. Changes in coronary perfusion pressure (CPP) were achieved by a pressure–regulated perfusion source. These experiments have yielded several observations:

1. The waveform morphology of CPP and the time–derivative of IMP (d(IMP)/dt) exhibited similar temporal features. Component of IMP is transduced across the vessel wall, demonstrating that IMP modulates coronary blood flow directly.
2. In the vented left ventricle (LV) (left ventricular pressure (LVP) $\approx$ 0), coronary inflow remained phasic. Thus, systolic inflow impediment is independent of developed LVP.
3. Systole only minimally effected the subsequent diastolic flow. That is, coronary inflow during long diastoles (diastasis) was shown to be similar to end–diastolic flow levels in the beating heart implying that reactive components (capacitative backflow) have very short time constants or have minimal influence, i.e. systolic volume changes in the arterial bed (compartment) are small. Flow measured during long diastoles at a given perfusion pressure was seen to be essentially independent of inotropic state, but dependent on vascular tone and passive distending transmural pressure. Clearly, diastolic flow levels are determined by the state of vascular tone and intramural hydraulic milieu.
4. Systolic flow impediment was made to increase with an increased inotropic state (isoproterenol); and decrease with a decreased myocardial inotropic state (Beta–adrenergic blockade). These results suggest that the systolic flow

inhibition is influenced by the myocardial active state. The contracting myocardium modulates diastolic flow; the source of systolic impediment is in the muscle–interstitium–microvessel interface.

ISOLATED RABBIT HEART EXPERIMENTS

Isolated, perfused hearts from New Zealand white rabbits (2.5–3.5 kg) were used. A Langendorff perfusion apparatus, modified to enable a working heart preparation, allowed precise control over coronary perfusion pressure, myocardial preload and afterload, LV volume, and inotropic state in the normal and maximally vasodilated coronary bed, all in an environment free of central nervous and humoral regulation. The protocol was designed to uncover the separate and combined effects of the various regulated parameters, all at a given inotropic state: perfusion pressure (CPP), intramyocardial pressure (IMP), LVP, and coronary blood flow (CBF). The perfusion system enabled three modes of operation: 1. Isobaric (LVP = 0), no–load (non–working heart) contractions under constant perfusion pressure; 2. Isovolumic contractions (working heart) with controlled LV volume; 3. Pumping LV (working ejecting heart) with controlled preload against a controlled afterload.

To elucidate the role of intraventricular pressure on the coronary flow dynamics, the LV chamber volume (VOL) was modulated using an external syringe–pump in beating and arrested states (Fig. 1). The response of the coronary system to large LV–pressure changes was most striking in the lack of any detectible change in flow pulse–amplitude or mean value. The evidence is most compelling, implicating the extravascular ("intramyocardial

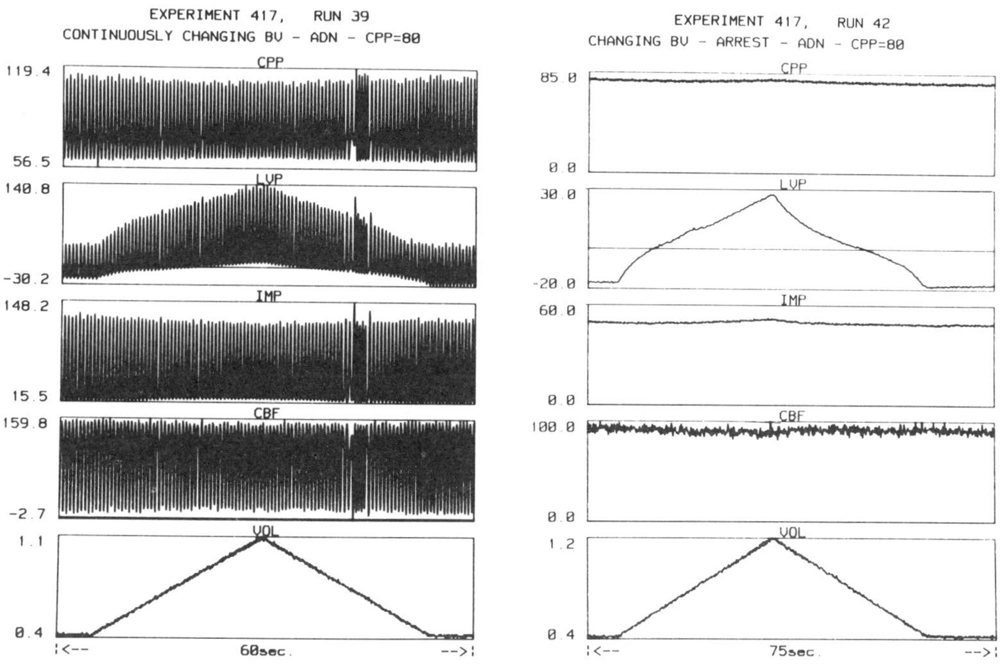

Figure 1. LV–chamber volume (VOL) modulation using an external pump in beating **(Left)** and arrested **(Right)** state. Coronary blood flow (CBF) and intra–myocardial pressure (IMP) are insensitive to VOL change.

pump") pressure as the primary mechanism of coronary inflow modulation, causing systolic inflow impediment. A prevailing view, based on elastic theory, relating intramyocardial pressure to a particular (radial) wall–stress component is misleading and inaccurate. In such a framework, intramyocardial pressure is taken to be proportional to LVP (monotonically decreasing from endocardium to epicardium). If this were the case, then measured coronary inflow (pulse–amplitude) would be a function of LVP, and if this pressure was reduced to zero (vented LV), flow would cease to have a phasic systolic decrease. Clearly, the existence of a phasic coronary flow when LVP $\approx$ 0 is proof in itself that the radial wall–stress alone can not account for the extravascular traction and retraction forces on the intramural vasculature. The energy source for the mechanical modulation is in the myocardium in the form of muscle fiber generated stress, manifested as intramyocardial interstitial pressure. The LVP is merely one (endocardial) boundary condition (see below).

To examine the mechanical coupling function of the myocardium to the imbedded circulation, coronary blood flow (CBF) – perfusion pressure (CPP) relations were studied in LV–unloaded (LVP $\leq$ 0) (Table 1), *beating* and *arrested* hearts [13]. Mean CBF–CPP relation was linear (r = 0.91 to 0.99) in both cases. The slope (average ± SD) of CBF–CPP did not change ($p>0.6$) with arrest. The elevated intramyocardial tissue pressure (IMP) induced by the high interstitial edema of K–H perfusion in the *arrested* hearts, resulted in a similar ($p>0.1$) mean–IMP, generated in the *beating* state; concurrent with an insignificant slope change ($p>0.1$) in mean IMP–CPP relation. Zero–flow (Z_f) – pressures (CPP @ Z_f and IMP @ Z_f) were minimally ($p>0.25$) affected by cardiac arrest.

Under these experimental conditions, similar flow–pressure responses in beating and arrested hearts reveal the dominant role of myocardial forces, manifested and magnified by the interstitial edema or generated by muscular contraction.

Table 1. Comparison of beating and arrested hearts.

	CBF vs CPP			IMP vs CPP		
	Slope	CPP@Z_f	r	Slope	IMP@Z_f	r
Beating	1.5 ± 0.3	3.9 ± 2.9	0.96	0.5 ± 0.1	6.3 ± 2.7	0.95
Arrested	1.4 ± 0.3	4.0 ± 3.9	0.94	0.4 ± 0.1	4.6 ± 3.4	0.92

To study the influence of the extravascular (interstitial) compartment, a hyper–osmolar stimulus (Dextran) was transiently infused. As seen in Fig. 2, the dramatic increase in flow and a concomitant decrease in IMP suggests that the intravascular compartment volume is increased, i.e. actively *retracted* into the interstitial space by collagen attachments; evidenced by a drop in CPP (decrease in microvascular resistance) and 50% increase in CBF.

Additional supporting evidence of this phenomenon is revealed in Fig. 3. A transient cardiac arrest with a calcium channel antagonist (LV–decompressed, LVP = 0) attenuated both phasic–flow amplitude and diastolic level, demonstrating a primary coupling between intramyocardial tissue pressure and intravascular response. In this study, despite the constancy of the coronary perfusion pressure, a phasic component of IMP is transduced across the vessel wall, superimposed on the CPP measurement.

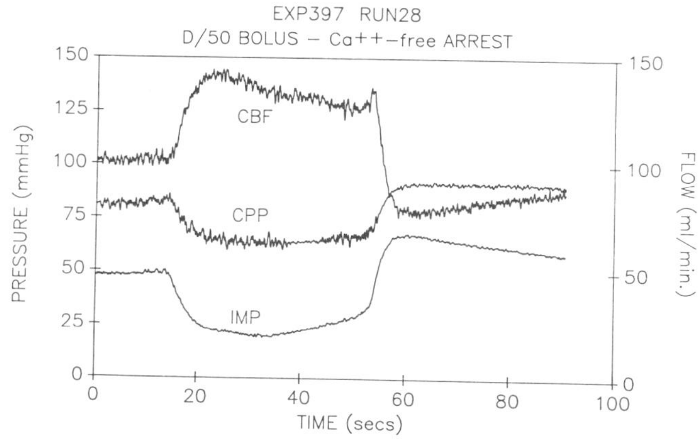

Figure 2. Effect of Osmotic Pressure Transient (50 mOsm): time–course of changes in perfusion pressure (CPP), Intramyocardial pressure (IMP) and coronary blood flow (CBF). The profound changes seen in CBF are direct reaction to changes in IMP.

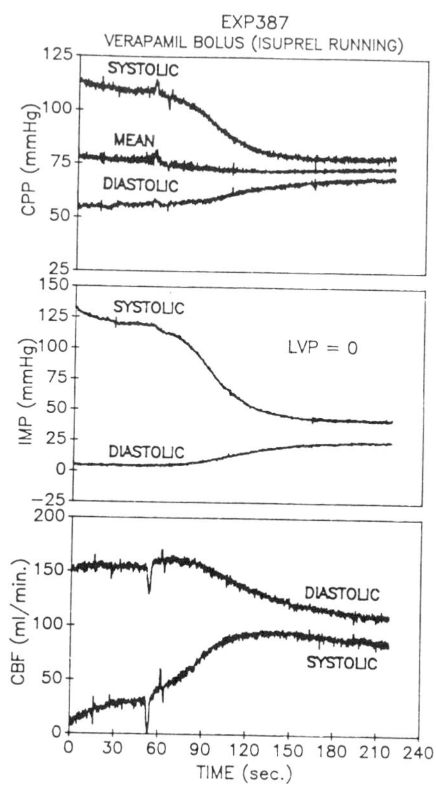

Figure 3. Transient cardiac arrest with Verapamil (LVP≈0). Note the prominent intramyocardial pressure (IMP) dependent response of the coronary blood flow–CBF (i.e. diastolic level, systolic inhibition, pulse amplitude). Despite the constancy of coronary perfusion pressure (CPP–80 mmHg.) a phasic component of IMP is transduced (superimposed) on the mean–CPP.

The two extremes of the intramyocardial tissue boundary conditions (passive arrest–systolic contracture) are best described in Fig. 4, where a pronounced rise in IMP (30 to 80 mmHg) gives rise to a striking reduction in flow (125 to 50 ml/min), thus substantiating the dominance of IMP in mechanically modulating CBF.

Coronary flow modulation depends on passive stresses exerted on the microcirculation by its surrounding environment. In particular (see Fig. 5), the extravascular matrix of collagen struts and weave has been proposed to maintain vascular patency when extravascular pressure exceeds intravascular. The loss of collagen attachments (lysis with DTNB) caused a striking reduction in CBF (mean/pulse) and markedly elevated diastolic–IMP (see Table 2). Scanning Electron Microscopy studies revealed degradation of the extracellular collagen matrix and an enlarged interstitial compartment [14].

Mechanically, collagen fibers can support a tensile stress but not a compressive stress. Consequently, increasing size of extravascular space should have differential effects in the presence or absence of the collagen matrix. In the former case, tensile stress in collagen fibers will be increased and vascular patency will be maintained despite the

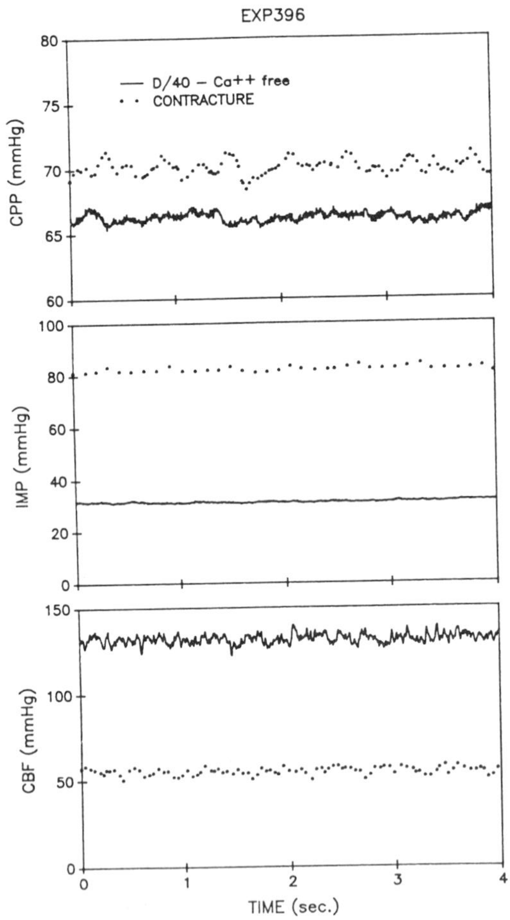

Figure 4. Response to a hyperosmolar (passive, Ca^{++}free) arrest and $BaCl_2$ induced (active arrest) contracture (LVP≈0, maximally dilated flow–CBF). Note the parallel changes in CBF and IMP. Similar response was observed with Ryanodine ("systolic–tetanus") arrest.

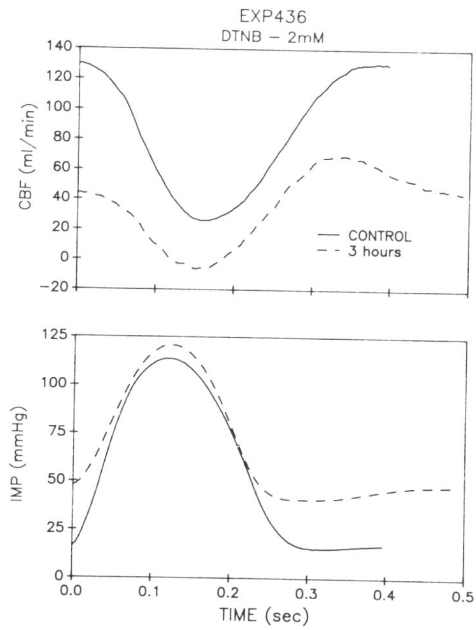

Figure 5. Acute dissolution of extravascular collagen (2 mM DTNB 3 hr infusion) resulted in an increased extravascular pressure and a significant inhibition of coronary flow amplitude; pulse excursion (max/min) was drastically altered.

increase in extravascular pressure accompanying an increased extravascular space. In the later case—i.e. following the acute dissolution of extravascular collagen (2 mM 5,5'–Dithio(2–Nitrobenzoic acid (DTNB) 2 hr infusion)—the increased extravascular pressure (diastolic from 15 to 40 mmHg) resulted in a significant inhibition of coronary flow by compressing the vascular space and hence increasing coronary resistance: change in mean value flow from 82 to 36 ml/min; pulse amplitude excursion (max./min.) was drastically altered (131/25 ml/min to 70/−6 ml/min). Compared to 2–hr. control perfusion, the heart was severely dilated; myocardial edema was present; water content increased from 79% to 83%.

Table 2. Effect of collagen lysis on flow parameters.

	$PEAK_d$	MIN_s	$AVRG_i$	RES	IMP_d
CONTROL	132 ± 12	21 ± 15	77 ± 11	1.1 ± 11	13 ± 5
DTNB	66 ± 20	3 ± 11	35 ± 11	2.3 ± 11	31 ± 11
P–value	< 0.001	< 0.03	< 0.001	< 0.001	< 0.001

$PEAK_d$ – Peak Diastolic Value (ml/min); MIN_s – Systolic Minimum (ml/min); $AVRG_i$ – Integrated Average (ml/min); RES – Flow Resistance (mmHg x min/ml); IMP_d – Intramyocardial Tissue Pressure (diastolic–mmHg).

Boundary Conditions Around Intramyocardial Vessels

The persistent pulsatile coronary flow in the decompressed heart (LVP = 0) accompanying phasic IMP, and the pulseless inflow into a region that is made akinetic (IMP is minimal) is evidence—albeit indirect—that the major determinant of the stress field surrounding the coronary circulation is manifested by the measured intramyocardial tissue pressure (IMP). When IMP was recorded in a dyskinetic region, a negative IMP component was noted, indicating that the interstitial space is actively expanded by the neighboring contracting muscle fibers. In addition, when interstitial edema is experimentally induced, the resulting elevated IMP is attended by a decrease in flow, providing supporting evidence that the transduction of this "stress–like" attribute is also revealing of the degree of structural dissociation in the extracellular matrix.

Ideally, it may be important to know the immediate extravascular–pressure surrounding a specific part of the vasculature. The IMP measurement technique as used here represents an index of the extravascular stress environment, which may or may not be quantitatively precise. The IMP measurement embodies a regional *spatial* average of a three–dimensional stress field. The methodological means for measuring direction–dependent solid stresses around a particular vessel are not currently available and would be prohibitively difficult to attain.

CONCLUSION

Contraction of the heart muscle exerts a constraining effect on the imbedded coronary microcirculation. This influence was shown to persist in the passive myocardium when a controlled deformation is imposed. Systolic and diastolic flow impediment is strongly influenced by passive and active properties of the muscle surrounding the coronary vasculature. The extravascular matrix provides mechanical coupling and a stress bearing function ("scaffolding effect") for muscle bundles and imbedded microvasculature. Selective remodeling of the extracellular collagen–matrix and partial uncoupling of the intramyocardial structure(s) causes profound functional alterations in the coronary circulation and interstitial compartment fluid–dynamics. Mechanical impediment to coronary inflow resides in the muscle fiber–interstitium–microvessel interface, functioning independently of the generated chamber pressure conditions.

By exploring systematically the spectrum (beating—isobaric/isovolumic; arrested—systolic/diastolic) of intramyocardial mechanical modulation states, an assessment of what constitutes mechanical regulation is made more evident. The systolic stiffening and/ or deformation and diastolic relaxation (stretching) effects of the myocardium were shown to be related to the coronary flow dynamics without invoking a unique, causal relationship between ventricular chamber pressure and intramyocardial stress–field distribution. An underlying theoretical/conceptual construct, supported by experimental observations, emphasizes the coupling of extravascular pressure to changes in microvascular resistive and capacitative properties. The dynamic interplay between microvascular distensibility (volume) and resultant resistance in response to extravascular changes, be they interstitial, connective tissue (collagen) dependent or intramyocardial tissue stress in origin underscore the tight coupling of the intravascular and extravascular compartments. The analysis of intramyocardial mechanical milieu in terms of solid elastic theory stresses can be misleading. Lumenal narrowing and patency of the coronary resistance vessels depend, in part, on the supporting (tethering) structure of the myocardium and interstitial fluid (hydraulic skeleton) matrix. The notion that the "extravascular–boundary" conditions remain constant during changes in arterial or venous pressure must be reexamined.

DISCUSSION

Dr. Y. Lanir: You state that intermyocardial pressure is primarily dependent on perfusion pressure. Is it independent of chamber pressure, so that the chamber pressure has no effect on it?

Dr. J.Y. Kresh: Very little effect. The modulation of the chamber pressure, in the rabbit heart, has very little effect on the measurement of intramyocardial pressure, in the location where it was measured, which is midwall.

Dr. Y. Lanir: I find it hard to reconcile this with mechanics because at the endocardium one must have a balance of forces between chamber pressure on one hand and intramyocardial pressure and solid fibers stress on the other.

Dr. J.Y. Kresh: That is right. If you look at this particular extraordinary state, something else has to take place once the intraventricular restraining boundary disappears, such as magnified wall deformation. The net effect on intramyocardial pressure may be that the modulation by LV pressure can not be measured, but it is not because there is no relationship, other enhanced deformational forces mask and/or compensate for it. The relationship would have been observed if one could maintain similar deformations or similar regional strains.

Dr. Y. Lanir: Can you suggest any mechanism by which myocyte contraction would affect intramyocardial pressure?

Dr. J.Y. Kresh: Essentially, you have to start with the assumption that the myocyte generates an intracellular pressure (the measurements were made in a barnacle muscle). This transmural pressure is transduced across the membrane (sarcolemma); if you assemble a number of these changes, concurrently, it would result in what we measure as intramyocardial tissue pressure, in some global way.

Dr. Y. Lanir: Say you have an isometric condition, and the myocyte does not change its volume..

Dr. J.Y. Kresh: Then you will not observe an intramyocyte (intracellular) pressure. Now you will ask how we observe intramyocardial pressure changes in the isovolumic contraction?

Dr. Y. Lanir: Lets put it more sharply – isometric contraction.

Dr. J.Y. Kresh: The heart muscle imposes an internal load to shortening. The regional contraction is never truly isometric under isovolumic global conditions. When restricted, the muscle undergoes isometric contractions, no changes in intramyocardial or intramyocyte pressure were observed. In a barnacle muscle, when shortening was not allowed to take place, no visible changes in intramyocyte pressure could be detected. One cannot experimentally (whole heart) create true isometric contraction because of the ongoing rearrangement within the muscle fibers. In affect an internal load persists, the myocytes are moving past each other, perhaps less than they would have with an isobaric or a "unloaded" contraction. There is no true state of isometric contraction in the myofibrils.

Dr. N. Westerhof: You are not perfusing during the heart beat with a constant perfusion pressure; it oscillates. Do you not know that no capacitance effect plays a role. Because if your perfusion pressure varies, then your epicardial vessels may empty and fill and that may give an apparent oscillation in coronary flow which has nothing to do with what happens in the periphery. You might fool yourself because you will find some changes but they will only be there because of the changes in the perfusion pressure.

A more or less related question: you give barium contracture and you see flow decrease. How do you know it is not the smooth muscle tone that changes, i.e. that the vessels get a smaller lumen?

Dr. J.Y. Kresh: When the heart was arrested with Verapamil we observed the same effect, the barium contracture (systolic arrest) was not a unique observation. About the pulsation/modulation: certainly, in the beating heart, one cannot separate–out or exclude the pulsatile component of flow. But if you look at the morphology of the coronary perfusion pressure modulation it resembles the time–derivative of the intramyocardial pressure. The transduction of the intramyocardial pressure is inherent to the intravascular pressure. There is no means of excluding it. One can regulate it upstream but not intramurally, it must persist. The mechanism of the intramyocardial pump dictates it so. You cannot get rid of it. That is simply not doable.

Dr. N. Westerhof: How do you know that the vessels do not change diameter?

Dr. J.Y. Kresh: I do not know that. The one thing we know is that we imposed maximum vasodilation with adenosine infusion, what may have resulted is a contest between apposing vasoactive forces: (micro)vascular contraction and vascular dilatation. I would like to think that these vessels were maximally dilated. Therefore, what we observed was due to the changes imposed by the external (extravascular) environment.

Dr. J. Janicki: In your preparation, it seems that you are "stacking the deck" in favor of your hypothesis. You effectively get rid of all autoregulation in the coronary bed and you have tremendous edema. Both of these events would favor an interaction between pressure in the interstitium and in the chamber and its effect on coronary flow. Would you expect to see this tight coupling in the normal heart?

Dr. J.Y. Kresh: All of the canine experiments were *in vivo* blood perfused studies. The observations are similar. The isolated hearts were perfused with Fluosol (a perfluorochemical emulsion), Krebs–Henseleit and rabbit donor blood. The magnitude of the transcapillary leakage is expected to be different, but surprisingly, the directional changes were identical in a blood–perfused rabbit isolated heart, in a Fluosol perfused rabbit heart and in all of the canine experiments.

As an aside, in the open–heart patient undergoing cardiopulmonary bypass we also measured intramyocardial tissue pressure along with "coronary" flow in the saphenous vein graft, the observation were essentially same. Changes in myocardial tissue pressure (increase) were noted in the patients with prolonged cardioplegic arrest, resulting from the overt tissue edema. Many of the same features were noted, it is a question of magnitude. In short, you are right –Fluosol/Krebs perfusate is extremely leaky; we used it to our advantage, stacking the cards as you say, to amplify this mechanism. I do not mean to suggest that the magnitudes are necessarily the same, the mech–anism –interaction of tissue pressure and coronary flow is tightly coupled under these conditions.

Dr. J. Janicki: Wouldn't autoregulation tend to override this effect?

Dr. J.Y. Kresh: Yes, it will. The purpose was to separate the mechanical effects from the metabolic effects. The premise for these experiments was to look at the mechanical boundary conditions and the intramyocardial structural environment; how it effects coronary perfusion. This is an ongoing argument: what are the physical determinants of coronary flow? Is the function and structure cooperative in the outcome?

REFERENCES

1. Spaan JAE, Breuls NPW, Laird JD. Diastolic–systolic flow differences are caused by intramyocardial pump action in the anaesthetized dog. *Circ Res* 1981; 49: 584–593.
2. Downey JM, Kirk ES. Inhibition of coronary blood flow by a vascular waterfall mechanism. *Circ Res* 1975; 36: 753–760.
3. Arts T, Reneman RS. Interaction between intramyocardial pressure (IMP) and myocardial circulation. *J Biomech Eng* 1985; 107: 51–56.

4. Hoffman JIE. The regulation of total regional coronary blood flow. In: Sideman S, Beyar R (eds) *Simulation and Control of the Cardiac System, Vol II*. Boca Raton: CRC Press, 1985, pp 133–141
5. Arts T, Reneman RS, Veenstra PC. A model of the mechanics of the left ventricle. *Ann Biomed. Eng* 1979; 7: 299–318.
6. Falsetti HL, Mates RE, Grant C, Greene DG, Bunnell JL. Left ventricular wall stress calculated from one-plane cineangiography. *Circ Res* 1970; 26: 71–83.
7. Mirsky I. Left ventricular stresses in intact human heart. *Biophys J* 1969; 9: 189–208.
8. Rabbany SY, Kresh JY, Noordergraaf A. Intramyocardial pressure: interaction of myocardial fluid pressure and fiber stress. *Am J Physiol* 1989; 257: H357–H364.
9. Caulfield JB, Borg TK. The collagen network of the heart. *Lab Invest* 1979; 40: 364–372.
10. Kresh JY, Fox M, Brockman SK, Noordergraaf A. Model based analysis of transmural vessel impedance and myocardial circulation dynamics. *Am J Physiol (Heart Circ Phys 27)* 1990; 258: H262–H276.
11. Kresh JY, Cobanoglu MA, Brockman SK. The intramyocardial pressure: a parameter of heart contractility. *J Heart Transplant* 1985; 4: 241–246.
12. Krams R, van Haelst ACTA, Sipkema P, Westerhof N. Can coronary systolic–diastolic flow differences be predicted by left ventricular pressure or time-varying intramyocardial elastance? *Basic Res Cardiol* 1989; 84: 149–159.
13. Kresh JY, Frasch HF, McVey M, Brockman SK, Noordergraaf A. Mechanical coupling of the myocardium with coronary circulation in the beating and arrested heart. *Circulation* 1991; 84(4): II–45.
14. Kresh JY, McVey M, Frasch HF, Brockman SK. Collagen–matrix dependent modulation of coronary circulation dynamics. *Circulation* 1992; 86(4): I–170.

CHAPTER 12

MYOCARDIAL MECHANICS AND CORONARY FLOW DYNAMICS

Rafael Beyar, Dan Manor and Samuel Sideman[1]

ABSTRACT

The interaction between cardiac mechanics and coronary flow is highlighted here. Left ventricular (LV) structure and geometry are related to coronary flow dynamics and used in the analysis of experimental coronary flow data. The important role of the collagen mesh in the generation of the intramyocardial pressure (IMP), the pressure in the interstitial fluid, at a wide range of loading conditions is emphasized. The calculated IMP, based on a structural model of the LV myocardium, can explain most of the observed coronary compression characteristics under a variety of loading and contractility conditions. A more general compression function, the extravascular compressive pressure (ECP), is suggested to define coronary compression and is presented here based on the dynamics of the coronary inflow under constant perfusion conditions. Coronary compression is shown to be affected by fluid transport and the bi-directional coupling of coronary hemodynamics and IMP dynamics.

INTRODUCTION

The mechanisms of interaction between myocardial function and coronary flow dynamics have been extensively investigated in numerous studies. The recorded coronary phasic flow is the outcome of complex interactions between the coronary perfusion pressure and factors associated with myocardial function, and the coronary network structure and function. The mechanisms involved in generating the phasic flow dynamics have been a subject of ongoing controversy. The waterfall [1] and the myocardial pump [2] theories are two classical concepts suggested to explain this controversy. The role of the IMP, the

---

[1]Heart System Research Center, The Julius Silver Institute, Department of Biomedical Engineering, Technion–Israel Institute of Technology, Haifa, 32000, Israel.

Interactive Phenomena in the Cardiac System, Edited by
S. Sideman and R. Beyar, Plenum Press, New York, 1993

driving force of coronary compression, has also been subject of controversy. An analysis of the dynamics of the coronary flow signal, based on an attempt to identify and integrate the major mechanisms involved in the coronary flow, is obviously needed.

THE PHASIC CORONARY FLOW SIGNAL

The phasic coronary flow signal results from the interaction of input conditions (aortic and right atrial pressures), the compressive function of the contracting myocardium and the properties of the coronary vascular bed. An example of a coronary flow signal, measured in our laboratory in an open chest anaesthetized dog with a transonic flowmeter, is given in Fig. 1. As also shown by Kowenhoven et al. [3], the coronary flow has a typical early-systolic flow decrease, with a recognizable early negative peak which occurs simultaneously with the build up of the LV pressure. Following this stage, there is a mid-systolic flow increase which is followed by a late-systolic flow decrease. A rapid rise in the coronary flow to diastolic levels occurs as the ventricular pressure relaxes. The diastolic flow then declines simultaneously with the decline in the aortic pressure.

The phasic coronary signal can be used to derive information about the mechanisms that may be involved in the interaction between the contracting myocardium and the coronary flow. The characterization and modulation of the phasic nature of the coronary arterial flow were obtained from the dynamic flow measurements at the level of the mid LAD in a series of 18 open chest dogs [4]. The parameters in Fig. 1 were related to the aortic and LV pressure waves, measured by Millar transducers, at steady state baseline conditions for all dogs. As summarized in Table 1, the normalized mid-systolic flow increase, F_{ms}/Q_m, correlates with both the aortic pressure amplitude and the aortic pressure derivative. The late systolic flow decrease, F_{ls}, correlates with the aortic pressure negative derivative. The relaxation flow increase rate correlates inversely with the LV cavity pressure relaxation time. In contrast, no correlation was found between the LV pressure derivative and the initial negative flow slope, neither was there a correlation with the early systolic normalized negative peak, F_{es}/Q_m.

While direct relationship between the flow at early systole with the LVP derivative could not be demonstrated, some relationship between relaxation time and flow increase

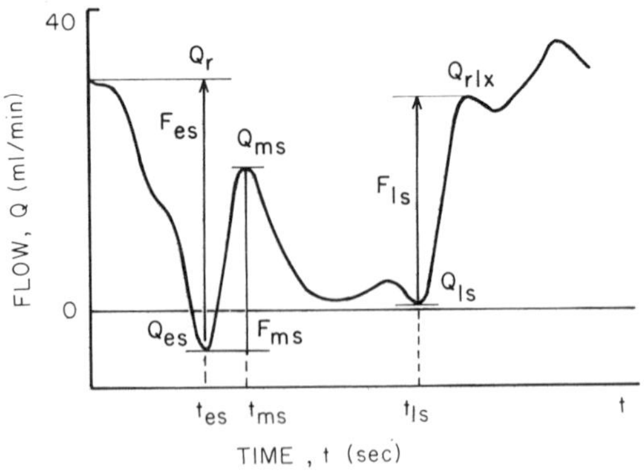

Figure 1. Mid-left anterior descending coronary phasic flow. F_{es}– early systolic flow decrease; F_{ms}– mid systolic flow increase; F_{ls}– late systolic flow increase. The corresponding absolute flow levels are denoted by Q and the time points by t.

Table 1. Correlation of coronary flow variables with ventricular and aortic pressure variables. (See Fig. 1 for notation.)

	Correlates With	Does Not Correlate With
$-dF/dt$		dLVP/dt
F_{es}/Q_m		IVC duration, dLVP/dt, LVPmax
F_{ms}/Q_m	amp(P_{ao}), dP_{ao}/dt	
F_{ls}/Q_m	P_{ao} decrease to EE$-dP_{ao}/dt$	
$+dF/dt$	I/RT$-$dPLV/dt	

IVC – isovolumic contraction; EE – end ejection; RT – relaxation time.

rate could be demonstrated in late–systole. Mid–systolic flow events were more consistently related to the aortic pressure waveform.

An analog model, Fig. 2, was used to explain the phasic coronary flow. A sharp decrease in coronary flow was obtained during the isovolumic relaxation phase; this decrease was affected by the rate of pressure increase. No relationship between the slope of the flow decrease to the LV pressure was noted under the experimental steady state conditions employed in this study [4], though this relationship was demonstrated by others [3]. The sharp increase in the aortic pressure upon opening the aortic valve reverses the coronary flow decrease and sets the early systolic negative peak. The mid–systolic flow increase is thereafter attributed to the aortic pressure increase, charging the epicardial and intramyocardial arterial capacitance. The decrease in coronary flow following the mid–systolic peak is similarly related to the fall in aortic pressure and the consequent discharge of the intramyocardial capacitance, which is continuously being squeezed by the contracting LV. The relaxation of the myocardium is immediately followed by a sharp increase in coronary flow, associated with recharging the intramyocardial compliance due to the rapidly falling vascular transmural pressure.

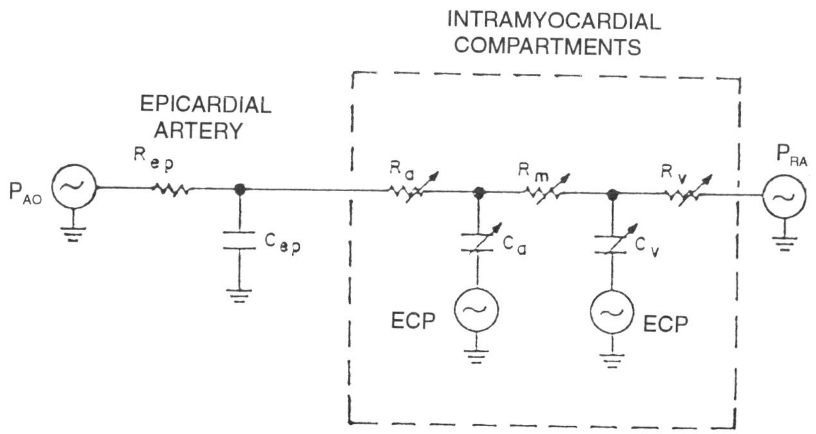

Figure 2. Perfusion line model—electrical representation of the coronary circulation. P_{ao} – perfusion pressure; R_{ep}, C_{ep} – epicardial artery resistance and compliance; R_a, C_a – arterial intramyocardial resistance and compliance; R_m – microcirculatory resistance; R_v, C_v – venous intramyocardial resistance and compliance; ECP – extravascular compressive pressure.

CORONARY FLOW DYNAMICS AND THE EXTRAVASCULAR COMPRESSIVE PRESSURE (ECP)

The magnitude of coronary compression was stipulated by Krams et al. [5] from the coronary flow signal under a variety of loading and contractility conditions. The oscillatory flow amplitude under *constant perfusion pressure* was used as an index of the magnitude of the coronary compression. Indeed, under such conditions, the changes in the coronary inflow reflect the external pressure acting on the intramyocardial circulation. This approach is used here to calculate the ECP that acts on the intramyocardial circulation, using the perfusion line model presented in Fig. 2. Employing parameter estimation techniques, the ECP function is determined so as to yield flow characteristics which fit the measured dynamic coronary flow under constant perfusion pressure. This analysis is based on a series of dogs [6] subjected to maximum vasodilatation and constant perfusion pressure. The normalized coronary flow signal is shown in Fig. 3, together with the calculated ECP for one of the dogs. Note that the normalized ECP is almost identical with the inverted normalzed coronary flow. The ECP function is compared in Fig. 4 to the LV cavity pressure and IMP functions measured by intramyocardial tip manometer. Note that the ECP function resembles the IMP more than the LVP function. The significant delay in the ECP and IMP functions, relative to the LVP relaxation, is further discussed below.

The load dependence of the ECP was also examined in these series of dogs. Load changes were caused by occluding both vena cavae, leading to acute reductions in venous return and the preload and afterload. While the ECP decreased as the LVP was reduced, the amount of reduction in ECP amplitude was less significant than the reduction in LVP; these findings are in discord to the study of Krams et al. [5] who showed the oscillatory flow amplitude in a cat's heart to be completely independent of ventricular pressure under similar conditions. It is speculated that these different results may be related to the experimental setup or the type of animal.

DEFINING THE ECP AND IMP

The intramyocardial vessels are subjected to external compression which is generated by myocardial contraction. Many factors may possibly affect an intramyocardial vessel. First, the vessels are surrounded by an interstitial fluid and the pressure in this fluid is commonly defined as the IMP. However, the hydrostatic pressure in the fluid around the

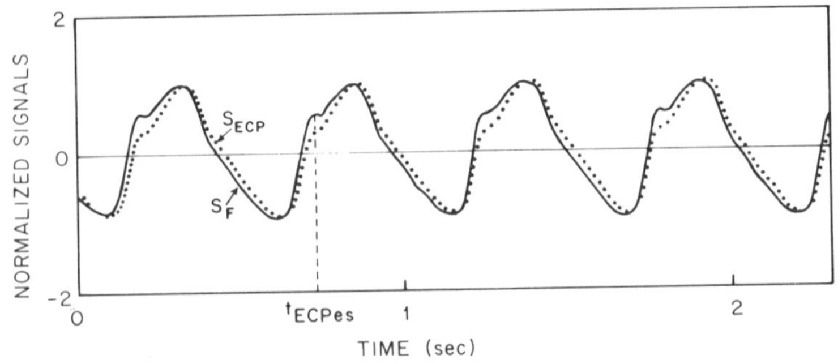

Figure 3. The calculated normalized ECP signal S_{ECP}, superimposed on the normalized epicardial flow signal S_F, under constant perfusion pressure conditions.

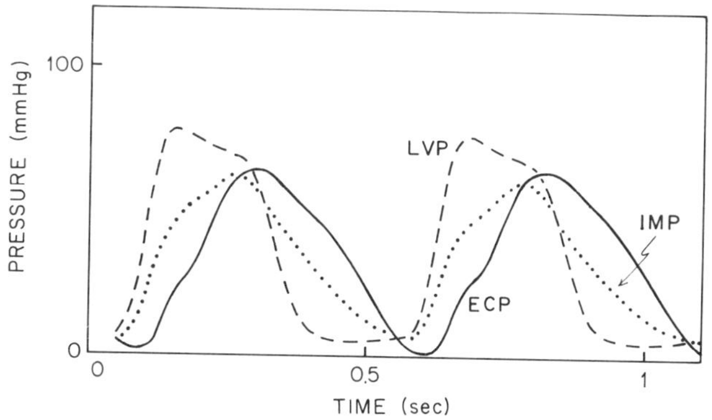

Figure 4. The calculated ECP compared to the measured (Millar micromanometer) LVP and IMP.

vessels is not the only factor effecting the compression. Attachments between collagen and muscle fibers and the blood vessels, as well as possible direct compression from adjacent contracting myocytes can modify this compression effect. Therefore, we define the ECP as the effective compressive pressure on the vessel, which changes throughout the cycle. While both the IMP and the ECP are transmural functions which change across the myocardium, it is not clear how much these functions differ quantitatively. It is conceivable that different kinds of vessels may be subjected to different ECP (even in the same location) due to differences in the local microstructure.

Our earlier model [7, 8], which accounts for the muscle fibers architecture across the LV wall, was used to calculate the coronary flow dynamics. This model was more recently modified to include the collagen fibers interconnecting the muscle fibers across the wall of the LV and to predict the flow across the myocardium, linked to a non–linear resistive capacitive coronary flow model [9]. The calculated transmural IMP results are shown in Fig. 5. When the LV preload is reduced while contractility is kept constant, the pressure in the interstitial fluid, i.e. the IMP, is almost unchanged while LV cavity pressure is reduced in proportion to the preload changes. This is due to stretching of the radial collagen fibers leading to increased fiber stresses in the radial direction with reduced afterload.

The calculations predict a dissociation between the LVP and the IMP. This is consistent with the measurements of Krams et al. [5] that have shown dissociation between coronary compression, indexed as the "oscillatory flow amplitude", and the LVP. The model also explains why the empty beating heart can generate high IMPs during myocardial contraction.

Another interesting prediction of the model which includes the radial stiffness elements is a delay in the relaxation of the IMP relative to the relaxation of the LV pressure (Fig 6). This delay is attributed to the contribution of the transverse collagen fibers which are considerably stretched due to systolic thickening until the diastolic filling of the LV. Therefore, at the isovolumic relaxation the LVP relaxes quickly while the IMP is delayed. From an energetic point of view, while most of the energy is transformed into hydraulic energy, some of the energy from the contracting myocytes is used to stretch the radial collagen fibers during active contraction. This energy contributes to the IMP and generates the ventricular restoring forces which help ventricular filling. The lower the afterload and the higher the wall thickening, the larger is the difference between the LVP and IMP during systole, the larger the restoring forces and the larger is the delay between the IMP and LVP relaxations.

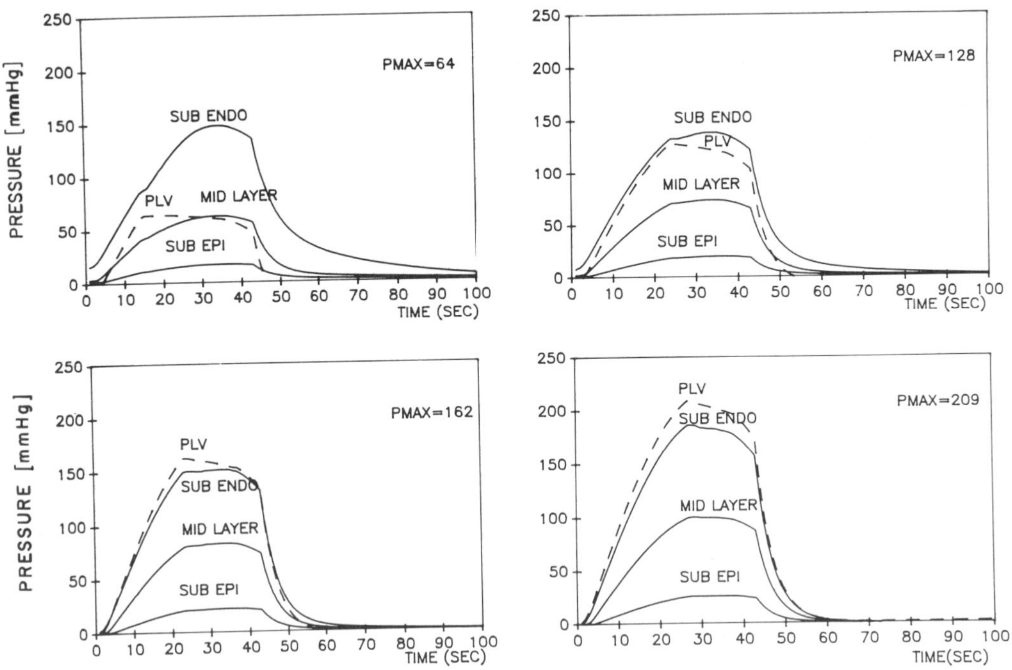

Figure 5. The IMP values predicted by the structural model for three myocardial layers in comparison to the left ventricular pressure (PLV) at four levels of preload volumes under near isovolumic conditions. The maximum LV pressure is denoted for each case.

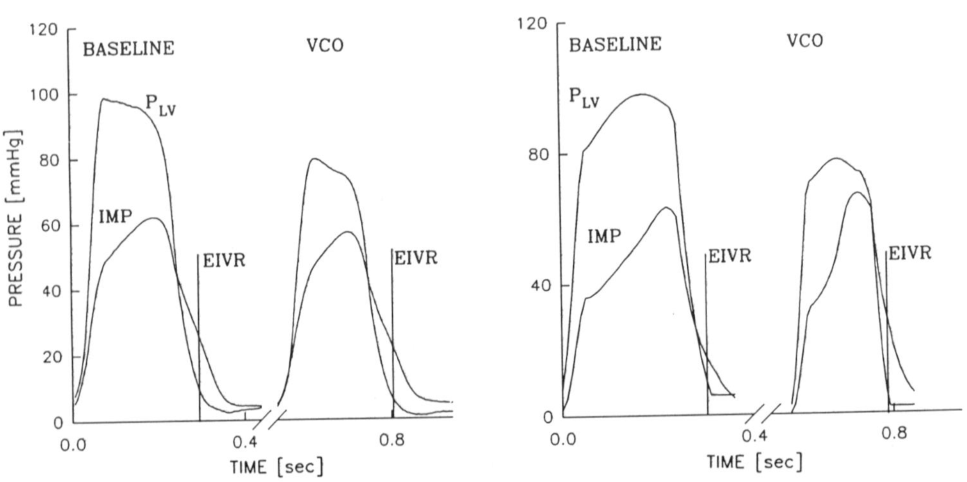

Figure 6. The predicted IMP and LVP tracings (right) vs the measured tracings (left). Note that the calculated delay in the IMP relaxation relative to LVP relaxation is similar for the model including transverse collagen fibers and the IMP measurements using a flat IMP Konigsberg disc transducer. EIVR – end of isovolumic relaxation; VCO – vena-cava occlusion.

LINKING THE ECP TO THE LV FUNCTION

The relationship between the ECP, the LVP and the radial stretching and thickening is approximated here by assuming that the net ECP is determined by two terms: 1) the LVP; and 2) a term relating the end-systolic (ES) wall thickness T_{ES} to an initial wall thickness, T_0. Thus,

$$ECP_{ES} = a\, LVP_{ES} + b\, [T_{ES} - T_o] / T_o \qquad (1)$$

where a and b are proportionality constants. Figure 7A shows the classical ES pressure–thickness relationship (ESPTR) for (1) the normal myocardium, (2) the passive myocardium, (3) the reduced contractility case. As demonstrated in Fig. 7B curve (4), the stress is built in the radial fibers steeply as they are stretched beyond their slack structure curve. This phenomenon occurs at a thickness T_o corresponding to the ES pressure P_o (or P_o' for the reduced contractility case). The radial ES thickening T_h above T_o is defined from these relationships by:

$$T_h = [P_o - P_{ES}]/E_{TES} \qquad (2)$$

where E_{TES} is the slope of the ESPTR curve. Substituting Eq. (2) into Eq. (1), the ES extravascular compression pressure is given by:

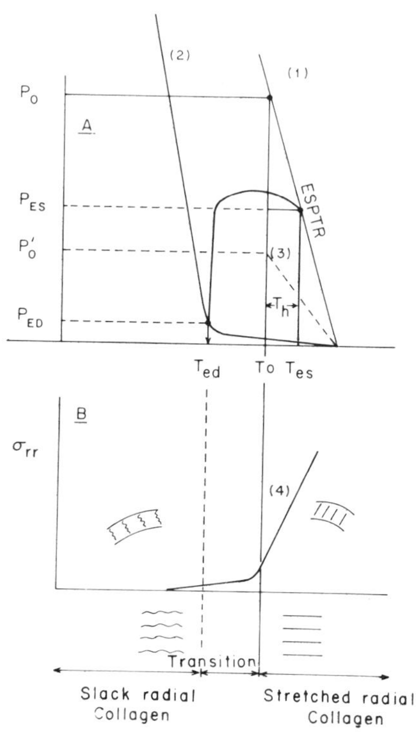

Figure 7. A: The pressure–wall thickness relationship at ES. (1) – normal LV; (2) – passive muscle; (3) – reduced contractility. **B:** The radial stress component vs thickness is shown by curve (4). T_o is the transition thickness from slack to tense collagen fibers in the radial direction. P_o is the corresponding ES pressure at an ES thickness of T_o. As shown, T_o changes linearly with the contractility, defined here based on the slope of the end-systolic pressure–thickness relationship (ESPTR).

$$ECP_{ES} = a \cdot LVP_{ES} + b\,[P_o - P_{ES}]/(E_{TES} \cdot T_o) \qquad (3)$$

Equation (3) relates the end–systolic ECP to the LV cavity pressure and to the combination of the pressure driving force and the contractility which leads to the radial stretch. Equation (3) is obviously a simplification of the real, non–linear, stress–strain relationship of the collagen elements that stretch from a slack position and approach a non–slacked position at the transition thickness T_o. However, this simplified formulation suffices at this point as it provides a clear framework for the parameters involved here, and allows to explain the reported controversial, apparently incompatible, experimental data.

In terms of Eq. (3), the experimental data [5] show that the ECP remains unchanged when LVP_{ES} is changed while E_{TES} is kept constant. Inspection of Eq. (3) reveals that under this situation $a = b / (E_{TES} \cdot T_o)$ and therefore

$$ECP_{ES} = b\,P_o/(E_{TES} \cdot T_o) \qquad (4)$$

indicating that the ECP_{ES} is constant for a constant contractility.

If, on the other hand, LVP_{ES} is changed by modulating the contractility, represented here by changing E_{TES}, both LVP_{ES} and the constant P_o change in parallel to the changes in the contractility. Since P_o, LVP_{ES} and E_{TES} change proportionally, the right hand term in Eq. (3) is constant and ECP_{ES} becomes linearly related to $a \cdot LVP_{ES}$. In this situation, the coronary compression in isovolumic contraction is proportional to the peak LVP, consistent with recent observations. It is also apparent that the right hand term in Eq. (3), which describes wall thickening, does not exist in models which do not account for the collagen related radial stiffness. For such models, Eq. (3) is expressed as $ECP_{ES} = a \cdot LVP_{ES}$, demonstrating the linear dependency of the ECP_{ES} on LVP_{ES} under all conditions.

The situation is somewhat different when regional function rather than global function is changed by, say, local paralysis by Lidocaine. Under these conditions, the cavity LVP is only slightly modified (due to blood pressure control mechanism) and therefore the first term in Eq. (2), $a \cdot LVP_{ES}$, remains practically constant. Furthermore, the artificially paralyzed region undergoes wall thinning instead of thickening in the normal myocardium, which is accompanied by the shortening of the radial elastic elements. This phenomenon leads to slack radial fibers with no significant radial stress generation in the fiber media. Consequently, only the first term of Eq. (3) is expressed and $ECP_{ES} = a \cdot LVP_{ES}$. Again, we see that under these special conditions the compression forces change linearly with the LVP_{ES}, or more generally, with LVP.

Having said all that, one still needs to explain why the systolic modulation of the coronary flow is only slightly modified, as compared to the normally functioning myocardium when Lidocaine is administered regionally, causing local muscle paralysis [11].

Assume that $P_o \approx 100$ mmHg and that $a = 0.5$. This means that for $LVP_{ES} = 100$ mmHg, the right hand term in Eq. (3) is zero. Consequently, when the second term is abolished by the Lidocaine infusion (thinning rather than thickening occurs and no radial stress is built in the radial fibers), we observe no change of the ECP and the systolic modulation of coronary flow is therefore unchanged. Suppose now that we let the ventricle contract against a decreased afterload, say 50 mmHg. Muscle paralysis which eliminates the right hand term in Eq. (3) must now reduce the coronary compression only by about 50%, from $0.5*50 + 0.5*(100 - 50) = 50$ mmHg for a functioning myocardium, to $0.5*50 = 25$ mmHg for the paralyzed myocardium. Consequently, this simple analysis suggests that while muscle paralysis at a given loading condition may result in a minimal change in systolic coronary flow modulation, it is possible that this would not be the case for different loads.

TRANSMURAL DISTRIBUTION OF FLOW BASED ON PRESSURE DEPENDENT RESISTANCE AND COMPLIANCE

Two conceptual models of the coronary circulation are the well known waterfall model developed by Downey and Kirk [1] and the intramyocardial pump model developed by Spaan [2]. These "isolated" models explain the systolic impediment in arterial flow, but only the pump model explains the systolic venous outflow. An attractive model which modifies the simplified intramyocardial pump concept and takes into account the compression of the intramyocardial compliance is the pressure dependent resistance and compliance model [9, 12–14]. This model assumes that the cross–sectional area of a vessel is a function of the local transmural pressure, i.e. the local intraluminal minus the external pressure. The vessel resistance and compliance are derived from the transmural pressure vs the cross–sectional area relationship of the artery, and are therefore modified dynamically throughout the cycle [9]. These models represent unidirectional interactions, i.e. the flow dynamics is affected by the IMP input value.

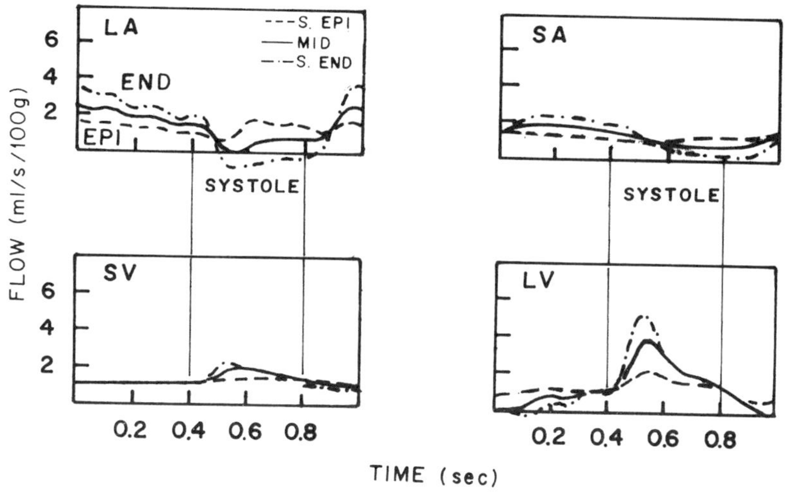

Figure 8. Flow patterns in the larger (>150 μ) and smaller (<150 μ) intramyocardial arteries and veins. L.A. – large arterieris; L.V. – large veins; S.A. – small arteries; S.V. small veins.

The transmural flow distribution in the LV wall is also of great interest [9]. Figure 8 depicts the flow distribution in a three–layered LV myocardium based on the pressure dependence of the resistance and compliance. Also shown in Fig. 9 are the cross–sectional areas and resistances of the different compartments. Note that the largest area reduction occurs at the larger (> 150 μ) intramyocardial veins, followed by the larger (>150 μ) intramyocardial arteries. The smaller vessels (<150 μ) are characterized by small area changes. Kajiya et al. [15] have developed an "endocardial microscope" capable of observing the area changes in small subendocardial vessels. They report that the arteriolar diameter in the subendocardium (117 μ) changes by 26.9% while the venular diameter (107 μ) decreased by 18.8%; this is in good agreement with the predictions of our model for the small subendocardial intramyocardial arteries and veins.

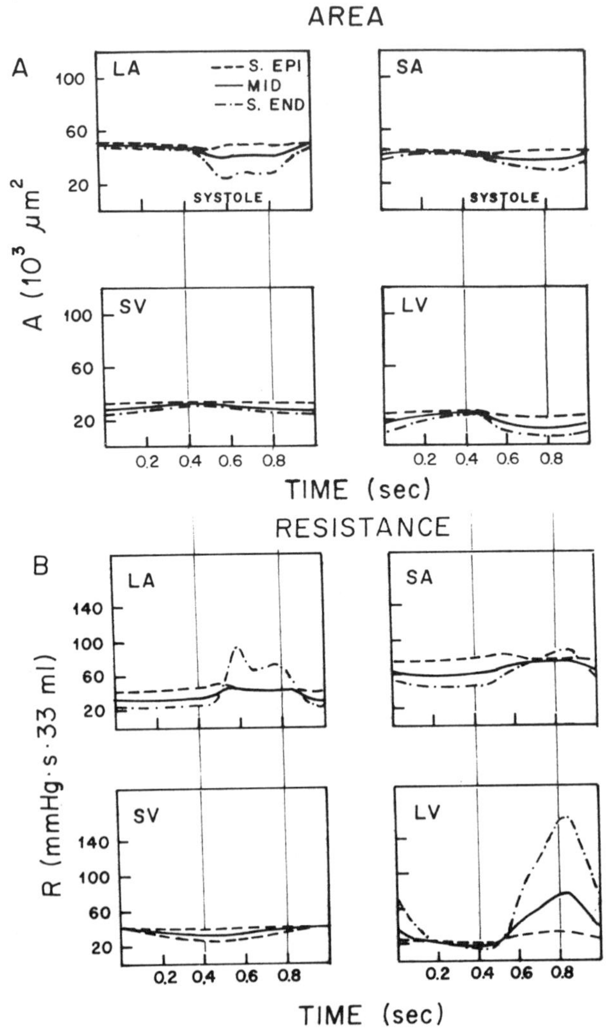

Figure 9. The corresponding changes in cross-sectional area (A) and resistance (B) for the different compartments during the cardiac cycle.

EFFECT OF INTRAMYOCARDIAL EXCAPILLARY FLUID TRANSPORT

An important factor, which has so far not been considered in the analysis of cardiac mechanics, is the intramyocardial fluid transport which both affects and is affected by the myocardial contraction. The myocardium stress–strain relationship is determined by the fibers and collagen mesh. The capillaries "leak" into the interstitial space and lymphatic flow is responsible for drainage. In addition, the pressure in the intramyocardial vasculature can, through the coronary compliance and the myocardial compliance, modify the tissue pressure. A detailed description of this model is presented in Chapter 21.

The two–directional interaction between the coronary hemodynamics and myocardial mechanics are essential to the comprehensive description of the physiological phenomena associated with coronary flow such as the Gregg effect, or the effect of coronary pressure on the myocardial function. In general, the coronary flow waveforms are affected by the IMP (or ECP) waveform by the laws of flow in elastic tubes subjected to external pressure. The coronary pressures and flows determine the fluid flux into the interstitial space, which in turn affects the fluid content of the myocardium and the IMPs throughout the cardiac cycle. The stresses in the fiber and fluid media of the heart are both determined by systolic and diastolic LV function. Bi–directional interaction between coronary pressure and myocardial function are thus manifested. The diastolic restoring forces are strongly dependent on the fluid balance in the myocardium and the coronary intravascular pressures, in addition to their dependence on muscle contractility. The local properties of the myocardium, in terms of the local (interstitial) pressure–volume relationship which may be defined as myocardial elastance, are determined by the muscle and collagen structure and properties, the instantaneous active force level, myocardial deformation, coronary pressure and fluid balance in the myocardium.

CONCLUSIONS

The dynamics of intramyocardial and epicardial coronary flows are determined by the interaction of the coronary perfusion pressure and the extravascular compressive pressure, with the coronary network which is composed of elastic tubes with a given pressure–cross–sectional geometry. The ECP is the driving force affecting the coronary circulation and is a complex function of myocardial structure and function, myocardial fluid transport and the loading conditions imposed on the heart.

Acknowledgement

This study was supported by grants from the Technion Fund for Promotion of Research, the Wolf Award, the Anna and George Ury Fund (Chicago, USA), Mr. Yochai Schneider (Las Vegas, USA), the Michael and Adelaide Kennedy–Leigh Fund (London, UK) and the numerous beautiful ladies of the Women's Division of the American Society for the Technion, NY, USA.

DISCUSSION

Dr. W. Welkowitz: I noticed that you do not have any effect of the inertance of the blood in your coronary model. Clearly, the blood has inertance. Why was this not included? We have studied a full coronary model with branches with inertance in all the sections as well as capacitance and resistance. We found that by feeding in the appropriate pressure from the ascending aorta, one also can duplicate the waveforms of the coronary flow. Thus, the fact that the waveforms are duplicated does not by itself validate a model, since there are a number of ways in which one can obtain the waveforms.

Dr. R. Beyar: I agree that inertia, especially in large coronary arteries, may have some effect. But it is our feeling, and the feeling of some other investigators, that these effects are not very large. The exact magnitude of these effects may obviously depend on the heart rate, on the rate of changes of dynamic events there, etc. We have not yet performed a study to determine these possible effects.

Dr. R. Mates: A comment on Dr. Welkowitz's remark. We tried, in a much simpler model shown in Chapter 14, to include inertial effects and they do not seem to have much of an effect. The question I have for Dr. Beyar is, can you explain a little bit more the difference between the IMP and the ECP in your model?

Dr. R. Beyar: We define the IMP as the hydrostatic pressure in the interstitial space, which, by definition is equal in all directions. It might be that this pressure is the only factor that effects the coronary vessels. But if the coronary vessel is attached to fibers in a muscle layer, this may affect what the coronary vessels "feel." So we define the ECP as the sum of the IMP and these other possible effects. The other effects can be collagen attachments, and direction and interaction between vessels and muscle cells, which I am not sure exist. All of the effects are lumped together in this ECP concept, the magnitude of which is still unclear.

REFERENCES

1. Downey JM, Kirk ES. Inhibition of coronary blood flow by vascular waterfall mechanism. *Circ Res* 1985; 36: 753–760.
2. Spaan JAE, Breuls NPW, Laird JD. Diastolic systolic coronary flow differences are caused by intramyocardial pump action in the un–anesthetized dog. *Circ Res* 1981; 49: 584–593.
3. Kouwenhoven E, Vergrossen I, Han Y, and Spaan JAE. Retrograde coronary flow is limited by time varying elastance. *Am J Physiol* (*Heart and Circ Physiol* 32) 1992; 263: H484–H490.
4. Manor D, Sideman S, Shofti R and Beyar R. Characterization and modulation of the phasic nature of the coronary arterial flow. Submitted, 1992.
5. Krams K, Sipkema P, Zegers J, Westerhof N. Contractility is the main determinant of coronary systolic flow impediment. *Am J Physiol (Heart Circ Physiol)* 1989; 26: H1936–H1944.
6. Manor D, Beyar R, Shofti R, Sideman S. Relating extravascular compressive pressure dynamics to the epicardial arterial coronary flow wave at constant perfusion pressures. *D.Sc. Thesis*, Technion, 1993.
7. Beyar R, Sideman S. A computer study of left ventricular performance based on fiber structure, sarcomere dynamics, and transmural electrical propagation velocity. *Circ Res* 1984; 55: 358–375.
8. Beyar R, Sideman S. Time dependent coronary blood flow distribution in the left ventricular wall. *Am J Physiol* (*Heart and Circ Physiol* 21) 1987; 252: H417–H433.
9. Beyar R, Caminker R, Manor D and Sideman S. Coronary flow patterns in normal and ischemic hearts: transmyocardial and artery to vein distribution. *Annals Biomed Eng* 1993; in press.
11. Doucette JW, Goto M, Flynn AE, Husseini WK, Hoffman JIE. Effect of left ventricular pressure and myocardial contraction on coronary flow (abstract). *Circulation* 1990; 82: Supp III, III–379.
12. Bruinsima P, Arts T, Dankelman J, Spaan JAE. Model of the coronary circulation based on pressure dependence of the coronary resistance and compliance. *Basic Res Cardiol* 1988; 83: 510–524.
13. Kresh JY, Fox M, Brockman SK, Noordergraaf. A Model–based analysis of transmural vessel impedance and myocardial circulation dynamics. *Am J Physiol* 1990; 258: H262–H276
14. Beyar R, Caminker R, Manor D, Ben Ari R, Sideman S. On the mechanism of transmural myocardial compression and perfusion. In: Sideman S, Beyar R, Kléber A (eds) *Cardiac Electrophysiology, Circulation and Transport.* Kluwer Academic Publ, Boston, 1991, pp 245–258.
15. Kajiya F, Goto M, Yada T, Ogasawara Y, Kimura A, Hiramasatu O, Tsujioka K. How does myocardial contraction affect intramyocardial microcirculation (abstract). *Heart and Vessels*, Supp 1992; 8: 129.

CHAPTER 13

Modeling of Coronary Capillary Flow

Gadi Fibich[1*], Yoram Lanir,[2] Nadav Liron,[1] and Mark Abovsky[2]

ABSTRACT

The coronary capillary flow is analyzed theoretically based on the laws of continuum mechanics. The capillary is considered as a long, elastic and permeable vessel loaded externally by tissue pressure. It is subjected to periodic length changes, together with adjacent myocytes. Capillary flow is driven by arteriolar–venular pressure differences. Ultrafiltration due to transmural hydrostatic and osmotic pressure gradients is included in the model. Consideration of mass conservation leads to a nonlinear flow equation. The results show that under stable physiological conditions ultrafiltration is of minor importance. The analysis of untethered capillaries predicts regional differences in capillary flow. In all regions, but more so in the subendocardium, capillaries undergo significant periodic volume changes, giving rise to intramyocardial pumping. In the deeper layers, capillary wall elasticity is of major importance. In the subepicardium, the possible capillary length-changes with adjacent myocytes tend to enhance systolic/diastolic volume differences. The predicted patterns of the overall capillary flow in the left ventricular (LV) wall are in good qualitative agreement with measured coronary phasic flow, showing systolic retrograde arterial inflow, accelerated venal outflow, and diastolic rapid filling accompanied by venal retrograde flow. Analysis of the flow in tethered capillary shows significant effect of the collagen attachments between the surrounding myocytes and the capillary wall. The advantage of the continuum analysis is demonstrated in the present study by its ability to elucidate and evaluate the role of flow controlling mechanisms and their complex interactions.

INTRODUCTION

Coronary circulation has several unique features. Amongst them are the phasic nature of the arterial inflow and of the venous return [1]; the occurrence of retrograde flow;

[1]Department of Mathematics and [2]Department of Biomedical Engineering, Technion–Israel Institute of Technology, Haifa 32000, Israel; *Current address: Courant Institute, New York University, New York, NY, 10012, USA.

Interactive Phenomena in the Cardiac System, Edited by
S. Sideman and R. Beyar, Plenum Press, New York, 1993

pronounced regional perfusion differences; the existence of a significant vascular compliance [2]; the vanishing of flow at pressure lower than the zero–flow pressure and the considerable autoregulatory capacity demonstrated by the coronary reserve [3]. Under constant autoregulation, the coronary flow is controlled by several passive mechanisms. Their nature and significance is not yet sufficiently clear.

The present study focuses attention on the capillary level, since capillaries occupy a major portion of the microvasculature volume [4] and approximately 30% of the total coronary volume, the largest fraction for a single compartment [5]. Thus, the characteristics of the capillary flow are expected to make a substantial contribution to the overall flow. The goals of the study are: Account for the observed features of the coronary flow by distributive simulation based on the laws of continuum mechanics; evaluate the relative significance of the mechanisms that control the flow; identify characteristic parameters of the flow and verify the model by contrasting it with available data. Note that the modeling process presented here can be used quite similarly for other coronary microvessels, using the appropriate structural and material data.

There are very few distributive models for the coronary system. Dinnar [6] studied the effect of varying tissue pressure and ultrafiltration in a rigid capillary. Schmid–Schonbein et al. [7] modeled the blood flow in a skeletal muscle capillary, taking into account the viscoelastic properties of the capillaries. Chadwick et al. [8] developed a model for the entire coronary microcirculation which began as a distributive model, by applying mechanical laws for the vessels and fluid. These were then reduced to a lumped model by a process of spatial averaging.

THE PHYSIOLOGICAL MODEL

Consider first an untethered capillary. The capillary system is shown in Fig. 1. It is a long circular vessel [9] with an elastic permeable wall. The capillary radius is determined by the dynamic transmural pressure difference between the internal blood and the external tissue. The flow is driven by the difference between the arterial supply pressure (P_A) and its venal outlet counterpart (P_V) at the capillary ends. Fluid filtrates through the capillary wall due to hydrostatic and osmotic transmural pressure gradients.

A mechanism that did not receive attention in previous models is the possible periodic length change of a coronary capillary. A coronary capillary runs parallel to the

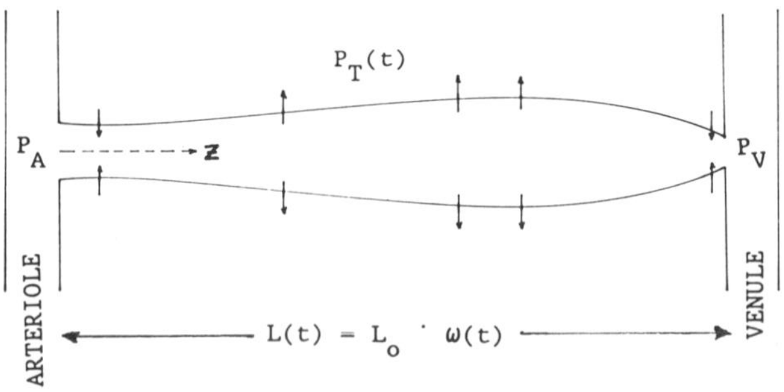

Figure 1. A scheme of the capillary model. The arterial and venular pressure P_A and P_V are boundary conditions acting at the capillary ends. The tissue pressure P_T and internal pressure P are acting on the capillary wall, which is elastic and permeable. The capillary length changes with time in accordance with the myocyte contraction.

adjacent myocytes [10] to which it is connected by a network of stiff and short collagen struts [11]. These observations lead intuitively to the possibility that the capillary changes its length in accordance with the neighboring myocytes to which it is connected. Such length–changes have been reported in skeletal muscle [12], where it was found that in the extensor digitorum muscle of a rat lengthening of the muscle fibers resulted in stretching the capillaries and in a reduction of their tortuosity. In the myocardium, Poole et al. [13] found that capillary length increases with increasing sarcomere length above 1.9 μm and decreases at short fiber lengths. This decrease in length is accompanied by little change in capillary tortuosity. Tortuosity was found to have only a small effect on the resistance to flow [14]. The present study is focused on the effects of the capillary length–changes by stretch. To study the effect of this hypothesized dynamic length change of coronary capillaries, we consider two extreme cases: capillary length–changes in accordance with neighboring muscle fibers, and a fixed capillary length.

THE ANALYTICAL MODEL

Basic Assumptions

The model of the flow in an untethered coronary capillary is based on the following assumptions [17]:

a. The level of autoregulation is constant.
b. The flow in a single capillary is radially symmetric and the capillary maintains a circular cross–section.
c. Blood is incompressible and homogeneous. Local effects due to interactions of blood cells with the capillary wall are not considered. This is a reasonable approximation for a long capillary (500–1000 μm [9]), since the local effects can be regarded as small deviations from an otherwise smooth flow pattern.
d. The capillary discharge is related to the pressure gradient by a Poiseuille-like equation with an apparent viscosity μ_{apar} of 5 cp [15]. Hence

$$Q = -\frac{\pi a^4}{8\mu_{apar}}\left(\frac{dP}{dz}\right) \tag{1}$$

where $a = a(z,t)$ is the dynamically varying radius, z is the axial coordinate, t, denotes time, and dP/dz is the pressure gradient inside the capillary.
e. The time dependent external tissue pressure (P_T) is constant along each capillary but varies transmurally in the LV wall. This follows from the observation that capillaries run along myocytes which are parallel to the endocardial and epicardial surfaces, while the tissue pressure varies normal to these surfaces.
f. Capillary distensibility is governed by [16]

$$\Delta P = \alpha E \tag{2}$$

where $\Delta P = P(z,t) - P_T(t)$ is the local instantaneous transmural pressure difference, i.e. the difference between the hydrostatic pressure in the capillary P and the external loading pressure represented by an intramyocardial tissue pressure P_T, α is the elasticity coefficient, and E is the strain measure defined as:

$$E = \frac{1}{2}\left[\left(\frac{a(z,t)}{a_0}\right)^2 - 1\right] \quad (3)$$

where a_0 is the reference radius at zero transmural pressure ($\Delta P = 0$). The measured value of α in the spinotrapezius muscle of the rat was α = 1250 ± 450 mmHg for the instantaneous elastic response [16]. In the heart, based on Spaan's [5] evaluation of distensibility, α is of the order 340 mmHg. In the present study, the range of α = 200 to 1250 mmHg is used in order to study the effect of elasticity on the flow.

g. Ultrafiltration is governed by Starling's law. Hence

$$q = k(\Delta P - \Delta\Pi) \quad (4)$$

where q is the outward fluid flux per unit area, k is the filtration coefficient and $\Delta\Pi$ is the colloid osmotic pressure difference between the plasma and the interstitial fluid.

Equation of Flow

The flow equation is based on consideration of mass conservation (Fig. 2); thus:

$$\frac{\partial}{\partial t}\left[\pi a^2(z,t)\right] = -\frac{\partial}{\partial z} Q(z,t) - 2\pi a(z,t)\cdot q(z,t) \quad (5)$$

Equation (5) can be expressed in a nondimensional form by introducing nondimensional variables [17]:

$$\tau = t/T_0 \quad ; \quad \zeta = z/L(t) \quad ; \quad h = a(z,t)/a_0 \quad ; \quad \omega = L(t)/L_0 \quad (6)$$

where τ, ζ, h and ω are, respectively, the nondimensional time, position, radius, and lengthening: $L(t)$ and L_0 are the time varying and reference length, respectively, and T_0 is the cardiac period. With these variables, Eq. (5) obtains the following form:

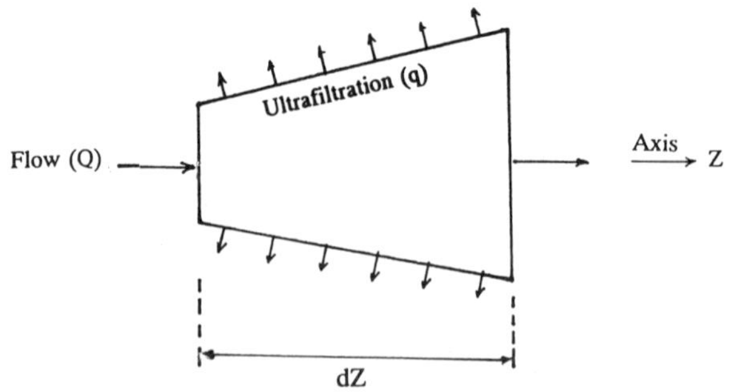

Figure 2. Mass conservation equation for a capillary section. The rate of change of the capillary volume between two fixed axial points is equal to the difference in axial discharges between these points minus ultrafiltration through to capillary wall.

$$(h^2)_\tau = \frac{\beta}{\omega^2(\tau)}(h^6)_{\zeta\zeta} - \frac{\omega'(\tau)}{\omega(\tau)}h^2 - \lambda(h^3 - h) + \eta h \tag{7}$$

where the subscripts τ and ζ denote partial derivatives with respect to these variables, and $\omega'(\tau)$ is the time derivative of $\omega(\tau)$.

The boundary conditions for $h(\zeta,\tau)$ are derived from Eqs. (2), (3) and (6). They are:

$$h^2(0,\tau) = 1 + \frac{2}{\alpha}(P_A(\tau) - P_T(\tau)) \quad \text{for the arterial end} \tag{8a}$$

$$h^2(1,\tau) = 1 + \frac{2}{\alpha}(P_V(\tau) - P_T(\tau)) \quad \text{for the venal end} \tag{8b}$$

where P_A, P_V are the blood pressure in the arterial and venal ends of the capillary, respectively.

There is no natural initial condition for the problem. Instead, there is a periodicity condition expressed by:

$$h(\zeta,\tau) = h(\zeta,\tau+1) \tag{8c}$$

Equation (7) shows that the flow is characterized by three nondimensional parameters β, λ and η, which are defined as:

$$\beta = \frac{T_0 \alpha a_0^2}{48\mu_{apar} L_0^2} \quad ; \quad \lambda = \frac{k\alpha T_0}{a_0} \quad ; \quad \eta = \frac{2\Delta\Pi k T_0}{a_0} \tag{9}$$

The values of these characteristic parameters for α = 1250 mmHg are (following Table 1):

$$\beta = 3.85 \quad ; \quad \lambda = 2 \quad ; \quad \eta = 0\ (\pm 0.03)$$

Subsequent analysis and calculations [17] indicate that β is an important parameter in determining the nature of the flow. The physical interpretation of β is as follows: β is the ratio of cardiac period (T_0) to the characteristic time constant (RC) of the vessel. It is a measure of the relative speed by which the flow can equilibrate, following a change in the external forces which drive the flow. For large values of β, the flow can reach equilibrium quickly, without significant volume changes. For small values of β, the flow reaches equilibrium slowly while large volume changes of the vessel occur in the process. This gives rise to pumping of blood out of the vessel during systole, and into the vessel during diastole.

The parameters λ and η describe ultrafiltration due to hydrostatic and osmotic pressure differences, respectively. Under normal physiological conditions, ultrafiltration has a secondary effect on the axial flow, and the effect of the colloid osmotic gradient is negligible.

Input Data

The pressures at the capillary ends, P_A and P_V, are input functions to the model, and are taken as *experimentally measured values*. Tillmanns et al. [23] measured the pressures in small subepicardial arterioles and venules of the rat left ventricle (LV). They reported peak systolic and diastolic pressures of 67 ± 12 mmHg and 45 ± 9 mmHg respectively for small arterioles, and 24 ± 5 mmHg and 5 ± 2 mmHg respectively for small venules. Chilian

Table 1. Values of Parameters and Their Sources

Parameter	Units	Source	Values in Literature	Values Used
a_0	μm	Ono et al. [18] Bassingthwaighte et al. [9]	5 – 7 5.6±1.3	5.5
L_0	μm	Bassingthwaighte et al. [9]	500–1000	750
μ	cP	Lipowsky et al. [15]	5	5
α	mmHg	Skalak & Schmid–Schonbein [16] Spaan [5]	1250±450 364	200÷1250
k	cm/sec·cm H_2O	Boseck [19] Baldwing and Gore [20]	$0.68{\cdot}10^{-6}$ $0.61{\pm}0.12{\cdot}10^{-6}$	$0.6{\cdot}10^{-6}$
ΔΠ	mmHg	Ruch and Patton [21] Hargens [22]	(–)5 ÷ 5 (–)13÷27	0±10
T_0	sec			0.5

et al. [24] reported peak systolic and diastolic pressures of 77 ± 5 mmHg and 68 ± 6 mmHg for arterioles and 11 ± 4 mmHg and 1 ± 1 mmHg for venules of the cat LV. Klassen et al. [25] reported that the pressure drops in the microcirculation and small veins in the dog LV during systole and diastole, were 16.4 ± 1.2 mmHg and 8.5 ± 0.8 mmHg, respectively. These pressure drops are much smaller than the ones between arterioles and venules reported by Tillmanns et al. [23] and Chilian et al. [24]. The differences in the pressure data were probably caused by the different locations along the arterioles where pressures have been measured, since the pressure gradient over the arteriole level is more than 50 mmHg [25]. The entrance pressure to the capillary should be lower than the above cited values since the arteriolar pressures in the studies of Tillmanns et al. [23] and Chilian et al. [24] were probably not measured near the entrance to the capillary.

In the absence of data on the pressures at the capillary ends that could serve as a basis for the present simulation, the data of Tillmanns et al. [23] for the waveform pattern in subepicardial arterioles and venules $P_A(t)$ and $P_V(t)$, were used after scaling them linearly so that the values of the peak systolic and diastolic pressures in subepicardium were 32 mmHg and 15 mmHg for $P_A(t)$, and 13.5 mmHg and 5 mmHg for $P_V(t)$. These values are in agreement with the data of Klassen et al. [25] on the pressure gradients. The resulting waveform (Fig. 3A) was used as input to the model.

There is no data on the coronary microcirculatory pressures in the deeper layers, and the values of $P_A(t)$ and $P_V(t)$ in these layers are a matter of speculation. There are two extreme cases: if the supplying and collecting vessels were rigid, then the intramyocardial tissue pressures would have no influence on $P_A(t)$ and $P_V(t)$ at all layers of the LV wall. A reasonable approximation would then be that $P_A(t)$ and $P_V(t)$ are the same for all myocardial layers. On the other hand, if these vessels were closed distensible compartments, then any change in the surrounding intramyocardial tissue pressure P_T would be followed by a similar change in arterial (P_A) and venular (P_V) pressures. This possibility was discussed in Hoffman et al. [3]. The realistic situation is in between these two extreme cases. In the present work, it is assumed that the levels of the pressures in the capillary inlet (P_A) and outlet (P_V) at the deeper layer, are the corresponding measured values at the

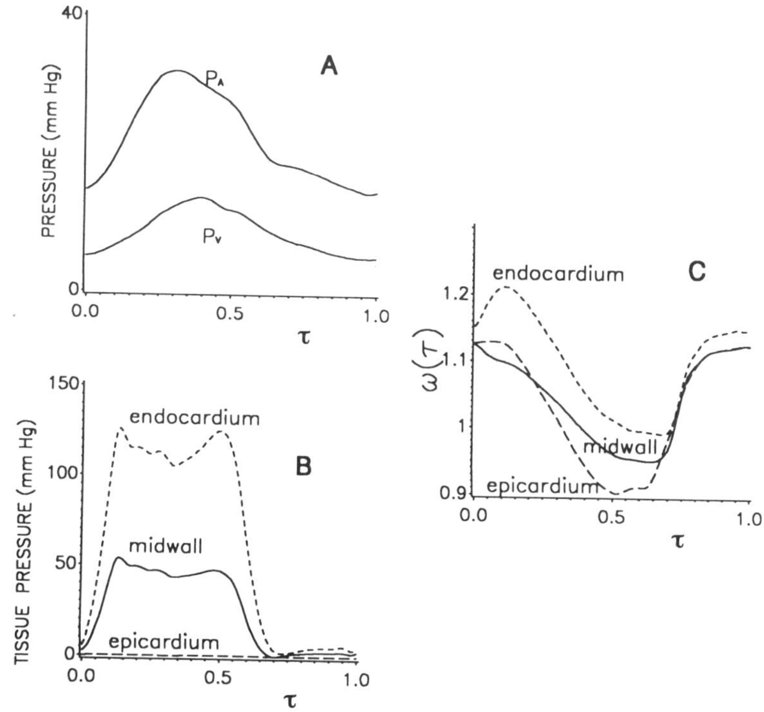

Figure 3. Data used in the numerical simulations. **A** – the time varying pressure input at the arterial and venular ends of a subepicardial capillary, P_A and P_V. Data was digitized from Tillmanns et al. [23], and adjusted as explained in the text. **B** – the time varying interstitial tissue pressure P_T at the epicardium, midwall and endocardium as determined from mechanical simulation of the LV [27]. **C** – the time varying relative length change, ω, of the muscle fibers at the epicardium, midwall and endocardium. From [17], with permission of the American Physiological Society (APS).

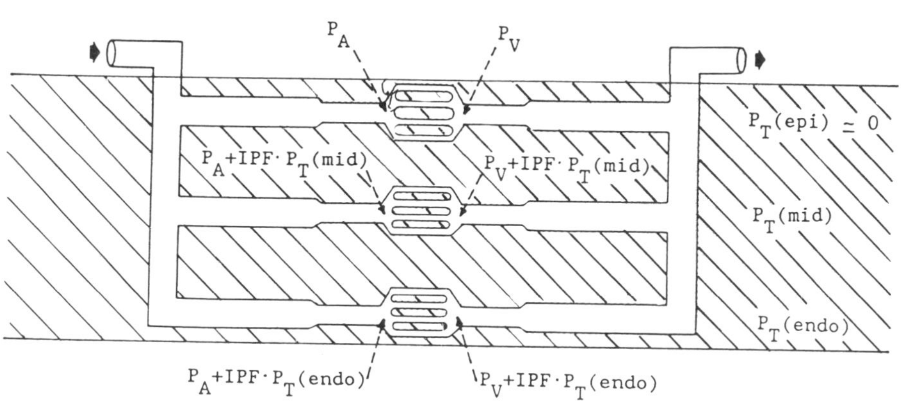

Figure 4. A scheme of the coronary system showing the regional difference in the inlet and outlet capillary pressures which are the boundary conditions for the flow equations. In the subepicardial capillaries these pressures were the measured values P_A and P_V. In deeper layers, there is an additional contribution of the tissue pressure (P_T) given by $IPF{\cdot}P_T$ where $0 \leq IPF \leq 1$. IPF – interstitial pressure factor.

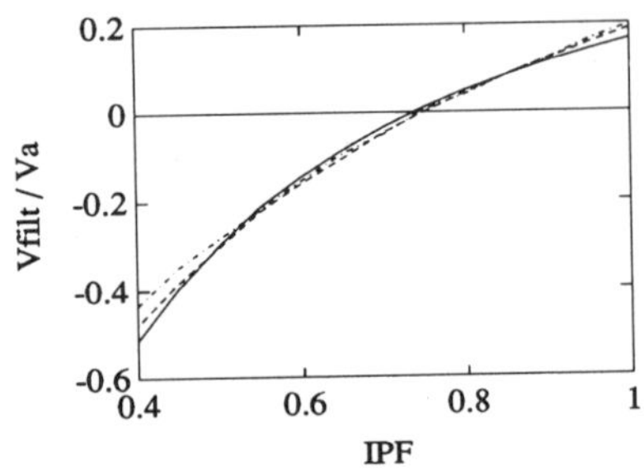

Figure 5. The ratio V_{filt}/V_a as a function of the interstitial pressure factor, *IPF*, for an endocardial capillary. The three curves correspond to three different values of the wall elasticity α (in mmHg): 200 (solid line), 500 (dashed line) and 1250 mmHg (dash dot line). Input data used are as shown in Fig. 3. From [17], with permission of the APS.

epicardium, augmented due to the interstitial pressure P_T by ($P_T \cdot IPF$), where *IPF* is the Interstitial Pressure Factor (Fig. 4). The value of *IPF* can vary between 0 (no effect) and 1 (full augmentation).

The level of *IPF* determines the value of V_{filt}, the net volume of fluid exchange per carciac cycle across the capillary wall due to ultrafiltration. Under stable conditions, V_{filt} corresponds to the fluid drainage to the lymphatic system. The latter is estimated to account for approximately 0.1% of the coronary flow [26]. Thus, the net ultrafiltration volume V_{filt} should be positive (i.e. in the outward direction), and the ratio of V_{filt} to V_a (V_a being the net volume of fluid that enters the capillary through the arteriolar end during one cardiac cycle) should be of the order of 0.001.

In a preliminary study, the model was used to calculate the ratio of the net filtration discharge during one cardiac cycle, V_{filt}, to the net arteriolar discharge into the capillary over that period, V_a, for three levels of the wall elasticity α, and for a range of values of the *IPF*. The results are presented in Fig. 5.

It can be seen that for these three values of α, the choice of *IPF* = 0.75 provides a small positive ratio (a fraction of one percent), which is compatible with the normal physiological level of the lymphatic drainage. Hence, IPF = 0.75 was used in the subsequent calculations, unless otherwise indicated.

Other input data required for the model are the time dependent transmural distribution of the tissue pressure (P_T) and myocyte lengthening (ω). Discrete values of the input functions ω(t) and $P_T(t)$ for different layers in the myocardium were supplied by E. Nevo (Fig. 3); they are the output of a model simulation of the LV in a dog [27].

RESULTS

The numerical results confirm the preliminary assessment as to the insignificant effects of the ultrafiltration and osmotic pressure on the capillary flow under stable physiological conditions. The error due to neglecting both, (i.e. $\lambda = 0$, $\eta = 0$) turns out to be less than 0.5%, for the normal cardiac cycle. Under abnormal situations such as long diastole or arrested heart [28], the effect of ultrafiltration may become more significant.

The calculated results show considerable differences between subendocardial, midwall and subepicardial capillaries. The differences are in both the pattern of their responses as well as in the role and relative importance of the participating mechanisms.

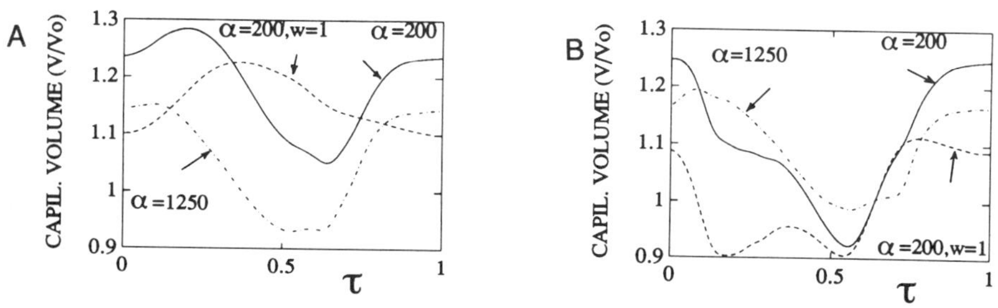

Figure 6. Relative capillary volume change during the cardiac cycle as affected by the capillary distensibility α and capillary length changes ω for *IPF* = 0.75. **A:** Subepicardial capillary; **B:** subendocardial capillary. The three curves in each figure correspond to the following cases: α = 200 mmHg and ω ≡ 1 (no length changes); α = 200 mmHg and ω as in Fig. 3C; α = 1250 mmHg and ω as in Fig. 3C. Note the regional differences and the considerable volume changes for all values of α. These volume changes result in a pumping effect. From [17], with permission of the APS.

Figure 6 is an example of the time–varying capillary volume for subepicardial (Fig. 6A) vs subendocardial (Fig. 6B) capillaries. The time variable in Figs. 6–9 is the normalized time, τ. The systolic and diastolic phases correspond roughly to τ between 0–0.5 and between 0.5–1, respectively.

The results in Fig. 6 show the effect of the wall distensibility α and that of the possible length–changes $\omega(t)$. This was done since α proved to be an important flow parameter and its value could vary under different conditions. The effect of possible capillary length–change can be evaluated from Fig. 6 by comparing results obtained using the input data (Fig. 3) with results obtained for the case of a fixed capillary length ($\omega(t) = 1$).

The most reliable data available at present on coronary flow are measurements in the epicardial arteries and veins. These represent the discharges in and out of the entire myocardial wall. It is instructive to compare these data with the pattern of combined discharges of myocardial capillaries from the three layers: epicardium, midwall and endocardium. The combined inflow and outflow are expressed here as wall averaged discharges $\bar{Q}_{in}$ and $\bar{Q}_{out}$. The phasic patterns of $\bar{Q}_{in}$ and $\bar{Q}_{out}$ and the effects of the elasticity coefficient α and length changes $\omega(t)$ on these discharges are presented in Figs. 7A ($\bar{Q}_{in}$) and 7B ($\bar{Q}_{out}$).

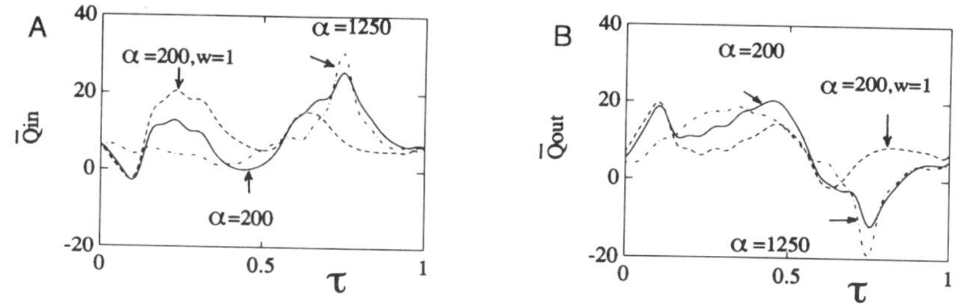

Figure 7. A: The time varying inflow $\bar{Q}_{in}$, averaged across the LV wall (average of subendocardium, midwall and subepicardium). **B:** The corresponding outflow, $\bar{Q}_{out}$. The three curves in each figure correspond to the cases in Fig. 6 with *IPF* = 0.75. The discharge units are $cm^3/sec \cdot 10^{-9}$. Note the rapid filling in **A** during diastole, except when there are no length changes. There is a retrograde diastolic flow $\bar{Q}_{out}$ in **B** and an increased systolic anterograde flow, except when there are no length changes. From [27], with permission of APS.

An important question relates to the dependence of the model results on the input data P_A and P_V. This question arises due to the uncertainty by which these data were obtained indirectly from data on the microcirculation (as already discussed). The sensitivity of the model results to two features of P_A and P_V has been studied: One feature is the absolute levels of both P_A and P_V, and the other is the pressure drop $P_A - P_V$. The results are shown in Figs. 8 and 9 for the wall averaged discharge $\bar{Q}_{in}$. It is important to indicate that each new set of P_A, P_V data as used in Figs. 8 and 9 required a new evaluation of the level of *IPF* so as to ensure a reasonable lymphatic discharge compared with the main capillary flow.

DISCUSSION

Capillary capacitance and the possible existence of an intramyocardial pump mechanism are closely related to capillary volume changes. From Fig. 6 it is seen that capillaries undergo substantial volume changes that are larger in the subendocardium (up to 30%) compared with the subepicardium (20%).

The results of Fig. 6 suggest that the influence of the elasticity coefficient α and lengthening $\omega(t)$ on the volumes of capillaries is different across the myocardial wall. In the subepicardium (Fig. 6A) higher elasticity coefficient (α) is associated with smaller capillary volume throughout the cardiac cycle, but has no effect on the systolic/diastolic volume difference. Capillary lengthening $\omega(t)$ changes the pattern of volume dynamics and increases systolic/diastolic volume differences.

In the subendocardium, higher elasticity coefficients reduce systolic/diastolic volume differences. In the absence of lengthening ($\omega(t) = 1$), the volumes reduce and so does the systolic/diastolic volume difference.

The predicted combined flow in the three wall layers (Fig. 7) exhibits similar patterns in all cases: The inflow ($\bar{Q}_{in}$) is small during early systole and is followed by rapid

Figure 8. Sensitivity of the average inflow ($\bar{Q}_{in}$) to the absolute values of the arterial and venal pressures P_A and P_V. Values of $\bar{Q}_{in}$ were calcu- lated for: (1) reference values of P_A and P_V used throughout the simulations (Fig. 3A), solid line; (2) P_A and P_V raised by 4 mmHg each, dashed line; (3) P_A and P_V lowered by 4 mmHg each, dash dot line. In all cases α = 200 mmHg. The factor *IPF* in Fig. 4 was recalculated for each case as in Fig. 5. *IPF* = 0.68 for $P_A + 4$, $P_V + 4$, and *IPF* = 0.82 for $P_A - 4$, $P_V - 4$.

Figure 9. Sensitivity of the averaged inflow Q_{in} to the pressure gradient $P_A - P_V$. Values of Q_{in} were calculated for the reference values of P_A and P_V (Fig. 3A), solid line; P_A raised by 4 mmHg and P_V lowered by 4 mmHg, dashed line; P_A lowered by 4 mmHg and P_V raised by 4 mmHg, dash–dot line. In all cases α = 200 mmHg, and *IPF* = 0.75.

filling in early diastole. A smaller value of α results in larger systolic/diastolic flow differences, with retrograde flow in early systole. Capillary length changes $\omega(t)$ tend to decrease the inflow during late systole and to increase it during late diastole.

The opposite behavior is seen for the combined outflow at the venular end $\bar{Q}_{out}$(Fig. 7B): there is a rapid venular emptying during early systole and retrograde filling during diastole. Higher elasticity α changes the phasic behavior of $\bar{Q}_{out}$and reduces the systolic/diastolic flow differences. The capillary's length change $\omega(t)$ increases both the systolic emptying and the diastolic retrograde filling.

The absolute levels of P_A and P_V have an effect (Fig. 8) on the combined inflow $\bar{Q}_{in}$ only during early systole (where lower levels of P_A, P_V increase retrograde flow) and during early diastole (where higher levels of P_A, P_V enhance diastolic filling). These results lead to the conclusion that the total inflow over a cardiac cycle is insensitive to the absolute levels of P_A, P_V. The same conclusion may hold for the sensitivity of the total flow to the level of the tissue pressure P_T since it is added to P_A, P_V (multiplied by *IPF*) in the boundary conditions (Eq. (8)).

Changes in the pressure drop (P_A–P_V) do not effect the phasic nature of the combined inflow (Fig. 9), but they do effect the level of the flow: Increased pressure drop increases the flow consistently throughout the cardiac cycle, and vice versa. This leads to the conclusion that the total inflow over the whole cycle will increase with increasing pressure drop (P_A–P_V).

Effect of Capillary Tethering

The capillary flow, Eq. (7), is found to depend primarily on the characteristic parameter β, which depends in turn on the wall elasticity, α. The analysis giving rise to the flow equation in the untethered capillary relies on the assumption that the wall elasticity α remains constant under all circumstances. This assumption can be disputed in view of morphological evidence [e.g. 29] that the capillary membrane is attached to surrounding myocytes by a network of collagen fibers. When these fibers are taut, the membrane resistance to transmural pressure is the result of the combined effects of membrane and collagen fibers which tether it. Hence, the apparent membrane elasticity may no longer be considered as constant when a more realistic morphology is considered.

The analysis of the effects of tethering is the subject of ongoing research. The first major question that arises is whether the response of tethered capillaries shows patterns of behavior which are sufficiently different form the untethered one, so as to justify the need for a more complex analysis. Borg and Caulfield [29] observed that a common feature of

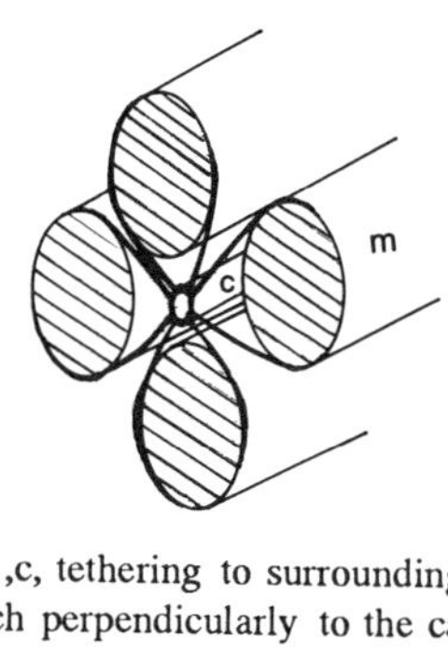

Figure 10. Schematic of the capillary ,c, tethering to surrounding myocytes, m, as proposed by Borg and Caulfield [29]. The collagen fibers attach perpendicularly to the capillary wall but tangent to the myocytes.

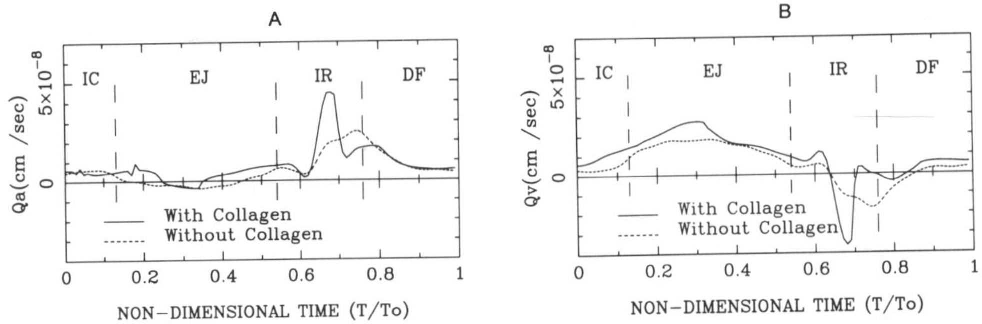

Figure 11. Effect of tethering on the flow in a subepicardial capillary. **A:** inflow at the arterial end (Q_a); **B:** outflow from the venular end (Q_V). Solid line – with collagen tethering; broken line – without tethering. α = 1250 mmHg.

the capillary tethering is that collagen fibers attach to the capillary perpendicular to its wall, but as tangentially to the myocyte wall. They proposed the simplified schematic model for this system shown in Fig. 10. This model is used here as a basis for a detailed structural analysis which considers mechanical equilibrium, and constitutive laws for the capillary membrane and collagen fibers. The tension in the fibers depends amongst others on the time-dependent myocyte to capillary distances in both directions (x,y) normal to their common axial direction. These distances are input data to the model. They are obtained from the same structural model of the LV mechanics [27] from which the input data, Fig. 3, was derived. The other input data used for the current analysis (P_A, P_V, P_T, ω) are the same as in the model of untethered capillaries.

The analysis is two dimensional and reduces to a set of 16 coupled nonlinear equations. It provides the relationship between capillary area and shape on one hand, and the transmural pressure difference, ΔP on the other, throughout the cardiac cycle. Hence, the tethering analysis replaces Eq. (2) in the untethered (no collagen attachments) model. Otherwise the methodology is the same (i.e. the flow is derived from mass conservation with the appropriate boundary conditions).

Without going into mathematical details, the inflows and outflows of a subepicardial capillary are presented in Fig. 11 for the tethered and the untethered models. The results show that the pattern of flow is affected by attachments of the collagen fibers. In the subepicardial capillary, the difference is significant during the isovolumic relaxation and early diastolic filling.

These results indicate that collagen tethering must be considered if one wishes to obtain a more realistic model of the coronary flow.

DISCUSSION

Dr. R. Chadwick: A question about the capillary volume changes. You report that there was a 25% volume change of a capillary. If you converted that to volume change per 100 gm tissue, would that agree with what Jos Spaan and others have measured, which is only a few percent.

Dr. Y. Lanir: We did not. We looked at a single capillary. The results for resilient (α = 200 mmHg) subepicardial capillaries show systolic/diastolic volume changes of 25% including lengthening. Without capillary length change it is about 12%.

Dr. R. Chadwick: When you assume lengthening to occur, do you assume anything about the change in cross-sectional area of the capillary wall? Is there a constant capillary wall?

Dr. Y. Lanir: The cross-sectional area, flow and volume of fluid within the capillary is governed by mass conservation. The question is, what would be the mechanical interaction between lengthening and area changes if lengthening occurs in an empty capillary. Lengthening of capillaries was observed. Their walls are not continuous membranes. They consist of interconnected endothelial cells and it has been shown that under certain circumstances these cells can fold and bulge during contraction. So this evidence does not point necessarily to a direct effect of lengthening on changes in the area. This question is, however, open and should be further studied. In our model there is a decoupling between lengthening and area.

Dr. J. Bassingthwaighte: I believe that Dr. Lanir is on the right track. In isolate rabbit hearts perfused with Krebs-Henseleit buffer, if you make a 30 milliosmol increase in osmolarity as a step change above a standard 300 milliosmol perfusate, you reduce the total vascular resistance in a totally vasodilated preparation by 80%. It is absolutely astounding how huge is this reduction in resistance. I believe it is all at the capillary level and it is via the mechanisms that you propose, the tethering of capillary walls to the myocytes. You need to push on with this.

REFERENCES

1. Chilian WM, Marcus ML. Phasic coronary blood flow velocity in intramural and epicardial coronary arteries. *Circ Res* 1982; 50: 775–781.
2. Hoffman JIE, Spaan JAE. Pressure flow relations in coronary circulation. *Physiological Rev* 1990; 70: 331–390.
3. Hoffman JIE, Baer RW, Mandey FL, Messina LM. Regulation of transmural myocardial blood flow. *ASME Trans J Biomechan Eng* 1985; 107: 3–9.
4. Levy BI, Samuel JL, Tedgui A, Kotelianski V, Marotte F, Poitevin P, Chadwick RS. Intramyocardial blood volume in the left ventricle of rat arrested hearts. In: Brun P, Chadwick RS, Levy BI (eds) *Cardiovascular Dynamics and Models* (Colloque INSERM 183). INSERM: Paris, pp 65–71, 1988.
5. Spaan JAE. Coronary diastolic pressure–flow relation and zero flow pressure explained on the basis of intramyocardial compliance. *Circ Res* 1985; 56: 293–309.
6. Dinnar U. Interaction between intramyocardial pressure and transcapillary exchange: A possible control of coronary circulation. In: Sideman S, Beyar R (eds) *Simulation and Control of the Cardiac System*, CRC Press: NY, pp 109–130, 1987.
7. Schmid-Schonbein GW, Lee SY, Sutton D. Dynamic viscous flow in distensible vessels of skeletal muscle microcirculation: application to pressure and flow transients. *Biorheology* 1989; 26: 215–227.
8. Chadwick RS, Tedgui A, Michel JB, Ohayon J, Levy BI. Phasic regional myocardial inflow and outflow: comparison of theory and experiments. *Am J Physiol* 1990; 258: H1687–H1698.
9. Bassingthwaighte JB, Yipintsoi T, Harvey RB. Microvasculature of the dog left ventricle myocardium. *Microvasc Res* 1974; 7: 729–249.
10. Berne RM, Rubio R. Coronary circulation. In: *Handbook of Physiology – The Heart* (section 2/1). Am Physiology Soc:MD, 1979; pp 873–952.
11. Caulfiled JB, Borg TK. The collagen network of the heart. *Lab Invest* 1979; 40: 364–372.
12. Ellis CG, Mathieu-Costello O, Potter RF, MacDonald IC, Groom AC. Effect of sarcomere length on total capillary length in skeletal muscle: *In vivo* evidence for longitudinal stretching of capillaries. *Microvasc Res* 1990; 40: 63–72.
13. Poole DC, Batra S, Mathieu-Costello O, Rakusan K. Capillary geometrical changes with fiber shortening in rat myocardium. *Circ Res* 1992; 70: 697–706.
14. Chadwick RS. Slow viscous flow inside a torus. The resistance of small tortuous blood vessels. *Quart Appl Math* 1985; 43: 317–323.
15. Lipowsky HH, Kovalcheck S, Zweifach BW. The distribution of blood rheological parameters in the microcirculation of cat mesentery. *Circ Res* 1978; 43: 738–749.
16. Skalak TC, Schmid-Schonbein GW. Viscoelastic properties of microvessels in rat spinotrapezius muscle. *ASME Trans J Biomech Eng* 1986; 108: 193–200.

17. Fibich G, Lanir Y, Liron N. Mathematical model of blood flow in a coronary capillary. *Am J Physiol* 1993; accepted for publication.
18. Ono T, Shimohara Y, Okada K, Irino S. Scanning electron microscopic studies on microvascular architecture on human coronary vessels by corrosion casts: Normal and focal necrosis. *Scanning Electron Microvasc* 1986; 1: 263–270.
19. Boseck GL. Transcapillary fluid exchange in rat spinotrapezius muscle. *Ph.D. Thesis*. Univ of California: La Jolla, CA, 1983.
20. Baldwin A, Gore RS. Simultaneous measurement of capillary distensibility and hydraulic conductance. *Microvasc Res* 1989; 38: 1–22.
21. Ruch TC, Patton HD. *Physiology and Biophysics*. WB Saunders Co: Philadelphia, 1966.
22. Hargens AR. Interstitial fluid pressure and lymph flow. In: Skalak R, Chien S (eds) *Handbook of Bioengineering*. McGraw-Hill:NY, pp 19.1–19.25, 1987.
23. Tillmanns H, Steinhausen M, Leinberger H, Thederan H, Kubler W. Pressure measurements in the terminal vascular bed of the epimyocardium of rats and cats. *Circ Res* 1981; 49: 1202–1211.
24. Chilian WM, Layne SM, Klausner EC, Eastham CL, Marcus ML. Redistribution of coronary microvascular resistance produced by dipyridamole. *Am J Physiol* (*Heart Circ Physiol* 25) 1989; 256: H383–H390.
25. Klassen GA, Armour JA, Garner JB. Coronary circulatory pressure gradients. *Can J Physiol Pharmacol* 1987; 65: 520–531.
26. Solti F, Jellinek H. *Cardiac Lymph Circulation and Cardiac Disorders*. Akademiai Kiado: Budapest, 1989.
27. Nevo E, Lanir Y. Structural finite deformation model of the left ventricle during diastole and systole. *ASME Trans J Biomech Eng* 1989; 3: 342–348.
28. Kresh YJ. Myocardial modulation of coronary circulation. *Am J Phsyiol* 1989; 257: H1934–H1935.
29. Borg TK, Caulfield JB. The collagen matrix of the heart. *Federation Proc* 1981; 40: 2037–2041.

MICROSTRUCTURE:

MECHANICS AND MICROCIRCULATION

CHAPTER 14

Models for Coronary Pressure–Flow Relationships

Robert E. Mates[1] and Robert M. Judd[2]

ABSTRACT

We have developed a mathematical model which describes pressure–inflow relationships in the coronary circulation. Model parameters have been identified during metabolic and pharmacologic vasodilation. These two stimuli appear to affect resistance and back pressure in different ways. A possible explanation involving myogenic and metabolic effects is suggested.

INTRODUCTION

The dynamics of coronary pressure–flow relationships have received considerable attention over the last decade. Improved medical and surgical techniques for the treatment of coronary artery disease have increased the motivation for more quantitative diagnostic methods, and these in turn have required an improved understanding of the control of coronary flow. It has become evident that coronary pressure–flow relationships are much more complex than the traditional Ohm's Law description.

Bellamy's observations in awake dogs that diastolic coronary inflow ceased at pressures well above right atrial pressure [1] suggested the need for more complex models to explain pressure–flow relationships. Two models were suggested to explain this phenomenon. The vascular waterfall concept postulates a pressure regulator in the coronary microcirculation which maintains intraluminal pressure at some level above right atrial pressure [2]. Spaan's intramyocardial pump model [3] suggests that a pressure regulator is not necessary to explain the observed high values of zero–flow pressure. Rather, Spaan has suggested that a large intramyocardial capacitance may maintain capillary perfusion even

[1]Departments of Mechanical and Aerospace Engineering and Medicine, State University of New York at Buffalo, Buffalo, NY 14215, USA. [2]Presently, Department of Radiology and Radiological Sciences, Johns Hopkins University, Balimore, MD 14260, USA.

Interactive Phenomena in the Cardiac System, Edited by
S. Sideman and R. Beyer, Plenum Press, New York, 1993

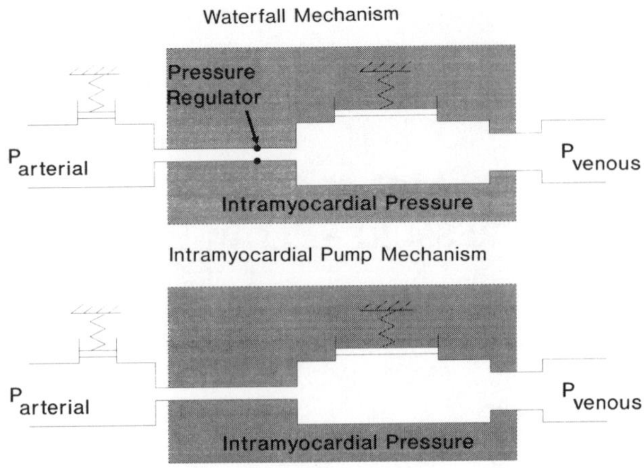

Figure 1. Comparison of waterfall and intramyocardial pump model.

though inflow has ceased. The two models are shown schematically in Fig. 1. The fact that phasic coronary outflow peaks during systole while inflow peaks during diastole shows that there is indeed a large intramyocardial capacitance as Spaan suggested. Whether a pressure regulator is needed in addition remains controversial. Unfortunately, methods are not yet available to measure detailed phasic pressure and flow fluctuations in the myocardium. Our laboratory, as well as others, has attempted to use mathematical models to explain the observed pressure–inflow relationships.

METHODS

We have used a lumped parameter model of the coronary circulation to identify parameters governing coronary pressure–inflow relationships under various conditions. The model, shown schematically in Fig. 2, includes a resistive element R and a Voigt visco-elastic compliance characterized by C and K [4]. The zero-flow pressure is shown as P_{IL}. A servovalve control system [5] has been used to apply various pressure waveforms to the left circumflex coronary artery of open chest, anesthetized dogs. Initially, we applied small amplitude sinusoidal pressure oscillations during prolonged diastoles to obtain values of the model components [6]. Subsequently, ramp waveforms were applied to show that diastolic model parameters were the same in prolonged and normal diastoles [7]. Based on the

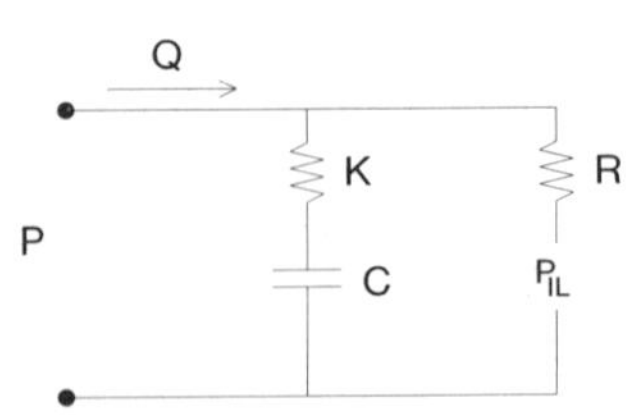

Figure 2. Schematic representation of the RC viscoelastic model of coronary inflow. R – resistance; K – viscoelasticity; C – capacitance (Voigt viscoelastic compliance constants); p – coronary perfusion pressure; P_{IL} – zero flow pressure.

suggestion of Van Huis et al. [8] that impedance is the same in systole and diastole, we used the same model to analyze pressure–inflow relationships in normal cardiac cycles [9]. It was assumed that R, C and K in Fig. 1 were constant throughout the cycle and that P_{IL} varied in proportion to left ventricular (LV) pressure P_{LV} with a diastolic value P_d when LV pressure is zero, i.e.: $P_{IL} = 0.5*P_{LV} + P_d$. Left ventricular and left circumflex (LC) coronary artery pressure and coronary inflow were measured at various heart rates with normal vascular tone and during adenosine vasodilation. The ordinary differential equations describing the model in the time domain were solved numerically for assumed values of the parameters R, C, K and P_d. An optimization algorithm [7] was used to adjust model parameters to obtain the best possible agreement with the data in a least–squares sense.

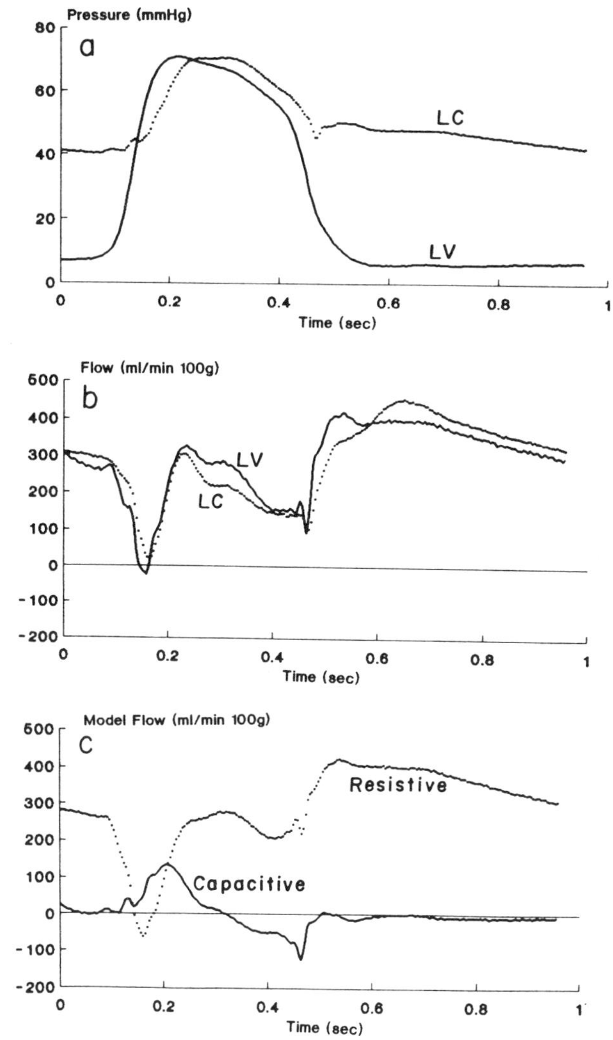

Figure 3. Comparison of measured and predicted inflows at 60 bpm. Redrawn from [9] with permission of the *Am J Physiol*. LC – left circumflex, LV – left ventricular.

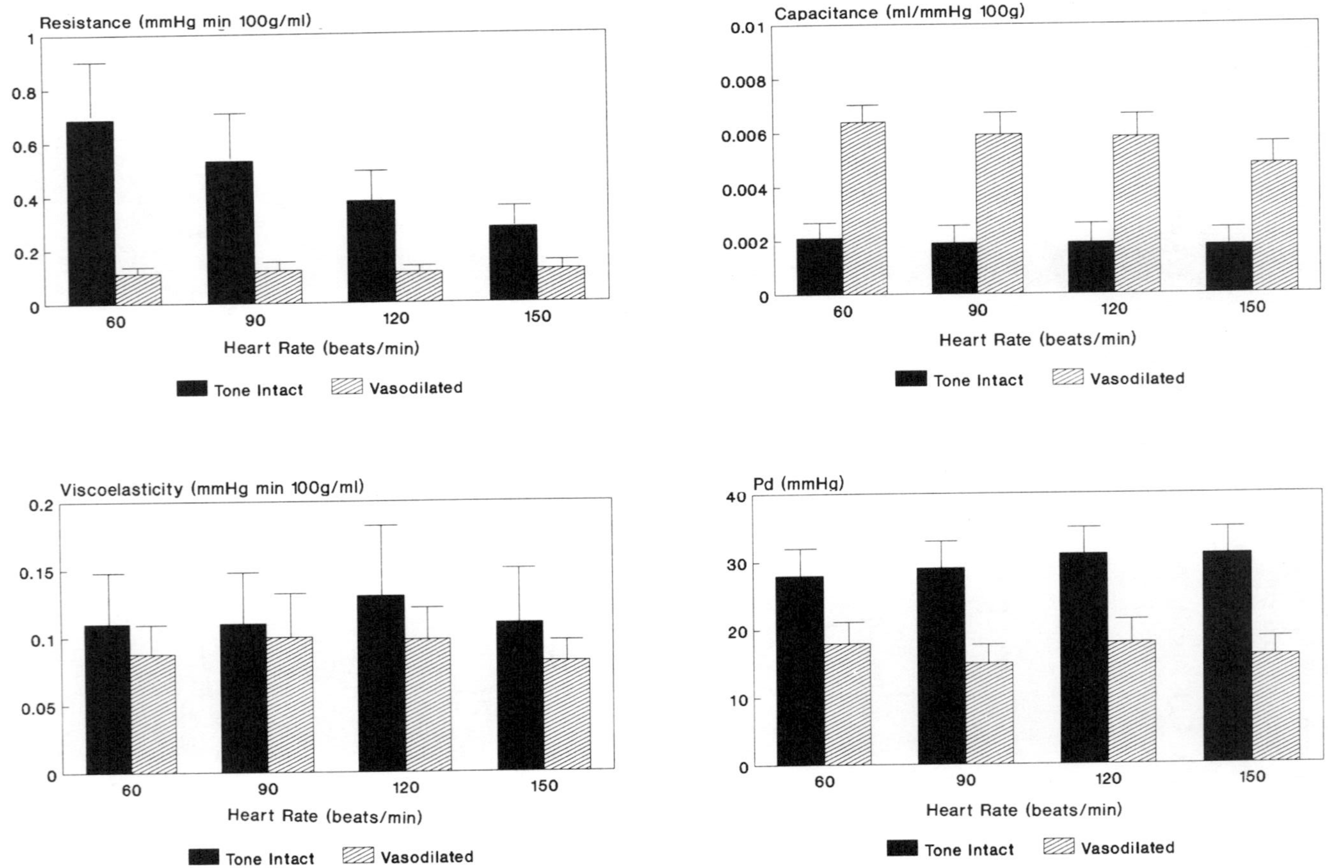

Figure 4. Summary of model parameters obtained during metabolic and pharmacologic vasodilation. Redrawn from [9] with permission of the *Am J Physiol*.

RESULTS

An example of the results is shown in Fig. 3 for a heart rate of 60 bpm during adenosine vasodilation. Panel (a) shows the measured LC and LV pressures as functions of time. In panel (b), the measured LC flow is shown by the dots while the solid line is the model–predicted flow. The agreement is quite good. Panel (c) shows the computed flows through the resistor (dots) and capacitor (solid line). Note that the capacitive flow predicted by the model is negligibly small during diastole. Similar agreement was obtained at higher heart rates and with normal vascular tone.

Figure 4 summarizes the four model parameter values under the various experimental conditions. R is shown in the upper left panel, K in the lower left, C in the upper right, and P_d in the lower right. The solid bars give values with tone intact and the shaded bars are the values during vasodilation. Heart rate is seen to affect primarily the value of R with tone intact. All of the variables except K are altered significantly by adenosine dilation. Adenosine reduces R and P_d and increases C. Diastolic pressure–flow relations (for $P_{LV} = 0$) for heart rates of 60 and 150 with tone intact and for adenosine vasodilation are shown in Fig. 5. The solid lines cover approximately the pressure range over which data was obtained. Metabolic vasodilation is accomplished with no change in P_d while adenosine causes a substantial reduction.

DISCUSSION

It seems remarkable that the effects of ventricular contraction can be explained by postulating variations in only one of the four model parameters, the zero–flow pressure P_{IL}. The force balance on a vessel embedded in the myocardium is shown schematically in Fig. 6. At equilibrium, the intraluminal pressure P_{IL} must balance the forces of extravascular pressure KP_{LV} and the wall tension T. For a thin–walled vessel, the effect of wall tension on intraluminal pressure is given by $P_d = 4T/d$ where d is the vessel diameter.

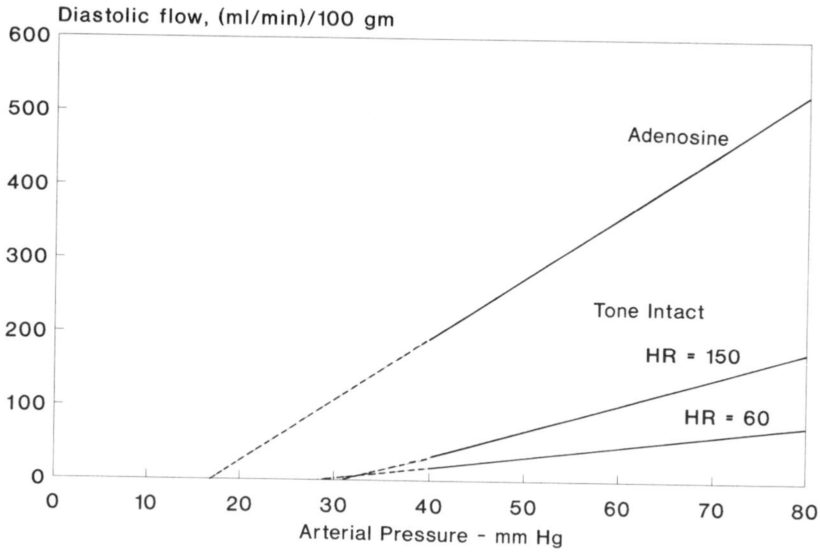

Figure 5. Diastolic pressure–flow relations during metabolic and pharmacologic vasodilation.

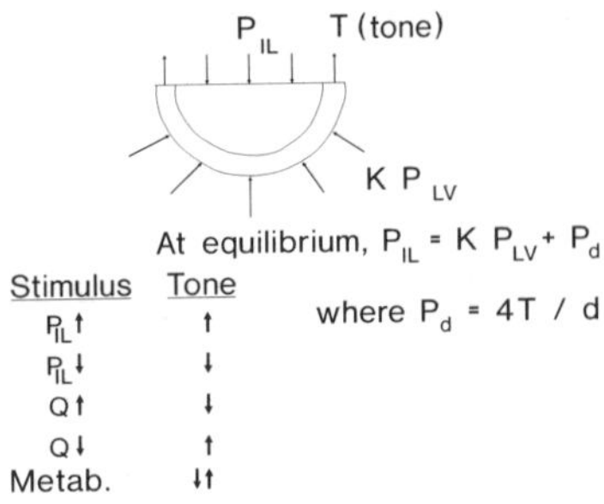

Figure 6. Force balance on an embedded blood vessel. T – wall tension, d – vessel diameter.

Krams et al. [10] have shown that systolic flow is impeded by muscle contractility even in the absence of developed ventricular pressure. In the intact heart, developed pressure is the only readily available index of myocardial contraction. Our results suggest that, at least under normal loading conditions, LV pressure is a reasonable index of effective intramyocardial stresses.

Wall tension is a function of vascular tone. In addition to metabolic effects, Kuo et al. [11] have shown that myogenic and flow–induced stimuli can both affect vascular tone. An increase in P_{IL} was shown to cause vasoconstriction, while a reduction induced vasodilation. Increasing the flow Q resulted in vasodilation, while flow reductions produced constriction. The two effects appear to be coupled. The flow–induced changes in tone, presumably related to changes in wall shear stress, are abolished by removal of the endothelial cells. Thus, there are at least three separate stimuli which can cause changes in vascular tone and hence P_d: metabolic, intraluminal pressure, and flow.

What could be the teleological reason for multiple feedback paths in the control of the coronary circulation? While most attention is focused on flow regulation, it is equally important that capillary pressure be closely regulated. Shifts in capillary pressure may result in transcapillary fluid shifts which can significantly affect the function of cardiac muscle. Fig. 7 shows schematically a possible role for myogenic regulation. The upper part is a schematic of the resistive components of the coronary circulation, lumped in three parts, the arteriolar R_a, the capillary R_c, and the venous R_v resistances. The regulated pressure P_{IL}

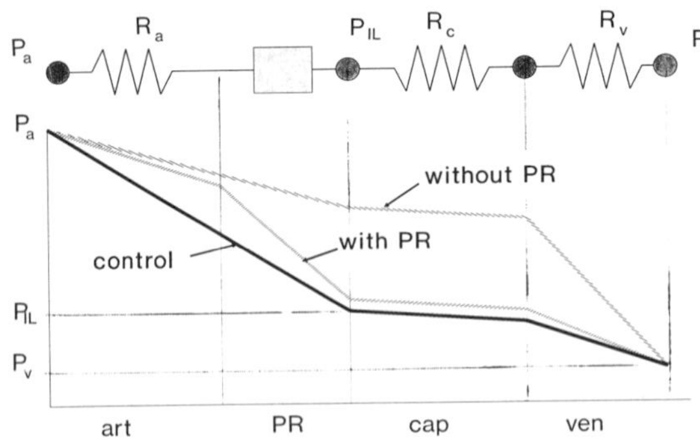

Figure 7. Hypothetical pressure distributions during normal flow and vasodilatation. P_a – arteriolar pressure; R_a – arteriolar resistance; R_c – capillary resistance; R_v – venular resistance; P_v – venular pressure; PR – pressure regulator.

is shown as the capillary entrance pressure. The lower part shows three hypothetical pressure distributions. The solid line represents the distribution at normal coronary flow, the lower hatched line the distribution at increased flow with pressure regulation, and the upper hatched line the distribution with increased flow without pressure regulation. In spite of a substantial reduction in R_a, capillary pressure can be maintained nearly constant by pre-capillary pressure regulation. As flow begins to increase, pre-capillary pressure will tend to rise as R_a is reduced. This will cause a myogenic response which will increase vascular tone, thereby decreasing vessel diameter, increasing the pressure drop through the regulator and hence limiting the rise in P_{IL}. There will, of course, be changes in R_c and R_v as well. Close regulation of capillary pressure would require that a venous pressure regulator be present as well. To the authors' knowledge, myogenic properties of venules have not been studied.

Can this myogenic mechanism explain the results shown in Fig. 4? With normal vascular tone, increasing metabolic demand by pacing reduced resistance with no appreciable reduction in zero–flow pressure P_d. This suggests that metabolic stimuli have little effect on P_d, or that metabolic dilation is overcome by myogenic constriction resulting in little or no change in vascular tone at the site of pressure regulation. On the other hand, adenosine vasodilation reduced both R and P_d appreciably. Adenosine was given in doses sufficient to abolish reactive hyperemia following 30 sec occlusion (9 μmol/min). At these high doses, it seems quite possible that the myogenic response may be blocked, thus explaining the drop in P_d.

A schematic diagram of the possible control paths is shown in Fig. 8. The dotted lines are the feedback loops, with K_Q, K_P and K_m the gains of the flow, pressure and metabolic paths, respectively. It is postulated that the myogenic response is concentrated on the pressure regulator, while both metabolic and flow–induced alterations in tone affect the arteriolar resistor. This is highly speculative and requires experimental confirmation. Chilian et al. showed that more than 50% of vascular resistance is located in arterioles <100–150 μm in diameter [12]. The myogenic and flow–induced effects mentioned above were demonstrated in arterioles 40–80 μm in diameter [11]. The latter studies were conducted on excised vessels, and it is difficult to study smaller vessels due to technical difficulties.

Why should adenosine affect capacitance, while heart rate appears to have no effect with tone intact? There appear to be two potential explanations for the effect of adenosine. The first is that adenosine directly influences vessel elasticity by altering smooth muscle

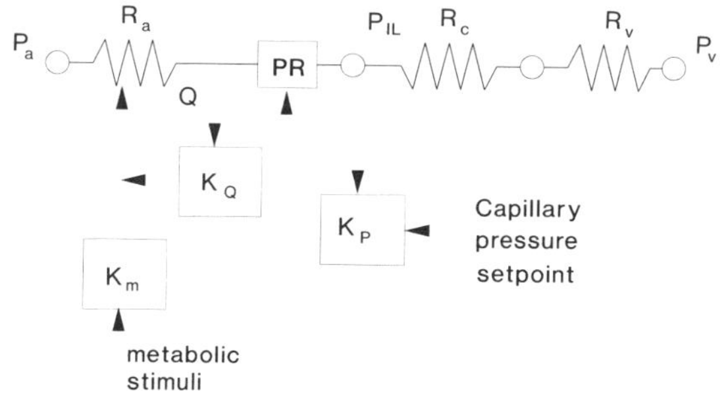

Figure 8. Possible control mechanisms governing coronary pressure and flow. R_a – arteriolar resistance; R_c – capillary resistance; R_v – venous resistance. K_Q, K_P, K_m – gains of flow, pressure, and metabolic paths, respectively.

tone. The second is that, by dilating small resistance vessels, adenosine exposes smaller vessels to phasic fluctuations in perfusion pressure. The circuit in Fig. 2 lumps all capacitance in a single parameter. Capacitance as well as resistance is distributed throughout the vasculature. It is not possible to distinguish between these effects from the available data. If, as suggested above, large doses of adenosine overwhelm other regulatory stimuli, the increases in capacitance shown in Fig. 4 may not occur during normal physiologic conditions.

Of necessity, most studies which focus on the detailed behavior of components of the coronary circulation utilize experimental models which do not replicate normal physiology. Particularly when control mechanisms are studied, it is important to keep in mind that responses may vary with the preparation. Anesthetics depress or block central nervous system responses, open–chest preparations differ from closed, and excised vessels are not subjected to neural or humoral influences. Thus, it is important to try to integrate findings from different experimental settings. Mathematical models are a useful vehicle in this effort.

Acknowledgements

This work was supported by National Heart, Lung and Blood Institute Program–Project Grant 2–PO1–HLB–15194.

DISCUSSION

Dr. W.M. Chilian: Muscular venules in the heart do have a very weak myogenic response. It is not as robust as in arterioles, but there is a weak myogenic response.

Dr. R. Mates: I know you have looked at a variety of different diameters. Were you able to identify the size of vessels in which the effects occur preferentially or is that too difficult to do?

Dr. W.M. Chilian: In part we have. This is discussed in Chapter 17. The other comment I would like to make is about the concept of a pressure regulating system. We have found that in isolated exchange vessels the convective flux of albumin, water and solute transport, is very sensitive to pressure perturbations. That is, for about 1 mmHg increase of pressure in an exchange vessel, there is approximately a 10% increase in the flux. That might be at least a teleological reason why this system might want to regulate pressure, because we do not want to have an overload of fluid and solute transport which could possibly cause edema.

Dr. E.O. Feigl: What is the difference between your back–pressure and Jos Spaan's pump?

Dr. R. Mates: We have been arguing about that for years and I don't know that we are in agreement yet. One difference, at least with this modification, is that the back–pressure becomes active rather than simply passive. It is a quantity which can be modulated separately from flow so there is an extra degree of active control which would not be in the myocardial pump. The real question is whether you need it and whether it is there. One bit of evidence in the vasodilated bed showed that there is a necessity for a pressure regulator to explain even flow regulation in these long diastoles. But, as Dr. Spaan has pointed out, maybe the vasodilated bed is different. One of the questions I said nothing about is, why, when you give adenosine, does the back–pressure stay constant, independent of heart rate. Part of the answer to that is that we give large doses of adenosine and we probably paralyze any response that would be there and it might be argued that the autoregulating bed is different. We do not have a really good way at this point of distinguishing these effects, except for those measurements in the microcirculation.

Dr. J. Spaan: I would like to point out that the coronary system is not linear. The data you show is again a linear model. What does compliance and resistance in a linear model mean for a nonlinear system? Could you comment on measurements from Frank Yin's lab on the septal system where he shows that volume in the microcirculation changes very slowly when you do a pressure step. You show that if you do a pressure step, the flow has a fast equilibrium, while volume in the microcirculation changes very slowly.

Dr. R. Mates: We would argue that this is evidence that there is a regulator somewhere upstream of where that volume change takes place. Otherwise, as volume changes you would expect to see a change in inflow as you charge the distal capacitor. The fact that we do not see that in the vasodilated bed is evidence for the pressure regulator.

Dr. J. Spaan: You can also explain that by saying that during the change of volume you have a change in resistance as well, affecting the dynamic change of flow, counteracting the capacitance effect. You may have a seemingly rapid response which is basically a response of a very slow volume change within the capillary bed. The question is, if we need the intramyocardial pump.

Dr. R. Mates: I do not think anybody questions the need for the intramyocardial pump. That is certainly the only way you can explain the output. I am asking if there is, in addition to that, a need for a pressure regulator. I am trying to suggest that perhaps there is a need for it.

Dr. J. Spaan: I suggest that if you do nonlinear analysis properly, you do not need a pressure regulator because it comes out of the system.

REFERENCES

1. Bellamy RF. Diastolic coronary artery pressure–flow relations in the dog. *Circ Res* 1978; 43: 92–101.
2. Klocke FJ, Mates RE, Canty JM Jr, Ellis AE. Coronary pressure–flow relationships - controversial issue and probable implications. *Circ Res* 1985; 56: 310–323.
3. Spaan JAE. Coronary diastolic pressure–flow relation and zero flow pressure explained on the basis of intramyocardial compliance. *Circ Res* 1985 56: 293–309.
4. Fung YC. *Biomechanics - Mechanical Properties of Living Tissue*. Springer Verlag: NY, 1982, p 41.
5. Canty JM Jr, Mates RE. A programmable pressure control system for coronary flow studies. *Am J Physiol* 1982 243: H796–H802.
6. Canty JM Jr, Klocke FJ, Mates RE. Pressure and tone dependence of coronary diastolic input impedance and capacitance. *Am J Physiol* 1985; 248: H700–H711.
7. Judd RM, Redberg DA, Mates RE. Diastolic coronary resistance and capacitance are independent of duration of diastole. *Am J Physiol* 1991; 260: H943–H952.
8. Van Huis GA, Sipkema P, Westerhoff N. Coronary input impedance during the cardiac cycle as determined by impulse response method. *Am J Physiol* 1987; 253: H317–H324.
9. Judd RM, Mates RE. Coronary input impedance is constant during systole and diastole. *Am J Physiol* 1991; 260: H1841-1851.
10. Krams R, Sipkema P, Westerhof N. Varying elastance concept may explain coronary systolic flow impediment. *Am J Physiol* 1989; 257: H1471–H1479.
11. Kuo L, Chilian WM, Davis MJ. Interaction of pressure– and flow–induced responses in porcine coronary resistance vessels. *Am J Physiol* 1991; 261: H1706–H1715.
12. Chilian WM, Eastham CL, Marcus ML. Redistribution of coronary microvascular resistance produced by dipyridamole *Am J Physiol* 1989; 256: H383–H390.

CHAPTER 15

In Vivo Myocardial Microcirculation: Evaluation with a Whole–Body X–Ray CT Method

Erik L. Ritman[1]

ABSTRACT

The detailed anatomic geometry of the myocardial microvasculature is unresolvable by current "whole body" imaging techniques. An index of microvascular patency can however be provided by monitoring the intramyocardial blood content by whole body imaging methods. Both spatial distribution and intracyclic changes of regional intramyocardial blood volume can be estimated by whole–body imaging techniques such as x–ray CT and SPECT. Examples of how these methods can be used are provided.

INTRODUCTION

Resolution of blood vessels less than 0.1 mm in cross– sectional diameter throughout much of the *in vivo* heart wall, at anyone time, is currently not possible because of both technical and physiological difficulties. Very high radiation exposures, invasion of the thoracic cavity and/or long duration of the scanning period would be needed to achieve adequate signal to noise in the images and hence the scanning procedure is likely to result in unstable hemodynamics. Even if we could image the microcirculation in a small region of the heart wall, we still have the problem of not knowing how representative this set is of the entire myocardial microcirculation. If, by some unknown method, we could image a large fraction of the microcirculation – we would have the severe logistic problem of analysis of the inevitably large volume of image data.

Despite these concerns, we need to explore to what extent we can obtain quantitative information about the microcirculation even though we cannot directly measure individual vessels. One method that does appear to have immediate promise is imaging of the intramyocardial blood content as an index of the microcirculatory intravascular blood

[1]Department of Physiology & Biophysics, Mayo Clinic, Rochester, MN 55905, USA.

Interactive Phenomena in the Cardiac System, Edited by
S. Sideman and R. Beyar, Plenum Press, New York, 1993

volume [1]. This value would appear to be an index of the total lumenal volume and/or the number of intramyocardial vessels that are open to blood flow, within a selected volume of myocardium.

This overview outlines evidence that this basic proposition is supported by experimental data, that its use as an index of microvascular patency may be useful in understanding pathophysiological responses to alterations of the coronary circulation and that it may give some insight into regionality of these microcirculatory responses. Although the results discussed in this presentation were obtained with the DSR x–ray tomography and a SPECT scanner, other x–ray CT scanners [2], ultrasound [3] and MRI scanners [4] have been used to estimate regional parenchymal blood volume.

METHODS

The Dynamic Spatial Reconstructor (DSR) has been described in detail elsewhere [5]. It is an x–ray CT scanner that scans a cylindrical volume that is 21 – 50 cm in trans–verse diameter and is 18.5 cm in axial height. It scans this volume 60 times per second for up to 1200 times in any one scanning sequence. These 3D images can be "added" retro–spectively in an ECG gated manner so as to provide increased signal to noise. From selected regions of interest, within these volume images, a time sequence of image bright–ness can be constructed from which intramyocardial blood volume and blood flow can be estimated [6,7].

Figure 1 illustrates a typical relationship between myocardial blood flow and blood volume. As discussed in [6] this quadratic relationship is quite reproducible and is consis–tent with Poiseuille's law describing the relationship between the flow and vessel lumen cross–sectional area. As also pointed out in [6], the values for intramyocardial blood volume match the values obtained by other, but more invasive, methods quite well. A more

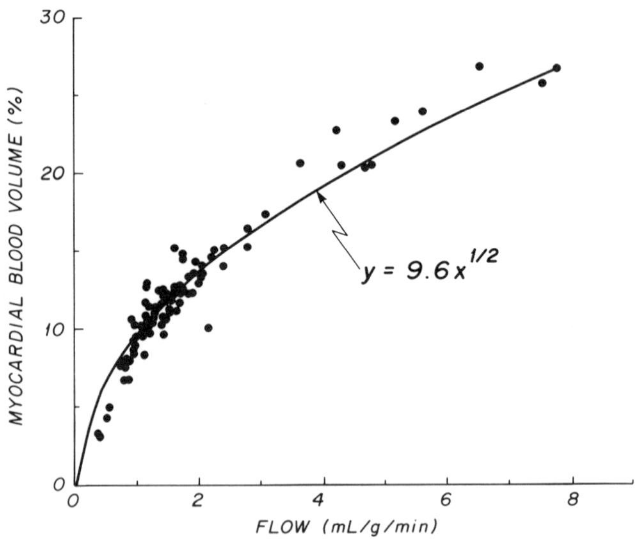

Figure 1. Scatterplot show curvilinear relations between intramyocardial blood volume (FMB) and flow (F) in the myocardium. Solid curve is the least–squares best fit of formula FMB = $a \cdot F^{1/2}$ to the experimental data points. (Reproduced with permission of the American Heart Association from [6].)

"direct" approach [8] shows that changes in myocardial blood volume are closely related to concurrent changes in myocardial volume.

The indicator dilution method for estimating intramyocardial blood volume is limited, however, in that it provides little intracycle temporal resolution. Two imaging methods have been developed to provide improved temporal resolution. One utilizes the volume encompassed by radiopaque markers attached to the epicardial and endocardial surfaces of the heart wall [9] and the other uses the alterations of intramyocardial image brightness in SPECT images of radiolabeled myocardium [10].

However, neither of these two methods provides an index of absolute intramyocardial blood volume, merely of changes. Consequently they would have to be used with the indicator dilution method if absolute responses to interventions are to be evaluated.

RESULTS

Indicator Dilution Based Method

a) Stenosis of the epicardial coronary artery [6]: Figure 2 illustrates how increasing stenosis of the epicardial coronary artery results in increasing intramyocardial blood volume. This is consistent with vasodilation of the microcirculation downstream to the stenosis. As a consequence, the downstream vascular resistance decreases and flow to the region remains essentially unchanged.

b) Embolization of microvascular vessels [6]: Figure 3 shows how progressive, selective, embolization of the myocardial arterioles with 15 micrometer microspheres results in essentially no change in the intramyocardial blood volume until 50% of the fatal dose

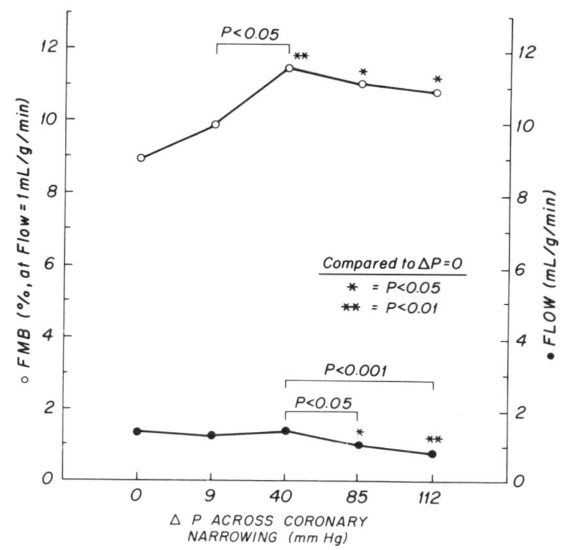

Figure 2. Figure shows myocardial perfusion characteristics in dogs with an intracoronary balloon. In resting state, the value at flow = 1 ml/g/min intramyocardial blood volume increased significantly at moderate narrowing (pressure gradient, across balloon, ΔP, ~40 mmHg), whereas flow was impaired only at more severe narrowing (ΔP ~85 mmHg). FMB – intramyocardial blood volume. (Reproduced with permission of the Americna Heart Association from [6].)

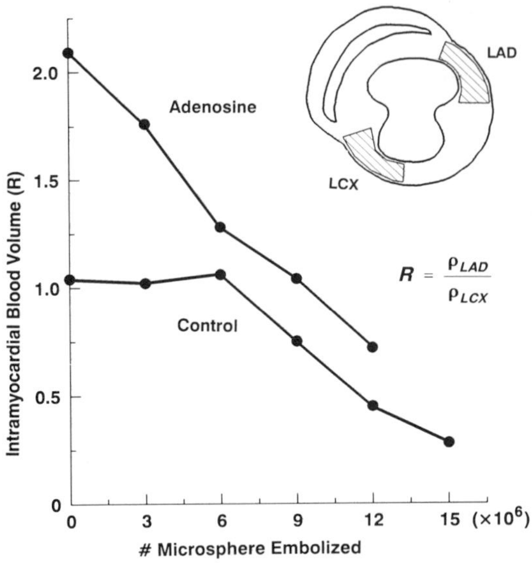

Figure 3. Increasing embolization of intramyocardial arterioles in the left anterior descending (LAD) coronary artery perfusion area results in progressive decrease in intramyocardial blood volume. Under control conditions almost 50% of the fatal dose of microspheres have to embolize before intramyocardial blood volume changes. Intramyocardial blood volume (ρ) in the embolized myocardium is expressed as the ratio R of the ρ in the LAD and the ρ in the left circumflex (LCX) arterial perfusion areas.

has been lodged. At greater doses there is a linear decrease in blood volume in proportion to the number of microspheres embolized. This observation is consistent with recruitment of microvessels in a way that maintains the constant blood volume at a particular level appropriate for the hemodynamic demands of the myocardium. This method, however, cannot distinguish between dilation and recruitment.

c) Myocardial hypertrophy [11]: Figure 4 shows the fraction of left ventricular myocardium that is intramyocardial blood estimated *in vivo* using fast CT.

One group of dogs ("adult" and "adolescents") were scanned before and after three to ten months of training, and another group was scanned without training. Following training the adolescents and adults increased LV mass over control. Adolescent training increased intramyocardial blood volume over control and decreased in adults. Consequently for adolescent hypertrophy, the total LV intramyocardial blood volume increased, whereas for adults hypertrophy intramyocardial blood volume decreased. These data suggest that training in adolescent dogs results in growth of total intramyocardial blood volume matching muscle growth but in adult dogs intramyocardial blood volume did not increase with myocardial hypertrophy.

d) Heterogeneity of myocardial perfusion [12]: If there is recruitment of microvessels, rather than vasodilation, then the heterogeneity of opacification should diminish with increase in blood volume. Such heterogeneity can be expressed via a fractal analysis of the sort illustrated in Fig. 5.

Indeed, if a statistically random recruitment of vessels occurs with increasing probability as blood flow increases then it should be possible to predict the fraction of available vessels that can be recruited [13].

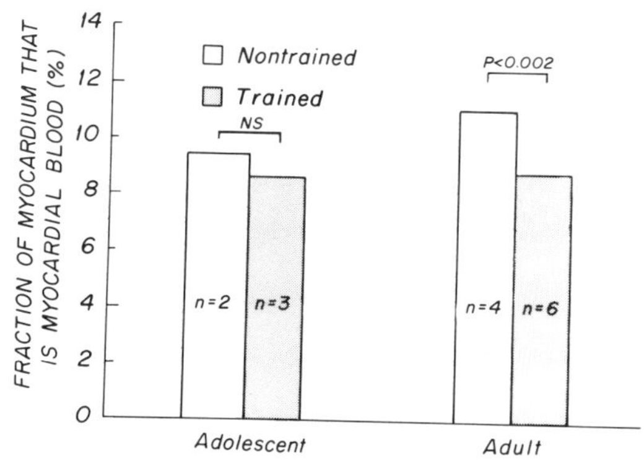

Figure 4. LV myocardial mass in nontrained and trained groups of dogs increased by a mean of 41% for adolescents and 26% for adults, respectively, over the control group. In the adolescents, the intramyocardial blood volume increased in proportion to the hypertrophy whereas in the adults it decreased with the hypertrophy.

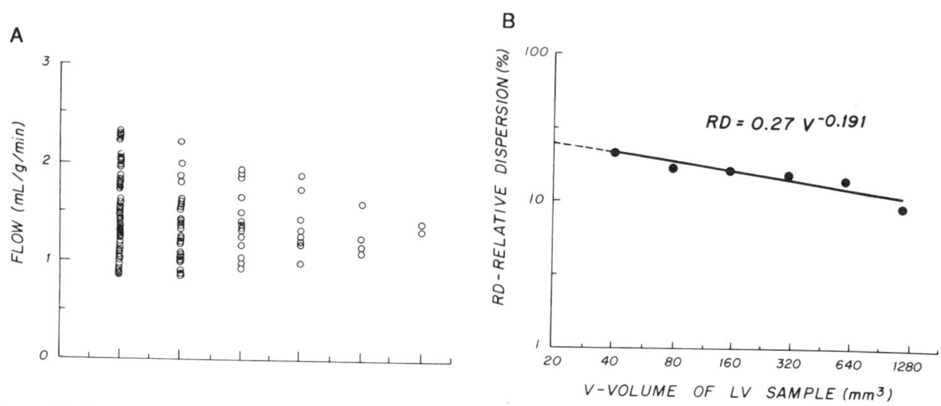

Figure 5. A sequence of fast CT images of a single, mid ventricle, slice was analyzed for myocardial perfusion—first two halves, then in four quadrants, etc. up to 64 equal size pieces around the circumference. Abscissa is same in both panels. **A:** As the volume of the region of interest decreases in size the range of the perfusion values increases but the mean value for the group remains unchanged. **B:** The log/log plot of the relative dispersion is well described by a power law relationship. (Reproduced with permission of the American Physiological Society from [13].)

Myocardial Marker–Based Methods

a) Radiopaque markers on LV wall – x–ray CT [9]: The volume encompassed by the radiopaque markers attached to the LV free wall and the CT indicator dilution method were used simultaneously from a single 3D scan sequence during anatomic root injection of roentgen contrast agent.

Using the marker–based volume of myocardium estimate of intramyocardial blood volume (V) and the simultaneous indicator dilution–based data (ρ) we have that

$$\rho = B/(B+M) \quad ; \quad V = B+M \tag{1}$$

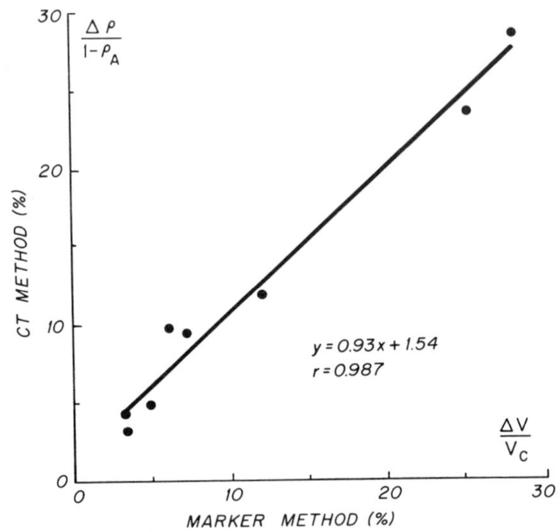

Figure 6. Comparison of computed tomography (CT) contrast dilution–based (ρ) vs. lead marker–based volume (V) methods for estimating change in intramyocardial blood volume. (Reproduced with permission from [9].)

where B is the volume of myocardium that is blood within volume V and M is the volume of myocardium that is muscle within volume V. Now

$$\Delta\rho = B_2/(B_2+M) - B_1/(B_1+M) \tag{2}$$

$$\Delta V/V_1 = (B_2-B_1)/(B_1+M) \tag{3}$$

Rearranging yields

$$\Delta\rho = M(B_2-B_1)/[(B_2+M)(B_1+M)] = (1-\rho_2)[\Delta V/V_1] \tag{4}$$

Hence

$$\Delta\rho/(1-\rho_2) = \Delta V/V_1 \tag{5}$$

The relationship between these two methods is illustrated in Fig. 6.

b) Radiolabeled microspheres – SPECT [10]: SPECT image average brightness results are illustrated in Fig. 7. Again, this method does not provide an absolute value for intramyocardial blood volume, but its change can be computed as illustrated by the following analysis:

$$Br = KN/(M+B) \quad V = (M+B)L \tag{6}$$

$$BR/BR_{max} = (M+B_{min})/(M+B) \quad V/V_{min} = (M+B)/(M+B_{min}) \tag{7}$$

hence

$$BR_{max}/Br = V/V_{min} \tag{8}$$

where Br is the image brightness/voxel over myocardium; V is the volume encompassed by lead beads; M is the volume of myocardium that is muscle; B is the volume of

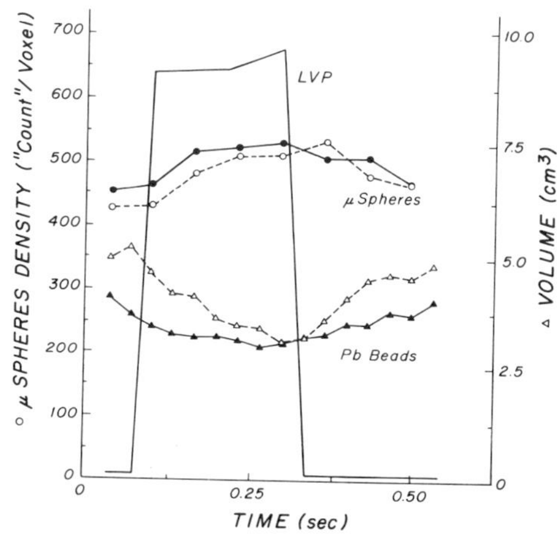

Figure 7. Comparison of myocardial volume changes during one cardiac cycle. Solid line is control condition and dashed line is adenosine (1 mg/kg/min) infusion. (LVP maintenance with inflation of intra aortic balloon.) The volume encompassed by eight lead beads on the epicardial and endocardial surface shows decrease in volume (i.e. expression of blood from) of the myocardium, and the SPECT data show an increase in myocardial count density. These results suggest blood is squeezed out of the myocardium during systole.

myocardium that is blood; K and L are constants; and N is the number of μ spheres in the heart wall.

It is of interest to note that both the lead marker and SPECT methods suggest that the blood volume at peak systole is essentially invariate whereas it changes at end diastole by an amount depending on the hemodynamics.

CONCLUSIONS

The fast x-ray CT tomographic imaging method permits analysis of average behavior of the intramyocardial microvascular vessels. Additional work needs to be done on the mathematical models used to translate the image data into the physiologically meaningful results.

Acknowledgements

I wish to thank Ms. Delories Darling for typing this manuscript and my colleagues for their work which I quoted. This work was supported in part by National Institutes of Health grants HL-04664 and HL-43025.

DISCUSSION

Dr. Y. Kresh: Is there recruitment of the microvasculature? Is there also recruitment of active myocytes? Are some myocytes sitting, blinking, waiting on-demand to respond to increased perfusion? The "idle" myocytes may be recruited; that may explain/suggest that the function is autoregulated.

Dr. E. Ritman: I am not quite sure. Others would know better than I do about entire myocytes. But I believe that within the myocytes there is some evidence that certain sarcomeres turn on and off, so it is not a homogeneous on or off type situation. Whether the perfusion turn on and off correlate exactly with, say, whatever part of the muscle it is turning on and off, I do not know, but that would be an interesting study.

Dr. E. Feigl: Your values are that the intramyocardial blood volume is about 8%. Is that correct?

Dr. E. Ritman: Yes, under the control conditions, which in my animals are anesthetized and are on their back with a closed chest.

Dr. E. Feigl: What are the numbers relative to 8% in the cardiac cycle?

Dr. E. Ritman: We have not been able to study the variation during the cardiac cycle with the indicator dilution method. So that is why we used the lead–bead or microsphere method. Both methods suggest that there are quite large changes in the intramyocardial volume, from 8% to 12%, for instance.

Dr. E. Feigl: Is it oscillating about 8%, 7–12 or 6–11? are those reasonable guesses?

Dr. E. Ritman: Yes.

Dr. E. Feigl: Where do you think that oscillation is occurring? Take a guess.

Dr. E. Ritman: The SPECT data suggests that the end–systolic minima in intramyocardial blood volume is independent of the systolic pressure. The changes therefore are in diastolic blood content, which suggest that changes depend very much on the diastolic hemodynamic conditions.

Dr. F. Prinzen: Can recruitment also include vasomotion? That means that every arteriole is closing and opening in a certain rhythm?

Dr. E. Ritman: Yes, I believe it is something like that and related perhaps to the "twinkling" that people have talked about for many years. For example, if there are 100 capillary beds, or arteriolar beds at any one time under control conditions, only 50% of them are open. Each one of the 100 would be opening and closing with a certain cycle, maybe minutes. Statistically it works out that only 50% are open at any one time.

Dr. J. Spaan: If it really goes from 6–11%, then you need to have much more versatility in arterial and venous flow to accommodate those volume changes. I feel those volume changes are at the high side. You find a relation between flow and volume but you expect volume to be at a site where there is a low resistance, so how do you explain that parabolic relationship?

R. E. Ritman: I was amazed when we put the lead markers on the myocardium, on the epicardium and endocardium, to see the large changes in volume we saw during the cardiac cycle. About a year ago, Leon Axel, of the Univ. of Pennsylvania, who has been working with the MRI striping method doing something very similar, also came up with very large volume changes in the myocardium and was concerned about that. He then used the same program to analyze our bead data and came up with similar answers. All I can say is that we find big changes in the volume of the myocardium. Now if that is all due to changes in intramyocardial coronary circulation, or to what extent that is at the endocardial trabeculation squeezing in and out, remains to be demonstrated. But there are large changes in volume.

As to the parabolic relationship between flow and volume. Poiseuille's Law says that the flow is proportional to the radius to the fourth power, which is the cross–sectional area squared. If the length of the microvessels does not change much, then volume that we estimate should be proportional to the sum of the cross-sectional areas, so that by Poiseuille's Law, flow would be proportional to the volumes squared. I can not tell you exactly what this volume measurement that we come up with means in the anatomic sequence from arteries to veins. That is why I am stimulated to look at the longitudinal problem, that is look at the entire circulation from epicardial vessel to the capillaries in continuity by high spatial resolution imaging methods.

REFERENCES

1. Iwasaki T, Ritman EL. Intramyocardial blood volume dynamics in the cardiac cycle (abstract). *Fed Proc* 1984; 43: 422.
2. Rumberger JA, Bell MR, Sheedy PF, Stanson AF. *in vivo* quantitation of intramyocardial blood volume by ultrafast computed tomography. *Circulation* 1988; 78: II-398.
3. Kaul S, Glasheen W, Ruddy TD, Pandian NG, Weyman AE, Okada RD. The importance of defining left ventricular area at risk *in vivo* during acute myocardial infarction: an experimental evaluation with myocardial contrast two-dimensional echocardiography. *Circulation* 1987; 75: 1249-1260.
4. Sandman CA, O'Halloran JP, Isenhart R. Is there an evoked vascular response? *Science* 1984; 224: -1355-1357.
5. Jorgensen SM, Whitlock SV, Thomas PJ, Roessler RW, Ritman EL. The dynamic spatial reconstructor: A high speed, stop action, 3-D, digital radiographic imager of moving internal organs and blood. *Proc SPIE, Ultrahigh- and High-Speed Photography, Videography, Photonics, and Velocimetry '90* 1990; 1346: 180-191.
6. Wu XS, Ewert DL, Liu YH, Ritman EL. *in vivo* relation of intramyocardial blood volume to myocardial perfusion: evidence supporting microvascular site for autoregulation. *Circulation* 1992; 85: 730-737.
7. Wang T, Wu X, Chung N, Ritman EL. Myocardial blood flow estimated by synchronous, multislice, high-speed computed tomography. *IEEE Trans Med Imaging* 1989; 8: 70-77.
8. Wu X, Chung N, Ritman EL. Phasic distribution of *in vivo* intramyocardial blood volume estimated using fast CT (abstract). *FASEB J* 1989; 3: A405.
9. Liu YH, Bahn RC, Ritman EL. Dynamic intramyocardial blood volume: evaluation with a radiological opaque marker method. *Am J Physiol* 1992; 263: H963-H967.
10. Behrenbeck T, Foley DA, O'Connor MK, Ritman EL. Cyclic variation of the intramyocardial blood volume/muscle mass ratio (BV/MM) in intact dog model (abstract). *FASEB J* 1993; 7:A319.
11. Wu X, Chung N, Stray-Gundersen J, Ritman EL. Intramyocardial blood volume in dogs with exercise hypertrophy (abstract). *The Physiol* 1988; 31: A218.
12. Shu NH, Haydock C, Ritman EL. Recruitment of myocardial arteriolar beds - estimation by fractal analysis of fast CT images (abstract). *FASEB J* 1990; 4: A587.
13. Liu YH, Shu NH, Ritman EL. A fast CT imaging method for indicator dilution analysis. *Am J Cardiac Imaging* 1993; in press.

CHAPTER 16

ENDOCARDIAL CORONARY MICROCIRCULATION OF THE BEATING HEART

Fumihiko Kajiya, Toyotaka Yada, Akihiro Kimura, Osamu Hiramatsu, Masami Goto, Yasuo Ogasawara, and Katsuhiko Tsujioka[1]

ABSTRACT

Direct and continuous observation of subendocardial (deep myocardial) microcirculation provides essential information on coronary circulation, since cardiac contraction affects subendocardial vessels most vigorously. To achieve this aim, we developed a portable needle–probe video–microscope with a charge–coupled–device (CCD) camera to visualize the subendocardial microcirculation. Images of the subendocardial microcirculation of a porcine beating heart were successfully observed in all cases. The vascular compression by cardiac contraction decreased the diameter of subendocardial arterioles and venules by about 20%.

INTRODUCTION

The phasic flows in the left coronary artery and vein are unlike those of other organs; the arterial flow is restricted to diastole, whereas the venous flow is restricted to systole [1–4]. Figure 1 shows an example of velocity waveforms in a small epicardial artery (150–400 μm) of the left ventricle just before its penetration into the myocardium, and in a small vein just after its emergence from the myocardium. These velocities were measured by a laser Doppler method with an optical fiber and the fiber tip (velocity sensor: core diameter 0.05 mm) was fixed on the outer surface of the vessel by a drop of cyano–acrylate. The measurement of small arteries and veins enables us to evaluate coronary artery inflow and venous outflow of myocardium without the capacitance effect of epicardial vessels.

---

[1]Department of Medical Engineering and Systems Cardiology, Kawasaki Medical School, Kurashiki 701–01, Japan.

Interactive Phenomena in the Cardiac System, Edited by
S. Sideman and R. Beyar, Plenum Press, New York, 1993

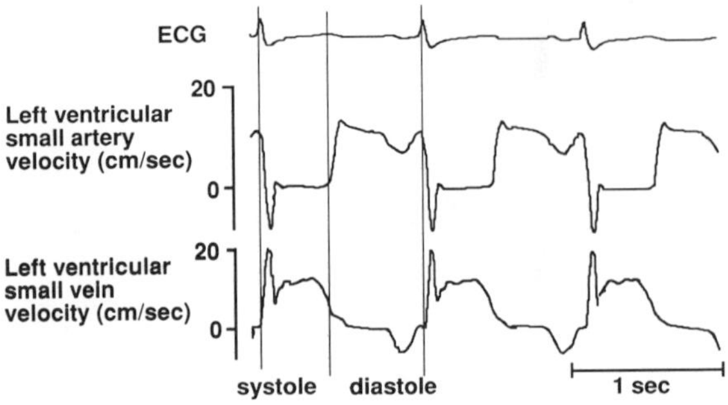

Figure 1. An example of velocity waveforms in a small epicardial artery of the left ventricle just before its penetration into the myocardium, and in a small vein just after its emergence from the myocardium. The velocity waveform of coronary arterial inflow into the left ventricular myocardium is almost exclusively diastolic, which is opposite to the arterial flows of other organs, i.e., systolic–predominant flow. Inversely, the coronary venous outflow from the myocardium is predominantly systolic. In addition, there were small reverse flows both in the arterial (systolic) and venous (diastolic) flows.

This unique pattern of coronary arterial and venous flow was already noticed in 1695 by Scaramucci [5] who today is considered as the founder of coronary physiology. He hypothesized that the deeper coronary vessels are squeezed by the contraction of the muscle fiber around them, which displaces the intramyocardial blood into the coronary veins, and that the vessels are refilled from the aorta during diastole. To prove the hypothesis directly, it is necessary to observe subendocardial (deep myocardial) micro–circulation in an *in vivo* beating heart. If such an observation is possible, it should also greatly contribute to the understanding of higher vulnerability of the subendocardial muscle to ischemia by giving a new information about the time sequential responses of subendocardial microcirculation to various interventions.

Direct *in vivo* observation of the subendomyocardial circulation has been hampered, however, mainly by the lack of appropriate optical technology to investigate subendo–myocardial vessels, and only subepimyocardial microcirculation has been analyzed by sophisticated microscopic systems [6–9]. To overcome this limitation, we developed a portable needle–probe video–microscope with a charge–coupled device (CCD) camera and succeeded to obtain an access to subendocardial microvessels [10, 11].

METHODS

Optical System

Figure 2 is the photograph of the needle–probe video–microscope. The system consists of a needle–probe, a camera body containing a CCD camera, a lens and light guides, a control unit, a light source, a monitor and a videocassette recorder (VCR). The camera body has a 1/2–inch CCD image sensor, about 250 thousand pixels and 330–line horizontal resolution.

The needle–probe (diameter: 4.5 mm) contains a gradient index (GRIN) lens surrounded by an annular light guide. One end of the needle–probe is attached to the camera body with a focusing system. The image passes through the GRIN lens and focuses on the CCD image sensor. This is monitored and recorded on a videotape. The tissue is

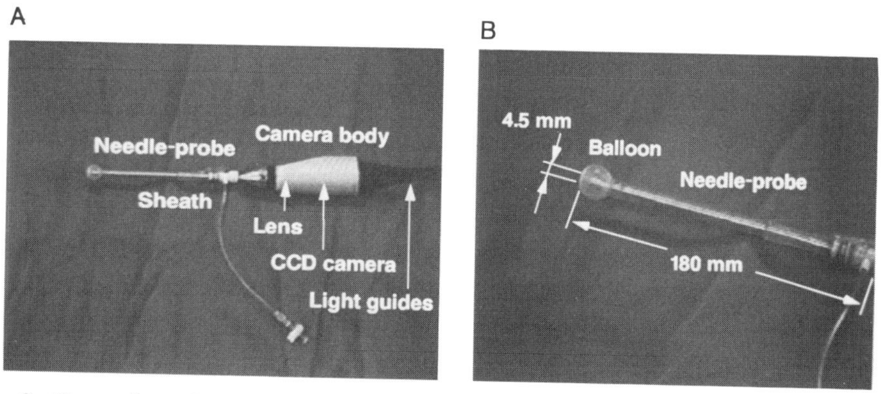

Figure 2. The needle–probe video–microscope with a CCD camera and a silastic double lumen sheath (A), and their expanded images (B). A needle–probe containing a gradient–index (GRIN) lens is used to obtain the images of the subendocardial microcirculation of the left ventricle.

illuminated by light from a halogen lamp, which is transmitted through light guides surrounding the GRIN lens. A green filter is used to accentuated the contrast between the image of the vessel and the surrounding tissue. Since both the vessel and the tissue have strong component of red, red does not provides good contrast and must be filtered from the image. The needle–probe is enclosed in a Silastic 14F double lumen sheath, with a doughnut–shaped balloon at its tip (See Fig. 2). Blood between the tip of the needle–probe and the endocardial surface inside the doughnut is flushed away with Krebs–Hensleit buffer solution injected through a microtube to obtain a clear image.

Animal Preparation

Eleven pigs were anesthetized with ketamine and sodium pentobarbital. The right carotid artery and the right jugular vein were catheterized for hemodynamic and arterial blood gas measurements and for fluid and drug administration. Blood pressures were measured in the ascending aorta and the left ventricle. Electrocardiograms were recorded by standard leads. Following a medium sternotomy and a left thoracotomy through the fifth intercostal space, the heart was exposed and suspended in a pericardial cradle. The proximal portions of the left anterior descending coronary artery was isolated so that brief occlusion could be made. The sheathed needle–probe was introduced into the left ventricle via an incision in the left atrial appendage and the mitral valve (Fig. 3). The inflated doughnut balloon was gently placed against the endocardial surface and the intervening blood was flushed away with Krebs–Hensleit buffer solution.

RESULTS

We have found subendocardial microvessels in all cases studied, although it has been difficult to find an appropriate vessel in some cases due to wide variation in vessel distribution in subendocardium.

Figure 4 shows typical images of a subendocardial arteriole and venule at end–systole and end–diastole. Arterioles and venules were differentiated by the direction of movement of blood cells and/or the sequence in which blood refilled the vessels following a transient occlusion of the anterior descending coronary arteries and/or an injection of indocyamine green. Although the diameters of subendocardial arterioles and venules decreased significantly from end–diastole to end–systole as can be seen in Fig. 4, we usually did not observe any collapse of these vessels during systole. Very rarely, segmental collapse was observed. Pinching, kinking and stretching of subendocardial vessels were observed partly in both arterioles and venules, although their degrees varied individually. The image density of both arterioles and venules decreased at end–systole in comparison with that at end–diastole in all cases. This may indicate that the diameter in the vertical direction also decreases from end–diastole to end–systole.

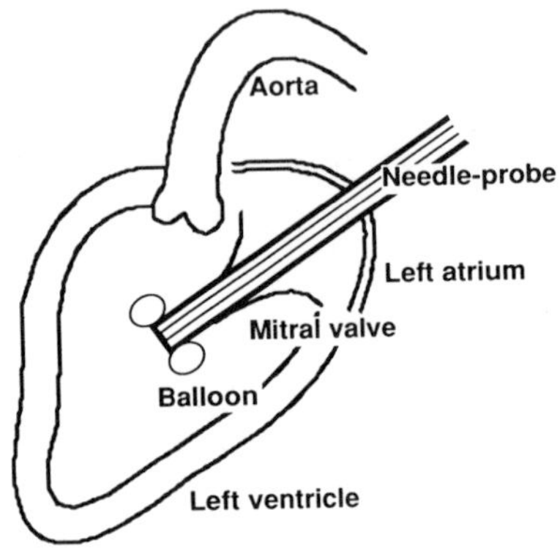

Figure 3. Experimental preparations carried out for the observation of subendocardial arterioles and venules of the porcine left ventricle with the needle–probe video–microscope. The sheathed needle–probe was introduced into the left ventricle via an incision in the left atrial appendage and the mitral valve. The balloon was inflated to prevent compression of the endocardial microcirculation by the needle–probe and the intervening blood between the needle–probe and endocardium was flushed away with a Krebs–Hensleit buffer solution.

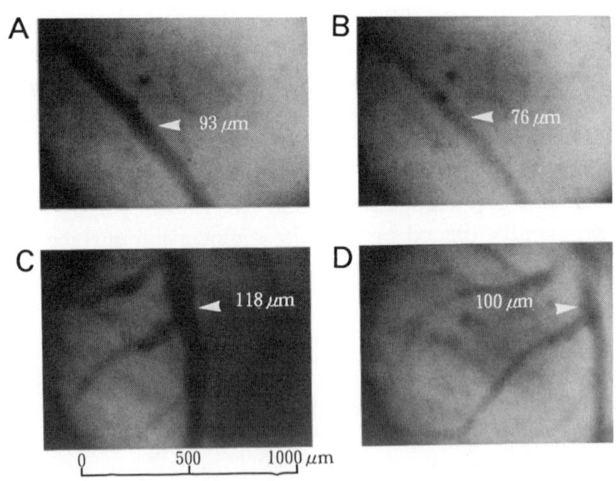

Figure 4. Images of a subendocardial arteriole and venule at end–systole and end–diastole. A green filter was used to contrast the images of the vessels against surrounding tissue. The diameter was measured by marking the branch portion of the vessel. **A:** Image of a subendocardial arteriole at end–diastole, **B:** Image of a subendocardial arteriole at end–systole, **C:** Image of a subendocardial venule at end–diastole, **D:** Image of a subendocardial venule at end–systole.

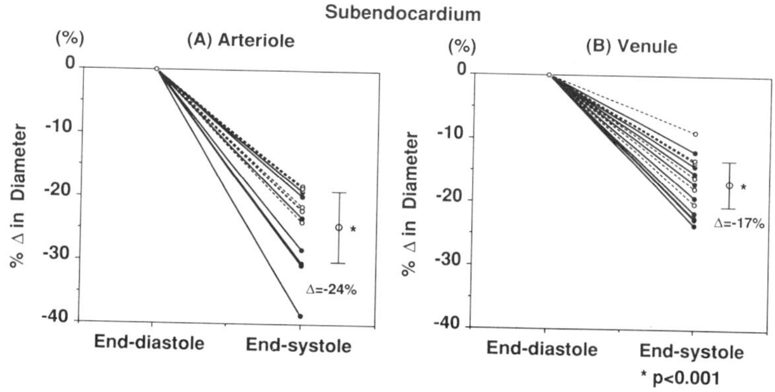

Figure 5. The percent diameter changes (%Δ) of subendocardial arterioles **(A)** and venules **(B)**. Solid lines indicate the vessels with diameter greater than 100 μm and dotted lines the vessels with diameter less than 100 μm. Subendocardial arteriolar diameter decreased by about 24% and venular diameter decreased by about 17%.

Figure 5 shows the percent diameter changes in arterioles and venules between end–diastole and end–systole. The diameter was measured for the vascular segment with a relatively uniform change along the vessels. Arteriole diameter decreased by about 24% and venule diameter decreased by about 17%. It seems that the vessels with smaller diameters are less pulsatile than larger vessels.

DISCUSSION

The changes in subendocardial arterioles and venules differ greatly from those of the epimyocardial microcirculation. Kanatsuka et al. [12] observed only 1.1% diameter change of the left ventricular epimyocardial arterioles during a cardiac cycle as measured by an intravital microscopic system. Nellis et al. [13] reported 20% *increase* in the right ventricular venular diameter just after end–systole as measured by a transillumination microscope with a cardiac cycle–synchronized light source. Using systolically and diastolically arrested hearts, Goto et al. [14] showed that cardiac contraction affects deep myocardial small arterioles and capillaries predominantly. Judd and Levy [15] used arrested hearts with several species under various experimental conditions, and found significant decrease in vascular volume by cardiac contraction. The results of both Goto et al. and Judd and Levy are consistent in showing a significantly smaller diameter of subendocardial vessels in the systolic arrest than that in the diastolic arrest, and they are consistent with our present findings. The degrees of the subendocardial arteriolar and venular diameter changes indicate that the vascular compression by myocardial contraction increased arteriolar resistance by about three times and venular resistance by about two times as compared with their diastolic resistance, assuming that Poiseulle's law holds for the calculation of resistance and that the change in diameter in the vertical direction is similar to that in the horizontal direction.

It was demonstrated that the novel portable needle–probe video–microscope with a CCD camera is a powerful tool for observing changes in the diameter of subendocardial small vessels during a cardiac cycle and on a beat–to–beat basis. The vascular compression by cardiac contraction decreased the diameters of subendocardial arteriole and venule remarkably with partial kinking and pinching of the vessels.

Acknowledgements

We thank Miss Chikako Tokuda and Mr. Hiroyuki Tachibana for excellent technical assistance and Miss Kazue Nishizaki for secretarial help. This work was supported by Grant–in–Aid 03454259 for Scientific Research (B) and Grant–in–Aid 03670471 for Scientific Research (C) from the Ministry of Education, Science, and Culture, Japan. We are grateful to the American Heart Association, Inc. for permission to reproduce part of our paper published in Circulation Research, vol. 72, 1993 "In Vivo Observation of Subendocardial Microvessels of the Beating Porcine Heart Using a Needle–probe Video–microscope with a CCD Camera."

DISCUSSION

Dr. R. Beyar: When comparing the results of our nonlinear modeling of the transmural distribution with your measurements, I see two things which are in common. As shown before, the range of compression of venules and arterioles, which are at the 100μ range, is about 20%; larger vessels show larger compression values. Our model shows the same feature, i.e. larger vessels have larger diameter changes. To me, at least, this is an indirect suggestion that the nonlinear RC modeling may be compatible with the observations and that it does not contradict the waterfall concept in general, because what happens is that the larger vessels undergo large diameter change, leading to larger changes in the resistance. That is in fact a waterfall, or a partial collapse, at the level of the veins exiting from the myocardium.

Dr. F. Kajiya: Concerning the change of the arterioles and venules, it was difficult to interpret that straightforward. As you know, there are many models or theories to explain the extravascular compressive forces but we cannot discriminate between each other, since each force can interact. So I do not think it is possible to discriminate what kind of force is dominant. As to the second point—We have observed the partial collapse of the subendocardial vessels in some cases. I think that in some place in the myocardium, waterfall–like phenomena can occur. But generally, we can not account for this kind of collapse.

Dr. J. Bassingthwaighte: In looking at microfil casted dog ventricle, we see relatively few large vessels toward the endocardium and they are not on the surface of the endocardium except for the four Thebesian veins. Would you comment on how many of these arterioles and venules you might be able to see from the ventricular cavity and how deeply you can see into the myocardium?

Dr. F. Kajiya: That is a very important question. The maximum depth of the field is about ±250 μ. So we can not focus the vessels deeper than 500 μ from the endocardial surface. Above that it is difficult to get clear images. The lower vascular density in subendocardium is true. Accordingly, it is very difficult to find arterioles and/or venules in the subendocardium. We searched very carefully to find appropriate size of vessels by changing the visual field. We started this experiment using pigs, but it was a little bit easier to find arterioles and/or venules in the dog than in pigs. Now we are studying mostly dogs. It is true that finding appropriate arterioles and venules is difficult.

Dr. N. Westerhof: When the LV pressure is 100 mmHg in the subendocardial area and you see a vein with a mean pressure of 20 mmHg, how do you explain that the diameter changes so little?

Dr. F. Kajiya: At first I was surprised. I expected that the venous diameter would change more, but actually the change was almost the same as that of arterioles. For explanation it is convenient to introduce the time–varying elastance model proposed by your group. The elastance model may explain the similar diameter changes in the arterioles and venules. But, as I explained earlier, it is difficult to differentiate each compressive force.

Dr. R. Chadwick: You were measuring one particular diameter, the one that is in the image plane. My question concerns the diameter perpendicular to that plane. Using optical density, were you making some statement about diameter changes perpendicular to the one you measured? I am concerned about converting diameter to area change.

Dr. F. Kajiya: The reason why we measured vascular green color density was to get some information about the diameter change in depth. At this moment it is difficult to convert the density information into diameter straight forwardly, but the diastolic increase in the vascular diameters in the horizontal plain was consistent with the increase in diastolic vascular green color density in depth.

Dr. T. Arts: This is more or less similar to the question Dr. Chadwick just asked. The circumference is shortening very much and I guess that the vessels are generally in parallel with the muscle fibers. I can imagine that the diameter projection decreases but in the other direction you have a very high wall thickening so I would expect that vessels are stretched along the thickness of the wall. You observed, or lets say you have an idea, that the opposite occurs. So, I have a problem.

Dr. F. Kajiya: No data is available other than vascular green color density. The density may be suitable for the diameter estimation in depth direction. It decreased during systole, indicating the diameter of the depth also decreased during systole. However, it is difficult to convert the density information into diameter change quantitatively at this moment.

Dr. S. Sideman: Does your method have the potential for measuring red cell velocity at some point?

Dr. F. Kajiya: The light illumination of the present system was not strong enough to observe fluorescent imaging. Accordingly, we need a more powerful way to visualize fluorescent particles to evaluate red cell velocity. Then it will be possible.

Dr. E. Feigl: I would just like to comment to all of the modelers that these are real measurements which you have to take into account. While we can argue about some of the fine points, there is clear evidence that the inner layer is squeezed much more than the outer layer and we have to have a model which shows that.

REFERENCES

1. Anrep GV, Cruickshank EWH, Downing AC, Subba Rau A. The coronary circulation in relation to the cardiac cycle. *Heart* 1927; 14: 111–133.
2. Wiggers CJ. The interplay of coronary vascular resistance and myocardial compression in regulating coronary flow. *Circ Res* 1954; 2: 271–279.
3. Gregg DE, Fisher LG. *Handbook of Physiology*. In: Hamilton WF, Dow P, eds. American Physiological Society. Washington DC 1963; 1517–1584.
4. Kajiya F, Hiramatsu O, Mito K, Tadaoka S, Ogasawara Y, Tsujioka K. Evaluation of coronary blood flow by fiber–optic laser Doppler velocimeter. In: Kajiya F, Klassen GA, Spaan JAE, Hoffman JIE, eds. *Coronary Circulation*, Basic mechanism and clinical relevance, Tokyo: Springer–Verlag 1990; 43–53.
5. Scaramucci J. Theoremata familiaria viros eruditos consulentia de variis physico–medicis lucubrationibus juxta leges mecanicas: *Apud Joannem Baptistam Bustum* 1695; 70–81.
6. Ashikawa K, Kanatsuka H, Suzuki T, Takishima T. Phasic blood flow velocity pattern in epimyocardial microvessels in the beating canine left ventricle. *Circ Res* 1986; 59: 704–711.
7. Nellis SH, Liedtke AJ, Whitesell L. Small coronary vessel pressure and diameter in an intact beating rabbit heart using fixed–position and free–motion techniques. *Circ Res* 1981; 48: 342–353.

8. Tillmanns H, Ikeda S, Hansen H, Sarma JSM, Fauvel JM, Bing RJ. Microcirculation in the ventricle of the dog and turtle. *Circ Res* 1974; 34: 561–569.
9. Chilian WM, Eastham CL, Marcus ML. Microvascular distribution of coronary vascular resistance in beating left ventricle. *Am J Physiol* 1986; 251: H779–H788.
10. Kajiya F, Goto M, Yada T, Kimura A, Yamamoto T, Hiramatsu O, Ogasawara Y, Tsujioka K, Yamamori S, Hosaka S. In-vivo evaluation blood vessels by a new needle type CCD microscope (Abstract). *Circulation* 1991; 84: II–271 (Suppl II).
11. Yada T, Kimura A, Yamamoto T, Hiramatsu O, Goto M, Ogasawara Y, Tsujioka K, Kajiya F. Nitroglycerin dilates larger coronary venules both in epicardium and endocardium (Abstract). *Circulation* 1991; 84: II–673 (Suppl II).
12. Kanatsuka H, Lamping KG, Eastham CL, Dellsperger KC, Marcus ML. Comparison of the effects of increased myocardial oxygen consumption and adenosine on the coronary microvascular resistance. *Circ Res* 1989; 65: 1296–1305.
13. Nellis SH, Whitesell L. Phasic pressures and diameters in small epicardial veins of the unrestrained heart. *Am J Physiol* 1989; 257: H1056–H1061.
14. Goto M, Flynn AE, Doucette JW, Jansen CMA, Stork MM, Coggins DL, Muehrcke DD, Husseini WK, Hoffman JIE. Cardiac contraction affects deep myocardial vessels predominantly. *Am J Physiol* 1991; 261: H1417–H1429.
15. Judd RM, Levy BI. Effects of barium-induced cardiac contraction on large- and small-vessel intramyocardial blood volume. *Circ Res* 1991; 68: 217–225.

CHAPTER 17

DISTRIBUTION AND CONTROL OF CORONARY MICROVASCULAR RESISTANCE

Christopher J. H. Jones[1], Lih Kuo[2], Michael J. Davis[2], and William M. Chilian[2]

ABSTRACT

Coronary blood flow depends upon the vascular resistance distributed non-uniformly within the coronary microcirculation. Coronary microvascular resistance is governed by metabolic, myogenic, endothelial and neurohumoral influences. A number of these control mechanisms interact locally within a microvascular segment. In addition, these control mechanisms occupy differing longitudinal response gradients, a feature which maximizes their potential for the synergistic control of flow.

INTRODUCTION

Coronary blood flow is determined by coronary microvascular resistance, which is normally closely matched to the metabolic demand posed by myocardial oxygen consumption. Resistance is non-uniformly distributed within the coronary microcirculation. Phasic coronary microvascular pressures measured at different levels within the microcirculation of the beating heart indicate that 95% of total coronary microvascular resistance resides in microvessels less than 300 μm in diameter, and that more than 50% resides in arterioles less than 100 μm in diameter [1]. Coronary dilatation by papaverine leads to a redistribution of resistance towards larger coronary arterioles and venules. The matching of coronary blood flow to myocardial metabolism is achieved by the concerted action of metabolic, myogenic, endothelial and neurohumoral influences on the tone of coronary microvessels. Whilst these controlling mechanisms operate throughout the coronary microcirculation, there is increasing evidence of segmental differences in their relative contributions to microvascular tone. We speculate that the combination of

[1]Department of Cardiology, University of Wales College of Medicine, Cardiff, UK and [2]Texas A&M University, Health Science Center, College Station, TX 77843-1114, USA.

Interactive Phenomena in the Cardiac System, Edited by
S. Sideman and R. Beyar, Plenum Press, New York, 1993

regionally varying resistance and control of resistance is an important factor underlying appropriate changes in coronary blood flow in response to altered demand.

METABOLIC CONTROL

Coronary microvascular dilatation by metabolites produced within the myocardial parenchyma constitutes the major mechanism controlling the rapid changes in coronary blood flow that follow a change in myocardial oxygen consumption [2]. An increase in myocardial work leads rapidly to the increased production of vasodilatory metabolites. This is a potentially autoregulatory mechanism, since an initial increase in coronary flow will be followed by an increase in microvascular tone and resistance due to the wash–out of metabolites. Conversely, resistance will tend to fall following an initial reduction in coronary blood flow, due to the accumulation of metabolites. Myocardial metabolites dilate coronary microvessels non–uniformly, changing the distribution of resistance with the microvascular network. Endogenously produced or exogenously administered adenosine, a putative major vasodilatory metabolite, preferentially dilates microvessels <150 μm in diameter [3, 4]. A similar pattern of microvascular dilatation has been observed during modest reductions in coronary perfusion pressure [5], during short coronary occlusions [6] and during an increase in myocardial oxygen consumption caused by rapid cardiac pacing [4]. Despite the similarity of these dilatory response gradients to that observed with adenosine, metabolic vasodilatation is undoubtedly a complex process, mediated by the action of other metabolites, and even perhaps hypoxia and acidosis. The cellular mechanism by which these mediators induce smooth muscle relaxation is currently a subject of uncertainty. Closure of ATP–sensitive K^+ channels by glibenclamide attenuates coronary arteriolar dilatation during reductions in coronary perfusion pressure *in vivo* [7], suggesting that these membrane bound channels play a role in the autoregulation of flow. Furthermore, hypoxia dilates coronary microvessels *in vitro*, due to the release of prostaglandins [8]. Whatever the mechanisms, the net result of predominantly distal arteriolar dilatation will be not only a reduction in total resistance, but also a substantial shift in the major site of resistance to larger coronary microvessels because these vessels do not dilate to the same extent as smaller ones during functional hyperemia. Evidence is accumulating that resistance in these larger microvessels is reduced by substantially different mechanisms, namely their myogenic responsiveness and their capacity for endothelium–dependent dilatation in response to flow.

MYOGENIC CONTROL

The myogenic responsiveness of vascular smooth muscle may be defined as its intrinsic tendency to contract in response to an increase in transmural pressure, or stretch, and to relax when transmural pressure, or stretch, is decreased [9]. In a microvascular network, myogenic responsiveness will contribute to autoregulation, since changes in coronary blood flow are often associated with changes in coronary perfusion pressure. The existence of the myogenic response in the coronary microcirculation remained unknown for many years due to the difficulties in separating the microvascular responses to pressure and flow, and to the difficulties in controlling coronary pressure independently of changes in myocardial oxygen consumption. These difficulties were overcome by the development of techniques enabling the study of coronary microvessels, isolated from surrounding microvessels and myocardium and perfused in a system allowing independent control of intravascular pressure and flow. Using these techniques, Kuo et al. showed in 1988 that porcine coronary arterioles between 80 and 100 μm in diameter exhibit myogenic responses to increases and decreases in transmural pressure [10]. The myogenic response in these vessels was subsequently shown to be independent of an intact endothelium, and therefore an intrinsic property of microvascular smooth muscle [11].

As in other microvascular networks, myogenic responses to pressure appear to play their greatest role in governing the tone of intermediate size coronary arterioles [12]. Since the major site of myogenic control of tone is different from that of metabolic control, which predominates in the smallest arterioles, myogenic responsiveness might play a synergistic role in amplifying a change in coronary microvascular resistance which occurs in response to a change in myocardial metabolic demand. Indeed, we have speculated previously that metabolic dilatation of terminal arterioles reduces local arteriolar pressure and by this means stimulates to a further reduction in resistance mediated by myogenic dilatation of slightly larger vessels [13]. An important consequence of the dilatation mediated by the synergistic action of metabolic and myogenic control mechanisms will be a further shift in the major site of coronary microvascular resistance towards larger microvessels. It has been suggested that further amplification of the initial metabolic signal may occur in these larger vessels, due to the influence of flow–dependent dilatation mediated by the vascular endothelium.

ENDOTHELIAL CONTROL

Flow–dependent dilatation occurs in coronary microvessels, as it does in large epicardial coronary arteries. Kuo et al. demonstrated that isolated porcine coronary arterioles between 40 and 80 μm in diameter exhibit graded dilatation in response to graded increases in flow with intraluminal pressure held constant [14]. Increases in flow but not pressure were achieved by adjusting the height of perfusion reservoirs attached to each cannulating micropipette. By moving the reservoirs by equal distances in opposite directions, a pressure gradient for flow was introduced with no change in mean arteriolar pressure. The flow–dependent dilatation of arterioles was abolished by mechanical removal of endothelium, indicating its endothelium–dependence. A microvascular bioassay technique was used subsequently to demonstrate that flow–dependent dilatation is mediated by a transferable substance released by endothelium [15]. Furthermore, flow–dependent arteriolar dilatation was shown to be unaffected by inhibition of prostaglandin synthesis by indomethacin, but to be abolished by incubation with N^G–monomethyl–L–arginine (L–NMMA), an inhibitor of nitric oxide synthase. These experiments indicated that flow–dependent dilatation in the coronary microcirculation was mediated by a nitrovasodilator or endothelium–derived relaxing factor (EDRF)–like substance.

Flow–dependent dilatation of coronary microvessels, mediated through endothelial transduction of wall shear stress, may play an important role in the segmental control of coronary microvascular resistance. Although endothelial responses to flow have not been shown to play a significant local role in microvascular dilatation by metabolites, flow–dependent dilatation does interact locally with myogenic responses [15]. Using the dual reservoir perfusion technique to independently control step changes in pressure and flow in isolated porcine coronary arterioles between 40 and 80 μm in diameter, Kuo et al. demonstrated that flow–dependent dilatation and myogenic responses may interact either competitively or additively. In general terms, myogenic dilatation and flow–dependent dilatation may summate locally, while myogenic constriction and flow–dependent dilatation may counteract each other. We have speculated that the former mechanism may be of particular importance during an increase in myocardial metabolic demand, when coronary arteriolar dilatation occurring in response to both a decrease in pressure and an increase in flow would summate, and so tend to maximize the final reduction in coronary microvascular resistance. However, despite the existence of these interactions in smaller microvessels, flow–dependent dilatation appears to be most pronounced in larger arterioles between 100 and 200 μm in diameter [16]. This supports the possibility that the primary role of flow–dependent dilatation during a change in metabolic demand may be to amplify the reduction in coronary microvascular resistance by recruitment of upstream microvessels in the process of dilatation. This will also be made possible by the upstream shift in coronary microvascular resistance following the metabolic and myogenic dilatation of downstream microvessels.

It seems likely that flow–dependent dilatation exerts a more complex influence on the distribution of coronary microvascular resistance than that expected just from the local dilatation of larger microvessels. In particular, flow–dependent dilatation of upstream microvessels will, by changing the transmission of pressure and flow to distal arterioles, modify the tone of distal arterioles through both metabolic and myogenic mechanisms. This hypothesis is based upon our own observations that an autoregulatory increase in tone in coronary arterioles occurs progressively during the administration of nitroglycerin, a cyclic GMP–dependent vasodilator with a similar mechanism of action to that of EDRF [17]. In the beating canine heart *in vivo*, nitroglycerin initially dilates microvessels of all sizes and increases coronary blood flow, but the dilatation of smaller (<100 μm diameter), but not larger (>100 μm diameter), microvessels diminishes with time and coronary flow returns to normal. The time–dependent loss of arteriolar dilatation during nitroglycerin is likely to be an autoregulatory adjustment in the intact coronary microcirculation, since dilatation by nitroglycerin is *sustained* in isolated coronary arterioles. It is currently unknown whether autoregulatory constriction of arterioles may similarly overcome the dilator action of EDRF released in response to flow. However, autoregulation of flow in the experiments with nitroglycerin will be associated with a shift downstream in the major site of coronary microvascular resistance. This in turn implies that the potential of a distal arteriolar segment to respond to a dilatory stimulus, i.e. its level of resting tone, may depend upon its pre–existing autoregulatory status. If this in turn depends upon the flow–dependent dilatation of upstream microvessels, then EDRF may contribute to metabolic vasodilatation by an indirect mechanism ultimately operating primarily in distal arterioles.

NEUROHUMORAL CONTROL

A major mechanism underlying the circulatory response to exercise is activation of the sympathetic nerve system. Norepinephrine is released locally from sympathetic nerve terminals in the medial–adventitial junction of blood vessels, and into the blood stream from the adrenal medulla. The net coronary blood flow response to norepinephrine is an increase, mediated by metabolic mechanisms following the increase in myocardial oxygen consumption caused by activation of myocardial β–adrenergic receptors. Despite this, norepinephrine constricts coronary microvessels by its action as an α–adrenergic agonist. α–adrenergic coronary constriction is of sufficient significance to attenuate the increase in coronary blood flow which follows the increase in myocardial work [18]. We have shown also that α–adrenergic constriction is opposed by endothelium–dependent dilatation, the constrictor responses to α–adrenergic activation by norepinephrine being accentuated following inhibition of nitric oxide synthesis in the beating canine heart *in vivo* [19]. Under baseline conditions, α_1– and α_2–adrenergic receptors occupy different functional distributions. α_1–adrenergic constrictions predominates in larger microvessels >100 μm in diameter, whereas α_2–adrenergic constriction predominates in microvessels <100 μm in diameter where it may be overcome by autoregulatory dilatation [19, 20]. After inhibition of nitric oxide synthesis, both α_1– and α_2–adrenergically mediated vasoconstriction occur throughout the coronary microcirculation, suggesting that both receptor subtypes are in fact widely distributed in considerably varying densities. Since the competitive interaction between α–adrenergic constriction and endothelium–dependent dilatation applies to activation of both the α_1– and α_2–adrenergic receptor subtypes, we have speculated that nitric oxide modulates coronary microvascular constriction by a non–specific mechanism, perhaps by increased nitric oxide release in response to increased shear stress through constricted microvessels. The pathophysiological importance of these findings is that they may explain the previously documented increased susceptibility to sympathetic coronary constriction in patients with atherosclerosis and associated endothelial dysfunction [21, 22]. A finding of potential therapeutic importance is that L–arginine, the precursor to nitric oxide, rapidly restores to normal the impaired endothelial responses to both flow and agonists which are present in coronary microvessels isolated from atherosclerotic pigs [23]. This implies that L–arginine might serve to maximize the coronary flow response to an increase in the metabolic demand, by restoring endothelium–dependent dilatation and diminishing α–adrenergic coronary microvascular constriction.

CONCLUSIONS

The heterogeneity of coronary microvascular control implies that the concerted action of the various mechanisms will lead to complex changes in the distribution of the coronary microvascular resistance. This in turn will exert an important influence on the total change in resistance in response to any given stimulus. The segmental distribution and control of coronary microvascular resistance are neglected in studies which treat the coronary microcirculation as a homogeneous resistance bed. Technology is available which allows the study of segmental coronary microvascular resistance, and should be utilized in studies addressing the mechanisms controlling coronary microvascular resistance in health and disease.

DISCUSSION

Dr. Tsujioka: You show that myogenic response is different in the subendocardial and subepicardial arterioles. Is there any theoretical reason for this difference, and what causes it? Did you find any morphological differences between subendocardial and subepicardial arterioles or venules?

Dr. W.M. Chilian: In terms of the physiological differences, we can only speculate. The speculation would be that it is part of the reason, not the total reason, why the subendocardium autoregulates less effectively than the subepicardium. In terms of morphological differences, we have not pursued that systematically. All we have done are a few electron micrographs of the vessels and there do not seem to be any gross morphological differences. I can not account for the mechanism of the difference, nor can I account for the precise mechanism or the myogenic response. That is indeed debated in 1992 and probably will be in 1993 as well.

Dr. Tsujioka: You showed that when you inhibited the release of nitric oxide by L–NAME you observed a decrease in the permeability of venule. Do you know whether it has a physiological significance or is it just some side effect of nitric oxide?

Dr. W.M. Chilian: We believe that there is a basal release of nitric oxide from coronary venules which modulates permeability. The decrease at baseline represents the fact that we make our initial measurement at a flow rate of 7 mm/sec. Under those conditions there would be production of nitric oxide. That is what I think it means. In terms of nitric oxide and its physiological effects on permeability, it is difficult to examine precisely. We have done some work on atherosclerotic swine which show that baseline permeability is decreased in venules; they do not respond to histamine in the same manner as venules from a normal pig and they do not respond to flow as well. Maybe that has implications with solute delivery, especially the fatty acid – albumin solute delivery, on which the myocardium is so dependent for energy.

Dr. R. Mates: When you studied flow–induced vasodilation, were you perfusing with saline? Did you make an attempt to correct for the difference in viscosity to think about what this would imply for blood perfusion?

Dr. W.M. Chilian: No, in saline we did not do that systematically. We used saline with albumin for the simple reason: red cells plugged the small micropipettes, but we did not pursue that. Some other people have beaten us to the punch, varying shear by changing viscosity using different dextrans. Those investigators find that when viscosity is changed, shear stress also changes and vessels do indeed show flow–induced vasodilation, or I should say shear stress–induced vasodilation.

Dr. J. De Mey: In your final conclusion, you highlight that the different control elements in the arterial tree are heterogeneously distributed. I understand that this is primarily based on isolated vessel work, a very elegant work by the way. I wonder how much of your conclusion holds for the intact coronary tree, where we suspect upstream and downstream communication and conduction. How much of the heterogeneity that you discussed really applies to the entire tree?

Dr. W.M. Chilian: I am not sure how to answer your question. Just to backtrack, or maybe sidestep for a second: We have been able to show heterogeneous reactions to a variety of things in the beating heart preparation as well. For instance, the administration of certain vasodilators or constrictors causes preferential constriction at one site or another. The coordination of responses via propagated vasodilation is another way in which the message can be communicated upstream and downstream. This is an oversimplification. But it is just one attempt to try to understand how different elements which appear to show different sensitivities can act in a coordinated manner.

Dr. A. Small (Heart Lung & Blood Inst, NIH): Have you seen anything in your system resembling the conducted vasomotor response that has been described in the peripheral microcirculation?

Dr. W.M. Chilian: No, we have not. We have not even attempted to look at that. Those studies would be extremely difficult to do in a beating heart.

Dr. L.E. Ford: For someone who does not work in the field, I would like to say these seem to be very elegant experiments indeed. It is curious that the flow through the regulatory vessel would increase the flow in such a way, that it was acting on itself. Furthermore, such an effect creates positive feedback, so that increased flow dilates the arteries, and vica–versa. If this is so, such a vessel should turn itself completely on or off.

Dr. W.M. Chilian: Flow–induced effects are modulated through shear stress. If we have arteriolar vasodilation which is initially triggered by flow, the shear stress becomes normalized or tends to become normalized and the error signal goes away.

Dr. R. Chadwick: Do you know if these microvessels shorten when you take them out? If they do, do you restretch them?

Dr. W.M. Chilian: They do shorten when you take them out. They retract. We tried to approximate their native length in a block of myocardium. That is rough, but we probably estimate this value within 5 microns or so. When the vessels are excised and retracted, they are pulled to the estimated native length.

REFERENCES

1. Chilian WM, Eastham CL, Marcus ML. Microvascular distribution of coronary vascular resistance in beating left ventricle. *Am J Physiol* 1986; 251: H779–H788.
2. Berne RM. Regulation of coronary blood flow. *Physiol Rev* 1964; 44: 1–29.
3. Chilian WM, Layne SM, Klausner EC, Eastham CL, Marcus ML. Redistribution of coronary microvascular resistance produced by dipyridamole. *Am J Physiol* 1989; 256: H383–H390.
4. Kanatsuka H, Lamping KG, Eastham CL, Dellsperger KC, Marcus ML. Comparison of the effects of increased myocardial oxygen consumption and adenosine on the coronary microvascular resistance. *Circ Res* 1989; 65: 1296–1305.
5. Chilian WM, Layne SM. Coronary microvascular responses to reductions in perfusion pressure. Evidence for persistent arteriolar vasomotor tone during coronary hypoperfusion. *Circ Res* 1990; 66: 1227–1238.
6. Kanatsuka H, Sekiguchi N, Sato K, Akai K, Wang Y, Komaru T, Ashikawa K, Takashima T. Microvascular sites and mechanisms responsible for reactive hyperaemia in the coronary circulation of the beating heart. *Circ Res* 1992; 71: 912–922.
7. Komaru T, Lamping KG, Eastham CL, Dellsperger KC. Role of ATP–sensitive potassium channels in coronary microvascular autoregulatory responses. *Circ Res* 1991; 69: 1146–1151.
8. Myers PR, Muller JM, Tanner M. Effects of oxygen tension on endothelium–dependent responses in canine coronary microvessels. *Cardiovasc Res* 1991; 25: 885–894.
9. Meininger GA, Davis MJ. Cellular mechanisms involved in the myogenic response. *Am J Physiol* 1992; 263: H647–H659.
10. Kuo L, Davis MJ, Chilian WM. Myogenic activity in isolated subepicardial and subendocardial coronary arterioles. *Am J Physiol* 1988; 255: H1558–H1562.
11. Kuo L, Chilian W, Davis MJ. Coronary arteriolar myogenic response is independent of endothelium. *Circ Res* 1990; 66: 860–866.
12. Davis MJ. Myogenic response gradient in an arteriolar network. In: Mulvaney MJ, Aalkjaer C, Heagerty AM, Nyborg NCB, Strandgaard S (eds): *Resistance Arteries: Structure and Function.* Amsterdam, Elsevier, 1991; pp 51–55.
13. Kuo L, Davis MJ, Chilian WM. Endothelial modulation of arteriolar tone. *NIPS* 1992; 7: 5–9.
14. Kuo L, Davis MJ, Chilian WM. Endothelium–dependent, flow–induced dilation of isolated coronary arterioles. *Am J Physiol* 1990; 259: H1063–H1070.
15. Kuo L, Chilian WM, Davis MJ. Interaction of pressure– and flow–induced responses in porcine coronary resistance vessels. *Am J Physiol* 1991; 258: H1706–H1715.
16. Kuo L, Davis MJ, Chilian WM. Response gradient for flow–induced dilation in the porcine coronary microvascular network. *FASEB J* 1992; 6: A2078.
17. Jones CJH, Kuo L, Davis MJ, Chilian WM. Coronary arteriolar escape from dilation by nitroglycerin. *Circulation* 1992; 86: I–509 (Abstract).
18. Mohrman DE, Feigl EO. Competition between sympathetic vasoconstriction and metabolic vasodilatation in the canine coronary circulation. *Circ Res* 1978; 42: 79–86.
19. Jones CJH, DeFily DV, Patterson J, Chilian WM. Endothelium–dependent relaxation competes with a_1– and α_2–adrenergic constriction in the canine epicardial coronary microcirculation. *Circulation* 1993 (in press).
20. Chilian WM. Functional distribution of α_1– and α_2–adrenergic receptors in the coronary microcirculation. *Circulation* 1991; 84: 2108–2122.
21. Winniford MD, Wheelan KR, Kremers MS, Ugolini V, Van Den Berg E, Niggeman EH, Jansen DE, Hillis LD. Smoking–induced coronary vasoconstriction in patients with atherosclerotic coronary artery disease: Evidence for adrenergically mediated alterations in coronary artery tone. *Circulation* 1986; 73: 662–667.

22. Zeiher AM, Drexler H, Wollschlager H, Just H. Endothelial dysfunction of the coronary micro–vasculature is associated with impaired coronary blood flow regulation in patients with early atherosclerosis. *Circulation* 1991; 84: 1984–1992.
23. Kuo L, Davis MJ, Cannon MS, Chilian WM. Pathophysiological consequences of atherosclerosis extend into the coronary microcirculation. Restoration of endothelium–dependent responses by L–arginine. *Circ Res* 1992; 70: 465–476.

CHAPTER 18

THEORETICAL ANALYSIS OF CORONARY BLOOD FLOW AND TISSUE OXYGEN PRESSURE–CONTROL

Jos A.E. Spaan[1,2] and Jenny Dankelman[2]

ABSTRACT

Coronary blood flow is tightly coupled to the myocardial oxygen consumption. We have presented a control model based on the assumption that the tissue oxygen pressure is the controlled variable. The coronary blood flow in itself is not a controlled variable but merely the result of a different control system: the tissue oxygen pressure. From our control equation there is no relation between the slope of the autoregulation curve and the gain of the tissue P_{O_2} control system. The slope is independent of the level of oxygen consumption.

INTRODUCTION

From experimental observations we know that coronary blood flow is tightly coupled to the myocardial oxygen consumption but is relatively independent of arterial pressure at constant oxygen consumption. The relation between oxygen consumption and flow at constant arterial pressure is further referred to as metabolic adjustment and the independence of flow of arterial pressure at constant oxygen consumption as autoregulation.

Typical autoregulation curves are shown in Fig. 1 in which data are used from a classical paper of Mosher et al. [1]. There are quite a few substances and physical mechanisms that are known to interfere with blood flow control [2–4]. However, there is not a consistent integrated picture of how all these mechanisms interact and in which way all these mechanisms are tuned. We have presented a control model based on the assumption that the tissue oxygen pressure is the controlled variable [5]. In this study we have

---

[1]Department of Medical Physics and Informatics, University of Amsterdam AMC, Meibergdreef 15, 1105 AZ Amsterdam, The Netherlands and [2]Laboratory for Measurement and Control, Delft University of Technology, Mekelweg 2, 2628 CD Delft, The Netherlands.

Interactive Phenomena in the Cardiac System, Edited by
S. Sideman and R. Beyar, Plenum Press, New York, 1993

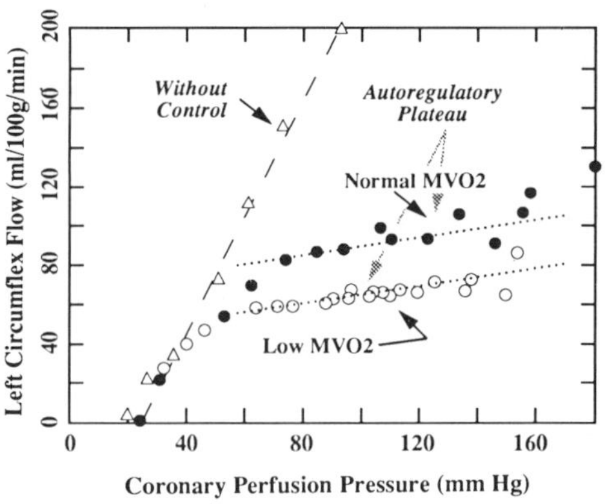

Figure 1. Illustration of autoregulation curves at two different levels of oxygen consumption of the heart. The working range of flow control is indicated by dotted curves. Figure based on data from Mosher et al. [1].

rewritten the model equations into a standard equation which is used in control theory which then allows us to speculate on the *gain* and *set point* of the tissue oxygen control system. Furthermore, the outcome of the study will be related to the observed distributions in blood flow and tissue oxygenation.

TISSUE OXYGEN CONTROL MODEL

The oxygen control–model is demonstrated in Fig. 2. Tissue is considered as a single compartment in which oxygen is consumed, with a tissue oxygen pressure which depends on the balance between oxygen supply and demand. Oxygen is supplied by the blood flow being controlled with a variable resistance. It is assumed that the variable resistance is under the influence of tissue oxygen pressure, $P_{O_2 tissue}$, in such a way that an increase in $P_{O_2 tissue}$ results in an increase of the resistance [5]. Metabolic flow adjustment is readily explained: An increase in oxygen consumption will decrease tissue P_{O_2} which in turn will lead to a reduction of the resistance and consequently to an increase of flow when perfusion pressure remains unaltered. Autoregulation is explained as well: As perfusion pressure is increased, flow increases, resulting in an increase in tissue oxygen pressure which then results in constriction until a new equilibrium is established.

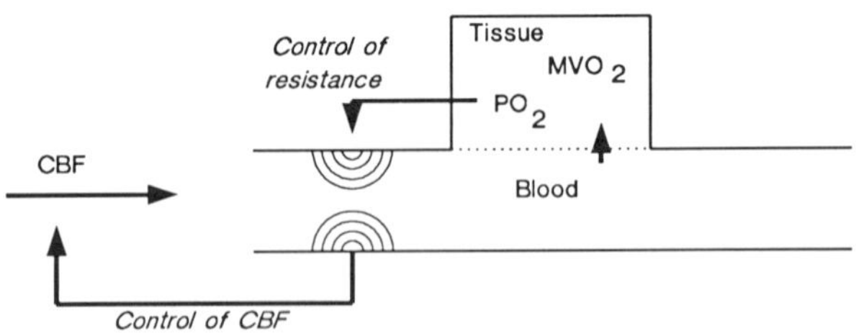

Figure 2. Model for oxygen control of coronary blood flow. Tissue–oxygen pressure is the controlled variable. Increase of $P_{O_2 tissue}$ results in vasoconstriction and reduces the oxygen supply by reducing the flow.

Model Equations

The oxygen supply and demand balance in the myocardium is given by [6]:

$$CBF \cdot K_3 \cdot \gamma \cdot [P_{O_2a} - P_{O_2v}] = MVO_2 \tag{1}$$

where CBF is the coronary blood flow; K_3 is the binding capacity of oxygen by haemoglobin; γ is the slope of the linearized oxygen–saturation curve of haemoglobin; P_{O_2a} is the coronary arterial oxygen pressure at full oxygen saturation of haemoglobin according to the linearized saturation curve; P_{O_2v} is the coronary venous oxygen pressure according to the linearized oxygen–saturation curve of haemoglobin; and MVO_2 is the myocardial oxygen consumption. Since the oxygen content of the arterial and venous blood is expressed in terms of oxygen pressure, the oxygen saturation curve is linearized and γ is the slope of the linearized part of the curve.

The resistance equation is given by:

$$R = K_4 \cdot P_{O_2tissue} \tag{2}$$

where K_4 is a constant.

Equation (2) reflects quite a few assumptions. In the first place it is assumed that the tissue pressure equals the coronary venous oxygen pressure used in Eq. (1). This is a consequence of the assumption of a well mixed compartment. Furthermore, it assumes that the arterial resistance is under the direct control of the tissue oxygen pressure. However, there need not to be a direct effect of oxygen on the arterioles.

The third equation relates coronary blood flow to perfusion pressure:

$$CBF = \frac{P_p}{R} \tag{3}$$

Again, Eq. (3) reflects some assumptions, namely that the driving pressure is equal to perfusion pressure and hence it is assumed that the back pressure for flow is zero. Moreover the effect of cardiac contraction on resistance is also neglected.

It is not difficult to see that the three equations yield an equation relating coronary blood flow to oxygen consumption and perfusion pressure [7]:

$$CBF = \frac{1}{K_3 \cdot \gamma \cdot P_{O_2a}} MVO_2 + \frac{1}{K_4 \cdot P_{O_2a}} P_p \tag{4}$$

Although Eq. (4) describes the characteristics of coronary blood flow control, the basis of the control principle being the tissue oxygen pressure can hardly be recognized.

It is not trivial to apply control theory to a biological system as the coronary circulation. A major uncertainty in a physiological system is the definition of the set point. In terms of our tissue pressure model one would have to define, on the basis of a certain criterium what the desired value for tissue pressure would be. This is quite an impossible task. Another approach is to try to force the model behavior, which is based on physiological principles expressed by the balance of factors involved in determining coronary blood flow into a mathematical form equivalent to that of the simple control model of Fig. 3. In this simple model the following equation holds:

$$y = \frac{K}{1 + K} x \tag{5}$$

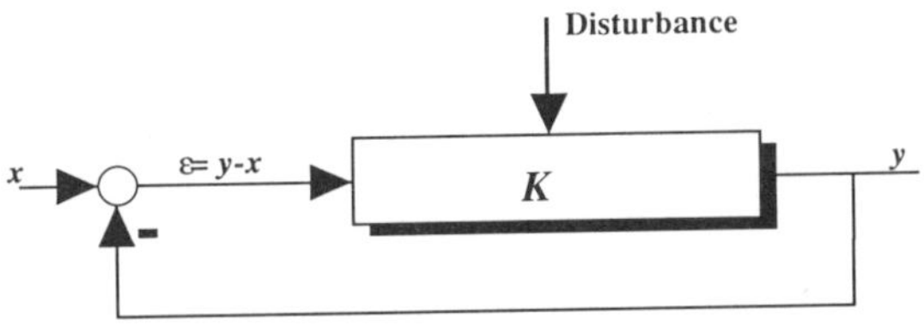

Figure 3. Illustration of a simple feedback control system. The output of the system is compared with the set point and the difference delivers a signal being the input to the process. Output to input is related by K / (1 + K).

where y is the controlled variable and x is the setpoint. K is known as the open loop gain and K / (1 + K) as the closed loop gain.

The importance of a control mechanism is clear from disturbances that will come into the process resulting in disturbances in K. The larger the K, the less these disturbances have an effect on the transfer function since the quotient will be closer to one. Therefore, the larger the open loop gain of the system, the better the control will be.

The output of the oxygen control model is, because of the assumption, the tissue oxygen pressure. If we make the tissue oxygen pressure explicit from the above equations then we arrive at the following equation:

$$P_{O_2 tissue} = \frac{\frac{P_p \cdot K_3 \cdot \gamma}{K_4 \cdot MVO_2}}{1 + \frac{P_p \cdot K_3 \cdot \gamma}{K_4 \cdot MVO_2}} \cdot P_{O_2 a} \qquad (6)$$

Comparison with Eq. (5) shows that the set point for tissue oxygen pressure is close to the arterial P_{O_2} as defined by the linearized saturation curve. The gain of the control loop is not constant but depends on perfusion pressure on the one hand and the oxygen consumption on the other. The real constant parameters in the system are the slope of the oxygen saturation curve, the sensitivity of resistance to oxygen and the oxygen hemoglobin content of the blood. Depending on the value of all these factors involved, the gain varies between 0.5 and 2.

DISCUSSION

The most important conclusion of this study is conceptual by nature. Although the coronary blood flow is tightly coupled to oxygen consumption on the one hand and quite independent of the coronary arterial pressure on the other, it does not necessarily imply that flow in itself is a controlled variable [8, 9]. The fact that coronary blood flow may depend on these factor as it does may just be the consequence of a control system designed to keep a total different variable at a more or less constant level, namely the tissue P_{O_2}. This conclusion seems counter–intuitive. The second counter intuitive conclusion is that the gain of the control system is so low, and the realized value of the control signal so far off from its possible setpoint, that one can hardly speak of a tight control system. These two conclusions may be counter–intuitive, but are consistent with several observations.

The heterogeneity in myocardial perfusion [10] and the tissue oxygen pressure are quite in agreement with the low gain of the oxygen control model. Additionally, the discrepancy between tissue pressure actually realized at the local level with respect to the desired value, the extrapolated arterial P_{O_2}, is consistent with the heterogeneity in the tissue oxygen pressure and venous oxygen saturations found in the myocardium [11].

A high gain control system would be difficult for controlling flow by the arterial tree. The coronary arterial tree has a very stochastic structure which in itself results, without control i.e. full coronary dilation, in a heterogeneous distribution of blood flow [12]. Hence the circulatory system to be controlled at the local level varies considerably throughout the myocardium. Also there is not a single site of flow control but control is distributed over vessels from 400 μm down to about 10 μm. Some parts of the capillary bed may be fed by a very few orders of short branching arteries while others by many orders of long vessels segments. Hence, the possibilities for local feedback to control vascular resistance are very heterogeneous as well.

The picture developed above must be placed in relation to the concept of oxygen usage by the myocardial cells. Oxygen is used by the mitochondria. This oxygen usage is related to the mechanical work of the myocytes which, per unit mass of myocardium, must be quite homogeneous. Because of heterogeneity of tissue P_{O_2} it is unlikely that there is a tight coupling between oxygen consumption and local tissue P_{O_2}. Most probable the mito–chondrial oxygen usage is independent of the level of tissue P_{O_2}. Oxygen consumption is regulated by intercellular mechanisms. The only task of the circulation is to maintain a minimal level of tissue P_{O_2}. This is consistent with the observations that in exercising dogs coronary sinus P_{O_2} is essentially decreasing at increasing flow rate and increasing myocardial oxygen consumption.

The conclusion of this study is that the coronary blood flow in itself is not a controlled variable but merely the result of a different control system: the tissue oxygen pressure. The slope of the autoregulation curve is often used as an index of the quality of coronary flow control [9]. As is clear from our control equation there is no relation between the slope of the autoregulation curve and the gain of the tissue P_{O_2} control system. Still, the slope of the autoregulation curve is, according to the model, independent of the level of oxygen consumption.

DISCUSSION

Dr. E.O. Feigl: I find your shift of gears a little confusing because in the mechanical model you have stressed the importance of nonlinearities, of compliance and so on, and now you have linear–ized a lot and you have come up with something which has a variable gain dependent on myo–cardial oxygen consumption. Of course it is terribly speculative to think that there is a sensor for oxygen consumption so I have a little trouble with the physiological mechanism which will do that.

Dr. J. Spaan: That is not the point I made. It is not the oxygen consumption but the tissue PO_2. If I were a biochemist I would look for something that affects the tissue PO_2, and not the myocardial oxygen consumption.

Dr. E.O. Feigl: Brosten et al. *[Circ Res 1991; 68:531–542]* found a nonlinear sensitivity to oxygen. There is a curved surface for coronary flow vs PO_2 and the steepness of that surface reflects the gain, the feedback regulatory gain, of the oxygen system. The gain gets very high at low PO_2 and wouldn't that be an equivalent statement?

Dr. J. Spaan: I do not think so. It all depends on the model one uses to apply the data. It should be noted that not only the slope of the curve you mentioned is the gain of the control system. It is just a part of it. The overall gain is the product of all those sensitivities involved in the loop. You may end up with a low gain when multiplying all sensitivities involved.

Dr. E.O. Feigl: We are talking here about where the nonlinearity lies. To introduce variable gain which is related in some way to myocardial oxygen consumption is a nonlinearity, if I may use the more general form. But there is a similar nonlinearity in the sensitivity to PO_2, that will give you the same effect.

Dr. J. Spaan: I did not introduce an MVO_2 dependent gain; it came out of the mathematics. It is not an assumption.

Dr. E.O. Feigl: Yes, but you introduced a very strange term with this autoregulation term.

Dr. J. Spaan: The amazing thing is that the autoregulation is the result of the same model that describe data well, but when interpreted in terms of control systems, comes up with striking conclusions.

Dr. R. Bünger: In a recent coronary flow autoregulation study on isolated perfused hearts *[Eur J Physiol 1992; 421: 188–199]* we also observed that venous pO_2 was correlated with coronary resistance. In a pO_2–coronary resistance plot, the shape and position of this correlation depended strongly on the energy state of the heart which was varied by perfusing with different metabolic substrates (e.g. pyruvate vs acetate vs octanoate). However, for any given metabolic state, the correlation was quite remarkable and also less complex than the one between venous adenosine concentration and coronary resistance. The pO_2–resistance correlations we observed could bear on the concept that you just presented.

Dr. Y. Kresh: There seems to be a disassociation between ATP–stores, metabolism and your proposed PO_2 regulation. There is considerable evidence that the absolute level of ATP is not a crucial regulator of cell function and survival. The source of ATP may vary; it can be glycolytic or oxidative. With this in mind, why would the PO_2 assume a primary regulator role if ultimately what is important to cell survival is its energy balance (metabolic state), which is very forgiving, so it seems.

Dr. J. Spaan: I do not know. There is quite a bit of heterogeneity in ATP too. I suggest that all the metabolic things in the myocytes are nicely homogeneous and only the flow and oxygen delivery are heterogeneous. But it may very well be that the control system is designed to bring everywhere at least a minimum of oxygen and is not really influenced by the amount of oxygen that is supplied.

REFERENCES

1. Mosher P, Ross Jr J, McFate PA, Shaw RF. Control of coronary blood flow by an autoregulatory mechanism. *Circ Res* 1964; 14: 250–259.
2. Broten TP, Feigl EO. Role of oxygen and carbon dioxide in coronary autoregulation. *FASEB J* 1990; 4: A403.
3. Mohrman DE, Feigl EO. Competition between sympathetic vasoconstriction and metabolic vasodilation in the canine coronary circulation. *Circ Res* 1987; 42: 79–86.
4. Nichols CG, Lederer WJ. Adenosine triphosphate–sensitive potassium channels in the cardiovascular system. *Am J Physiol* 1991; 261: H1675–H1686.
5. Dankelman J, Spaan JAE, Stassen HG, Vergroesen I. Dynamics of coronary adjustment to a change in heart rate in the anaesthetized goat. *J Physiol Lond* 1989; 408: 295–312.
6. Drake–Holland AJ, Laird JD, Noble MIM, Spaan JAE, Vergroesen I. Oxygen and coronary vascular resistance during autoregulation and metabolic vasodilation in the dog. *J Physiol Lond* 1984; 348: 285–299.
7. Vergroesen I, Noble MIM, Wieringa PA, Spaan JAE. Quantification of O_2 consumption and arterial pressure as independent determinants of coronary flow. *Am J Physiol (Heart Circ Physiol* 21) 1987; 252: H545–H553.

8. Broten TP, Romson JL, Fullerton DA, Van Winkle DM Feigl EO. Synergistic action of myocardial oxygen and carbon dioxide in controlling coronary blood flow. *Circ Res* 1991; 68: 531–542.
9. Dole WP, Nuno DW. Myocardial oxygen tension determines the degree and pressure range of coronary autoregulation. *Circ Res* 1986; 59: 202–215.
10. Yipintsoi T, Dobbs WA Jr, Scanlon PD, Knopp TJ, Bassingthwaighte JB. Regional distribution of diffusible tracers and carbonized microspheres in the left ventricle of isolated dog hearts. *Circ Res* 1973; 33: 573–587.
11. Weiss HR, Sinha AK. Regional oxygen saturation of small arteries and veins in the canine myocardium. *Circ Res* 1978; 42: 119–126.
12. VanBavel E, Spaan JAE. Branching patterns in the porcine coronary arterial tree. Estimation of flow heterogeneity. *Circ Res* 1992; 71: 1200–1212.

Microcirculation and Metabolic Transport

CHAPTER 19

Adenosine Coronary Vasodilation During Hypoxia Depends on Adrenergic Receptor Activation

Eric O. Feigl[1]

ABSTRACT

The adenosine hypothesis of coronary control was investigated during steady-state hypoxia by making measurements of coronary venous and epicardial well adenosine concentrations in adrenergically intact dogs and animals with α– and β–receptor blockade. The unexpected result was that a role for adenosine coronary vasodilation during hypoxia could only be found when adrenergic receptors were intact, but not during adrenergic blockade.

INTRODUCTION

The adenosine hypothesis proposes that adenosine is the physiological transmitter that couples coronary blood flow to myocardial oxygen metabolism. Information about the metabolic state of cardiac myocytes is transmitted across the interstitial space to coronary vascular smooth muscle by the diffusion of adenosine [1–3].

There are two forms of the adenosine hypothesis [4]. Form S (for Substrate) postulates that adenosine is released from cardiac myocytes in response to a low oxygen substrate level. Adenosine acts as the transmitter between cardiac myocytes and coronary vascular smooth muscle cells in a feedback control scheme whereby an incipient fall in oxygen tension (PO_2) is corrected by adenosine vasodilation that increases oxygen delivery, thus restoring oxygen tension to the operating point. This is the original form of the adenosine hypothesis proposed by Berne [5] and Gerlach [6]. The substrate form has been restated as the balance between oxygen supply and demand [7, 8]. A variation of the substrate hypothesis is that adenosine release from cardiomyocytes is correlated with the phosphorylation potential (ATP/ADP*Pi) [8–10].

---

[1]Department of Physiology and Biophysics, University of Washington, Seattle, WA 98195, USA.

Interactive Phenomena in the Cardiac System, Edited by
S. Sideman and R. Beyar, Plenum Press, New York, 1993

Berne and Rubio [11] later suggested that adenosine release from cardiac myocytes may be coupled to the *rate* of myocardial metabolism (MVO_2). That is, there is a stoichiometry between high–energy phosphate bonds consumed and adenosine released from the myocardial cell. This is a metabolite hypothesis, analogous to carbon dioxide production, where a vasodilator metabolite is produced in proportion to the rate of cardiac metabolism. This is form M (for Metabolite) of the hypothesis.

At the present time there is little support for the metabolite form of the hypothesis, and most research is directed to testing the substrate form [8, 10, 12].

A necessary prediction of the substrate form of the adenosine hypothesis is that myocardial hypoxia will lead to a sustained increase in interstitial adenosine concentration that causes the sustained increase in coronary blood flow. This aspect of the adenosine hypothesis was tested in two groups of animals: 1) nitrogen–breathing hypoxia with adrenergic receptors intact, 2) the same hypoxic stimulus but with α– and β–adrenergic receptor blockade. The unexpected result was that a role for adenosine coronary vasodilation during hypoxia could only be found when adrenergic receptors were intact, but not during adrenergic blockade [13].

METHODS

The methods have been described in detail elsewhere [13]. Briefly: dogs were anesthetized with morphine and chloralose, the chest opened and the heart suspended in a pericardial cradle. Left circumflex coronary blood flow was measured with a cannula tip flowmeter inserted via the right carotid artery. An epicardial well was attached to the surface of the left ventricle for measurement of epicardial adenosine concentration [14, 15]. A catheter was placed in the coronary sinus to obtain coronary venous samples for oxygen tension (PO_2) and plasma adenosine. Arterial and coronary venous adenosine levels were determined with a new HPLC method [16].

Hypoxia was induced by decreasing the fraction of inspired oxygen to between 7% and 10% by adding nitrogen to produce a coronary venous oxygen tension of about 8 mmHg. Two groups of animals were studied—one without adrenergic blockade and the other with combined α–receptor blockade (phenoxybenzamine 0.5 mg/kg iv) and β–receptor blockade (propranolol 2 mg/kg iv plus 0.2 mg/kg/hr iv). All animals received atropine (0.5 mg/kg iv) to prevent vagal bradycardia associated with hypoxia and reflex parasympathetic coronary vasodilation from chemoreceptor activation.

RESULTS

The major findings are summarized in Figs. 1 and 2. During an initial 18–min normoxic control period the hemodynamic variables were recorded. This was followed by an 18–min hypoxic period when the inspired oxygen was adjusted to give a coronary venous oxygen tension of about 8 mmHg in both the adrenergically unblocked and blocked groups. The intention was to subject the heart to the same degree of hypoxia, as indicated by the coronary venous PO_2, in both conditions.

In the adrenergically intact group, lowering arterial oxygen tension from 116 to 22 mmHg decreased coronary venous PO_2 from 23 to 9 mmHg. Coronary blood flow increased 243%, but myocardial oxygen consumption did not change significantly. The venous–arterial (v–a) adenosine concentration increased from 17 nM to 161 nM during hypoxia, and the epicardial well adenosine concentration increased from 221 to 358 nM.

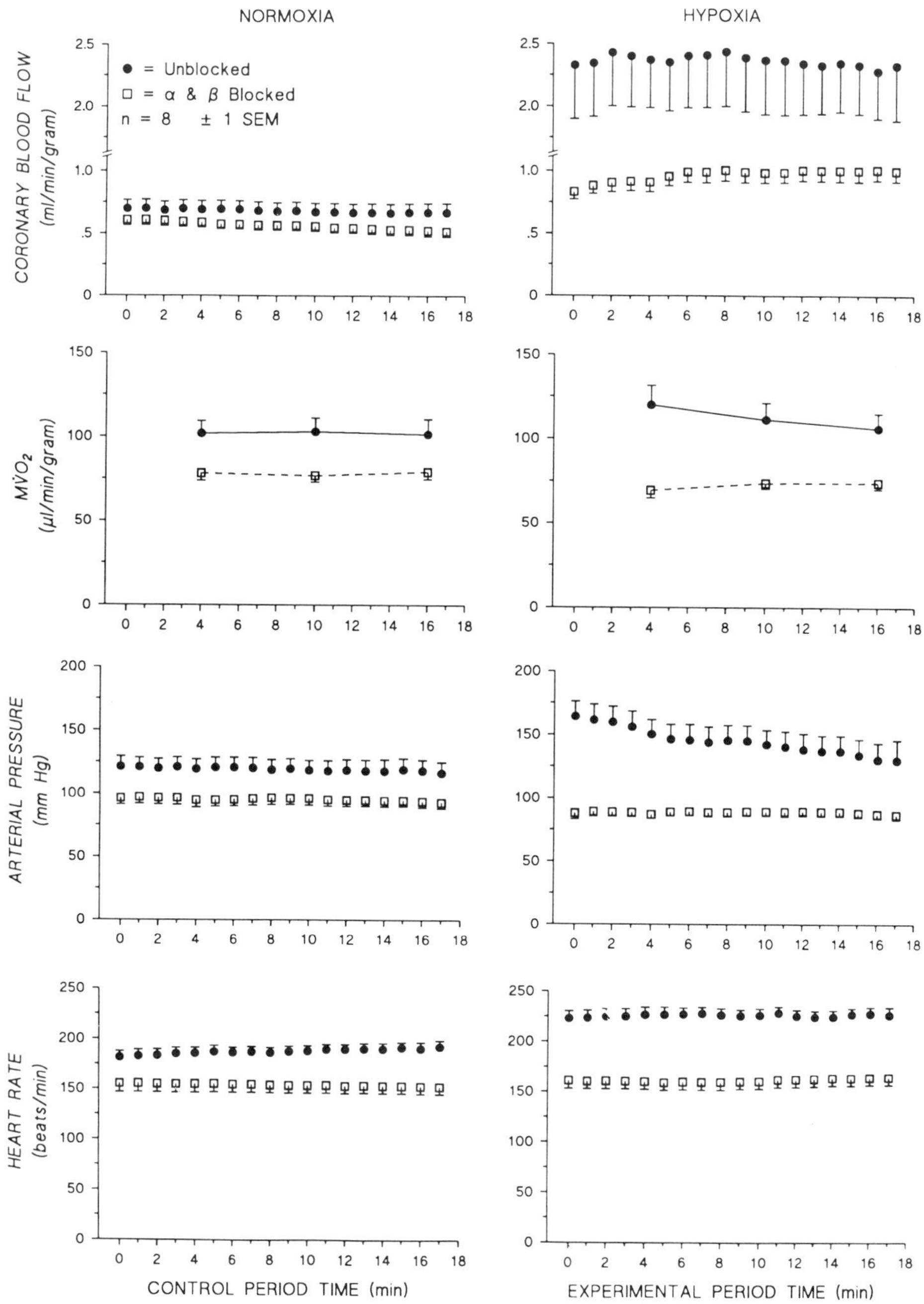

Figure 1. Comparison of the hypoxic response in adrenergically unblocked and blocked dogs. Coronary blood flow increased 243% in the unblocked group and only 75% in the α– and β–receptor blocked group (reproduced with permission [13], ©1992 American Heart Association).

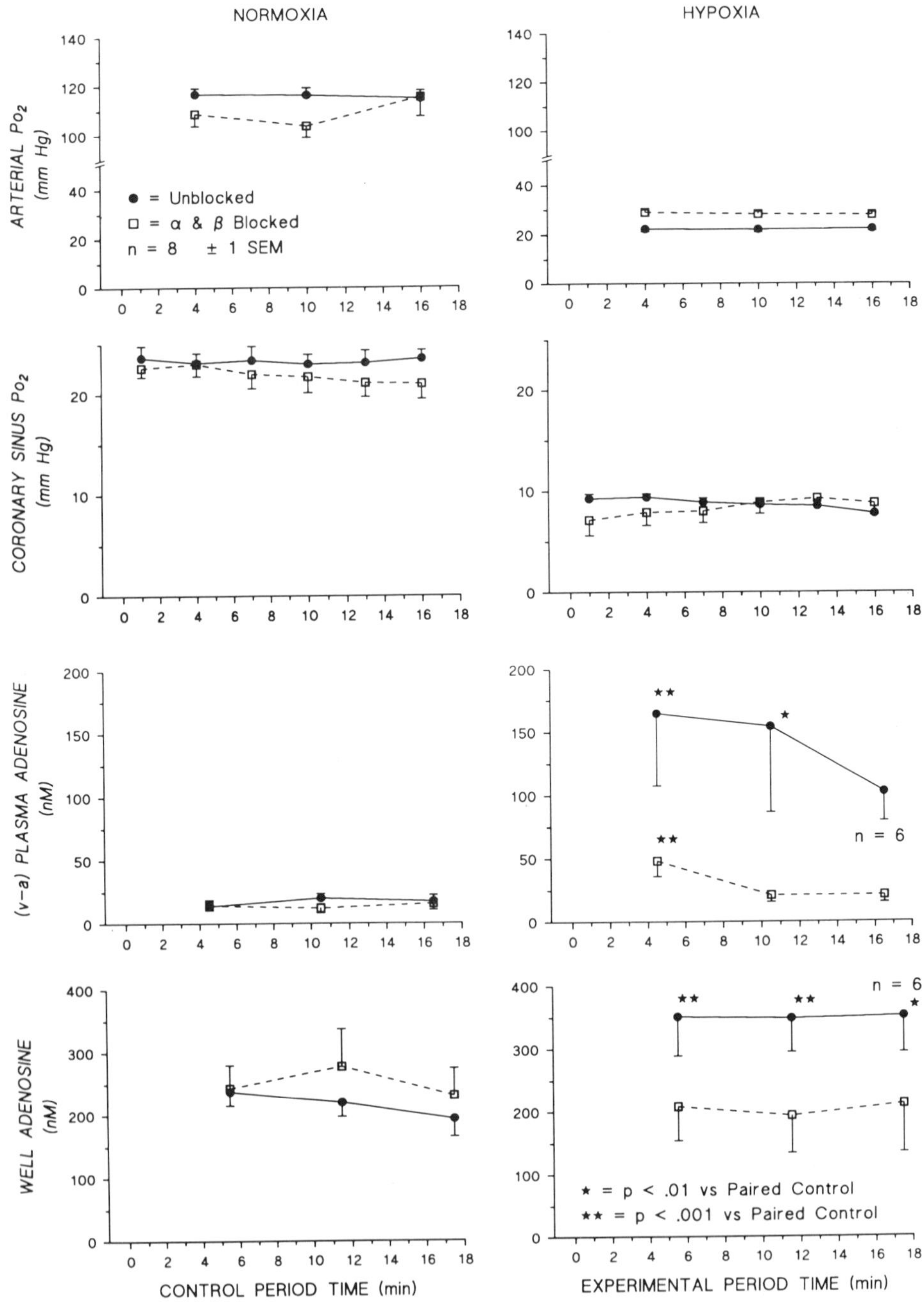

Figure 2. There was a sustained increase in the venous–arterial and epicardial well adenosine concentrations in the unblocked group during hypoxia but only a transient increase in v–a concentration in the α– and β–receptor blocked group (reproduced with permission [13], ©1992 American Heart Association).

In the group with combined α– and β–receptor blockade, lowering the arterial oxygen tension from 108 to 28 mmHg decreased coronary venous PO_2 from 22 to 8 mmHg. However, coronary blood flow only increased 75%, and myocardial oxygen consumption did not change significantly. The v–a adenosine increased transiently from 14 nM to 48 nM after 4 min of steady–state hypoxia, but was not significantly elevated during the rest of the hypoxic period. The epicardial well adenosine concentration *fell* insignificantly from 251 to 204 nM during hypoxia.

DISCUSSION

The unexpected finding in these experiments is that combined α– and β–receptor blockade blunts both the adenosine response and the coronary vasodilation that occurs during hypoxia. This result was not due to a difference in myocardial oxygen consumption, since oxygen consumption did not change significantly with hypoxia in either the adrenergically intact or blocked groups. The difference between the adrenergically blocked and unblocked groups was also not due to differing levels of myocardial hypoxia, since the coronary venous oxygen tension was very similar in both groups.

There was a positive correlation between the v–a adenosine concentration and coronary blood flow in both the adrenergically unblocked and blocked groups; however, only the data from the unblocked group support the hypothesis that adenosine causes the sustained coronary vasodilation observed during hypoxia. The usual forms of the adenosine hypothesis do not involve adrenergic receptors, and the interaction between adrenergic activation and adenosine adds a new level of complexity to the control of coronary blood flow.

The mechanism for the adrenergic–adenosine interaction found in the present experiments is unknown, although there are previous reports of related findings. Combined adrenergic α_1– and α_2–receptor blockade blunts the coronary vasodilating action of infused adenosine [17, 18]. Hori and co–workers have demonstrated that α_1–receptor activation augments adenosine release from ischemic myocardium, whereas α_2–receptor activation potentiates the coronary vasodilator action of adenosine [19,20]. Adrenergic β–receptor activation results in augmented levels in cyclic AMP which may be degraded to adenosine. However, Bardenheuer and Schrader [21] found that the cyclic AMP pathway contributed only a small amount to cardiac adenosine production. Thus, it is unclear how adrenergic and adenosine mechanisms interact in the myocardium to control coronary blood flow.

CONCLUSIONS

The adenosine hypothesis of adenosine–mediated coronary vasodilation during cardiac hypoxia was tested in two groups of dogs, one with adrenergic receptors unblocked and the other with α– and β–receptor blockade. In the adrenergically intact group, hypoxia resulted in a sustained increase in adenosine levels and coronary blood flow consistent with the adenosine hypothesis. In the adrenergically blocked group, the same level of cardiac hypoxia resulted in only a transient elevation of v–a adenosine concentration but a sustained hypoxic coronary vasodilation. This observation is inconsistent with the usual forms of the adenosine hypothesis and indicates that there is an unrecognized interaction between adrenergic receptors and adenosine mechanisms during hypoxia.

DISCUSSION

Dr. F. Kajiya: Is the interaction between α–adrenergic and adenosine receptors linear or nonlinear? Dr. Hori told me that the relation showed some nonlinear fashion interaction. Have you any comment about that?

Dr. E.O. Feigl: I have no data to describe whether the interaction is linear or nonlinear. Hori's data would certainly indicate that there is a nonlinear interaction. The α_2 mechanism is found at low doses but not at high doses. We do not have enough data to make a model of this yet.

Dr. J. Spaan: Nice experiments, and very difficult too. But why have you not done another experiment during normoxia, and changed the oxygen consumption to provoke the increase in adenosine, and then see what happens? Have you thought about it and not done it because it is too difficult?

Dr. E.O. Feigl: We are just beginning a campaign to do that with the improved methods that we now have. Of course the questions to be asked are if under normoxic conditions catecholamine increases adenosine and is this interactive mechanism involved? Many other experimenters have done this, particularly in isolated buffer perfused hearts, and there seems to be a transient effect. This may be related to the transient effects that you found with glibenclamide because the potassium–ATP channel and adenosine interact in curious ways. Thus, a possible working hypothesis is that adenosine is involved in transient effects but not in steady effects. That would be quite an amendment to the usual adenosine hypothesis, and I emphasize that this is a working hypothesis, no careful tests have been done yet.

Dr. J. Spaan: Are there certain mechanisms that are transient?

Dr. E.O. Feigl: Yes.

Dr. D. Kass: Have you done experiments selectively giving either the β–block or α–block to find out which of the two receptor pathways are more or less critical?

Dr. E.O. Feigl: We have not done that. Of course that is a very logical experiment to do and that is also planned. We did the combined blockade because the literature suggested that both might be involved and we were looking for the overall effect.

Dr. Y. Kresh: It is well accepted that adenosine acts as a "rescue" type of an agent, demonstrating cardioprotective effects. It may not have these overt effects on the coronary flow regulation but it has protective potent effects via the A_1 receptor, on preserving the myocyte. Would you comment on how that plays into your hypothesis?

Dr. E.O. Feigl: In ischemia, adenosine comes out of cardiac myocytes and that unquestionably has a cardioprotective role, producing autonomic effects, reducing contractility and so on. Ischemia is a different regime than we hope we were studying, which was control of physiologic coronary blood flow, albeit to hypoxia, but not to the point where we felt there was "ischemia". During ischemia adenosine probably has a more prominent role than these data would indicate for the control of oxygen tension within the myocardium.

REFERENCES

1. Berne RM. Regulation of coronary blood flow. *Physiol Rev* 1964; 44: 1–29.
2. Berne RM. The role of adenosine in the regulation of coronary blood flow. *Circ Res* 1980; 47: 807–813.

3. Olsson RA, Pearson JD. Cardiovascular purinoceptors. *Physiol Rev* 1990; 70: 761–845
4. Feigl EO. Coronary physiology. *Physiol Rev* 1983; 63: 1–205.
5. Berne RM. Cardiac nucleotides in hypoxia: possible role in regulation of coronary blood flow. *Am J Physiol* 1963; 204: 317–322.
6. Gerlach E, Deuticke B, Dreisbach RH. Der Nucleotid–Abbau im Herzmuskel bei Sauerstoffmangel und seine mögliche Bedeutung für die Coronardurchblutung. *Naturwissenschaften* 1963; 50: 228–229.
7. Sparks HV,Jr, Bardenheuer H. Regulation of adenosine formation by the heart. *Circ Res* 1986; 58: 193–201.
8. Olsson RA, Bünger R. Metabolic control of coronary blood flow. *Prog Cardiovasc Dis* 1987; 29: 369–387.
9. Nuutinen EM, Nishiki K, Erecinska M, Wilson DF. Role of mitochondrial oxidative phosphorylation in regulation of coronary blood flow. *Am J Physiol* 1982; 243: H159–H169.
10. Ning X–H, He M–X, Gorman MW, Romig GD, Sparks HV,Jr. Adenosine formation and energy status in isolated guinea pig hearts perfused with erythrocytes. *Am J Physiol* 1992; 262: H1075–H1080.
11. Rubio R, Berne RM. Localization of purine and pyrimidine nucleoside phosphorylases in heart, kidney, and liver. *Am J Physiol* 1980; 239: H721–H730.
12. Deussen A, Schrader J. Cardiac adenosine production is linked to myocardial pO_2. *J Mol Cell Cardiol* 1991; 23: 495–504.
13. Herrmann SC, Feigl EO. Adrenergic blockade blunts adenosine concentration and coronary vasodilation during hypoxia. *Circ Res* 1992; 70: 1203–1216.
14. Gidday JM, Hill HE, Rubio R, Berne RM. Estimates of left ventricular interstitial fluid adenosine during catecholamine stimulation. *Am J Physiol* 1988; 254: H207–H216.
15. Hanley F, Messina LM, Baer RW, Uhlig PN, Hoffman JIE. Direct measurement of left ventricular interstitial adenosine. *Am J Physiol* 1983; 245: H327–H335.
16. Herrmann SC, Feigl EO. Subtraction method for the high–performance liquid chromatographic measurement of plasma adenosine. *J Chromat* 1992; 574: 247–253.
17. Nayler WG, Price JM, Lowe TE. Inhibition of adenosine–induced coronary vasodilatation. *Cardiovasc Res* 1967; 1: 63–66.
18. Hori M, Inoue M, Kitakaze M, Koretsune Y, Iwai K, Tamai J, Ito H, Kitabatake A, Sato T, Kamada T. Role of adenosine in hyperemic response of coronary blood flow in microembolization. *Am J Physiol* 1986; 250: H509–H518.
19. Hori M, Kitakaze M, Tamai J, Iwakura K, Kitabatake A, Inoue M, Kamada T. α_2–Adrenoceptor stimulation can augment coronary vasodilation maximally induced by adenosine in dogs. *Am J Physiol* 1989; 257: H132–H140.
20. Kitakaze M, Hori M, Tamai J, Iwakura K, Koretsune Y, Kagiya T, Iwai K, Kitabatake A, Inoue M, Kamada T. α_1–Adrenoceptor activity regulates release of adenosine from the ischemic myocardium in dogs. *Circ Res* 1987; 60: 631–639.
21. Bardenheuer H, Schrader J. Supply–to–demand ratio for oxygen determines formation of adenosine by the heart. *Am J Physiol* 1986; 250: H173–H180.

CHAPTER 20

CHAOS IN CARDIAC SIGNALS

James B. Bassingthwaighte[1]

ABSTRACT

Chaotic dynamical systems analysis has become over the last two decades a standard tool for systems analysis in the hydrodynamics of turbulence, in mechanical systems, and in electrical signals. The label "chaotic" has summarized the lack of predictability of the weather and other complex systems. We can use "chaos" theory to enhance our understanding of cardiovascular pressures, flows, heart rates, and tracer exchanges. Explaining why we cannot predict exactly is an improvement over not understanding at all, and aids in taking the next steps toward deeper insight at the biochemical and electrophysiologic levels.

INTRODUCTION

"Homeostasis", the stability of the "milieu interieure" has been regarded as the *modus operandi* of physiological systems since the time of Claude Bernard [1]. The principle was that the body is designed so that concentrations and rates of processes tended toward a stable state, through multiple feedback mechanisms. This was not a passing idea, for it had many affirmations and was firmly positioned in the medical literature by Cannon [2], whose elegant experiments gave immense support. Now we question whether or not "homeostasis" ought to be replaced by the concept of "homeodynamics", allowing a more flexible view of how the systems work and making room for the concept of systems with complex responses, even to the point of inherent instability.

"Chaos", the new proposition, is the description applied to the state of a system which is unpredictable, even though bounded. Poincaré [3] observed that some simple differential equations resulted in unpredictable behavior. But, as brought forcefully to our attention in modern times by Lorenz [4], the unpredictability is not in the least equivalent to randomicity. There is no reason to think that biological systems must be chaotic, and

[1]Center for Bioengineering, University of Washington, WD-12, Seattle WA 98195, USA.

Interactive Phenomena in the Cardiac System, Edited by
S. Sideman and R. Beyar, Plenum Press, New York, 1993

Glass and Malta [5] argue that biochemical systems are in general not chaotic, so in this essay the focus is on the idea that consideration of chaotic and fractal aspects of systems augments our power to examine and interpret data, and perhaps to characterize the system. Most data on biological systems are in the form of time series, the measures of one or sometimes more variables taken at even intervals over time. Inevitably, most of the system variables are unmeasured, but a theorem by Takens points out that the influences of all of the unmeasured variables which are a part of the "system" are reflected in the dynamics of the one or two measured variables. Such a statement applies to both continuous systems and discrete systems [6]. This is the critical basis on which virtually all of the methods of analysis are based.

The features of *chaotic dynamics* can be summarized as follows:

1. *Unpredictability*, not randomicity.
2. *Sensitivity* to initial conditions (divergence), implying that small differences in initial state lead to dramatic differences in a later state because there is a divergence in the paths taken from two slightly different starting points.
3. *Boundedness* in the behavior, which implies that the functions reside within "basins of attraction", that there is an "attractor" toward which the function has some tendency to move, at least under some parametric conditions.
4. Rate dependence: At low rates the function may be stable, i.e. there is a stable attractor. At higher rates there may be periodic attractors or a series of 2, 4, 8, etc., settings as the rate of a process is increased. At high rates the process is "chaotic", meaning that while there is short term predictability, there is no long term precise predictability. The doubling of the attracting points of stability lengthens the period of the function accordingly, so this represents the "period doubling route to chaos".
5. *Insensitivity* to added noise: The function tends toward the attractor or remains in the basin of attraction in spite of random noise, and remains organized, chaotic, but not random.
6. *Susceptibility* to regulation, by external intervention. An external influence, properly applied can reduce a chaotic function to a stable, perhaps periodic, function.
7. *Efficiency:* A closed system may be cheaper to operate a little loosely in the chaotic mode than under tight control as a stable system. In a chaotic system "sloppy" control is merely cycling on the attractor, or within the basin of attraction. There is no mathematical need for "set points", and indeed so far as one can tell there are no such things as set points in the body; even so, the standard aspects of engineering control theory are applicable without change.
8. The power spectrum shows broad bands, rather than a few isolated stable *frequencies*. This is a reflection of the variation in frequency even in a system which demonstrates cycling.

DISTINGUISHING CHAOS FROM NOISE

The reasons for wanting to make the distinction between a truly chaotic signal and a merely noisy signal are both theoretical and practical: for description, for insight and prediction, or for providing a basis for intervention. If a signal is merely a constant summed with Gaussian noise, then the constant and the standard deviation of the noise constitute a full description. If it is chaotic, then the apparent dimension of the attractor provides a beginning of the description and a simple mathematical analog can augment this and provide some predictive capability that could not be reached for a noisy system. As we will see below, even an incomplete and insecure level of description and understanding can be sufficient to allow intervention and control. In the case of fatal cardiac arrhythmias, improving the capability for therapeutic intervention is a driving incentive for investigation, whether or not the signal is truly chaotic [7]. Also raised with respect to the cardiac rhythm is the question of the complexity of the variation in the signal: Goldberger makes the case that a healthy young person shows greater complexity than an older person, and that great loss of complexity (reduction to an almost constant rhythm) may be premonitory to a fatal arrhythmia [8, 9].

How to make the distinction is a deep and interesting question. Ideally the distinction between a coordinated signal emanating from a non–linear system and a purely random signal should be simple, but many complicating situations arise. Not at all the least of these is the need for extremely long times to acquire sufficient data on which to demonstrate the correlation inherent in the chaotic signal; with short data runs, the statistical methods currently developed do not have the power to make the distinction with assurance. This is an area of active research. Since there are enough conditions where a random signal can masquerade as a chaotic signal [10], and plenty of situations where low pass filtering of a random signal can produce short range correlation in the signal, even the distinction between a purely random and a purely chaotic signal is not easily assured. Considering that most natural signals are augmented with a combination of externally imposed noise and measurement error, easy distinction can be seen to be a will'o the wisp. The potential methods for distinguishing a chaotic from a noisy one–dimensional signal, e.g. one variable versus time at even intervals, are:

1. Standard methods of statistics:
   a. The probability density function of observed values over the whole observation period and over subsets of the whole.
   b. The power spectral density.
   c. The autocorrelation function.
2. Special methods for signals with correlation structure:
   a. Dispersional analysis.
   b. Rescaled range (Hurst) analysis.
   c. Visual analysis of phase plane plots.
3. Special methods suitable for low dimensional chaotic attractors:
   a. Grassberger–Procaccia correlation dimension and capacity dimension.
   b. Estimation of Lyapunov exponents.
   c. Variants on calculations of Kolmogorov–Smirnov entropy.
4. Special situations:
   a. Observations of changing states exhibiting bifurcations or changes of periodicities.
   b. Interventions that result in period doublings or changes in the apparent chaotic state.

A general principle to keep in mind when trying to make the distinction with these methods is that a very high order system such as that described by a dozen nonlinear differential equations, even though smooth and coordinated in a 12–dimensional domain, will not be distinguishable from noise unless the system is so dominated by a few variables that it behaves as a low dimensional attractor. This is not to recommend giving up, since most physiological and biochemical systems in block diagrams appear this complex, but rather to say that low dimensional systems are much easier to identify and characterize. But all is not lost for high dimensional systems; for example the chain of reactions in glycolysis is composed of sets of high velocity reversible reactions lying between relatively low velocity control reactions, and so the overall system behaves as a low order system. Such systems, even though inherently complex and seemingly naturally chaotic, often are locally more or less linear, and consequently stable [see 5].

Standard Methods of Statistics

Standard methods are useful. The probability density function may or may not be Gaussian, and one can be more suspicious about a highly skewed or markedly platykurtic or leptokurtic function than one that is normally distributed. The power density spectrum is somewhat more definitive, and a power spectrum that diminishes smoothly with frequency, f, as $1/f^{\beta}$ where the exponent β is between 0.2 and 1.8 is an indicator of a fractal that is different from noise. (The attractor may actually be a fractal in phase space, but this is not a requirement. A β of 0 is random, white noise; a β of 2.0 is Brownian motion, the integral of white noise, so the choice of 0.2 and 1.8 is merely to designate values different from noise.) The autocorrelation function is zero with noise, and extends only over a short range with filtered noise, but the autoregulation function for a fractally correlated function shows a slow fall–off and an extended range of positive correlation. (This statement applies to functions of time and also of space where the spatial range is very large; it has to be modified to account for negative correlation when there is a fractal relationship within an organ of finite size.)

Special Methods for Signals with Correlation Structure

The special methods are really general, and apply both to space–and time–based signals. Dispersional analysis is what we first used for looking at regional flow distributions [11, 12]. The basis of the method is to determine the spread of the probability density function (variance or standard deviation or coefficient of variation, relative dispersion) at the highest level of resolution, then to lump nearest neighbor elements of the signal together to obtain the local mean of the pair of elements and recalculate the dispersion at the reduced level of resolution, and to repeat this with successively larger lumpings of near neighbors. From this one calculates the slope of the log–log relationship between dispersion and level of resolution: a slope of 0.5 is obtained for a random signal, and a smaller slope indicates the internal correlation that allows us to call it "fractal" and to determine the degree of correlation between neighbors over a wide range of separations. The Hurst method likewise show the correlation structure by an analysis of the range of differences of the integral of the signal from the expected mean, making this estimate over subsets of the data set and using subsets of widely differing size [13–15].

The "visual" method is a serious one, based on Takens' theorem that says that information on all of the related variables is carried in the observed signal. For example, suppose that one has a pair of coupled differential equations in X and Y as a function of time, and that one has recorded only the X(t). The standard phase plane plot would be to plot Y(t) versus X(t), but without the Y(t), one can get an equivalent phase plane plot with dX(t)/dt versus X(t) since the derivative must be at least partially a function of Y(t). When the function has not been recorded continuously and one has only the series $X(t_i)$, for $i = 1, N$, at even intervals Δt, then the approximation to the derivative is $\Delta X/\Delta t$ or $(X(t_{i+1}) - X(t_i))/\Delta t$. In the special case where $dX(t)/dt = Y(t)$ the phase plane plot would be Y(t)

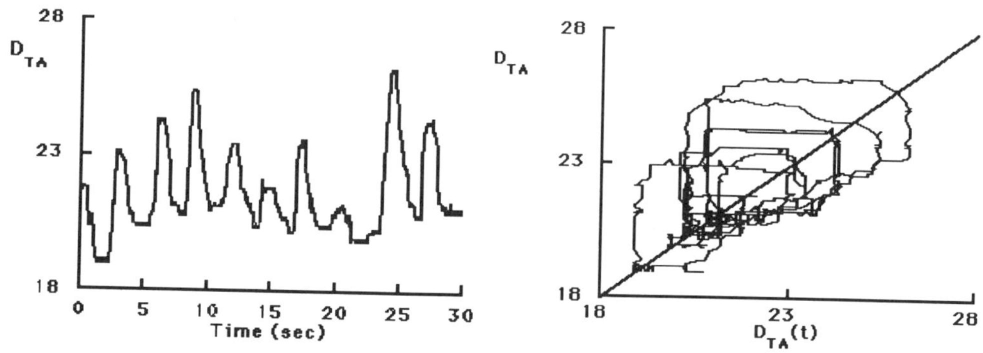

Figure 1. Vasomotion: **Left:** Diameter, X(t), versus time. **Right:** Delay plot of the diameter of a transverse arteriole from the rabbit tenuissimus muscle under physiological conditions. $\tau = 0.5$ seconds (From the studies of Oude Vrielink et al. [16] using the analysis of Yamashiro et al. [17]).

versus X(t), and in the more general case $X(t_{i+1}) - X(t_i)$ is taken as its representative. To be yet more general one may get a better approximation by using the time lead or lag to be j intervals rather than 1. This method is used for plotting the diameters (Fig. 1, left) of a small arteriole in the rabbit tenuissimus muscle in phase space, using a lag of 5 intervals or 0.5 second in the real signal (Fig. 1, right). This is a "delay plot". The data are from Oude Vrielink et al. [16]. The more or less smooth trajectory of the plot over successive intervals of time shows its continuity, or correlation, and the non-random coverage of the X,Y plane indicates that this is not a random signal. One looks in the plot for structure, different from just a jumble of points, and for some smoothness in the trajectory. The smoothness is dependent on the interval taken: with larger intervals the smoothness is less evident, but there will be nevertheless a characteristic pattern in the dot densities in the plane which distinguish chaos from noise. The quantitative techniques described next extend this idea to higher dimensions and to providing quantitating measures, not just the appearance.

Special Methods Suitable for Low Dimensional Chaotic Attractors

The method devised by Grassberger and Procaccia [18] has the strongest heritage and the longest usage, but should nevertheless be regarded as "under investigation". Its limitations and its accuracy are not yet well defined, nor is it clear how noise affects the estimates of the characterizing factor, the so-called correlation dimension, known as D_{corr} or D_{gp}, after the originators.

The basic idea of quantitative measures of the dimensionality of a chaotic signal is similar to that using fractal characterization, namely how much of the next dimension in N-space does it fill. There is a difficulty that is not so apparent for fractals: when one asks how much of a plane does an iterated line fractal fill, or how much of 3-space does a rough surface fill, one starts with a signal of known dimensionality, e.g. 1 for a line or 2 for the surface, and seeks a measure of the complexity of form by asking how much of the next dimension up is used. (So an infinitely recursive line segment algorithm gives a result with fractal D between 1 and 2, and a mountainous surface has for example a dimension 2.4 compared to hilly country with a dimension 2.2.) A signal from a chaotic attractor has clear dimensionality that is revealed when the trajectory in projected in a space where there are no intersections with itself: a ball of wool is fully expressed in 3–space but a 2–space silhouette will show intersection of the strand with itself. But we do not know from the signal or from a delay plot what this dimensionality might be. The delay plot (Fig. 1, right) is an attempt to display the signal as if it were the ball of wool in the appropriate dimension so that the next question (How much of space does it fill?) can be asked. The problem is that the delayed signal is not necessarily orthogonal to the original, as the derivative would be. If the chosen delay is too short then one or even a few delays will not unravel or prevent intersections. The embedding dimension is unrelated to the actual dimensions of the object, the complex signal. So a succession of embeddings must inevitably be used.

Methods for making a best guess at the most efficiently revealing delay time τ are to use the power spectrum and the autocorrelation function. From the power spectrum, take the reciprocal of 3 or 4 times the frequency in the middle of the lowest frequency broad peak; this attempts to capture the dominant period of the signal. (One can do this in the time domain also by picking a delay time τ about 1/4 of the period of a dominating cycle.) The autocorrelation function is 1.0 for zero lag and falls off with increasing distance between point pairs; the best choice of delay is the number of intervals for the autocorrelation to decrease to 1/e, about 0.37. It can be even a little longer, the number of intervals N to the first zero crossing or when the autocorrelation is close to zero. Now the delay τ is $N\Delta t$.

For a true three–dimensional signal, embedding in four or higher real dimensions reveals no more details of its structure, just as a sphere or cube is completely revealed in three–space. However, since the embedding dimension ε_m is usually less than real, dimension one often has to go to embedding spaces of 10 or more. The sum of the distances between all pairs of points is maximal when the embedding dimension (of the plotting space) is high enough to reveal all the true dimensionality of the signal. This is the basis for calculating the Grassberger–Procaccia [18] correlation dimension. The box dimension used by Liebovitch and Toth [19] is based on the same idea except that instead of measuring all of the individual lengths between point pairs to see how spread out the signal is, one puts N–dimensional boxes around the phase plot signal to determine the volume or number of boxes required to contain it. As one decreases the size of the boxes, the number of boxes required to enclose the signal increases while the total area or volume of the boxes decreases and tightens around the signal. An improved algorithm is available for workstations from Hou et al. [20].

The capacity or box fractal dimension is the logarithmic slope of the number of boxes required as a function of the box size. The strategy is to calculate the box fractal dimension, D_B, at successively higher embedding dimensions until D_B increases no further. This is a similar strategy to that used by Grassberger and Procaccia [18] for the correlation dimension while measuring lengths.The steps in calculating the box fractal dimension take advantage of the discretization of the signal, since the signal has lost its continuous nature to form a set of successive points in the embedding space. The steps are:

1. For embedding in two–dimensional (2D) space, use $X(t_i + \tau)$ versus $X(t_i)$ for each time point, t_i, in the original signal. Pick a length scale ΔX_1, and an arbitrary starting location for laying out a rectangular grid on the plane. Count N_1, the number of squares in which there are one or more points $X(t_i + \tau)$, $X(t_i)$. This provides one point N_1, versus ΔX_1, in two–space.
2. Repeat with a smaller length ΔX_2 and count the number N_2 of corresponding boxes. This gives a second point N_2, ΔX_2. Continue with successively smaller ΔX_i, to the limit of the smallest ΔX_i at which there is not more than one point per box. Going to this limit is not necessary for the next step. Now one has the set, N_i versus ΔX_i for embedding in 2–space, E_2.

3. Plot log N_i versus log ΔX_i, and determine the slope of the line. The slope $-d(\log N_i)/d(\log \Delta X_i) = D_B(2)$, the estimated box dimension for embedding in two-space. As the box size approaches the limit of one point per box, the curve reaches saturation so the slope should be estimated below this level as suggested by Liebovitch and Toth [19], for example between 25% and 75% of the maximum.
4. Repeat steps 1 to 3 using three-dimensional embedding, i.e., the original signal and two signals delayed by τ and 2τ. For E_3, plot log N_i versus log ΔX_i. The slope gives $D_B(3)$. Higher order embeddings are handled similarly.
5. The next step involves interpreting how D_B varies with embedding dimension, E_m. If enough data points are available D_B should reach a plateau as E_m is increased. This plateau level is taken to be the fractal dimension. With a limited number of data points, demonstration of a plateau may not be possible.
6. Randomize the ordering of the data set to create a surrogate data set with the same time-domain probability density function. (The power frequency spectrum may change. There are other methods for creating a surrogate data set with the same power spectrum.) Repeat steps 1 to 5. Plot D_B versus E_m as before and compare the estimates of D_B with the previous plot. The randomized set will give higher estimates at each embedding level and will not show a plateau.

The randomization of the data set should give a distinctly different result than does the original set, if the original set is chaotic or fractal. Methods for estimating D_B from the difference between the lines for D_B versus E_m with the two data sets are being attempted [21], but the critical point is that the lines are different, and therefore that measuring the chaotic dimension makes sense.

The dimension, D_B or D_{corr}, gives a measure of the complexity of the signal. For the Lorenz equations [4], D_B is 2.06 and D_{corr} is 2.05. For our vasomotion signals, D_B is less accurately defined, but about 1.5. For all signals, D_B is a little greater than D_{corr}.

The *Lyapunov exponent* measures the divergence of two trajectories originating from neighboring points. In general chaotic signals have three Lyapunov exponents, representing the eigenvalues of the system. For a chaotic system one exponent must be positive, representing a tendency toward expansion, one must be zero for there to be a stable limit cycle, and a third must be negative in order that the sum be negative, for this is the requirement that the signal tend toward the attractor and remain in the basin of attraction. From this it can be seen that a first or second order continuous system cannot be chaotic. Observation of a positive exponent in a signal on a limit cycle is diagnostic of chaos.

The Lyapunov exponent is notoriously difficult to calculate. Most methods involve picking points that are close, and then following their trajectories to see how fast they separate. But picking the points is tricky, and repetitions are required. The methods of Wolf et al. [22] paved the way. Parker and Chua [23] give a broad picture of the problems. This too is an active research area, so it may be that methods applicable to biological signals of limited length can be worked out.

Entropy calculations are based on the information content of the observed system. For example, while the box dimension gives a geometric measure of the space occupied by the signal on the attractor, there is an information dimension, D_I, which in addition accounts for the number of times a particular box is visited. D_I is slightly smaller than D_B; the entropy, H, is the amount of information needed to specify the system to an accuracy ε when the signal is on the attractor, $H(\varepsilon) = k\varepsilon^{-D_I}$ just as the number of boxes in the box counting method is $N(\varepsilon) = k\varepsilon^{-D_B}$. The usual problem is, as before, large amounts of data are needed to make the full calculations with any assurance of accuracy in estimating the dimension. Pincus [24] has developed a simplified variant on the entropy calculation that can really only be termed empirical, but it may prove useful because of its simplicity and applicability to short data sets.

Pincus' method [24] is called ApEn, approximate entropy. It is used somewhat in the style of the standard entropy calculations and its estimation has some similarity to that for D_{corr} but it uses only low embedding dimensions, typically $E_m = 2$ and 3. The steps for $E_m = 2$ are:

1. Calculate the mean and SD of the data set, X_i, i=1, N_x. Define a length r = 0.2 SD; this will be used as a tolerance limit to reduce the effects of noise.
2. Define a set of points in a 2D space from successive pairs of values in the one–dimensional signal. The pair X_i, X_{i+1} define a point in 2–space. For an X array of 1000 points, there are 999 points in 2D.
3. Obtain a measure of the distances between (X_i, X_{i+1}) and all other points (X_j, X_{j+1}). The distance may be the proper Euclidean distance, or may be simplified to be the $\mathrm{Max}[(X_j - X_i), (X_{j+1} - X_{i+1})]$, which makes the calculations faster and shortens the distances somewhat. (If Euclidean distance were calculated, one might use an r = 0.3 SD instead, for example.) There are N_x–2 distances for each X_i in 2–space.
4. For each of the data points, X_i, find the fraction of the distances to the other points which are less than r, and let this fraction be called $C_i(r)$. This fraction is a measure of the regularity or the frequency of similar patterns between successive points in the (phase plane) plot.
5. Find the average of the $C_i(r)$s for the N_x–1 fractions, and take the natural logarithm, so defining $\Phi(m{=}2, r{=}0.2)$ as this average.
6. Repeat steps 2 through 5 using $E_m = 3$, which means using triples (X_i, X_{i+1}, X_{i+2}) to define the point positions in 3–space. Again calculate the average fraction of distances less than r for N_x–2 triples. This gives $\Phi(m{=}3, r{=}0.2)$.
7. The measure, ApEn (m=2, r=0.2, N=1000) = $\Phi(m{=}2, r{=}0.2) - \Phi(m{=}3, r{=}0.2)$. Thus ApEn is a very specific example of a set of statistical measures that might be taken from the signal. Because it only uses small m and a particular r, its value does not approximate the formal entropy measures. (This is not a particular problem since the formal measures are not useful on mildly noisy signals.) Values of ApEn increase with increasing N_x. Therefore ApEn is used as a comparative statistic, with a fixed E_m, r, and N_x.

For heart rate variability ApEn (m = 2, r = 0.2, N = 1000) is around 1.0 for young adults and diminishes with age to around 0.7 at age 80 years [24]. The suspicion is that a diminution in ApEn may indicate an unhealthy degree of constancy of the heart rate, and research by Goldberger and others (e.g. Goldberger [25]) should determine whether or not ApEn can be used as a measure of risk of sudden death by arrhythmia.

Special Situations

Even low order process of generation and decay (chemical reaction networks, predator–prey relationships, etc.) can exhibit dependence on a rate coefficient. A cycling or periodic system in which an increase of this rate results in a bifurcation or period doubling is diagnosed as being potentially, if not actually, chaotic. A bifurcation is a doubling of the number of stable settings for the observed variable, which is equivalent to doubling the length of the period required to repeat the pattern. In an iterated system in which a rate increase causes a steady signal to take 2 alternating values, then 4, 8, and 16, and thereafter appears unpredictable at a higher value of the rate, the system is said to follow period–doubling bifurcations on the route to chaos. In continuously observable systems the same kind of thing can occur, a stable variable shifts to a single cycle (circular or elliptical in the phase plane), then to a two–cycle (two linked but distorted ellipses in the phase plane) and so on; at higher rates the signal may never be exactly repetitive and is called chaotic and even though the trajectories are nicely bounded and smooth they are not exactly predictable.

These kinds of shifting in periodicity can occur spontaneously in living systems or may sometimes be induced by temperature changes or other stimulus. Observations of jumps in behavior patterns should therefore raise one's suspicions that the system operates on a low dimension attractor in either a periodic or chaotic mode. The attractor, the region of phase space covered by the trajectories, is commonly fractal; like taking a slice through Saturn's rings, the distances between neighboring slices tends to show fractal variation in the intervals, which means the spacings show correlation structure, near neighbor spacings being more alike than spacings between N^{th} neighbors. Thus the spacings are neither random nor uniform.

CONTROL OF CHAOS, AND PERHAPS A LEAD TOWARD TREATING ARRHYTHMIAS

A recent study by Garfinkel and colleagues [26] illustrates the potential for incorporating the ideas of chaotic dynamics into therapeutic situations. The experiment was performed in an artificial situation, namely in the isolated perfused rabbit interventricular septum, in which chaotic cycling of excitation was induced by high dosage of oubain, blocking the sodium pump. The situation was found to be describable and understandable by using a 2D delay plot, plotting the duration of each interval against that of the preceding one. The trajectory of points revealed a saddle bifurcation: along one line in this plane the interval durations tended to go from alternating large or small values toward a middle point, moving closer to this point with successive iterations. This is like bouncing a ball in a bowl. In a second direction more or less at right angles to this line however the successive durations rapidly diverged, again oscillating from below to above this same middle point. (The line along which convergence occurred is the stable manifold, the other direction is the unstable manifold.) The divergence does not continue and ergodically there are shifts from the unstable toward the stable manifold, a truly chaotic behavior.

Control was attempted by stimulating the preparation at appropriate times. One must find the right time for the stimulus, since the only intervention that can be accomplished is to shorten the interbeat interval. The trick is to put the trajectory onto the stable manifold, more or less, and this is done by predicting from the trajectory the next long beat which will occur along the unstable manifold and then giving a stimulus to create a shorter interval that is closer to the stable manifold. The stimulus thus shortens the next interval, though it is longer than the preceding interval. Bring it closer to the stable manifold means that the interval will tend toward the intersection between the stable and unstable manifolds, but of course the basic instability remains and without repeated intervention the rhythm would return to the chaotic mode. In Fig. 2 is shown one example from Garfinkel et al. in which the control effected a triple rhythm with a mean interbeat interval longer

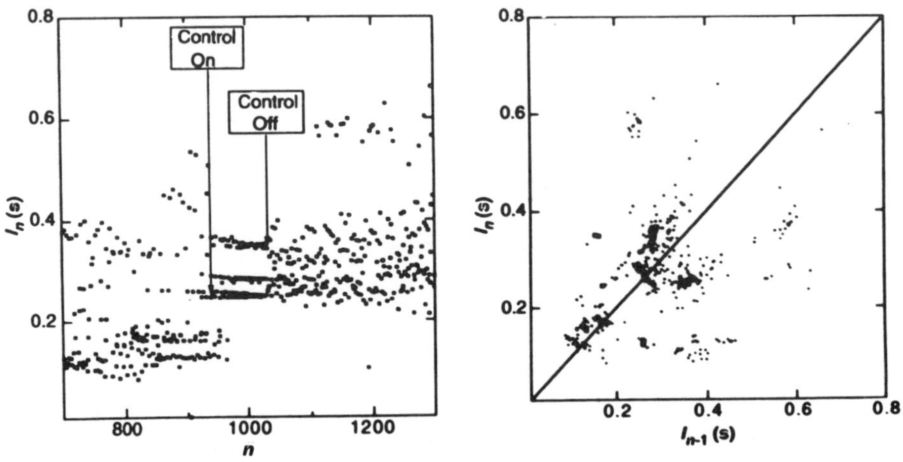

Figure 2. Controlling chaos in cardiac rhythm. Interbeat intervals in a oubain–treated rabbit septal preparation. **Left:** Interval length versus beat number for a 600 beat sequence. Computer control of a stimulus was started at "control on" and after some further cycling in the "chaotic" mode resulted in a stable 3–cycle. **Right:** Lag or phase plane plot of the intervals in the left panel. The period of control resulted in a 3–cycle with the middle interval probably representing points on the stable manifold and the other two points probably lying on either side of the stable manifold and approximately in the line of the unstable manifold. The larger dots represent data in the "controlled" period of data collection. (From [26] with permission, ©1992 by the AAAS.)

than that occurring in the chaotic state. We look on this as "effective treatment" in the sense that prolongation of the average interval length would give greater ventricular filling time. In this particular instance there also appeared to be some continuing benefit after the controlling stimulations were turned off, for the average interval was longer after the series of stimuli than it was before.

CONCLUSION

This is an introductory overview of chaotic dynamics and of the potential utility of using dynamical approaches for understanding and even controlling cardiovascular processes. The applications to biology are indeed very new, and the analytical techniques are a long way from being nicely defined or even thoroughly proven. The mammalian organism is composed of multiple nested loops of non–linear interacting systems, and so is of the sort susceptible to chaotic behavior. This is at the physiological level. How much greater are the possibilities for chaotic behavior at the psychological and societal levels!

Acknowledgment

The author is most appreciative of the efforts of Marguerita Jensen in the preparation of this manuscript.

DISCUSSION

Dr. R. Chadwick: You discuss three ways to analyze a signal. One is some kind of averaging in the time domain, another is doing a spectral analysis, and the third is using the phase plane. Is looking in the phase plane the only way you can distinguish a noisy nonchaotic signal from one that is chaotic?

Dr. J. Bassingthwaighte: The phase plane method is a prominent method and there are many variations on the theme of how to analyze these in terms of the correlation on Grassberger–Procaccia dimension, the information dimension, and so on. These are all various ways at getting at measures of the information content. Another way is the calculation of the so called "Lyapunov Exponent" which is a measure of the rate of divergence from a pair of nearby starting points; a high rate of divergence expresses something about that signal compared to another, lower Lyapunov exponent. There are several different ways of using successive embedding techniques. All of these beg the issue of what the underlying phenomenon really is.

You know what you need to do with smooth muscle. You need to measure the membrane potential, the calcium levels, the diameter measurement and the tension, for you know those are the real variables. All of the measures of the chaotic dimension or the Lyapunov exponent or whatever are only a statement that we have to go the next stage and get more data on the other variables. The huge gap in the whole field is to discover how to take the idea of a chaotic signal and then to try to understand it and put it into biological terms of what are the underlying phenomena. That is a big gap. Nobody has accomplished much in closing the gap. The closest are the electro–cardiographers.

REFERENCES

1. Bernard C. Leçons sur les phénomène de la vie communs aux animaux et aux végétaux. Paris: Bailliére, 1878.
2. Cannon WB. Organization for physiological homeostasis. *Physiol Rev* 1929; 9:399–431.
3. Poincaré H. *Mémoire sur les courbes définies par les equations différentielles, I–IV, Oevre I.* Paris: Gauthier–Villars, 1880.
4. Lorenz EN. Deterministic nonperiodic flows. *J Atmos Sci* 1963; 20: 130–141.
5. Glass L, Malta CP. Chaos in multi–looped negative feedback systems. *J Theor Biol* 1990; 145: 217–223.
6. Ruelle D. *Chaotic Evolution and Strange Attractors.* New York: Cambridge University Press. 1989.
7. Jalife J. *Mathematical Approaches to Cardiac Arrythmias.* New York, NY: New York Acad Sci 1990: 417.
8. Lipsitz LA, Mietus J, Moody GB, Goldberger AL. Spectral characteristics of heart rate variability before and during postural tilt. *Circulation* 1990; 81: 1803–1810.
9. Kaplan DT, Furman mi, Pincus SM, Ryan SM, Lipsitz LA, Goldberger AL. Aging and the complexity of cardiovascular dynamics. *Biophys J* 1991; 59: 945–949.
10. Osborne AR, Provenzale A. Finite correlation dimension for stochastic systems with power–law spectra. *Physica D* 1989; 35: 357–381.
11. Bassingthwaighte JB. Physiological heterogeneity: Fractals link determinism and randomness in structures and functions. *News Physiol Sci* 1988; 3: 5–10.
12. Bassingthwaighte JB, King RB, Roger SA. Fractal nature of regional myocardial blood flow heterogeneity. *Circ Res* 65:578–590, 1989.
13. Hurst HE. Long–term storage capacity of reservoirs. *Trans Am Soc Civ Engrs* 1951; 116: 770–808.
14. Mandelbrot BB, Wallis JR. Noah, Joseph, and operational hydrology. *Water Resour Res* 1968; 4: 909–918.
15. Feder J. *Fractals.* New York: Plenum Press, 1988).
16. Oude Vrielink HHE, Slaaf DW, Tangelder GJ, Weijmer–Van Velzen S, Reneman RS. Analysis of vasomotion waveform changes during pressure reduction and adenosine application. *Am J Physiol* (*Heart Circ Physiol* 27) 1990; 258: H29–H37.

17. Yamashiro SM, Slaaf DF, Reneman RS, Tangelder GJ, Bassingthwaighte JB. Fractal analysis of vasomotion. In: Jalife J (ed) *Mathematical Approaches to Cardiac Arrhythmias, vol. 591.* Ann NY Acad Sci 1990; 410–416.
18. Grassberger P, Procaccia I. Measuring the strangeness of strange attractors. *Physica* 1983; 9D: 189–208.
19. Liebovitch LS, Toth T. A fast algorithm to determine fractal dimensions by box counting. *Phys Lett A* 1989; 141: 386–390.
20. Hou XJ, Gilmore R, Mindlin GB, Solari HG. An efficient algorithm for fast O(N*1n(N)) box counting. *Phys Lett* 1990; A151: 43–46.
21. Theiler J, Galdrikian B, Longtin A, Eubank S, Farmer JS. Using surrogate data to detect nonlinearity in time series. *Los Alamos Preprint* 1991; LA–UR–91–2615.
22. Wolf A, Swift JB, Swinney HL, Vastano JA. Determining Lyapunov exponents from a time series. *Physica* 1985; 16D: 285–317.
23. Parker TS, Chua LO. *Practical Numerical Algorithms for Chaotic Systems*. New York: Springer–Verlag. 1989.
24. Pincus SM. Approximate entropy as a measure of system complexity. *Proc Natl Acad Sci* 1991; 88: 2297–2301.
25. Goldberger A L. Fractal mechanisms in the electrophysiology of the heart. *IEEE Eng Med Biol* 1992; 11: 47–52.
26. Garfinkel A, Spano ML, Ditto WL, Weiss JN. Controlling cardiac chaos. *Science* 1992; 257: 1230–1235.

CHAPTER 21

INTRAMYOCARDIAL FLUID TRANSPORT EFFECTS ON CORONARY FLOW AND LEFT VENTRICULAR MECHANICS

Daniel Zinemanas, Rafael Beyar and Samuel Sideman[1]

ABSTRACT

An integrated left ventricular (LV) model is used to solve, simultaneously and interactively, the LV mechanics, the coronary blood flow and capillary and interstitial fluid and mass transport, and to analyze the LV behavior under normal as well as pathological conditions. Accounting for the interstitial fluid mass balance in a LV flow–mechanical model allows to determine the LV wall volume in terms of the prevailing mechanical and flow conditions; it allows to uniquely define the flow–mechanical relationship and study pathologies, such as myocardial edema, which are directly related to changes in the myocardial fluid transport and content.

INTRODUCTION

Fluid transport and its content in the myocardium, as well as in other tissues, is integrally and functionally related to blood flow and muscle mechanics. This linkage is mainly due to the fact that the capillary wall is permeable to the transport of fluid and metabolites which are necessary for sustaining the myocardial activity.

A schematic description of the basic relevant elements in the myocardial tissue is shown in Fig. 1. These elements are part of the complex myocardial structure and include: 1) the muscle and collagen fiber matrices, with their particular orientation distribution; 2) the vascular network, which includes the various size levels of the circulation and accounts for 15% of the muscle volume [1], 3) the interstitial fluid, which fills the space between the fibers and the blood vessels, and occupies about 20% of the total muscle volume [1], and 4) the lymphatic circulation, which is responsible for the drainage of macromolecules to the venous return and plays an important role in the control of the tissue volume.

---

[1]Heart System Research Center, The Julius Silver Institute, Department of Biomedical Engineering, Technion–IIT, Haifa, 32000, Israel.

Interactive Phenomena in the Cardiac System, Edited by
S. Sideman and R. Beyar, Plenum Press, New York, 1993

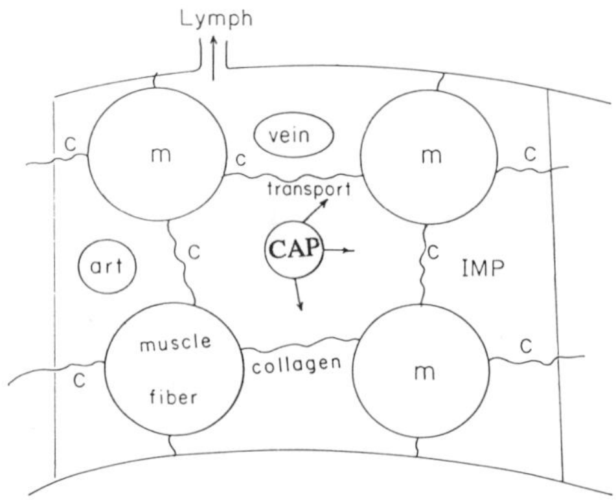

Figure 1. Schematic description of the basic elements of the myocardium. C – collagen; m – muscle fiber.

The interaction between the basic relationships that govern muscle mechanics, coronary flow and fluid transport is schematically depicted in Fig. 2. The myocardial stress tensor which determines, through the myocardial force balance, the mechanical behavior of the muscle is composed of the contribution of the muscle fiber and collagen stresses and the isotropic effect of the interstitial fluid pressure [2]. This fluid pressure is commonly denoted as the intramyocardial pressure (IMP). The coronary flow is determined by the perfusion pressure and the vascular impediment which depends on the vascular to intramyocardial hydrostatic pressure difference. Possible direct effects of the fiber stresses on the vessel impediment to flow [3] are still speculative and difficult to quantify and are not considered here. The fluid transport, and therefore the myocardial interstitial fluid content, is linked to the coronary flow and the mechanical variables since the fluid flux across the capillary wall is determined by the difference between the vascular capillary

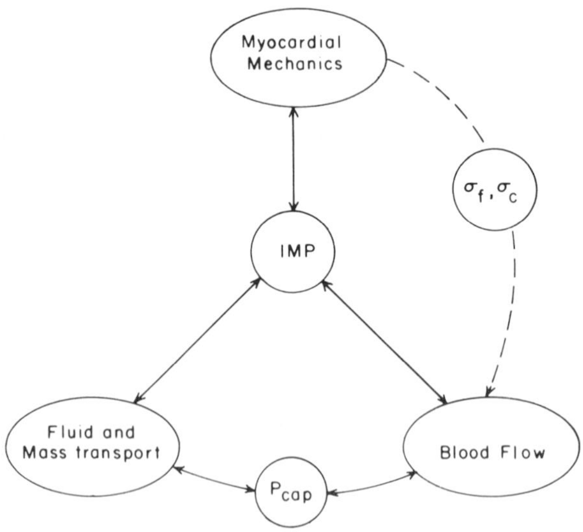

Figure 2. Schematic diagram of the mechanical—blood flow—interstitial fluid transport interactions. IMP – intramyocardial pressure = interstitial fluid pressure; P_{cap} – capillary pressure.

pressure and the IMP and by the vascular to interstitial osmotic pressure difference. Moreover, the lymphatic outflow also depends on the IMP.

Although the linkage between the fluid transport and the coronary flow and the muscle mechanics is self evident, there are no theoretical LV models that integrate these three elements together. For example, various LV models have concentrated on studying only mechanics [4–8], coronary flow [9–11] or fluid transport [12]. Others have integrated coronary flow and mechanical models [13, 14] to study the effects of the mechanics on the coronary flow. However, even modelling one, or two, of these phenomena is not a simple task and important information is lost due to the decoupling of the actual processes. The missing information has to be approximated or obtained experimentally. For example, the IMP or LVP are input data in various coronary flow models [9–11], and these values are usually obtained from experimental data. This approach is cumbersome since new guesses or experimental data must be provided for each different condition.

Flow–mechanical LV relationships, which are derived without considering fluid transport and mass balance, are usually inadequate since muscle mechanics is studied by solving the myocardial force balance constrained by the incompressibility condition, i.e., the wall volume is considered constant [4–8]. The limitation of this approach is that the incompressibility constrain does not provide the value of this "constant" volume, neither does it account for volume changes with changing conditions, such as variations in the coronary perfusion pressure, or under different arrested or beating heart conditions. The interstitial fluid mass conservation, together with an evaluation of the vascular volume from a coronary flow model, provide the additional and necessary linkage that uniquely defines the mechanical–flow relationship and allows to evaluate the LV wall volume according to the prevailing flow and mechanical conditions. This extra linkage thus substitutes the incompressibility constrain by a relationship requiring that the instantaneous LV wall volume equals the sum of the fibers (muscle + collagen), the vascular and the interstitial fluid volumes.

The integrated LV model that includes muscle mechanics, coronary flow and fluid transport and mass balance presented here allows to uniquely determine the flow–mechanical relationship and to explore the normal LV function. For example, the model allows to determine theoretically the value of the end–diastolic IMP in the normal beating heart and at other operating conditions of the heart. Thus, the integrated model helps to evaluate the basic role of the IMP in the heart as a function of the coronary perfusion pressure. In this situation the total wall volume changes due to vascular volume changes with the perfusion pressure and the shift in interstitial fluid content.

The model allows to determine the wall volume and fluid content from basic principles; it permits us to investigate and study the LV performance in pathological situations, which are directly related to changes in the myocardial fluid transport conditions such as myocardial edema. Edema may be caused by various factors, including lymphatic outflow blockage or increased perfusion pressure, and it is primarily linked to an increase in the interstitial fluid content and pressure.

This situation emphasizes the limitations of the incompressibility constrain which is insufficient and prohibits prediction of wall volume changes arising from changes in the flow conditions. McClough et al. [15] suggest that their experiments on the effects of coronary perfusion on the passive canine LV need a description of the myocardium that includes fluid transport, since small blood volume changes cannot explain the large changes observed in the LV compliance. Kresh [3] suggests that the myocardium should be considered as a composite material composed of connective tissue and contractile element (myocytes) vessel attachments, interposed by an interstitial fluid gel–like matrix. This is in fact the approach that is introduced here: a myocardium in which the muscle mechanics, the coronary flow and the fluid transport and mass balance are all considered simultaneously and interactively.

Obviously, the proposed model allows to calculate, as do earlier models [13–14], the effect of the mechanics on the coronary flow. However, unlike the earlier models, it permits to calculate the opposite effect, i.e., the effect of flow on myocardial mechanics, and also to evaluate any other interaction between these phenomena. Furthermore, the model is based on structural data and measurable physiological parameters, and does not require experimental or guessed values of the dependent variables such as the IMP or the LV cavity pressure.

BASIC ELEMENTS OF THE INTEGRATED MODEL

Muscle Mechanics

The LV wall is approximated by a thick cylindrical structure (Fig. 3). Muscle fibers are assumed to lie in the (θ–z) planes with changing orientation across the wall [16]. The collagen fibers are assumed to be distributed in the (θ–z) planes parallel and normal to the muscle fibers and are also radially oriented. The stress tensor in this configuration is described by [2]:

$$\boldsymbol{\sigma} = \boldsymbol{\sigma}_f + \boldsymbol{\sigma}_c - \text{IMP}\ \mathbf{I} \tag{1}$$

where $\boldsymbol{\sigma}_f$ and $\boldsymbol{\sigma}_c$ are the muscle and collagen fiber stresses, respectively, and IMP is the interstitial pressure. **I** is a unit tensor. The parametric data and constitutive equations for the muscle and collagen fibers stresses, used in this model, are taken from the mechanical models of Beyar and Sideman [5] and Nevo and Lanir [7]. The LV wall force balances are solved by using a transmural averaged stress analysis, i.e., the LV wall force balance is transformed into three (θ, z and r) force balances in terms of the transmural averaged wall stresses. From these three equations and the given wall volume, the mean wall stresses and

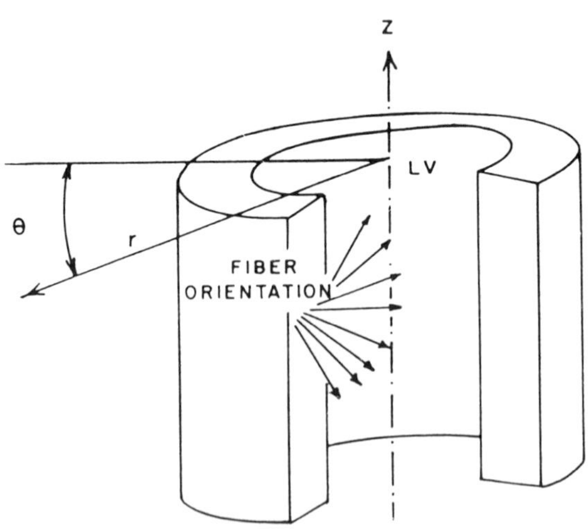

Figure 3. The assumed geometry of the LV wall.

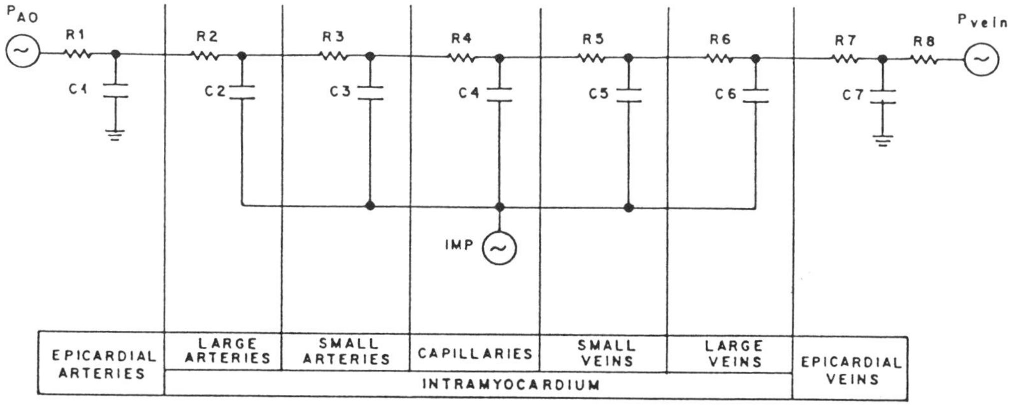

Figure 4. Electric analog of the coronary circulation.

the IMP are calculated. The IMP is then used as input data in the flow and fluid transport models [19].

The Coronary Blood Flow

The coronary circulation is simulated here by an electric analog composed of a series of capacitance–resistance elements representing the various levels of the circulation: large epicardial arteries, large and small intramural arteries, capillaries, small and large intramural veins, and epicardial veins. The model presented here is a modification of the transmural three–layered myocardial pressure dependent model of Beyar et al. [9], with only one averaged myocardial layer considered. A capillary compartment, necessary to evaluate the capillary fluid transport, is added. The components of the electric analog model depicted in Fig. 4 are assumed to depend on the transmural pressure difference, i.e., the resistance, R, and capacitance, C, of each compartment are functions of the cross sectional area of the vessel, A, which is in turn a function of the instantaneous difference between the vascular pressure, P_{vas}, and the extravascular interstitial (IMP) pressure. Thus,

$$R = R(A) \quad ; \quad C = C(A) \quad ; \quad A = A(P_{vas} - IMP) \tag{2}$$

The model thus allows to evaluate the instantaneous vascular flow, pressure and volume at each level of the circulation.

Fluid Transport

The total LV wall volume, V_{wall}, which is made up of the interstitial volume, V_{int}, the blood volume, V_{blood}, and the fiber volume, V_{fib}, has to be determined from the prevailing blood flow and mechanical conditions. The blood volume dynamics are evaluated by the blood mass balance. The myocardial interstitial fluid content is calculated by the mass conservation law, which states that the net rate of interstitial fluid mass accumulation equals to the net fluid influx across the capillary wall minus the net lymphatic outflow, i.e.

$$\frac{\partial V_{int}}{\partial t} = S_{cap} J_w - F_{lymph} \tag{3}$$

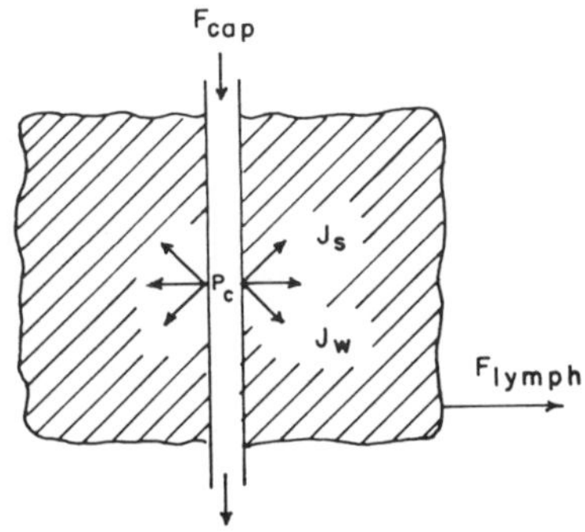

Figure 5. Interstitial fluid transport. J_w and J_s denote the fluid and solute (macromolecular) fluxes.

where S_{cap} denotes the total capillary wall surface area and J_w and F_{lymph} are the capillary fluid flux and the lymphatic outflow, respectively. The interstitial fluid mass balance is closely coupled to the blood circulation and the mechanical myocardial variables, and requires the simultaneous solution of the mechanical, fluid and blood flow models. The total interstitial fluid space is considered here as a single well mixed compartment (Fig. 5) and the capillary wall is assumed to be an ideal semipermeable membrane. In this case the fluid flux, J_w, across the capillary wall is given by [17]:

$$J_w = L_p\left[(P_{cap} - IMP) - \Delta\pi(c)\right] \tag{4}$$

where L_p is the hydraulic conductivity. P_{cap} denotes the capillary blood pressure, and $\Delta\pi(c)$ is the osmotic capillary to interstitial pressure difference which depends on the macromolecular concentrations, c, in the capillary and interstitial compartments. The capillary pressure is derived from the coronary flow model. The IMP is obtained from the mechanical model and the dynamics of the interstitial macromolecular concentration, c_{int}, is determined by a similar mass balance involving the capillary solute flux, J_s and the lymphatic transport of macromolecules:

$$V_{int}\frac{\partial c_{int}}{\partial t} = S_{cap}J_s - F_{lymph}c_{int} - c_{int}\frac{\partial V_{int}}{\partial t} \tag{5}$$

The lymphatic outflow, which drains the macromolecules that cannot return to the blood circulation by diffusion or convection across the capillary wall, is assumed here to be a linear function of the diastolic IMP in accordance to the experimental data of Laine and Granger [18], i.e.:

$$F_{lymph} = F_{lymph}\,(IMP) \tag{6}$$

Geometrical Constrains and the Reference State

Two geometrical constrains must be satisfied, in addition to the force, mass and flow relationships. The first relates to the instantaneous total wall volume, V_{wall}, which is necessary to calculate the wall stresses and the IMP, and is given by:

$$V_{wall}(t) = V_{blood}(P_{vas}, IMP) + V_{int}(P_{cap}, IMP, \Delta\pi) + V_{fib} \tag{7}$$

where V_{blood} and V_{int} are functions of the prevailing vascular and interstitial conditions. The fiber volume, V_{fib}, is considered constant. It is to be noted that in a steady state situation, this constrain is not much different from the incompressibility constrain, except that Eq. (7) yields the wall volume theoretically from its basic components.

The second geometric constraint states that the total LV cavity volume remains constant during the isovolumic, contracting and relaxing, stages.

The reference state is defined here as the unloaded (LVP = 0) LV with zero vascular pressure (P_{vas} = 0), zero intramyocardial pressure (IMP = 0) and zero osmotic pressure gradient ($\Delta\pi$ = 0).

The numerical procedure used to solve the mathematical representation of the integrated LV model is described in detail elsewhere [19] and involves the simultaneous and interactive solution of the force, balance, the interstitial fluid mass balance and the coronary flow.

RESULTS AND DISCUSSION

The effect of fluid transport in the LV wall is now demonstrated by some examples. First, we consider the simple cases of an isolated constant coronary perfused and empty (LVP = 0) beating and arrested hearts. Figure 6 shows the IMP dependence on the coronary perfusion pressure in both the arrested and beating hearts. In the beating heart case both the end–diastolic and mean IMP values are depicted. It is clearly seen, in agreement with experimental data [20], that the mean IMP increases with the perfusion pressure and that the mean IMP under beating conditions is larger than in the arrested heart. On the other hand, the end–diastolic IMP in the beating heart is smaller than the arrested heart IMP value. The increase of the IMP with coronary pressure is due to the increase in wall volume that comes from the corresponding changes in blood and interstitial fluid volumes, which increase with an increase in the coronary perfusion pressure. Evidently, larger wall volumes affect larger diastolic IMP, larger fiber stresses and larger fiber length, which lead to larger systolic and mean IMPs.

The smaller end–diastolic IMP value in the beating heart compared to the arrested heart value is due to the fact that the mean IMP in the beating heart is larger than in the arrested heart. Consequently, the wall volume in the beating case is smaller than in the arrested heart since with a larger mean IMP the fluid influx across the capillary wall is smaller and the lymphatic outflux is larger.

The results obtained here elucidate the experimental results of Kresh [3], of a constant perfused empty beating heart which is transiently paralyzed by a bolus injection

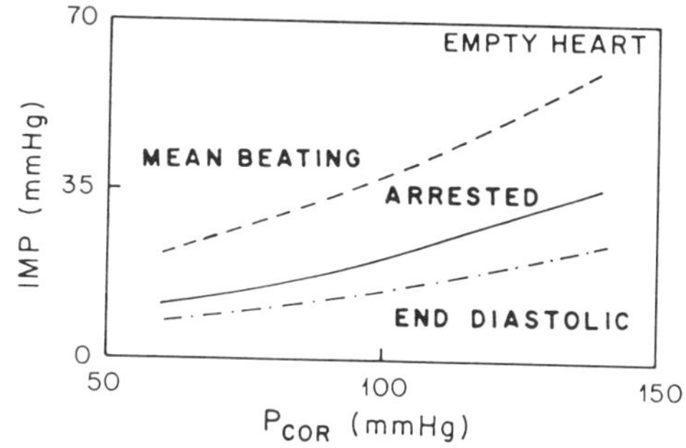

Figure 6. IMP vs coronary perfusion pressure in constant perfused empty beating and arrested hearts.

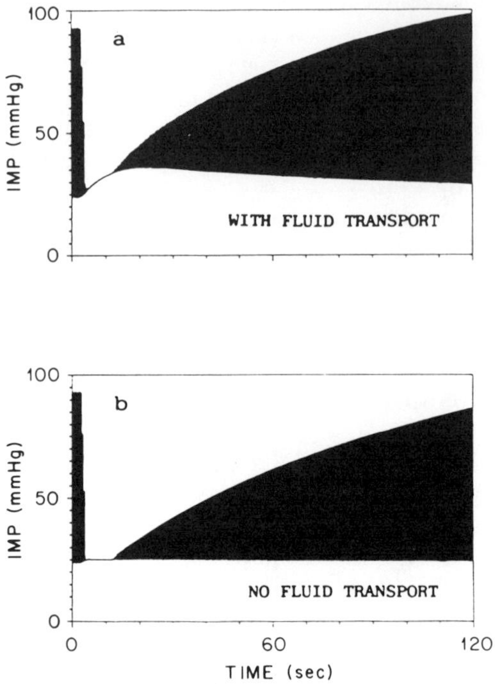

Figure 7. IMP dynamics in a transiently paralysed constant perfused empty beating heart. **a:** Calculated by the LV model with fluid transport, **b:** Calculated with no fluid transport, i.e., constant interstitial volume.

of pentobarbital. A simulation of such an experiment using the integrated LV model is shown in Fig. 7a. The results agree very well with the experimental data and show that immediately after the injection of pentobarbital the IMP remains at its end–diastolic value, which corresponds to the myocardial fluid content at that moment. When the muscle is paralyzed, the mean IMP becomes lower than during beating conditions; the fluid transport across the capillary wall increases and the lymphatic flow decreases. The consequent increase in the interstitial volume causes the IMP to rise toward the arrested heart value, consistent with the results depicted in Fig. 6. As the pentobarbital is washed out and the muscle slowly resumes its activity, the IMP returns to its beating heart values and the wall returns to its beating heart volume and fluid mass balance.

The effect of fluid transport in the situation described above is emphasized by comparison to a similar simulation carried out with no fluid transport, i.e., the interstitial volume was kept constant (Fig. 7b). As expected under these conditions, the IMP remains at the end–diastolic value during the transient paralysis, in disagreement with the experimental findings. It is perceived that the large changes in the IMP during the muscle paralysis cannot be explained in terms of blood volume changes only. A similar conclusion was reached by McCullogh et al. [15] who experimentally studied the mechanical effects of the coronary perfusion in the passive canine LV and proposed that the effects they have studied "may be modelled by treating the myocardium as a porous elastic medium swollen with an incompressible fluid rather than by an increase in ventricular wall thickness due to filling of the coronary vessels". They suggest that the large changes in the myocardial compliance cannot be explained in terms of the small changes in the vascular volume.

Another example where fluid transport is necessary to evaluate the LV performance is myocardial edema. One of the reasons for myocardial edema is blockage of the lymphatic outflow. This situation leads to myocardial dysfunction [21] and is simulated here by reducing the lymphatic conductivity, i.e., the proportionality constant giving the value of the ratio between the change of lymphatic flow with a change in IMP. Reducing the normal lymphatic flow and the lymphatic conductivity to a third of their normal value yields an increase of 24% in the mean IMP, a 14% decrease in the mean coronary flow and a 28% in the oscillatory flow amplitude (OFA) as compared to the normal lymphatic flow conditions. Not less important, it is predicted that the total wall volume increases by 4% and the interstitial volume increases by 40% (!).

These results demonstrate quite clearly why LV dysfunction follows myocardial edema: edema affects a decrease in the coronary flow due to an increase in the IMP which

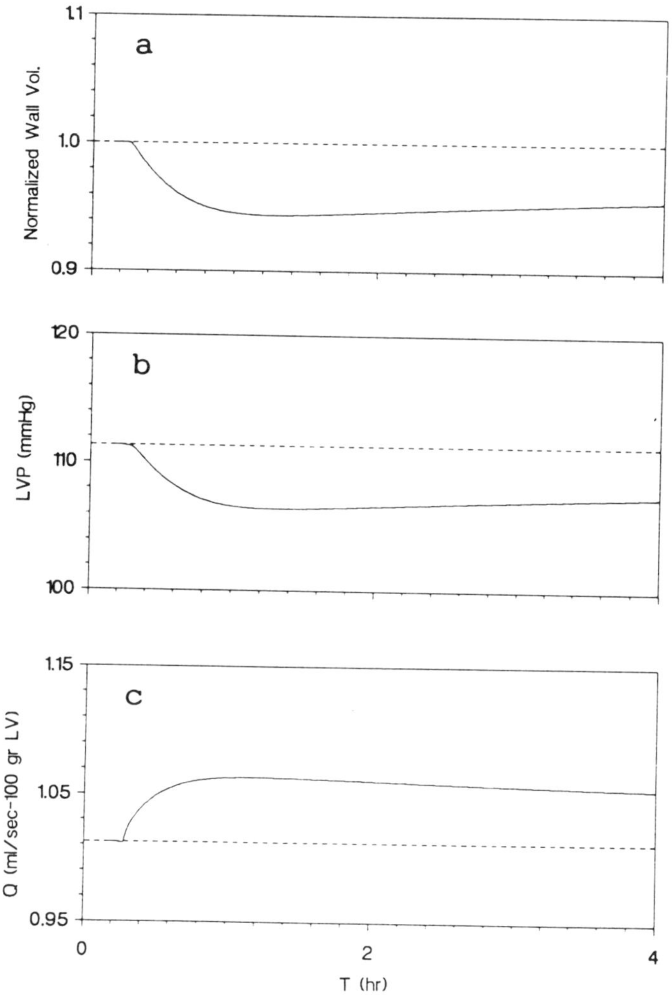

Figure 8. LV response to a step increase in albumin blood concentration in a normally beating heart. **a:** nondimensionalized LV wall volume, **b:** LV cavity pressure, **c:** mean coronary flow. The dashed lines denote the values of the variables previous to the step change in albumin concentration.

is caused by the increased wall volume and fluid content. It is important to note that although the total wall volume change is small, the corresponding changes of the IMP, blood flow and interstitial volume are significantly larger. Evidently, a smaller coronary flow which carries less nutrients for the muscle fiber, together with a larger diffusion distance due to the large increase in the interstitial volume, may significantly reduce the energy supply to the muscle and thus lead to a reduced LV activity.

Changes in the fluid content of the myocardium can also arise from variations in the blood macromolecular concentration. The response of a normal beating heart to a step increase in blood albumin concentration is depicted in Fig. 8. An increase in the albumin concentration produces an opposite effect to that noted during myocardial edema, i.e., the myocardial fluid content decreases. It can be observed that the wall volume decreases due to the suction of interstitial fluid caused by the change in the osmotic gradient at the capillary level (Fig. 8a). The reduced wall volume produces smaller LV pressures (Fig. 8b) due to a decrease in the diastolic IMP and sarcomere length. The reduction of the diastolic and systolic IMP values yields an increase in the mean coronary flow (Fig. 8c).

Last, we note the effect of the coronary perfusion pressure on the LV end–diastolic compliance of an isovolumic contracting heart. The results, summarized in Table 1, show that the LV compliance decreases with an increase in the perfusion pressure. This is in agreement with the experimental data [15, 22], and is due to the changes in myocardial fluid and blood content.

The foregoing examples emphasize the fluid and mean transport effects on the coronary flow and LV mechanics. Obviously, any one change in muscle mechanics, coronary flow or fluid transport, will consequently affect the other two.

Table 1. Effect of perfusion pressure on end–diastolic LV compliance.

P_{cor} [mmHg]	$C_{ED} = dV_{ED}/dP_{ED}$ [ml/mmHg]
60	1.62
100	1.25
150	0.89

CONCLUSIONS

The integrated approach to modeling the LV is shown to be helpful in analyzing natural (normal as well as pathological) and experimental situations. This approach differs from previous LV models since it requires that the myocardial interstitial fluid mass balance be satisfied simultaneously with the flow and mechanical relationships. The fluid mass balance provides an additional relationship between the flow and mechanical variables and allows to define uniquely the flow–mechanical relationship and to determine the LV wall volume from basic principles. Consequently, any case which involves changes in the LV fluid transport and content can be studied theoretically. For example, a change in heart rate will simultaneously affect the muscle mechanics, the coronary flow and the fluid transport and content. The analysis can then be performed with the integrated model presented here.

Although the principal characteristics of the LV mechanics, the coronary flow and the fluid transport are conserved in the present integrated model, some simplifying compromises have been introduced in describing the details of the system so that the mathematical description of the system can be handled with existing computational resources. Improved versions of this integrated model will have to take into account more realistic geometries, transmural heterogeneities, a more detailed lymphatic flow model, and the direct effects of fiber stresses on the coronary circulation.

Acknowledgment

This study was sponsored by the Women's Division of the American Technion Society, the Anna and Gorge Ury Research Fund (Chicago, USA), the Al and Phyllis Newman and the Joseph and Edith Jackier Research Funds (Detroit, USA).

DISCUSSION

Dr. R. Chadwick: It seems that the time constant for capillary transport is such that you should not have to worry about it. If one is operating in the steady state, without a long diastole, do you have to worry about the capillary transport?

Dr. D. Zinemanas: You need to consider the myocardial fluid transport even under steady state conditions. It must be noted that we not only consider the capillary fluid transport but we solve, simultaneously with the coronary flow and LV mechanics, the interstitial fluid mass balance. In other words, we assume that the interstitial fluid mass balance is satisfied in addition to the muscle mechanics and blood flow relationships. In a steady state situation this balance states that the net fluid flow across the capillary wall is equal to the lymphatic outflow. This balance determines the myocardial fluid content and provides another linkage between the mechanical and flow variables that allows to calculate, from basic principles, the LV wall volume and fluid content and the diastolic and systolic IMPs, according to the prevailing conditions. Even if the wall volume is constant in steady state conditions, you need to know the wall volume and diastolic IMP values since these values change with different conditions. While in other LV models these variables are input parameters and usually have to be guessed, or obtained experimentally, these variables are theoretically calculated here and are outputs of the model.

Dr. R. Mates: Do you have any numerical estimates of how different your intramyocardial pressure values are with and without the capillary transport?

Dr. D. Zinemanas: The difference can be of the order of 10 mmHg. The difference is, however, not only numerical but conceptual as well. When you use a mechanical LV model without fluid transport and mass balance, the diastolic IMP and LV wall volume should be provided as input data and must be guessed or obtained from experimental data. Thus, your results depend on your guess. Solving simultaneously the muscle mechanics, the coronary flow and fluid transport and mass balance, these values are obtained theoretically. The differences can be clearly observed in the simulations of Dr. Kresh's experiment (Fig. 7a,b) during the transient myocardial paralysis. It must be noted that in the simulation without fluid mass balance, the end–diastolic IMP value obtained in the simulation with fluid transport, was used prior to the pentobarbital injection. However, when you do not consider the interstitial fluid mass balance, the end–diastolic IMP is in fact unknown *a priori*. If you use another end–diastolic value, the differences may be larger. For example, some studies use an end–diastolic IMP equal to zero in their LV mechanical models.

Dr. Y. Kresh: Since you are using my data, I ought to comment on what it represents. The relationship between coronary perfusion pressure and intramyocardial pressure is not merely a by–product of capillary fluid transport. The relationship is an expression of the mechanical activity of the myocardium, that is to say, it is not simply a result of fluid transport at the capillary level. It represents the force generation capability of the myocardial cell, and specifically, the myofibril, as it is relates to the "quality" of the muscle perfusion. Part of the modulation resulting from verapamil infusion or sodium pentobarbital induced arrest (paralysis of the machinery of contraction) is related to the level of perfusion pressure. The diastolic part is indeed what you said: it represents the degree of leakage in the absence muscle pumping, from the capillaries into the interstitial space, increasing the fluid interstitial pressure. Most of the magnitude (perfusion pressure–intramyocardial pressure slope) has little to do with fluid transport per se.

Dr. D. Zinemanas: I agree. The flow, the IMP and the fluid transport are all passive events arising from the active muscle activity and stresses. That is the approach we describe here. Our integrated model solves simultaneously and interactively the muscle mechanics, the coronary flow and the interstitial fluid mass balance. This approach is required since these three phenomena are functionally interrelated and therefore cannot be considered separately without loosing important information. Briefly, the active muscle stresses generate the IMP which consequently affects the blood flow and the wall fluid interstitial content. On the other hand, these last two parameters determine the LV wall volume which in turn affects the muscle mechanics and the IMP. It must also be noted that it is not only the capillary fluid transport that is considered here but the interstitial fluid mass balance; the former is only a part of the latter. Moreover, fluid transport is not only important in transient cases, as in the transient LV paralysis, but also during normal steady state conditions. The interstitial fluid mass balance should also be observed in such cases. This balance, together with the blood flow and muscle mechanics, determines what is the myocardial fluid content and therefore also determines other variables such as the end-diastolic IMP.

Dr. R. Beyar: I agree with Dr. Kresh's comment, that the force of the muscle is a very important parameter which modulates the systolic IMP. The diastolic IMP is very much affected by fluid transport. But obviously there is a different time scale to these effects; it changes within minutes, maybe in many beats as in your experiment, but it is there and we have to account for it and that is the main purpose, of this presentation.

REFERENCES

1. Gonzalez F, Bassingthwaighte JB. Heterogeneities in regional volumes of distribution and flows in rabbit heart. *Am J Physiol* 1990; 258: H1012–H1024.
2. Ohayon J, Chadwick RS. Effects of collagen microstructure on the mechanics of the left ventricle. *Biophys J* 1988; 54: 1077–1088.
3. Kresh JY. Myocardial modulation of coronary circulation (letter). *Am J Physiol* 1989; 257: H1934–H1935.
4. Arts T, Veenstra PC, Reneman RS. Transmural course of stress and sarcomere length in the left ventricle under normal hemodynamic circumstances. In: Baan J, Arntsenius AC, Yellin EL (eds), *Cardiac Dynamics*, Martinus Nijhoff: The Hague, 1980; pp 115–122.
5. Beyar R, Sideman S. A computer study of the left ventricular performance based on fiber structure, sarcomere dynamics and transmural electrical propagation velocity. *Circ Res* 1984; 55: 358–375.
6. Chadwick RS. Mechanics of the left ventricle. *Biophys J* 1980; 39: 279–288.
7. Nevo E, Lanir Y. Structural finite deformation model of the left ventricle during diastole and systole. *J Biomed Eng* 1989; 111: 342–349.
8. Tozeren A. Static analysis of the left ventricle. J. Biomed. Eng. 1983; 105: 39–46;
9. Beyar R, Caminker R, Manor D, Sideman S. Coronary flow patterns in normal and ischemic hearts: Transmyocardial and artery to vein distribution. *Ann Biom Eng* 1993; in press.
10. Chadwick RS, Tedgui A, Michel JB, Ohayon J, Levy BI. Phasic regional myocardial inflow and outflow: comparison of theory and experiments. *Am J Physiol* 1990; 258: H1687–H1698.
11. Kresh JY, Fox M, Brockman SK, Noordergraaf A. Model-based analysis of transmural vessel impedance and myocardial circulation dynamics. *Am J Physiol* 1990; 258: H262–H276.
12. Bassingthwaighte JB, Goresky CA. Modeling in the analysis of solute and water exchange in the microvasculature. In: Renking EM, Michel CC (eds), *Handbook of Physiology*, American Physiological Society, Bethesda, U.S.A. 1984; pp. 549–626.

13. Arts T, Reneman RS. Interaction between intramyocardial pressure and myocardial circulation. *J Biomed Eng* 1985; 107: 51–56.
14. Beyar R, Sideman S. Time dependent coronary blood flow distribution in the left ventricular wall. *Am J Physiol* 1987; 252: H417–H433.
15. McCulloch AD, Hunter PH, Samill BH. Mechanical effects of coronary perfusion in the passive canine left ventricle. *Am J Physiol* 1992; 262: H523–530.
16. Streeter DD, Spotnitz HM, Patel DP, Ross J, Sonnenblick EH. Fiber orientation in the canine left ventricle during diastole and systole. *Circ Res* 1969;24: 339–347.
17. Kedem O, Katchalsky A. Thermodynamic analysis of the permeability of biological membranes to non–electrolytes. *Biochim Biophys Acta* 1958; 27: 229–246.
18. Laine GA, Granger HJ. Microvascular, interstitial and lymphatic interactions in normal heart. *Am J Physiol* 1985; 249: H834–H842.
19. Zinemanas D, Beyar R, Sideman S. A model study of muscle mechanics, blood flow and mass transport interactions in the LV wall. 1993; submitted.
20. Kresh JY, Frash F, Mcvey M, Brockman SK, Noordergraaf A. Mechanical coupling of the myocardium with coronary circulation in the beating and arrested heart (abstract). *64th Scientific Sessions AHA*, 1990.
21. Miller AJ. *Lymphatics of the Heart*, Raven Press: New York, 1982.
22. Fukui A, Yamaguchi S, Tamada Y, Miyawaki H, Baniya G, Shirakabe M. Different effects of coronary perfusion pressure on diastolic properties of left and right ventricles (abstract). *64th Scientific Sessions AHA*, 1992.

CHAPTER 22

METABOLIC PROTECTION OF POST–ISCHEMIC PHOSPHORYLATION POTENTIAL AND VENTRICULAR PERFORMANCE

Robert T. Mallet[1] and Rolf Bünger[2]

ABSTRACT

Relationships between cytosolic phosphorylation potential, low–flow ischemic purine release and post–ischemic left ventricular developed pressure were examined in perfused working guinea–pig heart. During moderate ischemic acidification, metabolic intervention by pyruvate attenuated cytosolic NADH accumulation and (ATP+ADP+AMP) degradation. In reperfusion, spontaneously developed ventricular pressure increased in parallel with the phosphorylation potential (R^2 = 0.71), but forced restoration of function by inotropic measures occurred at the expense of the phosphorylation potential.

INTRODUCTION

Myocardial contractile and hydraulic work requires high rates of energy consumption and oxidative metabolism. Endogenous energy reserves are limited; therefore, the working myocardium depends on exogenous energy–yielding substrates and oxygen. Thus, ventricular performance is acutely impaired during ischemic energy depletion but may be enhanced by metabolic substrate after coronary flow and O_2 supply are reestablished.

The present study tested whether acute metabolic measures could conserve myocardial adenylates during 45 min periods of ischemic stress. Also, the effects of metabolic vs. inotropic interventions on ventricular function were delineated in reversibly injured but reperfused hearts. The experimental model was the preload–controlled isolated guinea–pig heart performing external work and pressure development at physiologic levels.

---

[1]Department of Physiology, Texas College of Osteopathic Medicine, Fort Worth 76107–2699, TX and [2]Department of Physiology, Uniformed Services University of the Health Sciences, Bethesda, MD 20814–4799, USA.

Interactive Phenomena in the Cardiac System, Edited by S. Sideman and R. Beyar, Plenum Press, New York, 1993

METHODS

The Norepinephrine–Ischemia/Reperfusion Protocol in the Isolated Working Heart

Hearts, isolated from guinea pigs (400–600 g body mass) and beating at intrinsic sinus rhythm, were perfused as preload–controlled working hearts [1, 2] (mean left atrial filling pressure was 10 – 12 cm H_2O). Perfusion medium was a modified Krebs–Henseleit bicarbonate buffer [2], equilibrated with 95% O_2: 5% CO_2 at 37°C (pH 7.4–7.45) containing 5 U/l bovine insulin at physiologic free Ca^{2+}, Mg^{2+}, and inorganic phosphate concentrations (1.0, 0.6, and 1.2 mM, respectively). Myocardial energy state was varied by metabolic substrate supply [2, 3] as detailed in figure and table legends. Heart rate, left atrial filling pressure, phasic and mean aortic pressures, and coronary and aortic flows were continuously monitored [2, 3].

To induce global myocardial ischemia coronary flow was reduced to 15–20% of pre–ischemic control for 25 to 45 min by lowering the hydrostatic aortic pressure below the autoregulatory reserve [4]. In an attempt to mimic the known excessive adrenergic discharge triggered by acute myocardial ischemia and circulatory shock *in vivo*, *L*–norepinephrine was infused concurrently to maximally effective concentrations (0.7–1.1 μM). Intracellular pH judged from coronary venous PCO_2 [2] fell by 0.3 pH unit during ischemic perfusion, indicating moderate cellular acidosis. Active left ventricular pressure development ceased after 20–30 min ischemia [2]. Intensity of ischemic stress was standardized by controlling ischemic coronary flow and coronary venous PCO_2 (cellular acidification [2]); these indices of ischemic stress did not differ among the various metabolic conditions tested.

Reperfusion was effected by restoring hydrostatic aortic pressure to pre–ischemic level within 15 s and discontinuing norepinephrine infusion. Following a reactive hyper–emic period, new hemodynamic and metabolic steady states were established within 10 to 15 min reperfusion [2, 3]. Under this reperfusion protocol, developed left ventricular pressure reflected the spontaneous contractile capabilities of the reperfused myocardium. Metabolic substrate supply was constant throughout the protocols, except in some reperfu–sions with pyruvate as sole substrate; here, 5 mM glucose was supplied throughout ischemia to prevent irreversible contracture [3]. In other experiments a high concentration of 2–deoxyglucose was applied to disable glycolysis during reperfusion [3]. In experiments with inotropic agents (1 μM *L*–norepinephrine, 1 μM BayK 8644, 3.5 mM Ca^{2+}) drug infu–sion was commenced when new hemodynamic steady states were established after 10 min reperfusion.

Analytical Procedures

Coronary venous purines (adenosine, inosine, (hypo)xanthine, urate) were quantitated by C_{18} reverse–phase HPLC [3, 4]. Extracellular space was measured as [^{14}C]mannitol distribution space [3]. Lactate, pyruvate, and inorganic phosphate in arterial perfusion medium and coronary venous effluent were determined enzymatically [2, 3]. Hearts were stop–frozen with Wollenberger tongs cooled to the temperature of liquid N_2. Myocardial metabolites (ATP, ADP, AMP, creatine phosphate (CrP), creatine (Cr), inorganic phosphate (P_i), lactate, pyruvate) were measured in neutralized perchloric acid extracts [2, 3]. Intracellular concentrations of inorganic phosphate, lactate, and pyruvate were obtained by subtracting measured extracellular amounts from respective total tissue contents.

Statistics

Data are presented as means ± SE. Single comparisons of means were accomplished by two-tailed Student's *t* test. Multiple comparisons were accomplished by analysis of variance in combination with Tukey's test. $P \leq 0.05$ was considered statistically significant. Non-linear logistic or power fits as well as specific residual analyses were obtained using the Gauss-software as recently described [4].

RESULTS AND DISCUSSION

Pyruvate Attenuates Ischemic NADH Accumulation and ATP Degradation

The effects of the low-flow adrenergic ischemic stress and 5 mM pyruvate treatment on cytosolic redox state, cellular pH, and myocardial energy state are summarized in Table 1. In normoxia, pyruvate raised $[CrP]/[P_i]$ and $[CrP]/([Cr]\cdot[P_i])$ ratios (indices of the cytosolic ATP phosphorylation potential [2, 3]) by about 50 to 65% at constant cellular pH, filling pressure, and heart rate·pressure product. Ischemic perfusion produced large decrements in heart function, all indices of the phosphorylation potential, and the ATP concentration as well. Intracellular pH moderately but progressively decreased from near 7.2 in preischemia to 6.9 after 45 min ischemia. Pyruvate had no effects on ischemic $[CrP]/[P_i]$ and $[CrP]/([Cr]\cdot[P_i])$ ratios or cellular acidification. In contrast, pyruvate blunted the ischemic rise in the intracellular [lactate]/[pyruvate] ratio and hence accumulation of cytoplasmic NADH; also the [α-glycerophosphate]/[dihydroxyacetone phosphate] ratio confirmed the marked attenuation by pyruvate of ischemic accumulation of cytoplasmic NADH [2]. Further, after 45 min ischemic perfusion, the residual ATP concentration was higher with than without pyruvate (Table 1).

Figure 1 depicts the effects of ischemic perfusion with and without pyruvate on the net release of adenylate degradatives (Σ(adenosine + inosine + (hypo)- xanthine + urate)). Purine release increased rapidly at the onset of ischemia, peaking within 5 min at nearly two orders of magnitude above the pre-ischemic rate (in the absence of pyruvate) and subsequently declining to a relatively stable rate which was only moderately above the pre-ischemic level. Pyruvate markedly attenuated early peak purine release, while in the steady state during late ischemia pyruvate was less effective. Indeed, at 45 min ischemia, the total adenylate pool (Σ (ATP+ADP+AMP)) was less depleted in presence of pyruvate (Fig. 1, inset), even though ischemic residual coronary flow, acidification, and $[CrP]/([Cr]\cdot[P_i])$ were virtually identical with and without pyruvate. As expected, measured attenuation of ischemic purine release by pyruvate (Fig. 1, shaded area) accounted for 88% of the observed difference in Σ(ATP+ADP+AMP) at 45 min ischemia (Fig. 1, inset). Obviously, pyruvate de-accelerated adenylate depletion during ischemia without enhancing $[CrP]/([Cr]\cdot[P_i])$, the phosphorylation potential. Such a pyruvate effect could be due to improved salvage of adenosine and/or hypoxanthine, possibly resulting from the improved cytosolic redox state (Table 1). In pre-ischemia (normal redox state) purine release was minimal and total adenylate content was not measurably affected by pyruvate treatment (control: 3.55 ± 0.14, pyruvate: 3.69 ± 0.07 μmol/g wet mass).

Reciprocity between $[CrP]/([Cr]\cdot[P_i])$ and purine release has been reported in isolated but normoxic hearts [4-6]. When such hearts are perfused at their natural coronary flows adrenergic stimulation is associated with reduced $[CrP]/([Cr]\cdot[P_i])$ [2, 6] and a biphasic adenosine release [7]; however, these non-ischemically deenergized hearts are hemodynamically stable and perform at near-maximum levels [2]. In the present low-flow

Table 1. Effects of pyruvate on heart rate-pressure product and cytosolic energy and redox metabolites in pre–ischemic and low–flow–ischemic hearts

	HR·ΔP $\frac{cm\,H_2O}{min \cdot 10^3}$	[CrP]/[Cr]	[CrP]/[P_i]	$\frac{[CrP]}{[Cr]\cdot[P_i]}$ M^{-1}	[ATP] mM	$\frac{[Lactate]}{[Pyruvate]}$	pH_i
Pre–ischemia							
G+L	18.6 ± 0.7	2.47 ± 0.17	2.63 ± 0.16	325 ± 19	9.0 ± 0.4	17	7.21 ± 0.01
G+L+P	17.9 ± 0.4	2.65 ± 0.12	4.00 ± 0.18*	535 ± 36*	9.7 ± 0.3	–	7.19 ± 0.01
5 min ischemia							
G+L	5.4 ± 0.9	0.48 ± 0.05	0.58 ± 0.02	23 ± 4	6.2 ± 0.2	–	7.05 ± 0.01
G+L+P	2.2 ± 0.5*	0.30 ± 0.05	0.34 ± 0.05*	18 ± 3	6.0 ± 0.2	–	7.04 ± 0.01
45 min ischemia							
G+L	0	0.41 ± 0.04	0.30 ± 0.03	17 ± 3	4.9 ± 0.1	168	6.93 ± 0.01
G+L+P	0	0.47 ± 0.03	0.32 ± 0.02	19 ± 1	5.7 ± 0.3*	7	6.94 ± 0.02

Values are means ± SE, n = 5–8. Perfusion medium contained 5 mM glucose (G) + 5 mM lactate (L) ± 5 mM pyruvate (P). HR·ΔP = heart rate times developed pressure (ΔP = mean aortic pressure – mean left atrial filling pressure); CrP = creatine phosphate; Cr = creatine; P_i = inorganic phosphate; pH_i = intracellular pH. [ ]: intracellular concentration; – : not determined; *: $P < 0.05$ vs. respective (G + L) controls. Portion of data from reference [2].

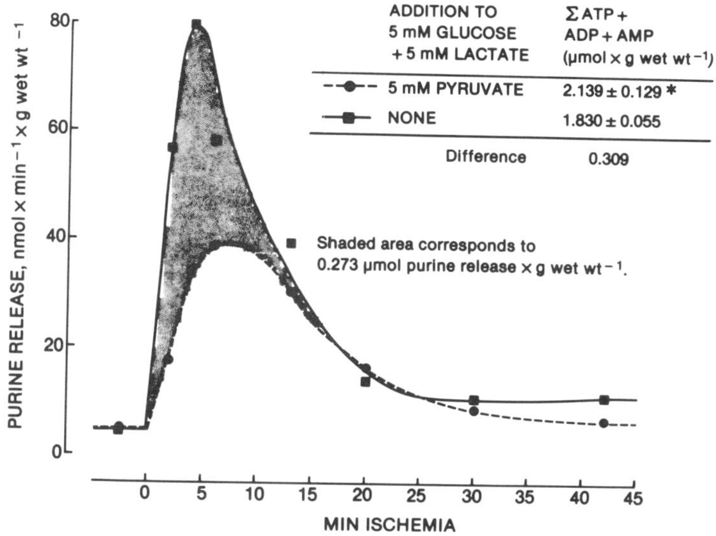

Figure 1. Myocardial purine release during low–flow adrenergic ischemia. Hearts received 5 mM glucose + 5 mM lactate alone (n = 20) or with additional 5 mM pyruvate (n = 13). Ischemic coronary flow declined from 4 ml/min/g wet mass at peak release to near 1 ml/min/g wet mass at 45 min ischemia [2]. Myocardial adenylates were measured at 45 min. ischemia in stop–frozen myocardium. Points represent mean values.

ischemia which was exacerbated by adrenergic stress, the cytosolic deenergization produced a massive albeit only transitory increase in purine release, although $[CrP]/([Cr]\cdot[P_i])$ remained decreased (Table 1). The [CrP]/[Cr] ratios also remained very low throughout ischemia (with only small changes in pH), which suggested sustained accumulation of free ADP and hence free AMP [2, 6]. The observed decays in purine release despite persisting ischemia (Fig. 1) could reflect impaired purine washout due to declining (limiting) coronary flow [2]; however, allosteric inhibition of *endo*–5'–nucleotidase by accumulated free ADP [8] and other as yet undefined allosteric factors may also have contributed. Conversely, the early massive peak release could reflect, besides high levels of free AMP [7], additional stimulation of *endo*–5'–nucleotidase by an acute increase in the cytosolic free Mg^{2+} level [8, 9]; an acute release of intracellularly bound Mg^{2+} is consistent with the precipitous fall in ATP (Table 1), the main physiologic chelator of Mg^{2+} [10].

Metabolic vs. Inotropic Intervention in Post–Ischemic Heart

Post–ischemic ventricular function was highly responsive to the metabolic state of the myocardium as manipulated by exogenous substrate. Thus, reperfusion left ventricular developed pressure varied over the full range from complete failure with pyruvate as sole substrate (no glucose) to poor recovery with glucose alone or in combination with acetate, to near–complete recovery with pyruvate plus glucose (Fig. 2A, [3]). Using all available single values (n = 45), reperfusion developed pressure could be fitted to a sigmoidal function [4] with $[CrP]/([Cr]\cdot[P_i])$ as the independent variable. Residual analysis of the fit yielded $R^2 = 0.71$ with acceptable Durban–Watson statistic (DW = 1.61) at moderate precision (SEEst = 33%). Thus, metabolic enhancement of reperfusion function appeared to be linked to, if not partially mediated by the cytosolic ATP phosphorylation potential. On the other hand, reperfusion ATP *per se* poorly correlated (power fit) with developed pressure (R^2 = 0.2; Fig. 2B) at unacceptable Durban–Watson statistic (DW < 1.0). This was not unexpected because residual ATP concentrations were all > 1.5 mM, i.e. near one order of magnitude above the $K_{m, ATP}$ values for, e.g., Na^+/K^+–ATPase, sarcoplasmic reticulum (SR) Ca^{2+}–ATPase, ATP–stimulated Ca^{2+}release from cardiac SR [11] or actomyosin ATPase (for review see [12]).

Pyruvate required the presence of glucose to effect near–complete restoration of CrP potential and left ventricular developed pressure (Fig. 2A, [3]). Glucose, but especially pyruvate as sole reperfusion substrate, only poorly or not at all restored CrP potential and left ventricular function (Fig. 2A). Other metabolic interventions (glucose present) with lactate, acetate, or β–hydroxybutyrate as well as phosphofructokinase and pyruvate dehydrogenase stimulations by dichloroacetate [3] did also not support sufficient cytosolic re–energization and hence functional restoration during reperfusion (Fig. 2A). Pyruvate–enhancement of reperfusion function (glucose present) did probably not stem from a primary improvement coronary perfusion, since pyruvate, unlike adenosine, is not a vasodilator metabolite; also, early reperfusion reactive hyperemic coronary flow did not differ among hearts that received additional pyruvate, lactate, or acetate; yet, only pyruvate (glucose present) supported near–complete recovery of ventricular function.

The energetics of metabolic intervention by pyruvate plus glucose contrasted sharply with those of traditional inotropic interventions without pyruvate (Fig. 2A, triangles). Thus, inotropic stimulation by norepinephrine, hypercalcemia or BayK 8644 (a stimulator of transsarcolemmal Ca^{2+} influx [13]) also completely restored reperfusion developed pressure in presence of glucose plus lactate (Fig. 2); this demonstrated complete reversibility of the partial reperfusion failure (pyruvate absent), a hallmark of cardiac "stunning" (for review see [14]). However, all inotropic measures tested produced cytosolic de–energization in

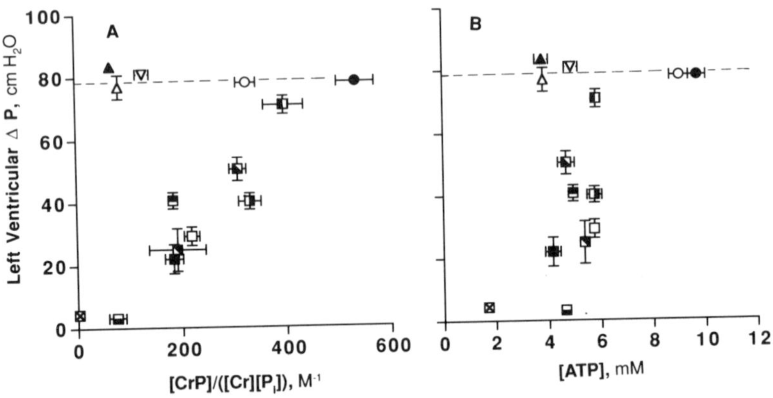

Figure 2. Plots of left ventricular developed pressure (ΔP) versus $[CrP]/([Cr]\cdot[P_i])$ **(Panel A)** or ATP concentration **(Panel B)**. Data are means ± SE (n = 5–7) from pre–ischemic hearts (circles) or from reperfused hearts in steady states (triangles, squares). Dashed line: ΔP = (mean aortic pressure minus mean atrial filling pressure) of normoxic controls. *Normoxia:* ○ 5 mM glucose + 5 mM lactate; ● 5 mM glucose + 5 mM lactate + 5 mM pyruvate. *Reperfusion inotropic intervention:* ▲ 5 mM glucose + 5 mM lactate + 1 μM *L*–norepinephrine or △ 3.5 mM Ca^{2+} or ∇ 1 μM BayK 8644. *Metabolic intervention with glucose:* □ no additional substrate; ■ + 5 mM lactate; ◧ + 5 mM pyruvate; ◨ + 10 mM DL–β– hydroxybutyrate; ◩ + 10 mM acetate; ⬒ + 2 mM dichloroacetate; ◪ + 5 mM lactate (+ 5 mM pyruvate in reperfusion). *Metabolic intervention without glucose:* ⬓ 5 mM pyruvate sole reperfusion substrate; ⊠ 5 mM pyruvate + 10 mM 2–deoxyglucose.

previously ischemic and only poorly recovered hearts (Fig. 2A). Obviously, these inotropic interventions restored reperfusion function at the expense of $[CrP]/([Cr]\cdot[P_i])$, while metabolic interventions, especially pyruvate treatment (glucose present), restored post–ischemic $[CrP]/([Cr]\cdot[P_i])$ and ventricular function in parallel.

CONCLUSIONS

Metabolic intervention by pyruvate (glucose present) can attenuate NADH accumulation in the cytoplasm during experimental myocardial ischemia; this "clamping" of the near–normoxic redox state during ischemia could attenuate reductive release of free Fe^{2+} from ferritin [15], which in turn could attenuate catalytic formation of cytotoxic hydroxyl radicals (Fenton reaction) upon subsequent reperfusion [15, 16]. Also, adenylate degradation and purine release is diminished by pyruvate during ischemic perfusion. Reperfusion metabolic measures including pyruvate (plus glucose), but not inotropic interventions by catecholamines or calcium agonists *per se*, can support virtually complete recovery of $[CrP]/([Cr]\cdot[P_i])$ in parallel with developed ventricular pressure at minor changes in cellular pH [2, 3]. These observations combined with the known stoichiometries of cellular ATPases suggest that the described metabolic–functional improvements could reflect a sensitivity of the ATPases to the ATP phosphorylation potential [2, 17] rather than to the ATP level *per se*. This interpretation of the energy–linked ventricular function in reperfused myocardium is novel and differs from the current practice of dobutaminergic treatment of cardiac patients with terminal heart failure.

Acknowledgement

This study was supported by a grant–in–aid to RTM from the American Heart Association, Texas Affiliate (92G–155) and by grants to RB from the National Institutes of Health (RO1 HL–36067) and the Uniformed Services University of the Health Sciences (RO7638).

DISCUSSION

Dr. F. Prinzen: You have shown pyruvate effects in the isolated pig heart which is perfused with pyruvate all the time. Then you have shown the results of adding pyruvate three times in the pigs. I am surprised to see that pyruvate also has a positive effect after reperfusion, although during ischemia there was no pyruvate. Do you have the same improvement after reperfusion as by keeping the pyruvate present all the time?

Dr. R. Bünger: Yes, pyruvate improves reperfusion function also if administered during reperfusion only (perfused guinea pig heart experiments). Also, even when pyruvate is administered after an initial period of pyruvate–free reperfusion, it has marked beneficial effects on cellular energy state and myocardial wall–thickening; the latter observation was made in the *in vivo* swine heart [our unpublished results]. When pyruvate is present throughout ischemia it can maintain the cytosolic NADH/NAD ratio close to that in normoxic hearts not receiving pyruvate treatment. Such a redox effect by pyruvate could be responsible, in part, for the observed attenuation of ATP + ADP + AMP depletion during low–flow ischemia (Fig. 1). Another consequence of the pyruvate attenuation of the ischemic NADH accumulation could be that the reductive release of ferritin–Fe^{2+} is minimized; this transition element catalyzes the Fenton reaction which has been implicated in the production of cytotoxic hydroxyl radicals during early reperfusion.

Dr. D. Allen: Another difficulty in interpreting your experiments is that in the presence of pyruvate there will be less acidosis. Clearly if acidosis is important in some way in loading the calcium, then you have two possible explanations. You obviously like the free radical explanation but there are others. The general problem with these experiments, and this applies to my experiments as well as anybody elses, is that there are a lot of variables that are important in reperfusion and unless you keep some of the other ones constant, it is very hard to interpret your experiment unequivocally.

Dr. R. Bünger: During the low–flow ischemia, coronary venous pCO_2, a quantitative index of the intracellular pH at constant cellular bicarbonate *[Eur J Biochem 1989; 180: 221–233]* was periodically checked. The experiments were conducted in such a way that already from 5 min ischemia on the intracellular pH was not different between pyruvate and non–pyruvate–treated hearts (Table 1). In the studies described here an effect of pyruvate on intracellular pH was not obtained. I agree that an unequivocal interpretation of our reperfusion data is difficult; besides the phosphorylation potential, sodium–calcium exchange and sarcoplasmic reticulum calcium handling may be involved. Indeed, the creatine phosphorylation potential parameter explained only 71%, not 100%, of the reperfusion function with only moderate precision. Regardless of the exact causal explanation of the beneficial pyruvate effect, there were consistent and clear–cut correlations between cytosolic creatine phosphate potential and reperfusion functional recovery.

Dr. J. Bassingthwaighte: A general question concerning lactate. Dr. Feigl mentioned that he used the absence of net lactate production as an indication of a healthy heart. But that is obviously dependent on what the incoming lactate concentration might be and if there is none you always produce lactate. How do you look at the pyruvate–lactate balances or net lactate production in a general way and would you advocate having pyruvate in our preparations always?

Dr. R. Bünger: Yes. Pyruvate has consistently proved beneficial for function and energetics of perfused hearts. One aspect of the pyruvate mechanism appears to be related to the cytosolic phosphorylation potential *[Eur J Biochem 1989; 180: 221–233]*. Regarding the myocardial pyruvate–lactate balance, lactate enters the cell via the specific monocarboxylate transporter with a Km about 5–10 mM. The transport capacity is very high so that even at 1 mM lactate, the physiological concentration, one observes a substantial lactate uptake by the heart. Pyruvate probably uses the same carrier as lactate to enter the cell, but with a lower Km of near about 1 mM *[Eur J Biochem 1990; 188: 481–493]*. At equimolar concentrations, pyruvate will be preferentially taken up, or released from, the heart. I agree with Dr. Feigl to view the absence of lactate production in the heart *in vivo* as an indication of a healthy heart; for the normal blood–lactate perfused heart and for the lactate–perfused isolated heart as well, net lactate production indicates oxygen–deficiency or extreme metabolic stress (maximum adrenergic stimulation resulting in glycogen depletion) in the presence of normoxia. A healthy heart can always pick up lactate as an energy substrate. However, when the pyruvate level of the blood or perfusion medium is raised sufficiently, pyruvate will increasingly compete with lactate for uptake, a situation that may be desirable under pathological conditions with intracellular acidosis since pyruvate oxidation, in contrast to lactate oxidation, does not generate intracellular hydrogen ions via lactate dehydrogenase.

REFERENCES

1. Bünger R, Sommer O, Walter G, Stiegler H, Gerlach E. Functional and metabolic features of an isolated perfused guinea pig heart performing pressure–volume work. *Pflügers Arch* 1979; 380: 259–266.
2. Bünger R, Mallet RT, Hartman DA. Pyruvate–enhanced phosphorylation potential and inotropism in normoxic and postischemic isolated working heart. *Eur J Biochem* 1989; 180: 221–233.
3. Mallet RT, Hartman DA, Bünger R. Glucose requirement for postischemic recovery of perfused working heart. *Eur J Biochem* 1990; 188: 481–493.
4. Kang Y–H, Mallet RT, Bünger R. Coronary autoregulation and purine release in normoxic heart at various cytosolic phosphorylation potentials: disparate effects of adenosine. *Pflügers Arch* 1992; 421: 188–199.

5. Headrick J, Clarke K, Willis RJ. Adenosine production and energy metabolism in ischaemic and metabolically stimulated rat heart. *J Mol Cell Cardiol* 1989; 21: 1089–1100.
6. Bünger R, Soboll S. Cytosolic adenylates and adenosine release in perfused working heart. *Eur J Biochem* 1986; 159: 203–213.
7. He M–X, Wangler RD, Dillon PF, Romig GD, Sparks HV. Phosphorylation potential and adenosine release during norepinephrine infusion in guinea pig heart. *Am J Physiol* 1987; 253: H1184–H1191.
8. Naito Y, Lowenstein JM. 5'–Nucleotidase from rat heart. *Biochemistry* 1981; 20: 5188–5194.
9. Murphy E, Steenbergen C, Levy LA, Raju B, London RE. Cytosolic free magnesium levels in ischemic heart. *J Biol Chem* 1989; 264: 5622–5627.
10. Mallet RT, Kang Y–H, Mukohara N, Bünger R. Use of cytosolic metabolite patterns to estimate free magnesium in normoxic myocardium. *Biochim Biophys Acta* 1992; 1139: 239–247.
11. Meissner G, Henderson JS. Rapid calcium release from cardiac sarcoplasmic reticulum vesicles is dependent on Ca^{2+} and is modulated by Mg^{2+}, adenine nucleotide, and calmodulin. *J Biol Chem* 1987; 262: 3065–3073.
12. Allen DG, Orchard CH. Myocardial contractile function during ischemia and hypoxia. *Circ Res* 1987; 60: 153–168.
13. Schramm M, Thomas G, Toward R, Franckowiak G. Novel dihydropyridines with positive inotropic action through activation of Ca^{2+} channels. *Nature* 1983; 303: 535–537.
14. Marban E. Myocardial stunning and hibernation. The physiology behind the colloquialisms. *Circulation* 1991; 83: 681–688.
15. Voogd A, Sluiter W, van Eijk HG, Koster JF. Low molecular iron and the oxygen paradox in isolated rat hearts. *J Clin Invest* 1993, in press.
16. Bolli R. Postischemic myocardial "stunning": pathogenesis, pathophysiology, and clinical relevance; In: Yellon DM, Jennings RB (eds) *Myocardial Protection*. New York, Raven Press 1992, pp 105–149.
17. Wimsatt DK, Hohl, CM, Brierley, GP, Altschuld, RA. Calcium accumulation and release by the sarcoplasmic reticulum of digitonin–lysed adult mammalian ventricular cardiomyocytes. *J Biol Chem* 1990; 265: 14849–14857.

CHAPTER 23

Metabolic and Mechanical Control of The Microcirculation

Uri Dinnar[1]

ABSTRACT

Existing models of the microcirculatory control usually assume a single mechanical parameter which in an unspecified way relates to the oxygen levels or to the metabolic demand. This parameter changes the mechanical properties of the microvascular bed upstream of where the change is needed, and in most cases affect a very wide region of the myocardium, rather than a number of cells at a specific location. The model presented here suggests a control mechanism which relates to the metabolic demand of a single cell, or a small number of cells. The analysis shows that each specific structure has a potential for a different change, and that these changes can occur with a minimal change in the energy demand. The model shows that these specific changes can affect a 300–500% change in rate of flow. This range of change is consistent with experimental evidence which is hitherto unexplained by current existing models.

INTRODUCTION

Although there is a general agreement that the major task of the microcirculation is to provide adequate supply of oxygen and nutrients to every single cell upon demand, almost all of the existing explanations and models do not attribute the task of circulatory, or microcirculatory, control to the oxygen level, or to metabolic demand, and relate them to several types of mechanical control.

There are some different schools of thought concerning the microcirculatory control; all assign the control to a single parameter that in an unspecified way relates to the oxygen

[1]The Julius Silver Institute, Department of Biomedical Engineering, Technion–Israel Institute of Technology, Haifa, 32000, Israel.

Interactive Phenomena in the Cardiac System, Edited by
S. Sideman and R. Beyar, Plenum Press, New York, 1993

level or to the metabolic demand, but all fail to give a reasonable explanation as to how this phenomenon relates to a single cell or a small tissue structure. Some of these mechanisms are generated upstream of the specific tissue location, while the other takes place in the microcirculation of the specific tissue.

The most popular control mechanism is based on the rate of flow. In this type of control model the oxygen demand changes the rate of flow by one of several mechanisms that affect the distribution and values of *the hydraulic resistances to flow*. Obviously, the changes in these models are not generated locally, but come from a higher controller that generates vasodilation in one, or more, of the larger blood vessels leading to the specific microcirculatory bed. There are different models that assign the vasodilation action to different locations in the arterial system, all of them upstream of the specific region of the tissue to be controlled.

Inspection of the distribution of the pressures along the arterial system in Fig. 1 shows that it is arranged so that the capillary perfusion pressure is set at a level of about 30–35 mmHg, and the pressure drop along the capillaries is set to agree well with the optimal values for transcapillary exchange of oxygen, nutrients, carbon dioxide and other metabolic substances, according to the well know Starling equation of exchange. We also see that the major drop in pressure occurs in the arterioles, and this is the location of the bulk of systemic hydraulic resistance. It is therefore not surprising that most of the reported models suggest the arterioles as the location of microcirculatory control. Clearly, the maximum change will take place, theoretically, if the arteriolar resistance is reduced to zero. Making the changes according to the appropriate values that generated the data shown in Fig. 1 yields the pressure distribution shown in Fig. 2. This figure shows that the total possible resistance decrease leads to a higher value of flow; the capillary perfusion pressure is now at a level which increases the transcapillary flow rate to an undesired value and completely eliminates the absorption of wastes from the cells. The appropriate compensation for such extreme values, such as increased hydraulic resistance in the capillaries or a decreased permeability coefficient, is found to be unable to correct for this situation. It is not conceivable that a central "command" will affect a decreased resistance in the arterioles and simultaneously increase the resistance in the capillaries. Yet, even at this extreme situation the change in capillary perfusion will only amount to twice the flow rate, whereas the increase in total flow can be fivefold or more in the extreme case of reactive hyperemia.

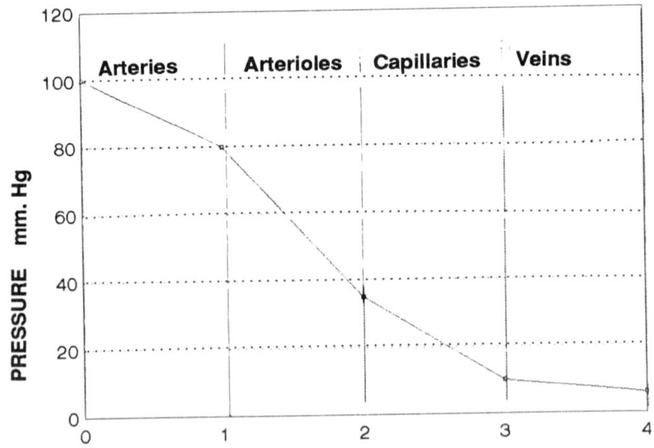

Figure 1. Pressure distribution along the cardiovascular system under normal conditions.

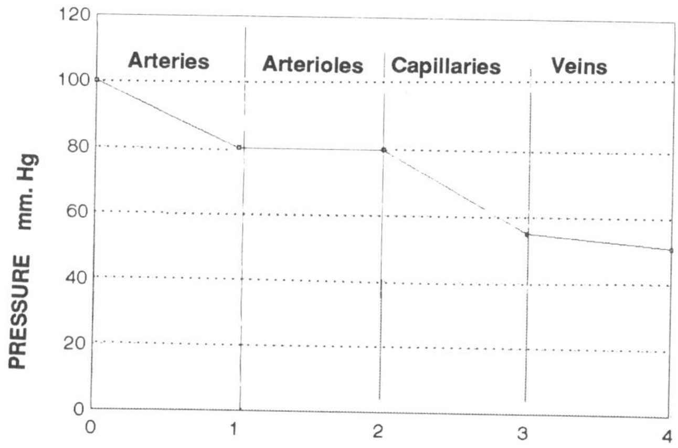

Figure 2. Pressure distribution along the cardiovascular system, for the extreme case of maximal theoretical vasodilation, without any other control compensation.

Moreover, the increased flow will lead to the shortening of the mean transit time of the red blood cells and thus make it harder to release oxygen and capture the waste materials from the tissue. In reality, the maximal vasomotion changes which take place during reactive hyperemia are much smaller and the amount of diameter changes is 16% in arterioles and 17% in venules [1], which affects a 50% decrease in the resistance and a 27% increase in flow. This is a much smaller change than the known 5–fold change and therefore cannot explain this phenomena. Note that the "mathematical" compensation of a reduction in the perfusion pressure is rather unphysiological.

Another popular control parameter is the *capillary perfusion pressure* [2]. Again, this parameter requires an upstream change which affects the entire microcirculatory bed and not the specific cells demanding more oxygen. If we assume that the response to demand is an increased pressure, we see, as discussed above, that the balanced pressure system of transcapillary exchange is disturbed, leading to edema and tissue swelling, and that the total blood pressures will have to yield unphysiological levels. Even if we accept this type of control, it will fall short of providing adequate local control of a single cell.

The third proposed mechanism of control was suggested as early as 1919 by Krogh [3], but was not accepted by the majority of researchers and remained highly controversial. This mechanism of *capillary recruitment* is assumed to increase the number of open capillaries upon demand. This is the only mechanism suggested to act within the desired microcirculatory bed and it is still the most controversial. It is believed that such mechanism can act in extreme cases, and only after prolonged time of oxygen deficiency. Part of the reason for the disagreement is due to difficulties in the measurements of capillary recruitment. Most techniques measure red blood cells, or number of capillaries in a given volume (Capillary Count), but fail to show if all the capillaries are open at the same time. This point is further discussed below.

THE MODEL

Looking at the anatomy of the microcirculation we see, Fig. 3, that there is an overlapping supply of vessels in almost every immediate neighborhood of individual cells. This points out to a possibility of oxygen supply through different blood vessels at different times. Despite the introduction of new and highly sophisticated measuring techniques there is still a lack of reliable information of the exact architectural structure of the microcirculatory bed in different beds, or different organs.

If we look carefully into the microstructure of the microvasculature we see that the arterioles have more than one layer of smooth muscle, which makes them capable of vaso–motion control. As we go further downstream to terminal arterioles, which are vessels with diameter smaller than 50 μ, we can see that the number of smooth muscle layers is reduced to a single layer, hence less capable of control. However, going further downstream we find *precapillary sphincters* with, again, 1–3 layers of smooth muscle. The precapillary sphinc–ters which are located at the entrance regions to almost any single capillary or small group of capillaries, Fig. 4, were first observed in 1925 by Tannenberg [5], who assigned these gate–keepers the task of sphincter–like controllers of the capillary flow. This idea was further investigated by Fulton and Lutz [6], Chambers and Zweifach [7, 8], Clark and Clark [9], Nicoll and Webb [4], Folkow and Mellander [10], Weidman et al. [11] and others.

While there is no agreement about the specific task of the precapillary sphincters, it is generally stated that they control the flow in an undefined manner, and that there is a lack of information about the triggering mechanism of the precapillary sphincters control. Some consider them to be another mechanism of hydraulic resistance, controlled by the sympathetic nervous system, while others assume that they can control the permeability conditions. A most common definition of the role of the precapillary sphincters is that they are the effector regulating capillary density, with the power to open and close specific capillaries. This idea is used in the present analysis, assuming that a specific precapillary is controlled by the local oxygen tension or, more precisely, by the oxygen tension in the cells lying downstream of its immediate supply route. To show the efficiency and controllability of such a structure is demonstrated by a few examples based on published anatomical data. However, in reality the microcirculatory structure can reach higher levels of complexity than those presented here.

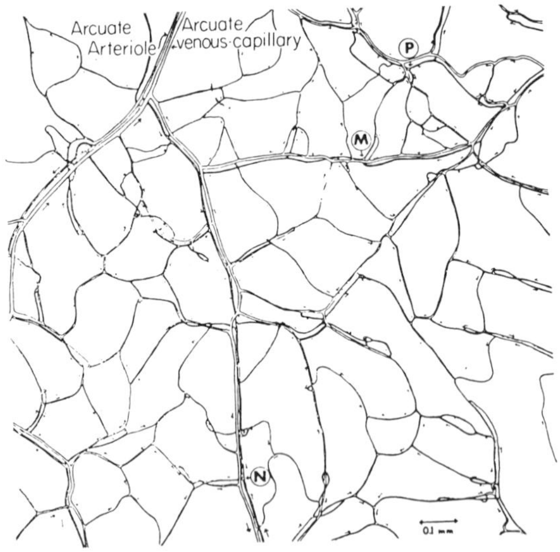

Figure 3. Arcuate patterns of arterioles and venous capillaries, terminal arterioles and capillaries.The arrows represent observed direction of flow. Points M, N and P have flow coming from two directions. From Nicoll and Webb [4], with permission.

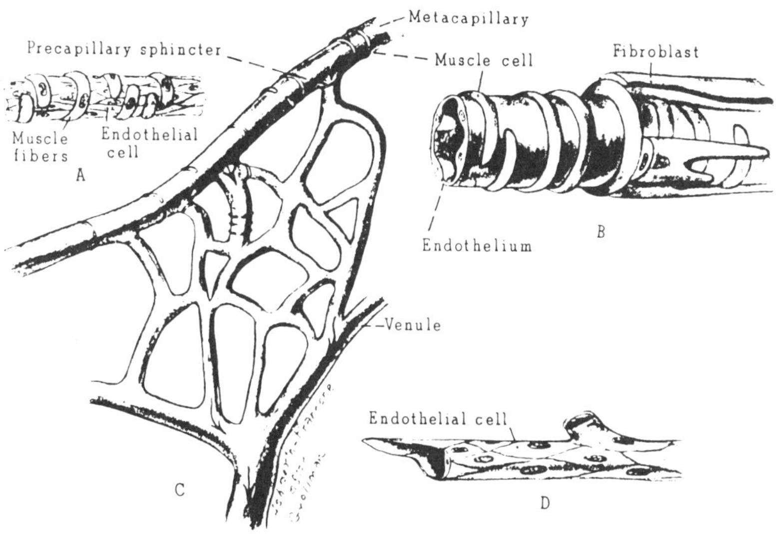

Figure 4. Schematic representation of a capillary bed. **A:** Some muscle fibers of the proximal part of a metacapillary. **B:** An arteriole. **D:** A true capillary. From [12], with permission.

Figure 5 shows a part of a microvasculature which has two branches leading from the arterioles to the venules. There are three possible modes of operation: either branches 1 or 2 are closed, or both of them are open. If we assume that the system is purely resistive (neglecting diameter changes leading to compliance), we can assume that the resistances are a linear combination of their length, and we can solve for the pressure distribution and the flow in each of the three situations. The results are given in Table 1, where the value of pressures are based on 100% of the arteriole–venule pressure difference, which depends upon the specific conditions in the cardiovascular system. The values for the flow are nondimensional and do not represent real values; they are used for comparison only. The

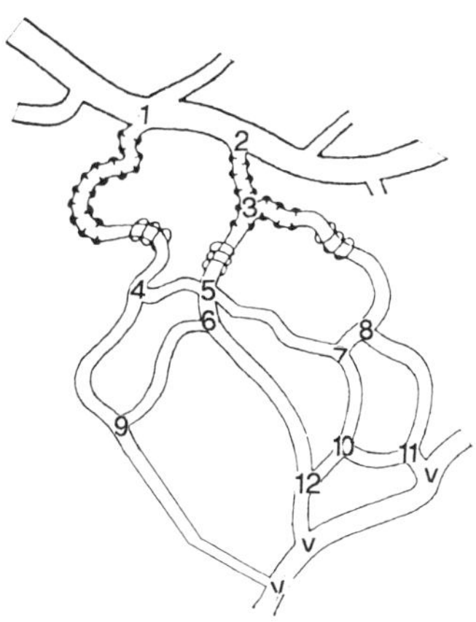

Figure 5. A schematic representation of a simple microvasculature which consist of two branches leading from the arteriole to the venules.

data show that flow can change directions in this structure (branch I–5, for example); it can be very small or relatively high (I–7, for example), and that the pressure at specific junctions change from high to low values (as in junction 9, for example). The overall change in the total flow rate to this specific branch is 230%, a relatively high value which is obtained without a change in the perfusion pressure, without affecting other vascular beds and without a significant change in the required power (which in related to the product of pressure and flow). If we accept this idea of a "blinking," alternating, flow network, where branches 1 and 2 alternate between the open and closed situations, we have a mechanism of varying flow directions and varying pressures in the junctions, which assist to remove or redirect larger particles (WBC or other) that may be stuck at a given junction. Yet, if the need arises, both branches 1 and 2 can open during the entire period, leading to capillary enhancement which increases the flow rate to the specific bed. Since the regulation here is based upon a specific demand of a single, or a small number of cells, the changes will be local and hardly measurable upstream. When the need arises, and the increased demand is in a larger region, or in an entire organ, the entire circulatory bed can change its rate of flow; many small changes will take place and the total change can be measurable upstream.

Table 1. Pressure and flow in the simple case of two intel branches.

	Pressure			Branch	Flow		
Node	Case 1 1 Open	Case 2 2 Open	Case 3 All Open		Case 1 1 Open	Case 2 2 Open	Case 3 All Open
1	100.00	100.00	100.00	I–1 1 to 4	2.19	0.00	1.53
2	100.00	100.00	100.00	I–2 2 to 3	0.00	4.03	3.50
3	18.91	67.76	72.02	I–3 3 to 5	−0.31	2.52	1.98
4	34.32	34.80	54.16	I–4 3 to 8	0.31	1.51	1.52
5	22.44	38.76	49.30	I–5 4 to 5	1.49	−0.49	0.61
6	19.40	32.00	41.31	I–6 4 to 9	0.70	0.49	0.92
7	11.02	25.24	29.60	I–7 9 to 6	0.01	−0.38	−0.32
8	10.63	27.06	30.90	I–8 5 to 7	0.57	0.68	0.98
9	19.53	24.43	34.84	I–9 7 to 10	0.47	1.13	1.31
10	4.39	9.44	11.26	I–10 8 to 11	0.40	1.05	1.20
11	2.54	5.96	6.95	I–11 6 to 12	0.61	0.97	1.27
12	3.43	6.67	8.18	I–12 10 to 11	0.23	0.44	0.54
				I–13 11 to v	0.64	1.49	1.74
				I–14 12 to v	0.86	1.67	2.04
				I–15 9 to v	0.70	0.87	1.24
Flow				I–16 5 to 6	0.61	1.35	1.60
I–1	2.90	0.00	1.53	I–17 10 to 12	0.24	0.69	0.77
I–2	0.00	4.03	3.50	I–18 8 to 7	−0.10	0.45	0.33
Total	2.19	4.03	5.03				

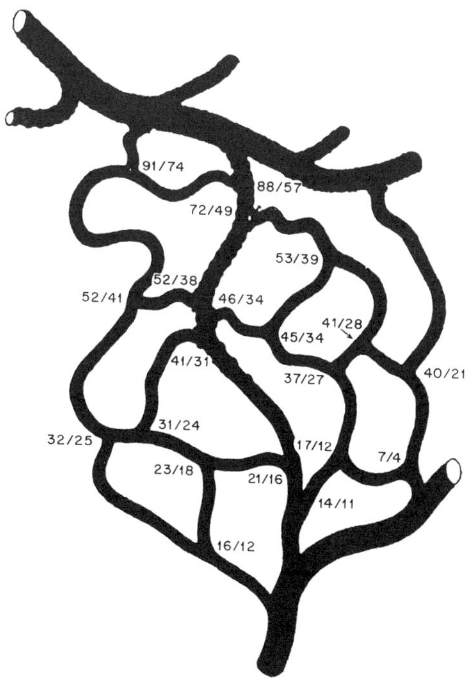

Figure 6. Pressure changes in a portion of the capillary bed shown in Fig. 7. The numbers represent high and low values of relative pressure between arteriole and venule, based on 100% of the existing pressure drop.

In the case of three inlet branches [7], we have a higher number of possible modes of operation. The rate of flow when one branch is open at a time amounts to nearly 20%. When two branches are open, the rate of flow doubles the original flow rate, and the maximal increase with maximal enhancement results in 235% of the original flow. In all these possibilities the pressure variations are minimal, but, as shown in Fig. 6, they are sufficient to open problematic junctions and to redistribute flow in different directions.

Figure 7 represents multiple branches, which have two levels of precapillary control. The first mechanism controls the two primary entrances, while the secondary

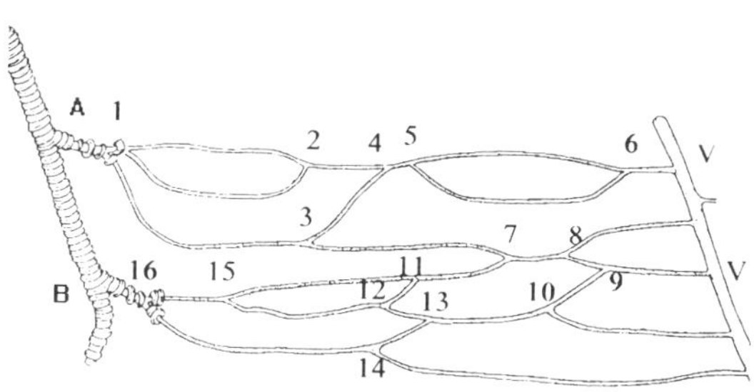

Figure 7. A microvascular unit built of a capillary network with multiple branches having two levels of precapillary control, **A** and **B**. Reprinted by permission of the publishers from [13], *The Pathway for Oxygen: Structure and Fuction in the Mammalian Respiratory System*, by E.R. Weibel, Cambridge, MA: Harvard University Press, ©1984 by the President and Fellows of Harvard College.

Table 2. Results of the pressure and flow for the microvasculature of Fig. 8.

Node	Pressure (Relative Units) Case 1 All Open	2 A$^+$	3 B$^+$	4 1–2$^+$	5 1–2$^+$	6 1–3$^+$	7 16–15$^+$	8 16–14$^+$
1	100.00	100.00	100.00	100.00	100.00	100.00	100.00	100.00
2	77.14	10.25	75.25	64.64	66.47	72.77	75.96	76.81
3	62.00	15.87	54.30	57.99	58.58	44.22	57.18	60.66
4	57.84	10.25	54.34	50.49	51.57	49.77	55.65	57.23
5	45.14	8.00	42.41	39.41	40.25	38.84	43.44	44.67
6	15.08	2.67	14.16	13.16	13.44	12.97	14.51	14.92
7	38.47	26.41	16.54	37.43	37.58	33.83	24.77	34.67
8	22.02	15.96	8.57	21.50	21.57	19.69	14.07	19.27
9	18.20	14.10	6.11	17.85	17.90	16.62	11.51	15.31
10	23.28	20.08	5.65	23.00	23.04	22.05	14.47	18.19
11	54.44	48.11	12.33	53.89	53.97	52.00	27.39	47.81
12	55.32	50.57	10.68	54.91	54.97	53.49	28.42	46.66
13	48.44	44.76	8.58	48.12	48.17	47.02	29.73	35.83
14	51.69	49.09	7.34	51.47	51.50	50.69	38.47	30.67
15	80.77	78.43	11.45	80.57	80.60	79.87	27.94	77.48
16	100.00	100.00	100.00	100.00	100.00	100.00	100.00	100.00
	Flow							
I–A	1.11	0.00	1.25	0.97	0.99	0.82	1.20	1.13
I–B	1.44	1.58	0.00	1.45	1.45	1.50	0.72	1.02
Total	2.55	1.58	1.25	2.42	2.44	2.32	1.92	2.16

Branch	Flow (Relative Units) Case 1 All Open	2 A$^+$	3 B$^+$	4 1–2$^+$	5 1–2$^+$	6 1–3$^+$	7 16–15$^+$	8 16–14$^+$
I–1 1 to 2	0.36	0.00	0.39	0.00	0.53	0.43	0.38	0.37
I–2 1 to 2	0.33	0.00	0.35	0.51	0.00	0.39	0.34	0.33
I–3 2 to 4	0.69	0.00	0.75	0.51	0.53	0.82	0.73	0.70
I–4 1 to 3	0.42	0.00	0.50	0.46	0.46	0.00	0.47	0.43
I–5 3 to 4	0.10	0.14	–0.00	0.19	0.18	–0.14	0.04	0.09
I–6 4 to 5	0.79	0.14	0.75	0.69	0.71	0.68	0.76	0.79
I–7 5 to 6	0.42	0.07	0.39	0.36	0.37	0.36	0.40	0.41
I–8 5 to 6	0.38	0.07	0.35	0.33	0.34	0.32	0.36	0.37
I–9 5 to 6	0.79	0.14	0.75	0.69	0.71	0.68	0.76	0.79
I–10 3 to 7	0.31	–0.14	0.50	0.27	0.28	0.14	0.43	0.35
I–11 7 to 8	0.78	0.50	0.38	0.76	0.76	0.67	0.51	0.73
I–12 8 to v	0.49	0.35	0.19	0.48	0.48	0.44	0.31	0.43
I–13 16 to 15	0.87	0.98	0.00	0.88	0.88	0.92	0.00	1.02
I–14 16 to 14	0.57	0.60	0.00	0.57	0.57	0.58	0.72	0.00
I–15 15 to 11	0.41	0.47	–0.01	0.42	0.42	0.44	0.01	0.46
I–16 15 to 11	0.46	0.51	0.01	0.47	0.47	0.48	–0.01	0.56
I–17 15 to 12	0.06	0.16	–0.11	0.07	0.07	0.10	0.07	–0.08
I–18 11 to 7	0.47	0.64	–0.12	0.48	0.48	0.53	0.08	0.39
I–19 9 to v	0.51	0.39	0.17	0.50	0.50	0.46	0.32	0.43
I–20 13 to 10	0.56	0.55	0.07	0.56	0.56	0.56	0.34	0.39
I–21 14 to 13	0.15	0.21	–0.06	0.16	0.16	0.17	0.42	–0.25
I–22 10 to 9	0.21	0.25	–0.02	0.21	0.21	0.23	0.12	0.12
I–23 10 to v	0.35	0.30	0.08	0.34	0.34	0.33	0.22	0.27
I–24 14 to v	0.41	0.39	0.06	0.41	0.41	0.41	0.31	0.25
I–258 to 9	0.29	0.14	0.19	0.28	0.28	0.24	0.20	0.30
I–26 12 to 13	0.40	0.34	0.12	0.40	0.40	0.38	–0.08	0.64

$^+$ denotes closed branch

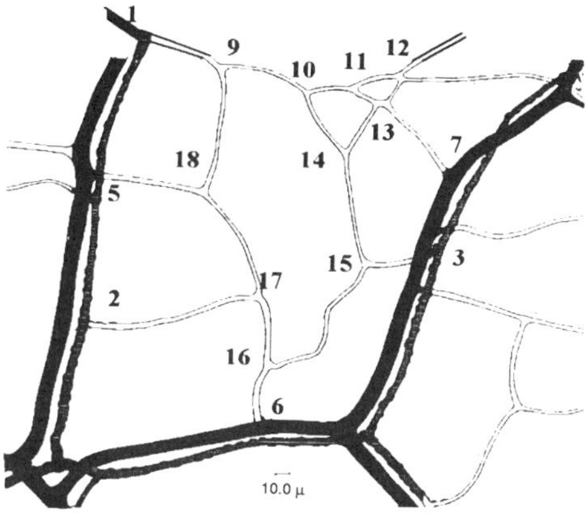

Figure 8. A microvascular unit built of a capillary network with four arterial inlets and four venous outlet, capable of generating multiple levels of precapillary control.

changes the local distribution of each of the branches. The results, summarized in Table 2, shows very similar changes in pressures, with a maximal value of capillary enhancement of 204%.

Obviously, the number of possibilities increases in a microstructure that has a large number of inlets and outlets; a wider range of flow rates can be achieved with different degrees of capillary enhancement, which will results from the specific demands of the interstitial oxygen tension. In the example shown in Fig. 8, the change can reach 210% if two inlets are open and 365% if all four inlets are open. Pressures can change from 28 mmHg to 19 mmHg with the variation of the open inlets.

DISCUSSION

The model presented here assumes that the microcirculatory bed works with capillary enhancement by alternating (blinking) inlet conditions. The microvasculature is controlled by local oxygen tension and can, under condition of insufficient oxygen supply or extensive oxygen demand, open more than one inlet at a time. This enhancement can increase the flow rates by 200–500% without any significant changes in the total arterial flow rates or arterial pressures. Since the power required for the flow is proportional to the product of pressure and flow rate, this increase in oxygen supply is achieved with a small increase in power. It is believed that only when the entire capillary bed in a specific region is at maximal flow conditions, will the "higher level" control centers become operative and the well known changes in arteriolar diameter will take place. To investigate this possibility it is necessary to identify the response of precapillary sphincters to various stimulus and to compare them to those of the arterioles and the venules. Unfortunately, there is very little information about the behavior of microcirculatory components to various hormonal substances or to vasoactive stimulus. Altura [14] showed, Fig. 9, that precapillary sphincters of rat mesentery is sensitive to various catecholamines in concentrations that are more than 1/1000 of the minimal thresholds that will cause any measurable effect in arterioles. It is thus assumed that precapillary sphincters respond to the slightest change in humoral composition, and can change local flow conditions. Only at a second stage, when the initial

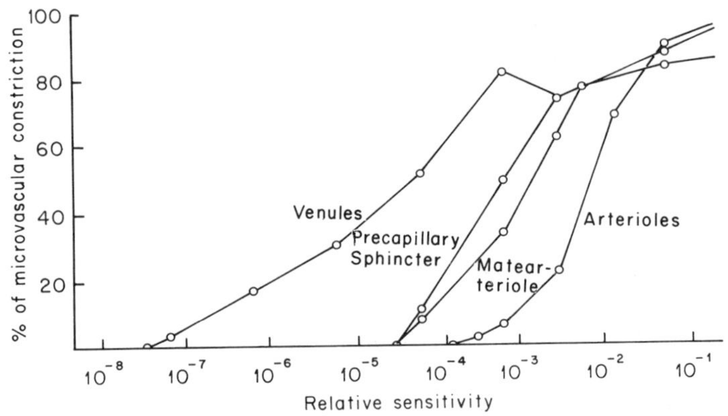

Figure 9. Relative sensitivity of rat mesenteric microvessels to activity of 2–phenylalanine–8–ornithine–vasopressin (From [14], with permission.)

changes cannot adapt to the new situation, will the humoral changes become sufficiently high to trigger arteriolar control mechanisms.

Finally, it should be noted that the capillary enhancement blinking mechanism is completely different from the well known capillary recruitment model [3], and can not be observed with the current measurement techniques for capillary count.

Acknowledgment

This research was supported by funds from the Berman Philanthropic Foundation, Michigan, USA, the Gerson family Foundation, Michigan, USA and the Fund for the Promotion of Research at the Technion. The author wish to express his many thanks for those foundation for their continuous support of research at the Technion.

DISCUSSION

Dr. N. Westerhof: How do you suggest that the signals from peripheral muscles or muscle cells go to the sphincters so that the sphincters know whether they have to open or close?

Dr. U. Dinnar: The data of Altura [14] shows that less than 1/1000 of the concentration of the active substance in the area of the free capillary will effect the free capillary and will not effect arterioles. The local concentration changes of some substances, maybe oxygen, adenosine, cate–cholamine, will affect the adjacent capillary. The data suggests that it is not an on/off mechanism; maybe there is a gradual change. But because of these biochemical changes (10^{-6} relative to the 10^{-2}), the flow changes are local at the capillary level. Only if the concentration is higher does it get to the arterioles.

Dr. W.M. Chilian: Do you have any idea whether the myocardium, more specifically, the microcirculation in the myocardium, has the appropriate network to account for the changes you have described.

Dr. U. Dinnar: I am looking into it.

Dr. R. Bünger: There is a recent review article by Kuschinsky and Paulson *[Cerebrovasc. Brain Metab. Rev. 1992; 4: 261–286]*, where they discuss the concept that there is no true closing or opening of brain capillaries, no stop–and–go–flow situation at any time. These authors conclude that what might actually happen is that upon increased demand the normal heterogeneity becomes relatively more homogenous, which can theoretically account for the observed increase in the overall brain flow. Is that what you are saying?

Dr. U. Dinnar: In a way. There is a lot of argument about whether recruitment exists or does not exist in brain and other tissue. If you take this blinking idea then it is very hard to measure recruitment because if you measure red blood cells at all times, you see red blood cells. It is not a mechanism where these capillaries are not perfused and others are perfused and when a crisis is started all of them are perfused. So all of the measurements are not appropriate. What I suggest here is that there is a flow through the capillaries at all times. We need more modeling to try and get to the parameters because we do not know what the time scale of the capillary blinking is.

Dr. R. Bünger: The flow exists at all times; that is what they concluded in that article.

Dr. F. Kajiya: I am not so familiar with the capillary flow. According to some biorheology textbooks, when capillary flow increases, red blood cell density increases in the capillary. The increase in red blood cell density causes viscosity increase, flow decrease and vice versa. Could you introduce such kind of rheological factors in your model?

Dr. U. Dinnar: What you just said helps my argument. I am saying that it is very hard to increase the flow 5–fold because the red blood cells will have to flow much faster, with higher viscosity and other higher properties. I am saying that flow remains about the same, but more avenues are open. The changes that you say are prevented this way.

Dr. E.O. Feigl: First of all I think that the language has to be cleaned up a little here. There is little anatomical evidence for precapillary sphincters in the coronary circulation.

Dr. U. Dinnar: Yes, that is why I have used two definitions.

Dr. E.O. Feigl: I do not think it is useful to use the word sphincter, even functional sphincter, because a sphincter is a well defined term, like an anal sphincter. What you mean by recruitment is subject to definition. We can talk about a PS product which certainly has been demonstrated to be recruitable, and that would fit in with what you want. The next comment is that models like Dr. Mates', which include no extra channels or no diversion of channels and thus argue for a pressure regulator which is a very difficult concept, are made unnecessary if we follow this path. Last, a better word than recruitment is wanted. Perhaps capillary augmentation or capillary enhancement would be suitable.

Dr. U. Dinnar: I agree, we should look for better wording.

REFERENCES

1. Yada T, Hiramatsu O, Tachibana H, Kimura A, Yamamoto T, Goto M, Ogasawara Y, Tsujioka K, Kajiya F. Reactive hyperemic response of subendocardial microvessels. *Heart & Vessels* 1992; supp 9: 144.
2. Bruinsma P, Arts T, Dankelman J, Spaan JAE. Model of the coronary circulation based on pressure dependence of coronary resistance and compliance. *Basic Res Card* 1988; 83: 510–524.
3. Krogh A. The supply of oxygen to the tissue and the regulation of the capillary circulation. *J Physiol (London)* 1919; 52: 457–474.
4. Nicoll PA, Webb RL. Vascular patterns and active vasomotion as determiners of flow through minute vessels. *Angiology* 1955; 6: 291–308.

5. Tannenberg J. Uber die Kapillartatigkeit. *Vehr Dtsch Ges Vil* 1925; 20: 374.
6. Fulton GP, Lutz BR. The neuro–motor mechanism of the small blood vessels of the frog. *Science* 1940; 92: 223–224.
7. Chambers R, Zweifach BW. Caliber changes of the capillary bed. *Fed Proc* 1942; 1: 14.
8. Chambers R, Zweifach BW. The topography and function of the mesenteric capillary circulation. *Am J Anatomy* 1944; 75: 173–205.
9. Clark ER, Clark EC. Caliber changes in minute vessels observed in the living mammal. *Am J Anatomy* 1943; 73: 215–250.
10. Folkow B, Mellander S. Aspects of the nervous control of the precapillary sphincters with regard to the capillary exchange. *Acta Phys Scand* 1960; 50, Suppl. 175: 52–54.
11. Wiedman MP, Tuma RF, Myrovitz HN. Defining the precapillary sphincter. *Microvasc Res* 1976; 12: 71–75.
12. Jacob SW, Francone CA, Lossow WJ. *Structure and Function in Man*, fourth edition. W.B. Saunders Co.:NY, 1978.
13. Weibel ER. *The Pathway for Oxygen. Structure and Function in Mammalian Respiratory System*. Harvard University Press: Cambridge, MA, 1984.
14. Altura BM. Pharmacology of the microcirculation. In: Effros EM, Dietzel J, Schmidt–Schonbein H (eds) *Microcirculation: Current Physiologic, Medical and Surgical Concepts*. Academic Press:NY, 1981: 51–105.

Remodeling of Muscle and Vessels

CHAPTER 24

ASYMMETRICAL CHANGES IN VENTRICULAR WALL MASS BY ASYNCHRONOUS ELECTRICAL ACTIVATION OF THE HEART

Frits W. Prinzen, Tammo Delhaas, Theo Arts, and Robert S. Reneman[1]

ABSTRACT

Ventricular pacing causes asynchronous electrical activation of the ventricular wall, because impulse conduction occurs via muscle fibers rather than via the Purkinje system. Chronic (up to 3 months) ventricular pacing caused about 30% decrease of wall mass in early activated regions but did not change wall mass in late activated regions. These are the first data indicating that chronic asynchronous activation induces asymmetrical structural adaptations. This asymmetry is likely to be evoked by regional differences in contractile work, as demonstrated in previous experiments from our laboratory. The nature of the structural adaptation as well as its clinical implications deserve more detailed investigation.

INTRODUCTION

Ventricular pacing, impulse conduction disorders and ventricular extrasystolic beats are associated with abnormal, slow electrical activation, since the conduction of the electrical wavefront occurs initially via myocardial muscle cells rather than via the Purkinje system. This causes asynchrony of contraction in the various regions of the ventricular wall [1, 2] and a decrease in global ventricular pump function [3]. The pattern of regional fiber strain is severely affected [4, 5]. In relatively early activated regions, fibers shorten considerably already during the isovolumic contraction phase, thereby stretching later activated fibers. During the ejection phase for the early activated fibers strain is small (less than −0.05) as compared to this strain during sinus rhythm (approximately −0.10), whereas fiber

[1]Departments of Physiology and Biophysics, Cardiovascular Research Institute Maastricht, University of Limburg, The Netherlands.

Interactive Phenomena in the Cardiac System, Edited by
S. Sideman and R. Beyar, Plenum Press, New York, 1993

strain was more pronounced in the late activated fibers (to more than −0.15, Fig. 1). These changes in the amount of fiber strain during the ejection phase are likely to be explained by local differences in sarcomere length at the time of electrical activation of the fibers [6]. Furthermore, during ventricular pacing the distribution of regional myocardial blood flow was similar to the distribution of fiber strain during the ejection phase [5] (Fig. 1).

The differences in fiber strain are likely to be associated with differences in workload, while regional blood flow is adjusted through metabolic regulation to meet the altered oxygen demand [5]. This hypothesis is supported by recent findings from our laboratory, showing that regional contractile work, defined as the time integral of the fiber stress–fiber strain diagram, was approximately 30% lower in early activated regions than

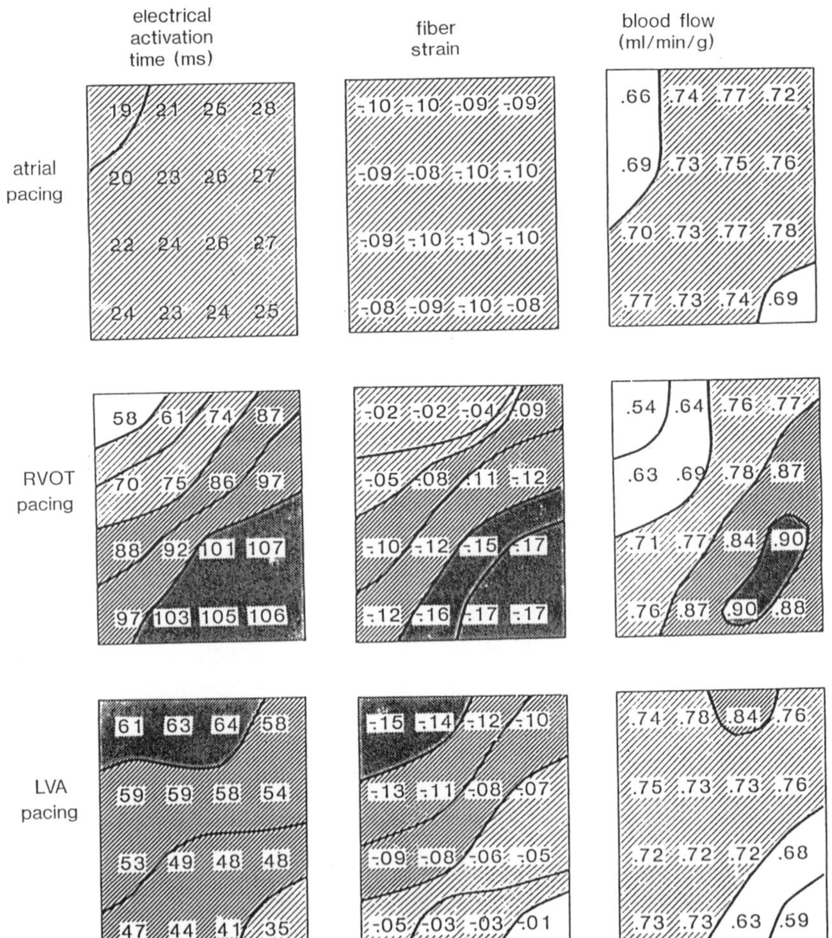

Figure 1. Mean maps of epicardial electrical activation time, fiber strain and blood flow. The rectangles represent a part of the anterior wall of the left ventricle, with the basal part at the top and the left anterior descending coronary artery on the left side. The part was divided in 16 regions using a 4 x 4 matrix. For the construction of the mean maps, the data from 8 – 10 experiments were used, in which all three variables were determined in the same regions. Isochrone, "isostrain" and "isoperfusion" lines were drawn to facilitate interpretation of the maps. Modified from [5], with permission of the American Physiological Society.

during atrial pacing. In contrast, in the late activated region contractile work was approximately 15% larger than during synchronous activation [7].

Mass and composition of cardiac muscle are known to adapt in response to altered external conditions. Sustained elevated ventricular cavity pressure causes an increase in wall thickness without major changes in cavity volume (concentric hypertrophy). In contrast, volume overload induces an increase of both ventricular wall mass and cavity volume (eccentric hypertrophy). Beside these adaptations of the whole heart to altered global loading conditions, also regional adaptations have been demonstrated, as a result of regionally abnormal loading. The best known example is ventricular remodeling after myocardial infarction. The entire ventricular wall is stretched and wall stress is increased. In the infarcted zone this may lead to infarct extension. In the surviving part hypertrophy occurs to compensate for the larger regional pump work. The structural adaptation in non-infarcted myocardium can be characterized as regional eccentric hypertrophy [8].

The goal of the present study was to investigate to what extent the regional differences in contractile work, induced by ventricular pacing, result in changes in the geometry of the left ventricular wall. To this purpose serial two dimensional (2D) echocardiographic measurements of regional ventricular wall mass were made in a group of dogs at various time intervals during chronic ventricular pacing.

METHODS

Implantation Procedure

Four mongrel dogs were used for this study. The pacemaker and pacing electrodes were implanted during a sterile surgical procedure. A Medtronic 4057 unipolar endocardial screw–in lead was introduced into the atrial cavity through the wall of the right atrial appendix and screwed into the endocardial surface of the right atrial wall. The ventricular lead was a Medtronic 6917A–35T sutureless lead. This lead was attached to the epicardium of the free wall of the left ventricle, 1 cm below the base, using its screw–in device. A pacemaker (Medtronic Synergist H7027) was implanted subcutaneously over the left lower thoracic region and the leads were guided subcutaneously towards the pacemaker pocket. After fixation of the leads into the pacemaker and checking proper electrical contact between pacemaker and lead, the pacemaker was introduced into its subcutaneous pocket and the skin over the pocket was closed. The animals were allowed to recover from anesthesia and from the surgical procedure, while the pacemaker was not in function yet.

Ventricular pacing was started approximately two weeks after implantation. Pacing was performed in the DDD–mode (dual chamber, dual sensing, dual pacing, with a maximal rate of 175 beats/min), so that the heart was paced at its natural rhythm. The A–V stimulation interval was 25 ms to assure that the whole ventricle was activated from the ectopic focus rather than through conduction via the A–V node.

Measurement of Ventricular Wall Mass

Ultrasound images of the left ventricle were made by 2D echocardiography using a Hewlett Packard Ultrasound System (77020A) with a 3.5 MHz transducer (21206A). The images were recorded on video–tape. One week before and 1, 2 and 3 months after onset of pacing measurements were made while the conscious animals were standing in the upright position. Cross–sectional images were made, taking care that the top of the papillary muscles and the pacing lead were visible and that the ventricular cross–section was as circular as possible.

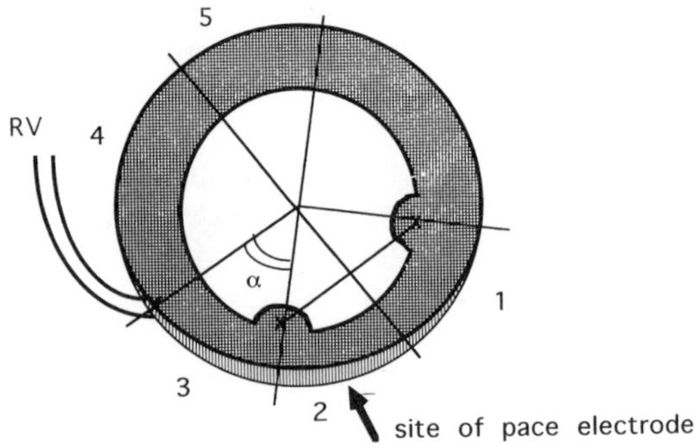

Figure 2. Division of a ventricular cross–section on a 2D echocardiographic image into six regions using three anatomical landmarks: the papillary muscles (crosses) and the attachment of the right ventricle to the left ventricle at the anterior wall. The center of the cavity was positioned midway the line perpendicular to the line connecting the two papillary muscles. The sector angles of regions 1, 2 and 5 are equal.

Measurements were made on videoprints (10 x 15 cm using a videoprinter) of end–diastolic images. Of each image, endocardial and epicardial contours were drawn on overhead sheets. Subsequently, the left ventricular cross–section of the pre–pacing image was divided into 6 regions, using the following anatomical landmarks: the anterior and posterior papillary muscles and the anterior attachment of the right ventricular wall to the left ventricular wall (see Fig. 2). The three anatomical landmarks in the images obtained at various time intervals during ventricular pacing were localized, by optimal superposition of templates of the endocardial (papillary muscles) and epicardial contour (RV–LV attachment) of the pre–pacing image. Thereafter, also the ventricular cross section of the images of paced beats was divided into 6 regions. Usually, in the echocardiographic images section 6 was incomplete. In all animals the pacing lead was located in wall section 2. Consequently, sections 1 and 3 were adjacent to the pacing electrode and section 5, located in the ventricular septum, was the most remote region.

The area of the wall sections (in case of regions 1, 2 and 3: including papillary muscle) as well as the area of the ventricular cavity was determined by planimetry. The sector angles of the various wall sections were determined as well. Regional wall mass was quantified by the ratio of the wall area and the sector angle of a particular wall section, and expressed as a percentage of the pre–pacing wall mass. Using these measurements an indication is obtained about the size of the ventricular cavity, and of the length and mass of the various wall sections. Using relatively large wall sections inaccuracies in determining the endocardial and epicardial boundary at a particular point were averaged out. Measurements on videoframes from end–diastole of subsequent cardiac cycles indicated a variation of ±5% (s.d.) in wall mass and ±5° in sector angle.

RESULTS

In three animals sensing and stimulation thresholds increased slightly. In these cases pacing was continued at higher amplitude or with longer duration of the stimulus. However, in one animal sensing and stimulation thresholds increased to such an extent within two weeks after onset of pacing, that ventricular pacing failed. Therefore, it was decided to program the pacemaker to its lowest, subliminal, values. This animal served as a sham animal.

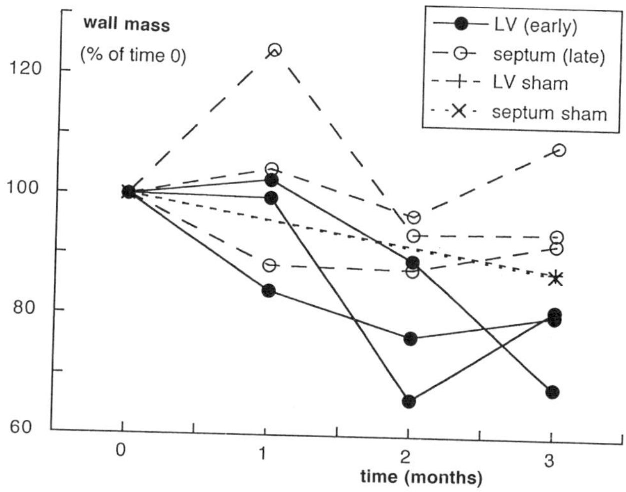

Figure 3. Time course of the change in local wall mass during chronic ventricular pacing. The values of the three paced dogs (circles) and the one sham dog (+ and x) are presented as % of the mass at time 0. Closed circles denote the early activated region 2 on the free wall of the left ventricle. Open circles denote the late activated region 5 in the ventricular septum (see Fig. 2).

Figure 3 depicts the time course of the changes in wall mass in regions 2 and 5. Although the individual patterns of the three paced dogs varied to some extent, the results indicate that wall mass at the left ventricular wall close to the pacing lead (region 2) gradually decreased during the 3 months of pacing, whereas it remained approximately constant in the late activated septal region (region 5).

After 3 months of ventricular pacing wall mass of region 2 decreased to 60, 61 and 83 % of the initial values in the three animals. Wall mass in section 5 was 96, 99 and 106% of its initial value. Also, no consistent change was observed in ventricular cavity area and in the angles of the 5 wall regions studied. In the sham animal the mass in regions 2 and 5 decreased to the same extent (11%) .

DISCUSSION

The data in the present study indicate that chronic ventricular pacing can induce a reduction in left ventricular wall mass in early activated regions. This reduction occurred in regions where, in acute experiments, fiber strain, contractile work and blood flow were found to be reduced compared with atrial pacing [5, 7]. Therefore, it seems likely, that the reduction in contractile work, induced by early electrical activation, results in the relative atrophy.

In the same studies, we also observed an increase in fiber strain [5] and contractile work [7] in late activated regions. Nevertheless, no consistent increase in wall mass was found in the late activated septum in the chronic pacing study. This may be due to the fact that the increase in contractile work in late activated regions was smaller than its decrease in early activated regions. Consequently, it can be expected, that the stimulus for hyper–trophy in late activated regions was smaller than the stimulus for atrophy in early activated regions. It is possible that such a hypertrophy can be demonstrated using either a larger number of observations or prolonged ventricular pacing. The latter possibility is supported by the observation, that in the early activated regions the reduction in wall mass had not yet reached a stable level after 3 months (Fig. 3).

The relation between sequence of electrical activation, fiber strain and blood flow, depicted in Fig. 1, was established in the epicardial layers of the left ventricular wall. Because of technical limitations to perform direct measurements of fiber strain in the deeper layers of the wall, we were not yet able to demonstrate the same relationship in the deeper layers. However, we hypothesized, that the inhomogeneity in contractile work as a function of the sequence of electrical activation would not be limited to the epicardial layers, since the differences in contractile work during ventricular pacing are most likely due to differences in the fiber (sarcomere) length at the beginning of the ejection phase, one of the basic myocardial material properties. Because the changes in wall mass during chronic pacing are too large to be located in a single layer, and because during volume–overload hypertrophy the distribution of tissue growth is homogeneous across the wall [9], the altered wall mass in early activated regions supports the idea, that the dependency of regional contractile work on the sequence of electrical activation also holds for deeper layers.

The present findings are interesting from a basic scientific point of view, but may also have implications for some cardiac abnormalities. Ventricular pacing appears to be a means to induce different levels of workload within the same heart, which may be useful in studying cardiac adaptive processes. This may, however, also imply, that ventricular pacing, and presumably also idiopathically originated impulse propagation can give rise to asymmetrical hypertrophy. No conclusive evidence for this hypothesis was found in literature so far.

Abnormal wall motion patterns are well known in patients with for example ventricular pacing, left bundle branch block and Wolfe–Parkinson–White syndrome [10, 11], but information on absolute wall thickness was lacking. In a recent retrospective study in patients with left bundle branch block [12], using M–mode echocardiography, wall thickness was found to be significantly less in the early activated septum than in the late activated posterior wall. These data support the idea from the present study, that asynchronous electrical activation may cause asymmetrical hypertrophy.

Consequence of the impact of asynchronous activation on the geometry of the ventricular wall may be the search for optimal positioning of ventricular pace electrodes. In case of patients with A–V block or sick–sinus syndrome this optimization should lead to the least asynchronous activation. In case of septal hypertrophy in patients with hypertrophic obstructive cardiomyopathy, positioning of the lead in the septal wall may be feasible, since this may lead to reduction of the regional hypertrophy. Interestingly, recent trials with pacing in the right ventricular apex in these patients showed significant reduction in ventriculo–aortic pressure gradients and subjective improvements [13, 14]. However, no reduction in hypertrophy occurred within 4 years [13]. It seems worthwhile to investigate, whether septal pacing rather than right ventricular apex pacing could further improve the results of the pacemaker therapy in these patients.

CONCLUSIONS

Prolonged (3 months) ventricular pacing reduced wall mass in early activated regions by approximately 30% and did not induce significant changes in wall mass in late activated regions. This indicates that asynchronous activation causes asymmetrical structural adaptations in the ventricular wall. These findings may have important implications for the use of pacemakers and the treatment of patients with abnormal impulse propagation.

Acknowledgements

This study has been supported by NWO/grant 900–516–091 and the Bakken Research Center, Medtronic. The authors thank Vincent Schouten (Bakken Research Center, Medtronic) for his technical support and scientific interest during this study.

DISCUSSION

Dr. E. Yellin: Your speculation that you could reduce hypertrophy by pacing is really intriguing. You are subjecting the paced region to a volume overload. Is it being pre–stretched?

Dr. F. Prinzen: The late activated region is pre–stretched, not the early one. The early one is contracting early, so its fiber length, at which major stress development occurs, is less than normal.

Dr. E. Yellin: Does the late activated region exhibit more force development because it is pre–stretched and does it hypertrophy?

Dr. F. Prinzen: We have not measured significant hypertrophy yet. But when we looked more closely at the numbers of contractile work in early and late activated regions the decrease in work in the early regions was larger than the increase in the later regions. There may be an increase in the late activated regions, but this could take more time because the changes are relatively smaller. We will have to extend to a longer period of pacing.

Dr. H. Halperin: It is a very elegant study. How do you deal with the fact that the fiber directions are different in the interlayers and you are looking at the epicardial fiber strains and then you are calculating a kind of stress and comparing that with regional blood flow?

Dr. F. Prinzen: In our acute studies [7] we limited ourselves to the epicardial layer. We measured the activation electrically on the epicardium. We measured epicardial deformation and epicardial blood flow. But we assumed that the abnormal electrical activation induces a kind of length shift in these regions and that the increase in the later regions is due to a local Starling effect. Since this is a general myocardial property, we believe that if this happens in the epicardium, it will also happen in the endocardium. We were glad to see the decrease in wall thickness after chronic pacing, because this decrease is more likely due to the change in all the myocardial layers.

Dr. H. Halperin: Did your studies with needles add any insight?

Dr. F. Prinzen: We did not use the needle technique *[J Biomechan 1984; 17: 801–811]* here.

Dr. J. Janicki: Did you take into account changes in ventricular volume when you were measuring thickness? Did your volume change at all with changing wall thickness by pacing?

Dr. F. Prinzen: We did not see any volume change of the cavity.

Dr. E. Hoffman: How did you choose your V_o points in the calculation of the total work from your loops?

Dr. F. Prinzen: The stress we calculated [7] is dependent on ventricular cavity pressure and the ratio of cavity volume to wall volume. For the V_o (according to Suga), we used cavity volume V =

0. This seems a reasonable assumption, because values of V_d are usually close to zero. Moreover, measurements of the cavity to wall volume ratio in excited hearts by Dr. Delhaas and comparison with sarcomere lengths in these hearts reported in literature, indicated that at cavity volume = 0, sarcomere length is about 1.6 μm, at which length, according to papillary muscle measurements, there is no active force development.

Dr. K. Tsujioka: Did you find any difference in regional efficiency between different regions?

Dr. F. Prinzen: This requires accurate measurement of regional oxygen consumption. Until now we do not think that the required accuracy is high enough to say something about regional differences in efficiency.

Dr. K. Tsujioka: In your chronic experiment, even in late–activated area, you observed a relatively large wall thickness. Have you observed some difference in total heart work between paced hearts and natural hearts?

Dr. F. Prinzen: We did not measure total heart work.

REFERENCES

1. Hotta S. The sequence of mechanical activation of the ventricle. *Jap Circ J* 1967; 31: 1568–1572.
2. Prinzen FW, Augustijn CH, Allessie MA, Arts T, Delhaas T, Reneman RS. The time sequence of electrical and mechanical activation during spontaneous beating and ectopic stimulation. *Eur Heart J* 1992; 13: 535–543.
3. Lister JW, Klotz DH, Jomain SL, Stuckey JH, Hoffman BF. Effect of pacemaker site on cardiac output and ventricular activation in dogs with complete heart block. *Am J Cardiol* 1964; 14: 494–503.
4. Badke FR, Boinay P, Covell JW. Effect of ventricular pacing on regional left ventricular performance in the dog. *Am J Physiol* 1980; 238, H858–H867.
5. Prinzen FW, Augustijn CH, Arts T, Allessie MA, Reneman RS. Redistribution of myocardial fiber strain and blood flow by asynchronous activation. *Am J Physiol* 1990; 259, H300–H308.
6. Delhaas T, Arts T, Prinzen F. W, Reneman, R.S. Relation between regional electrical activation time and subepicardial fiber strain in the canine left ventricle. *Pfluegers Arch* 1993; 423: 78–87.
7. Delhaas T, Arts T, Prinzen FW, Reneman, RS. Regional contractile work and electrical activation in the canine left ventricle during asynchronous electrical activation. *Pfluegers Arch* 1992; 420 (Suppl. 1): R110.
8. Pfeffer MA, Braunwald E. Ventricular remodeling after myocardial infarction. Experimental observations and clinical implications. *Circulation* 1990; 81, 1161–1172.
9. Omens JH, Covell JW. Transmural distribution of myocardial tissue growth induced by volume overload hypertrophy in the dog. *Circulation* 1991; 84, 1235–1245.
10. Boucher CA, Pohost GM, Okada RD, Levine FH, Strauss HW, Warren Harthorne J. Effect of ventricular pacing on left ventricular function assessed by radionuclide angiography. *Am Heart J* 1983; 106: 1105–1111.
11. Frais MA, Botvinick EH, Shosa DW, O'Connell WJ, Scheinman MM, Hattner RS, Morady F. Phase image analysis of ventricular contraction in left and right bundle branch block. *Am J Cardiol* 1982; 50: 95–105.
12. Prinzen FW, Cheriex EC, Arts T, Delhaas T, Reneman RS. Changes in ventricular diastolic wall thickness induced by chronic asynchronous electrical activation. *J Mol Cell Cardiol* 1992; 24 (Suppl. V): S.50.
13. Jeanrenaud X, Goy JJ, Kappenberger L. Effects of dual–chamber pacing in hypertrophic obstructive cardiomyopathy. *Lancet* 1992; 339; 1318–1823.
14. Fananapazir L, Cannon RO, Tripodi DJ, Panza JA. Impact of dual–chamber permanent pacing in patients with obstructive cardiomyopathy with symptoms refractory to verapamil and beta–adrenergic blocker therapy. *Circulation* 1992; 85: 2149–2161.

CHAPTER 25

Ventricular Remodeling after Myocardial Infarction

Gary F. Mitchell, Gervasio A. Lamas, and Marc A. Pfeffer[1]

ABSTRACT

Acute transmural myocardial infarction initiates a series of changes in left ventricular (LV) volume, regional function and geometry. This process, known as post–infarction LV remodeling, may continue for months or years following the initial ischemic event. To characterize the components of late ventricular remodeling, biplane left ventriculography was performed in 52 patients at 3 weeks and repeated at 1 year after first anterior myocardial infarction. Biplane circumference and contractile and noncontractile segment lengths were measured. Global geometry was evaluated by calculating a sphericity index and regional geometry was assessed by measurement of endocardial curvature. End–diastolic (ED) volume was increased at 3 weeks and enlarged further at one year. This late enlargement was accompanied by an increase in the length of the contractile segment and an increase in sphericity, whereas the length of the noncontractile segment decreased. Curvature analysis revealed that this late increase in sphericity resulted from flattening of regions of presumably high tension negative curvature at the infarct border zone and from less bulging of the infarcted anterior wall. Even in patients selected for late ventricular enlargement (change in ED volume > 20 ml, n = 19), this increase in volume resulted from both lengthening of the contractile segment and an increase in sphericity without a change in the noncontractile segment length. Thus, late ventricular enlargement after anterior myocardial infarction results from an increase in contractile segment length and a change in ventricular geometry and is not a result of progressive infarct expansion.

INTRODUCTION

Myocardial infarct expansion, the acute process of lengthening and thinning of the infarct zone in the absence of additional necrosis, is known to contribute significantly to

---

[1]Cardiovascular Division, Department of Medicine, Brigham and Women's Hospital, Harvard Medical School, Boston, MA 02115, USA.

Interactive Phenomena in the Cardiac System, Edited by
S. Sideman and R. Beyar, Plenum Press, New York, 1993

the marked early ventricular chamber enlargement and geometric distortion that may accompany myocardial infarction in certain settings. There is evidence to suggest that these early changes in ventricular topography [1–5] may predispose to the late ventricular enlargement that is known to occur in some patients following myocardial infarction [6–11]. However, the precise regional components of this late ventricular remodeling are not well understood. The goals of the analyses reviewed in this chapter were to examine the characteristics of late ventricular enlargement and to determine the role of changes in the lengths of contractile and noncontractile myocardial segments in the process of LV remodeling after myocardial infarction [12]. Further, the contributions of early and late alterations in ventricular geometry to the process of LV enlargement were explored.

METHODS

Patient Population

This analysis of the components of ventricular enlargement utilized the quantitative left ventriculograms from a randomized, double-blind, placebo-controlled trial designed to evaluate the effects of captopril on late ventricular chamber enlargement in the year following first anterior Q-wave myocardial infarction [10]. Other inclusion criteria for participation in the study were documented infarction within 30 days prior to randomization, radionuclide LV ejection fraction of 45% or less, age between 21 and 75 years, and freedom from symptoms of ischemia or congestive heart failure. The study protocol was approved by the Human Subjects Committee of the Brigham and Women's Hospital and each patient gave informed consent to participate in the study. Of the 59 patients who participated in the study, 52 had baseline and one year ventriculograms of adequate technical quality for the quantitative analyses required for this report. Clinical characteristics of the patients and reasons for failure to complete the study (7 patients) have been previously reported [10].

Catheterization Protocol

Biplane left ventriculography was performed in the 30 degrees right anterior oblique and 60 degrees left anterior oblique projections at a rate of 30 frames per second per view. The baseline study, 12 to 31 days after infarction, included coronary angiography with multiple views. One year (364 ± 11 days) after the baseline catheterization, repeat ventriculography was performed by the same investigators. Blinded study medication (captopril or placebo) was discontinued one day prior to the follow-up catheterization.

Data Analysis

Ventricular silhouettes were traced onto transparency film then digitized at a resolution of 10 points per millimeter using a digitizing tablet interfaced to a personal computer. Corrections for magnification and pincushion distortion were made and LV volumes were determined by the area/length method (ellipsoidal model) using a regression equation developed at this institution [13].

Wall motion was analyzed at 100 chords (Fig. 1A) by a modification of the centerline method [12, 14]. The percentage of each silhouette that was either akinetic (uncorrected wall motion 0.0 ± 1.0 mm) or dyskinetic (more negative than −1.0 mm) was calculated and multiplied by the magnification-corrected diastolic circumference to obtain

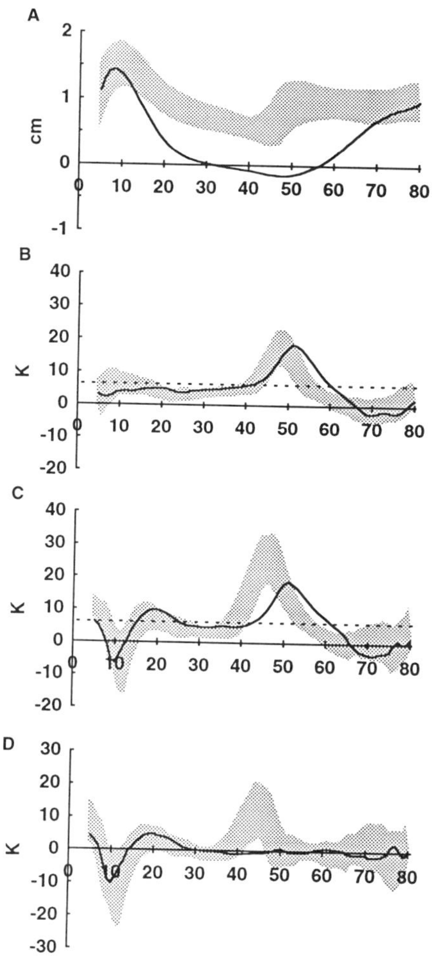

Figure 1. Baseline regional wall motion **(A)**, diastolic **(B)** and systolic **(C)** curvature and change in curvature during ejection **(D)** in 52 patients 11 to 31 days after anterior myocardial infarction (solid lines) and in 76 patients without coronary artery disease or history of infarction (shaded areas = normal means ± 1 SD). Dotted lines in panels **B** and **C** represent the spherical curvature value of 2p. (Adapted from [12].)

the absolute noncontractile segment length in centimeters. The length of the contractile segment was similarly obtained using the sum of the remaining chords. The aortic outflow tract was excluded from either of these determinations of contractile status but was included in the total circumference. Values obtained from right anterior oblique and left anterior oblique views were summed to give the biplane circumference and its component contractile and noncontractile endocardial segment lengths.

To evaluate changes in global LV shape, a circumference–based sphericity index [15] was defined that expresses the measured diastolic or systolic volume of the ventricle (ellipsoidal model) as a fraction of the volume of a hypothetical spherical left ventricle with the same biplane diastolic or systolic endocardial circumference, respectively.

Regional shape was assessed by measurement of local major axis (right anterior oblique) curvature (Fig. 1B–D) [16]. Following smoothing of the silhouettes as detailed elsewhere [12], curvature (K), which is the reciprocal of radius (R) of curvature, $K = 1/R$, was calculated at 100 points corresponding to the centerline wall motion chord intersections on each silhouette (Fig. 1). This reference system allows for direct comparisons between local shape and wall motion. Curvature, which has units of cm^{-1}, was normalized to ventricular size and made unitless by multiplying each value by the circumference ($2\pi R$) of the silhouette (diastolic or systolic) being analyzed. As a result of this normalization procedure, the hypothetical spherical ventricle noted above (sphericity index of one) would have a corrected curvature value of $(2\pi R)(1/R) = 2\pi$ at every point along its perimeter regardless of its size. Convexity is denoted by positive curvature whereas a negative value indicates concavity of the endocardial silhouette.

The important features of systolic endocardial curvature plots were summarized by searching each of four anatomic and functional LV regions and finding the contiguous 50% of the points within each region that characterize the geometry of that region (Fig. 1C). Thus, in the anterobasal region (points 5 to 17) a curvature minimum is found, in the infarcted anterior region (points 13 to 34) a maximum is found, at the apex (points 35 to 65) the maximum value is found and in the inferior region (points 60 to 80) a minimum is found. This approach eliminates the hazards of using fixed reference points to describe variable anatomic landmarks. For example, the apex may shift to the right or left but maintain its normal peak curvature following infarction or during recovery or as a variant of normal. Such a shift will have no effect on this system of dynamic localization of peak apical curvature.

Normal Values

Noninfarcted reference values for all hemodynamic data and for right anterior oblique curvature were obtained from the left ventriculograms of 76 patients without coronary artery disease or a history of myocardial infarction. Normal values for biplane ventriculographic parameters were obtained from the 37 of these patients who had biplane studies.

Statistical Analysis

Changes (baseline to one year) in hemodynamic variables and derived ventriculographic parameters (volume, contractile and noncontractile segment lengths, regional wall motion, sphericity, and curvature) in the entire study group ($n = 52$) regardless of drug therapy were analyzed with a paired t–test. Since late ventricular enlargement is a heterogeneous process, we defined significant enlargement as an increase in ED volume of greater than 20 ml. The subgroup of patients with marked late ventricular dilation ($n = 19$) were then analyzed to determine the components of this late change in ventricular volume, again without regard to drug therapy. Differences were considered significant if a two–tailed test gave a p value < 0.05. All values are presented as the mean ± SD.

RESULTS

Baseline Catheterization

At the time of the baseline cardiac catheterization, all patients were found to have disease of the left anterior descending coronary artery. Total occlusion of this artery was present in 36 (67%) of the 52 patients. On initial catheterization, mildly elevated LV ED pressure (20 ± 6 mmHg) was associated with marked elevation of both ED and end-systolic (ES) volume compared to "normal" noninfarcted patients, consistent with substantial early LV enlargement (Table 1). Baseline diastolic circumference and sphericity index were both increased in the study group indicating that early ventricular enlargement resulted from a combination of increased biplane endocardial circumference and sphericity of the ventricle.

One Year Catheterization

In the year following infarction the overall group exhibited a further increase in ED volume despite a reduction in ED pressure (20 ± 6 to 18 ± 7 mmHg, $p < 0.02$). This ventricular remodeling was a consequence of further distortion of the shape of the ventricle to a more spherical configuration, as the biplane circumference did not change significantly (Table 1).

Table 1. Paired ventriculographic data for patients with anterior myocardial infarction (N = 52) compared to normal noninfarcted patients. Values are mean ± SD. (Adapted from [12].)

	Normal	3 Weeks	1 Year	P
End–diastolic volume	142 ± 31 ml	230 ± 42	244 ± 55	0.010
End–systolic volume	40 ± 14 ml	136 ± 40	142 ± 54	–
Ejection fraction	0.72 ± 0.08	0.42 ± 0.10	0.43 ± 0.11	–
Diastolic sphericity index	0.663 ± 0.082	0.74 ± 0.07	0.76 ± 0.08	0.001
Systolic sphericity index	0.493 ± 0.108	0.62 ± 0.10	0.65 ± 0.10	0.001
Diastolic circumference	47.3 ± 3.8 cm	53.4 ± 3.3	53.8 ± 3.9	–
Systolic circumference	34.9 ± 3.7 cm	47.6 ± 4.0	47.0 ± 4.8	–
Contractile segment	42.6 ± 3.5 cm	34.4 ± 5.1	37.2 ± 5.0	<0.001
Noncontractile segment	0.0 ± 0.1 cm	14.6 ± 6.1	12.3 ± 6.3	0.003
Akinetic		8.2 ± 4.6	5.8 ± 3.7	<0.001
Dyskinetic		6.4 ± 4.2	6.5 ± 4.4	–

p = paired t–test.

Wall Motion Analysis

Overall, 14.6 ± 6.1 cm of the 53.4 ± 3.3 cm biplane ED circumference (27 ± 11%) was either akinetic or dyskinetic at baseline. At one year, despite no further change in the total circumference, there was a 2.7 ± 4.9 cm elongation of the contractile endocardial segment ($p < 0.001$) and a concomitant 2.3 ± 5.3 cm decrease in the length of the noncontractile segment ($p < 0.005$). Division of the noncontractile segment into akinetic and dyskinetic components revealed that the decrease was confined to the akinetic segment, which was 2.4 ± 4.6 cm shorter at one year ($p < 0.001$), whereas the dyskinetic segment remained unchanged.

As anticipated, centerline wall motion in the anterior (infarct) zone was severely depressed at baseline while wall motion in the noninfarcted inferior zone (the most vigorously contracting contiguous 50% of the chords in the inferior region) was not hyperkinetic as might be expected, but rather was mildly depressed. The one year catheterization revealed a slightly improved score in the anterior zone (from −3.4 ± 0.6 to −3.2 ± 0.8 SD/chord, $p < 0.02$) with mild deterioration in the inferior region (from −0.2 ± 1.0 to −0.6 ± 1.0 SD/chord, $p < 0.05$).

Left Ventricular Geometry

In conjunction with abnormal LV regional wall motion and global shape, we found severe abnormalities in endocardial curvature at baseline in these anterior Q–wave infarction patients when compared to the noninfarcted patients (Fig. 1). Specifically, at end–systole (Fig. 1C), when changes induced by heterogeneous ventricular contraction are most marked, adjacent to the negative curvature (concavity) associated with anterobasal contraction (points 5 to 17), there was excessive curvature (bulging) of the anterior wall (points 13 to 34). There was diminished curvature (blunting) and rightward or clockwise shifting of the apex (points 35 to 65), and excessively negative curvature (concavity) of the inferior region (points 60 to 80). When the curvature change from diastole to systole was analyzed (Fig. 1D) the normal systolic increase in curvature in the apical region was absent.

Regional systolic curvature averages in the patient group at baseline and at one year summarize the findings presented in the curvature plots. At one year, concavity became less prominent in the anterobasal (−6.0 ± 4.0 vs −4.5 ± 3.7, $p < 0.01$) and inferior (−4.5 ± 2.0 vs −3.6 ± 2.1, $p < 0.005$) regions while bulging of the anterior wall decreased (9.4 ± 2.5 vs 8.2 ± 2.3, $p < 0.001$) and blunting of the apex did not change (14.0 ± 1.4 vs 14.1 ± 1.4, p = NS). Each of the late changes in regional curvature is in the direction of the spherical value of 2 π, which is consistent with the observed increase in global sphericity index (Table 1).

Table 2. Paired Ventriculographic Data in Patients with Change in End–Diastolic Volume ≥ 20 ml at One Year (N = 19). Comparison to normal, noninfarcted patients. Mean ± SD. (Adapted from [12].)

	Normal	3 Weeks	1 Year	P
End–diastolic volume	142 ± 31 ml	236 ± 45	287 ± 54	<0.001
End–systolic volume	40 ± 14 ml	150 ± 43	182 ± 57	0.001
Ejection fraction	0.72 ± 0.08	0.37 ± 0.10	0.38 ± 0.10	–
Diastolic sphericity index	0.663 ± 0.082	0.75 ± 0.05	0.80 ± 0.08	0.004
Systolic sphericity index	0.493 ± 0.108	0.63 ± 0.09	0.71 ± 0.10	<0.001
Diastolic circumference	47.3 ± 3.8 cm	53.5 ± 3.2	56.0 ± 3.8	<0.001
Systolic circumference	34.9 ± 3.7 cm	48.7 ± 3.7	50.0 ± 4.7	–
Contractile segment	42.6 ± 3.5 cm	32.3 ± 3.7	36.3 ± 4.4	0.001
Noncontractile segment	0.0 ± 0.1 cm	16.9 ± 5.6	15.5 ± 6.4	–
Akinetic		10.0 ± 5.2	6.8 ± 4.1	0.012
Dyskinetic		6.9 ± 4.1	8.6 ± 4.5	–

p = paired t–test.

Late Enlargers

In those patients (n = 19) selected for late diastolic chamber enlargement, the 50 ± 27 ml increase above their already elevated baseline occurred with no change in distending pressure (22 ± 8 vs 20 ± 6 mmHg) (Table 2). This late increase in volume was due to a combination of increased circumference and increased sphericity. Associated with this diastolic enlargement was a 33 ± 38 ml ($p = 0.001$) increase in ES volume.

The 2.5 ± 2.2 cm increase in biplane ED circumference ($p < 0.001$) was a result of a 4.0 ± 4.4 cm elongation of the contractile segment ($p = 0.001$) with a concomitant 1.5 ± 5.0 cm shortening of the noncontractile segment (p = NS). In this group of volume enlargers, centerline wall motion was severely depressed in the anterior region (−3.7 ± 0.6 SD/chord) and mildly depressed in the inferior region (−0.5 ± 1.1 SD/chord) at baseline and did not change significantly over time. Analysis of local shape revealed marked accentuation of the normal concavity in the anterobasal region (−7.8 ± 3.2). As in the overall group, there was bulging of the anterior wall (10.1 ± 2.6), blunting of the apex (13.9 ± 1.6) and excessive concavity of the inferior wall (−4.7 ± 1.9). On follow–up evaluation, the same pattern of decreased concavity in the anterobasal (to −5.4 ± 2.9, $p < 0.005$) and inferior (−3.4 ± 2.3, $p < 0.01$) regions and less bulging in the anterior region (9.0 ± 2.6, $p < 0.02$) was observed (Fig. 2).

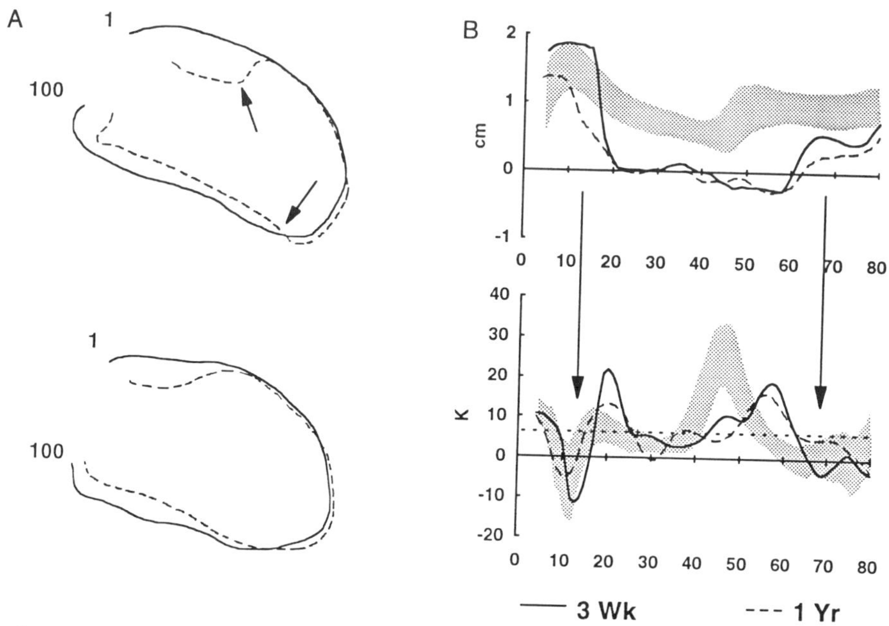

Figure 2. Adverse late ventricular remodeling in a patient with anterior myocardial infarction and marked abnormalities of ventricular volume and geometry. **A:** Diastolic (solid line) and systolic (broken line) silhouettes at 3 wk (above) and 1 yr (below). Volume (diastolic 302, systolic 186 ml) and sphericity (diastolic 0.70, systolic 0.60) are both markedly increased at baseline and increase further at one year. Biplane contractile segment length increased (30.5 to 33.8 cm) but noncontractile segment length did not change (23.7 to 23.5 cm). **B:** Changes in centerline wall motion (above) and curvature (below) at 3 wks (solid lines) and 1 yr (broken lines). The dotted line in the curvature plot represents the spherical curvature value of 2π. Arrows indicate the areas of negative or "anticlastic" curvature produced by the juxtaposition of functioning and nonfunctioning tissue at the infarct border zone. In this example of unfavorable remodeling, flattening in the anterobasal and inferior regions is due to a loss of contractile function of residual tissue in these regions.

DISCUSSION

Volume Enlargement

Prior observations have clearly established that marked early LV enlargement may be seen following myocardial infarction. In the present group of patients with large anterior Q–wave infarctions, this early increase in volume was present when compared to noninfarcted patients, and presumably occurred between the time of the myocardial infarction and the baseline (3 wk) catheterization. This early volume enlargement resulted from a combination of both increased endocardial circumference and sphericity of the ventricle. In the ensuing year, additional chamber enlargement occurred. This late ventricular enlargement was associated with significant lengthening of the contractile segment and with increasing sphericity of the ventricle despite a reduction in filling pressure. The noncontractile segment length decreased during this chronic phase suggesting that infarct expansion did not contribute to late ventricular enlargement in this patient population. Even in the subgroup selected for significant late volume enlargement, lengthening of the noncontractile segment was not observed. In contrast, in this group of volume "enlargers" there was substantial lengthening of the contractile segment at a constant LV filling pressure suggesting true hypertrophy rather than passive distention of residual, functioning tissue.

Contractile/Noncontractile Segment Lengths

There are several potential explanations for the observation that the length of the noncontractile segment decreases with time following a myocardial infarction. The most straightforward possibility is that a peri–infarct rim of noncontractile but perfused tissue regains function in the chronic phase of recovery. However, at least two additional possibilities merit consideration. In the dog model, Theroux has shown that acute infarction is associated with initial diastolic lengthening and paradoxical motion of the infarcted zone [17]. At four weeks, when scar formation is complete in the dog, the scar contracts to about 30% of its original diastolic length. The length of the noncontractile segment might be expected to decrease to a comparable degree in patients. Similar results have been reported in echocardiographic [18] and histologic [19] analyses of infarct size during the acute and convalescent phases of myocardial infarction. Additionally, Theroux demonstrated that the compliance of infarcted tissue decreases significantly as a function of time [17]. This decrease in regional compliance may influence the apparent length of the noncontractile segment because of improved tethering and passive inward motion of the scar. Inability to distinguish these mechanisms using angiographic data prevents a precise analysis of the degree to which the present observations represent a reclaiming of function along the rim of the infarction versus scar contraction accompanied by proportionate hypertrophy of the contractile segment.

Ventricular Geometry

Curvature analysis confirmed that juxtaposition of viable and akinetic or dyskinetic myocardium following a large anterior myocardial infarction created a rim of negative curvature encircling the infarct during systole. Although most models of ventricular regional wall stress have not been generalized to the case where one of the principal radii of curvature is negative, analyses of circumferential variability in aortic medial thickness suggest that such an "anticlastic" configuration imparts elevated local wall tension [20]. Bogen et al. [21] predicted a four–fold increase in circumferential stresses in the border zone following acute infarction in their model of the infarcted dog heart. Pouleur et al. [22] have shown that this peri–infarct zone has high ES and residual (early diastolic) wall stresses in humans and Anversa [23] has demonstrated a reduced oxygenation potential in this critical zone of perfused, viable but hypocontractile myocardium [24]. Thus, this zone may be at high risk for further ischemic insults. This local shape abnormality also may relate to the observation in the rat model of a rim of maximal hypertrophy at the interface between healing scar and viable myocardium [25]. Together, these observations suggest that in the infarcted ventricle, marked abnormalities of local LV geometry make a regional, rather than global, analysis of wall stress imperative.

In the year following infarction, global increases in ventricular chamber volume and sphericity are associated with regional flattening of the presumably high–tension rim of functioning anticlastic tissue that surrounds the infarct zone. This is accompanied by a decrease in the degree of bulging of the infarcted anterior wall. These changes could be interpreted as a redistribution of wall tension as the peri–infarct tissue, including any stunned myocardium, hypertrophies and/or regains function and the infarcted tissue forms a contracted, less compliant fibrous scar which yields less to high intracavitary pressures in systole [17, 21]. Histologic scar contraction and stiffening coupled with lengthening (eccentric hypertrophy) of the contractile myocardial segment will result in less of a size and compliance mismatch between functioning and nonfunctioning tissue in systole, leading to a reduction in the degree of local curvature abnormality at the interface between the two. Similarly, regained contractile function at this crucial interface will tend to reduce the local shape abnormality. However, the distinction between regained function improving shape or improved shape augmenting function (due to lower wall stress) becomes difficult to make in this region. Lessick et al. [26] have demonstrated that, despite these changes over time, curvature and wall motion remain abnormal in this border zone even after the development of a fibrous scar in those patients with aneurysms. Thus, rather than a cause of increased global wall stress [27], late increases in global sphericity may be viewed as an adaptation to abnormal regional wall stress, with increased sphericity (movement toward the spherical value of 2π on curvature plots) affording a redistribution of wall stress away from the critical border zone of viable myocardium. There may, however, be a limit beyond which these adaptations are inadequate, leading to loss of function, progressive volume enlargement and deterioration in chamber geometry (Fig. 2).

CONCLUSION

Late ventricular enlargement following a large first anterior myocardial infarction is associated with lengthening of the contractile segment rather than progressive infarct expansion. Further, we have quantitatively assessed the abnormalities in ventricular shape that accompany anterior infarction and confirm that severe abnormalities of global and regional LV shape are present three weeks following infarction and that further changes in geometry contribute significantly to late volume enlargement, suggesting that chamber geometry may play an important role in progressive ventricular remodeling following myocardial infarction.

DISCUSSION

Dr. M. Gotsman: Is there a difference between patent arteries and closed arteries after myocardial infarction? We have similar data that shows that when the artery is open, the ventricle remodels to a smaller volume. If the artery is closed, the ventricle enlarges. Do you think that remodelling occurs within days or weeks and is thus due to increased contractility? What is the nature of the change of the increasing curvature between an open and unopened artery?

Dr. G.F. Mitchell: We could not do a direct comparison between patients with patent and occluded vessels in this small study. However, patients with occluded vessels experienced late volume enlargement whereas patients with patent vessels did not. Furthermore, this late enlargement in the occluded group was prevented by captopril therapy. We have done a preliminary analysis of the effects of the infarct–related vessel in the SAVE study and found a similar effect on combined cardiovascular morbidity and mortality. That is to say, the patients with an occluded vessel did worse than those with a patent vessel, and either group did better if on captopril than if on placebo, to the extent that patients with an occluded vessel randomized to captopril did as well as patients with a patent vessel randomized to placebo.

Dr. F. Prinzen: Your analogies are based on the contour of the cavity. How did the muscle mass of the heart, either entirely or locally, change? The decrease in curvature in the border zone could suggest that there is a change in muscle mass there; the surviving fibers are increasing their mass. Do you have any indication for this?

Dr. G.F. Mitchell: We could not do that analysis on this angiographic data because you cannot see wall thickness well enough. However, Anversa et al. [23] have looked at this issue in the rat model of myocardial infarction and they have demonstrated a zone of hypertrophy at the border zone, which corresponds to the region of negative curvature. This suggests that the hypertrophy was in response to abnormal local stresses. There are over 500 patients in the SAVE study who have had serial echocardiograms. This will allow us to measure long and short axis curvature and wall thickness and address this issue.

Dr. G. Hasenfuss: Is there any evidence that late reopening of initially occluded vessels, and even after thrombolytic therapy of occluded vessels, reduces the risk of ventricular enlargement?

Dr. G.F. Mitchell: There is no evidence that I am aware of. There have been several attempts to demonstrate in retrospective analyses. However, there are obvious flaws with such studies where a clinical decision determined whether a patient was revascularized or not. For example, the decision to refer a patient for angioplasty may have been persistent chest pain, possibly due to a "less complete" infarction. The latter may have a greater influence on remodeling than the decision to revascularize. We are looking at these issues in the SAVE study patient population.

Dr. D. Kass: Your hypothesis seems to require a bulging shape of the aneurysm. One would speculate that aneurysm resection would potentially markedly change the outcome and the contractile region expansion over time. Traditional experience with aneurysm resection has shown it to be a very mixed bag and so I wonder how your data fits in?

Dr. G.F. Mitchell: There was a study done at Johns–Hopkins by Dr. Hutchins *[Am J Pathol 1980; 99: 221–230]* who looked at the effects of aneurysm resection techniques on clinical outcome. They found that everting the edges of the ventriculotomy led to an abnormal region of negative curvature at the site, whereas inversion of the edges produced a more normal convex curvature at the scar site. Patients with negative or anticlastic curvature were more likely to experience severe hemodynamic compromise post–op, while those patients with a convex anterior wall did a little better. This was a small study with only 18 patients.

Dr. E.O. Feigl: In one word: is remodeling good or bad?

Dr. G.F. Mitchell: Both.

REFERENCES

1. Eaton LW, Weiss JL, Bulkley BH, Garrison JB, Weisfeldt ML. Regional cardiac dilatation after acute myocardial infarction. Recognition by two-dimensional echocardiography. *N Engl J Med* 1979; 300: 57–62.
2. Erlebacher JA, Weiss JL, Weisfeldt ML, Bulkley BH. Early dilation of the infarcted segment in acute transmural myocardial infarction: Role of infarct expansion in acute left ventricular enlargement. *J Am Coll Cardiol* 1984; 4: 201–208.
3. Erlebacher JA, Weiss JL, Eaton LW, Kallman C, Weisfeldt ML, Bulkley BH. Late effects of acute infarct dilatation on heart size: A two dimensional echocardiographic study. *Am J Cardiol* 1982; 49: 1120–1126.
4. McKay RG, Pfeffer MA, Pasternak RC, et al. Left ventricular remodeling following myocardial infarction: a corollary to infarct expansion. *Circulation* 1986; 74: 693–702.
5. Weisman HF, Bush DE, Mannisi JA, Weisfeldt ML, Healy B. Cellular mechanisms of myocardial infarct expansion. *Circulation* 1988; 78: 186–201.
6. Pfeffer JM, Pfeffer MA, Braunwald E. Influence of chronic captopril therapy on the infarcted left ventricle of the rat. *Circ Res* 1985; 57: 84–95.
7. Jeremy RW, Hackworthy RA, Bautovich G, Hutton BF, Harris PJ. Infarct artery perfusion and changes in left ventricular volume in the month after acute myocardial infarction. *J Am Coll Cardiol* 1987; 9: 989–995.
8. Warren SE, Royal HD, Markis JE, Grossman W, McKay RL. Time course of left ventricular dilation after myocardial infarction: Influence of infarct–related artery and success of coronary thrombolysis. *J Am Coll Cardiol* 1988; 11: 12–19.
9. Lamas GA, Pfeffer MA. Increased left ventricular volume following myocardial infarction in man. *Am Heart J* 1986; 111: 30–35.
10. Pfeffer MA, Lamas GA, Vaughan DE, Parisi AF, Braunwald E. Effect of captopril on progressive ventricular dilatation after anterior myocardial infarction. *N Engl J Med* 1988; 319: 80–86.
11. Gadsboll N, Hoilund–Carlsen PF, Badsberg JH, Stage P, Marving J, Lonborg–Jensen H. Late ventricular dilatation in survivors of acute myocardial infarction. *Am J Cardiol* 1989; 64: 961–966.
12. Mitchell GF, Lamas GA, Vaughan DE, Pfeffer MA. Left ventricular remodeling in the year after first anterior myocardial infarction: a quantitative analysis of contractile segment lengths and ventricular shape. *J Am Coll Cardiol* 1992; 19: 1136–1144.
13. Wynne J, Green LH, Mann T, Levin D, Grossman W. Estimation of left ventricular volumes in man from biplane cineangiograms filmed in oblique projections. *Am J Cardiol* 1978; 41: 726–732.
14. Sheehan FH, Bolson EL, Dodge HT, Mathey DG, Schofer J, Woo H. Advantages and applications of the centerline method for characterizing regional ventricular function. *Circulation* 1986; 74: 293–305.
15. Lamas GA, Vaughan DE, Parisi AF, Pfeffer MA. Effects of left ventricular shape and captopril therapy on exercise capacity after anterior wall acute myocardial infarction. *Am J Cardiol* 1989; 63: 1167–1173.
16. Mancini GBJ, DeBoe SF, Anselmo E, Simon SB, LeFree MT, Vogel RA. Quantitative regional curvature analysis: an application of shape determination for the assessment of segmental left ventricular function in man. *Am Heart J* 1987; 113: 326–334.
17. Theroux P, Ross J,Jr., Franklin D, Covell JW, Bloor CM, Sasayama S. Regional myocardial function and dimensions early and late after myocardial infarction in the unanesthetized dog. *Circ Res* 1977; 40: 158–165.
18. Gibbons EF, Hogan RD, Franklin TD, Nolting M, Weyman AE. The natural history of regional dysfunction in a canine preparation of chronic infarction. *Circulation* 1985; 71: 394–402.
19. Reimer KA, Jennings RB. The changing anatomic reference base of evolving myocardial infarction. Underestimation of myocardial collateral blood flow and overestimation of experimental anatomic infarct size due to tissue edema, hemmorrhage and acute inflammation. *Circulation* 1979; 60: 866–876.
20. Burton AC. The importance of the shape and size of the heart. *Am Heart J* 1957; 54: 801–810.
21. Bogen DK, Rabinowitz SA, Needleman A, McMahon TA, Abelmann WH. An analysis of the mechanical disadvantage of myocardial infarction in the canine left ventricle. *Circ Res* 1980; 47: 728–741.
22. Pouleur H, Rousseau MF, van Eyll C, Charlier AA. Assessment of regional left ventricular relaxation in patients with coronary artery disease: importance of geometric factors and changes in wall thickness. *Circulation* 1984; 69: 696–702.

23. Anversa P, Beghi C, Kikkawa Y, Olivetti G. Myocardial infarction in rats. Infarct size, myocyte hypertrophy, and capillary growth. *Circ Res* 1986; 58: 26–37.
24. Cox DA, Vatner SF. Myocardial function in areas of heterogeneous perfusion after coronary artery occlusion in conscious dogs. *Circulation* 1982; 66: 1154–1158.
25. Olivetti G, Ricci R, Beghi C, Guideri G, Anversa P. Response of the border zone to myocardial infarction in rats. *Am J Pathol* 1986; 125: 476–483.
26. Lessick J, Sideman S, Azhari H, Marcus M, Grenadier E, Beyar R. Regional three–dimensional geometry and function of left ventricles with fibrous aneurysms––a cine–computed tomography study. *Circulation* 1991; 84: 1072–1086.
27. Gould KL, Lipscomb K, Hamilton GW, Kennedy JW. Relation of left ventricular shape, function and wall stress in man. *Am J Cardiol* 1974; 34: 627–634.

CHAPTER 26

ARTERIAL REMODELLING AFTER PERCUTANEOUS TRANSLUMINAL BALLOGN ANGIOPLASTY

Yoseph Rozenman, Chaim Lotan, Dan Gilon, Morris Mosseri, Dan Sapoznikov, Sima Welber, and Mervyn S. Gotsman[1]

ABSTRACT

Atheromatous coronary artery disease progresses by atheroma accretion, plaque rupture and thrombus formation, with or without spontaneous fibrinolysis [1–3]. The natural history may be altered by modifying risk factors in an attempt to induce regression [4], or treated by mechanical means such as balloon angioplasty, directional coronary atherectomy or drills, or flow modulated by the insertion of an aorto coronary bypass graft with or without endarterectomy [5, 6].

Here we discuss the natural history of the atheromatous disease in a series of 355 patients who underwent at least one PTCA procedure and then underwent a second angiographic study to determine the changes in the dilated and nondilated arteries.

MECHANICAL MECHANISMS OF ANGIOPLASTY

Balloon angioplasty stretches the intima, media and adventia of the artery. Marked stretching of the muscular media may cause paralysis of the muscle cells due to overstretching or organic disorganization of the myocytes with muscle cell lysis and twisting of the nuclei [7]. The intima is often cracked, and the crack or fissure may extend into the media and rarely into the adventia. The atheromatous material may be compressed, possibly with extrusion of fluid contents. The entire artery is remodelled into its new shape [8–10].

Deflation of the balloon may be followed by immediate recoil of the artery. Rensing et al. have shown that immediate recoil is responsible for a reduction of 50% of the luminal cross–sectional area [7]. This occurs more frequently in asymmetrical lesions,

[1]Department of Cardiology, Hadassah University Hospital, Ein–Kerem, Jerusalem, Israel.

Interactive Phenomena in the Cardiac System, Edited by
S. Sideman and R. Beyar, Plenum Press, New York, 1993

located in less angulated segments and those with a lower plaque content. Elastic recoil can be prevented by inserting an appropriately sized stent.

After removal of the balloon, a response to injury occurs [11]. Endothelium has been denuded and the intimal tear stretches into the media for a variable depth and length. Exposure of collagen and the liberation of van Willebrand factor initiates the thrombotic cascade and attracts and activates platelets. Fresh thrombus forms and propagates, but simultaneously undergoes spontaneous lysis and is washed away by good flow [2, 3]. Poor rheological conditions may cause abrupt closure of the artery due to an obstructive thrombus. The artery can occlude at this stage from acute thrombosis, due either to an intimal flap or severe intimal injury, marked reduction of blood flow or failure of adequate thrombolysis. In practice, good dilatation of the artery, adhesion of the intima to the media by balloon compression and effective anticoagulant therapy with heparin and aspirin prevent this tragic complication which occurs in less than 2% of patients [12].

In most patients only a thin layer of thrombus forms on the denuded surface. This attracts tissue plasminogen activator which converts plasminogen into plasmin. The tissue plasminogen activator contains growth factors which cause endothelial healing.

Heparin sulphate is a natural substance produced by intact endothelium. It prevents the replication of medial muscle myocytes and maintains their normal muscular phenotype. Lack of heparin sulphate, due to intimal denudation and the liberation from the alpha granules of the platelet, of platelet derived growth factor, a powerful mitogen, stimulates the stable muscle cells with its myocytic phenotype which are latent in the phase G0 of the cell cycle (1–2 days after PTCA). The cell rapidly enters the G1 phase and changes its phenotype to a fibroblastic form; it contains less actin and myosin but has more protein synthetic and secretory potential [11, 13]. It then enters the S and M phases. Other growth factors including interleukin I (from macrophages), epidermal growth factor (EGF) and insulin-like growth factor (IGF) and probably endothelin, together with other growth factors and also loss of the intact basement membrane, permit the multiplying cells to migrate into the subintima, where they bulge into the lumen of the artery and cause obstruction (2 weeks–2 months) [14]. The new fibroblastic cells also produce extracellular matrix—collagen, fibronectin and proteoglycans—under the influence of transforming growth factor beta (TGF beta). Multiplication and migration of the myocytes is slowed and halted by mechanical and rheological factors and also by TGF beta. At the same time endothelial repair is taking place, and unless the denudation is very extensive, repair is complete within a fortnight. The process progresses through the three phases of wound healing - inflammation (cells and growth factors), granulation (smooth muscle cell proliferation) and matrix remodeling with extracellular matrix deposition and proteoglycan synthesis [14].

In the final stage, the medial muscle myocyte returns to its muscular phenotype (3–6 months) [15].

The remodeling process may also be modulated and modified by the flow characteristics of the artery. Low shear stress prevents turbulence, but in its wake more platelets and macrophages adhere to the intima and may be responsible for initiating and secreting large quantities of the progression factors [11].

RESTENOSIS

Loss of luminal cross-sectional area after successful angioplasty is a random process with a single Gaussian distribution [16]. Significant restenosis occurs in 30% of patients after successful dilatation and may be higher after atherectomy and rotablation.

The clinical outcome depends on the final severity of the stenotic lesion which may be sufficient to induce flow limitation, with or without clinical symptoms. The reported incidence of restenosis depends on the criteria of the investigating group. Cellular restenosis starts after 14 days and is completed by 120 days [15].

CLINICAL STUDY

During a two year period 1,385 patients underwent coronary angioplasty for significant narrowing of a major coronary artery. Each patient had important angina pectoris or another form of symptomatic ischemic heart disease. Three hundred and fifty five had a second angiogram for recurrent clinical symptoms. Details of the angiographic technique are described in previous publications [17, 18].

The 355 patients studied twice form the basis of this study. In these 355 patients, 970 atheromatous lesions (>20% luminal diameter narrowing) were identified: 501 were dilated and 469 were not dilated. The mean diameter stenosis of the dilated lesion was 73 ± 18% compared to the nondilated lesions 53 ± 47% (p<0.001). Restenosis (defined as >50% in diameter stenosis) occurred in 37%.

Restenosis occurred in more severe lesions (80 ± 18 vs 69 ± 19% initial diameter stenosis) and after less complete dilatation (post dilatation stenosis 22 ± 26 vs 13 ± 17%). It occurred more commonly in long lesions (11 ± 8 mm vs 9 ± 4 mm) and was not influenced by the diameter of the adjacent normal artery.

We also examined the progression or regression of other lesions in the dilated and nondilated vessels. In the dilated artery there were 117 other lesions which were not dilated: 8 progressed, 10 regressed and 62 new lesions appeared. In the nondilated arteries, there were 352 additional lesions, 55 progressed, 7 regressed and 87 new lesions appeared.

This data suggests that progression of established lesions is slow, but new lesions occur frequently. The disease appears to progress in a step–wise fashion due, probably, to rupture of a previously otherwise normal arterial wall or an insignificant plaque [19, 20].

CONCLUSIONS

Our study has shown two interesting facts:

1. Progression of established lesion is slow and regression is very rare. Progression is more common in the non–intubated artery. On the other hand, the sudden appearance of new lesions is very common suggesting that plaque rupture occurs in small angiographically insignificant lesions.
2. Restenosis after PTCA is common and appears to occur in longer, more severe lesions which are less adequately dilated. It would seem that in these lesions more damage is induced and the damage is responsible for the liberation of growth factors which cause more intense healing.

Acknowledgement

This work was supported by a grant from the National Council for Research and Development, Israel, and GSF, Munchen, Germany.

DISCUSSION

Dr. L.E. Ford: It is possible that the probability of restenosis is directly proportional to the extent of the lesion, i.e. a sort of probability per millimeter. If this were so, the longer the lesion the higher the probability of the stenosis reoccurring at some region.

Dr. M.S. Gotsman: You are correct. The more severe the damage you inflict on the endothelium, the more factors you release and the more likely the stenosis is to recur.

Dr. Y. Kresh: I am curious, why is a patient subjected to multiple PTCA attempts? Do you think we are approaching a time we when we will you know when not to attempt a PTCA procedure on a given patient?

Dr. M.S. Gotsman: Let me present the other side of the argument. If 37% of patients return, then 63% of the patients are asymptomatic and do not return; 63% of the patients have a successful PTCA. Why did the patients return and why did we reinvestigate them? Three subsets. The first subset of patients were controls whom we simply reexamined 3 months after the initial angioplasty to determine our results. This was a very small group. The second subset, most of the patients, returned because of recurrent symptomatology, and the third subset of patients are patients who had had a PTCA, but returned with a new clinical syndrome later. Part of the subset returned because of new onset of angina. These are the patients who have sudden rupture of the atheromatous plaques and brand new lesions.

Dr. E. Ritman: You said that the myocytes proliferate locally. Is it known for sure that they come from a local source rather than from somewhere more remote? That would have great impact on treatment.

Dr. M.S. Gotsman: There are two major sources of the fibroblastic cells which develop in the intima. Some are true fibroblastic cells. Most have markers of medial muscle myocytes. They change their phenotypic profile. You can do this in cell culture. If you add growth factors to a cell culture of myocytes, you alter their phenotype and convert them into fibroblast like cells. Instead of producing actin and myosin, they develop more Golgi apparatus and coarse sarcoplasmic reticulum and then produce collagen. The production of collagen might either strangulate them or turn them off. Transforming growth factor beta is another substance which prevents cell multiplication. Biopsies were taken at atherectomy from these areas. The initial biopsies at the time of initial atherectomy show classical atheroma; ones made later, when restenosis is established usually contain fibrous tissue cells, but those in the intermediate or early stage are myocytes which have a fibrocytic phenotype. These fibrocytic phenotypic cells then return to their original profile and if examined 1 to 2 years later resemble myocytes located in the intima below the basement membrane of the artery.

Dr. Y. Lanir: Did you try to analyze your data to see if those factors that you have checked, like length and severity, are the only factors which determine the outcome; perhaps there is an additional variable that you have not looked at?

Dr. M.S. Gostman: There may well be additional variables that we have not examined, but we looked at many factors. Only three emerged as being statistically significant: the degree of initial stenosis, the degree of lack of improvement, and the length of the lesion.

Dr. D. Kass: I am interested in your patient who received a stent which seemed to resolve a lot of his problems. Given the pathophysiology of intimal proliferation, I would be somewhat surprised that you can prevent restenosis. You crack plaque and activate all the endothelial factors. Whether you insert a spring mesh against the wall or not, one would imagine that the process could now form in and around this mesh and should continue to form restenosis. Naturally elastic recoil is prevented.

Dr. M.S. Gotsman: Agreed: I took this patient to demonstrate the particular excellent result.

Dr. D. Kass: What do you think about the likelihood of success of stents, given the fact that elastic recoil plays less of a role?

Dr. M.S. Gotsman: Stents are used widely in the United States when the artery collapses and there is the need to reinforce its inner structure. The group in Tolouse implants stents routinely in virtually every patient with a larger artery and the restenosis rate is much lower. It prevents recoil and recoil is important. In some of our patients we reexamined the artery the day after angioplasty: the arteries looked quite horrific with mild restenosis due either to elastic recoil or to platelet aggregation and adhesion.

Dr. F. Kajiya: Have you any observations about the relationship between regression of atherosclerosis and reduction of risk factors, for example reducing blood cholesterol level?

Dr. M.S. Gotsman: We looked at the risk factor profile, but could not find any relationship to the degree of restenosis.

REFERENCES

1. Ross R. The pathogenesis of atherosclerosis – an update. *N Engl J Med* 1986; 314: 488–500.
2. Fuster V, Badimon L, Badimon JJ, Chesebro JH. The pathogenesis of coronary artery disease and the acute coronary syndromes (first of two parts). *N Engl J Med* 1991; 326: 242–250.
3. Fuster V, Badimon L, Badimon JJ, Chesebro JH. The pathogenesis of coronary artery disease and the acute coronary syndromes (second of two parts). *N Engl J Med* 1991; 326: 310–318.
4. Blankenhorn DH, Nessim SA, Johnson RL, Sanmarco ME, Azen SP, Cashen–Hemphill L. Beneficial effects of combined colestipol–niacin therapy on coronary atherosclerosis and coronary venous bypass grafts. *JAMA* 1987; 257: 3233–3240.
5. Holmes DR Jr, Vliestra RE, Smith HC, Vetrovec GW, Kent KM, Cowley MJ, Faxon DP, Gruentzig AR, Kelsey SF, Detre KM, Van Raden MJ, Mock MB. Restenosis after percutaneous transluminal coronary angioplasty: A report from the PTCA Registry of National Heart, Lung, and Blood Institute. *Am J Cardiol* 1984; 53: 77C–81C.
6. Kuntz RE, Safian RD, Levine MJ, Reis GJ, Diver DJ, Baim DS. Novel approach to the analysis of restenosis after the use of three new coronary devices. *J Am Coll Cardiol* 1992; 19: 1493–1499.
7. Rensing BJ, Hermans WR, Strauss BH, Serruys PW. Regional differences in elastic recoil after percutaneous transluminal coronary angioplasty. A quantitative angiographic study. *J Am Coll Cardiol* 1991; 17: 34B–38B.
8. Waller BF. Morphologic correlates of coronary angiographic patterns at the site of percutaneous transluminal coronary angioplasty. *Clin Cardiol* 1988; 11: 827–823.
9. Waller BF, Pinkerton CA, Orr CM, Slack JD, VanTassel JW, Peters T. Restenosis 1 to 24 months after clinically successful coronary balloon angioplasty. A necropsy study of 20 patients. *JACC* 1991; 17: 58B–70B.
10. Waller BF. "Crackers, breakers, stretchers, drillers, scrapers, shavers, burners, welders, melters" – the future treatment of atherosclerotic coronary artery disease? A clinical – morphologic assessment. *J Am Coll Cardiol* 1989; 13: 969–987.
11. Liu MW, Roubin GS, King SB III. Restenosis after coronary angioplasty – potential biologic determinants and role of intimal hyperplasia. *Circulation* 1989; 79: 1374–1387.
12. Ellis SG, Roubin GS, King SB, Douglas JS, Weintraub WS, Thomas RG, Cox W. Angiographic and clinical predictors of acute closure after native vessel coronary angioplasty. *Circulation* 1988; 77: 372–379.

13. Muller DWM, Ellis SG, Topol EJ. Colchicine and antineoplastic therapy for the prevention of restenosis after percutaneous coronary interventions. *JACC* 1991; 17: 126B–31B.
14. Forrester JS, Fishbein M, Helfant R, Fagin J. A paradigm for restenosis based on cell biology: Clues for the development of new preventive therapies. *J Am Coll Cardiol* 1991; 17: 758–69.
15. Serruys PW, Luijten HE, Batt KJ, Geuskens R, deFeyter PJ, van den Brand M, Reiber JHC, ten Katen HJ, vanEs GA and Hugenholtz PG. Incidence of restenosis after successful coronary angioplasty: A time–related phenomenon. *Circulation* 1988; 77: 361–371.
16. Rensing BJ, Hermans WRM, Deckers JW, deFeyter PJ, Tijssen JGP, Serruys PW. Lumen narrowing after percutaneous transluminal coronary balloon angioplasty follows a near gaussian distribution: a quantitative angiographic study in 1445 successfully dilated lesions. *J Am Coll Cardiol* 1992; 19: 939–945.
17. Halov DA, Sapoznikov D, Lewis BS, Gotsman MS. Localization of lesions in the coronary circulation. *Am J Cardiol* 1983; 52: 921–926.
18. Gotsman MS, Rosenheck S, Nassar H, Welber S, Sapoznikov D, Mosseri M, Weiss A, Lotan C, Rozenman Y. Angiographic findings in the coronary arteries after thrombolysis in acute myocardial infarction. *Am J Cardiol* 1992; 70: 715–723.
19. Ambrose JA, Tannenbaum MA, Alexopoulos D, Hjemdahl–Monsen CE, Leavy J, Weiss M, Borrico S, Gorlin R, Fuster V. Angiographic progression of coronary artery disease and the development of myocardial infarction. *J Am Coll Cardiol* 1988; 12: 56–62.
20. Lichtlen PR, Hugenholtz PG, Rafflenbeul W, Hecker H, Jost S, Deckers JW, on behalf of the INTACT Study Group Investigators. Retardation of angiographic progression of coronary artery disease by nifedipine. Results of the International Nifedipine Trial on Antiatherosclerotic Therapy (INTACT). *Lancet* 1990; 335: 1109–13.
21. Hwang MH, Sihdu P, Pacold I, Johnson S, Scanlon PJ, Loeb HS. Progression of coronary artery disease after percutaneous transluminal coronary angioplasty. *Am Heart J* 1988; 115: 297–301.

CHAPTER 27

Structural and Functional Remodeling of Poststenotic Arteries in the Rat

Jo G.R. De Mey, Harry Van Der Heijden, Ger Janssen, and Gregorio Fazzi[1]

ABSTRACT

In rat femoral arteries situated distally from a unilateral partial iliac artery obstruction, we observed: (i) 30% reduction of media cross sectional area, without alteration of arterial DNA content, (ii) a steeper relationship between strain and circumferential wall stress at rest, (iii) 12% reduction of the diameter at which maximal active wall tension was observed, (iv) reduction (25%) of maximal active wall tension, but not maximal active wall stress, and (v) a leftward shift of the relationship between diameter and sensitivity for contractile stimuli. Chronic flow reduction at constant pressure, did not modify arterial properties. These findings indicate that (pulse) pressure, influences arterial structure and function primarily by an effect on arterial smooth muscle cell volume. Vascular remodeling may thus result from disproportionate effects on vessel wall components.

INTRODUCTION

Chronic hypertension alters structure and mechanics of blood vessels [1, 2]. Hypertrophy and structural narrowing of the vascular wall are involved herein [3]. Arterial pressure, neural stimuli, humoral factors and genetic factors all may contribute to the development of hypertrophy [1, 4–6]. Determinants of arterial diameter are less clear. Folkow et al. [7] found that regional hypotension attenuated the increase in minimal resistance in the hind limb of spontaneously hypertensive rats (SHR). In a similar setting Bund et al. [5] observed that protection from pressure elevation prevented resistance artery structural changes. These findings suggest a role for hemodynamic forces but do not dissociate between mean pressure, pulse pressure and flow. Interventions that lower

---

[1]Vascular Biology Laboratory, Department of Pharmacology and Cardiovascular Research Institute Maastricht, University of Limburg, Maastricht, The Netherlands.

Interactive Phenomena in the Cardiac System, Edited by
S. Sideman and R. Beyar, Plenum Press, New York, 1993

systemic pressure yielded conflicting results with respect to prevention of both hypertrophy [8, 9] and remodeling [10]. This seems to be due to neurohumoral changes that accompany some types of antihypertensive therapy [9, 11] and on disproportionate effects on the different vascular wall components [12]. There is even less consensus in the literature concerning the role of variables and factors in the *maintenance* of vascular structure and on the possibility to reverse rather than prevent structural vascular changes. This may be of interest from a therapeutic point of view.

The goal of this study was to evaluate whether reduction of pressure or flow changes arterial wall structure in the adult and whether arterial smooth muscle cells and extracellular matrix components are equally affected. For this purpose we recorded structural and mechanical properties in femoral artery segments situated distally or proximally from a pressure and flow limiting stenosis.

METHODS

Our approach was inspired by a study by Bund et al. [5]. But rather than on preventing changes we focused on their reversal. We used adult WKY rats in which the left common iliac artery was equipped with a 0.3 mm stenosis (n = 10) or in which several side branches of the femoral artery were ligated (n = 10, Fig. 1). 4 Weeks later, intra–arterial pressure and flow were measured. Poststenotic and prestenotic femoral arteries were isolated along with contralateral control vessels.

From each vessel, a 2 mm segments was cut and the remainder was used for determination of DNA content [13]. The segment was chemically sympathectomized, connected to a force transducer and a displacement device and mounted in an organ chamber [14, 15]. Following 60 min equilibration these preparations were subjected to a sequential stimulation protocol. It consisted of activation at 5 min interval with 30 mM potassium (K^+), 125 mM K^+ and 125 mM K^+ plus 10 μM serotonin (5HT) in the presence of 2.5 mM calcium chloride. This was repeated over a range of imposed diameters (0.45 – 1.05 mm). Between stimulations, the vessels were maintained in Ca^{2+} –free solution. Tension levels in this situation were not modified by 10 μM Na–nitroprusside indicating resting conditions. Tension development induced by K^+ plus 5HT could not be enhanced by other vasoconstrictors, indicating maximal activation of the contractile machinery. Tension–diameter curves were constructed under these resting and activating conditions. The former resting wall tension (RWT) – diameter (D) curves could be fitted by RWT = $Ae^{-ßD}$ in which ß stands for a stiffness factor [16]. The latter active wall tension (AWT) –

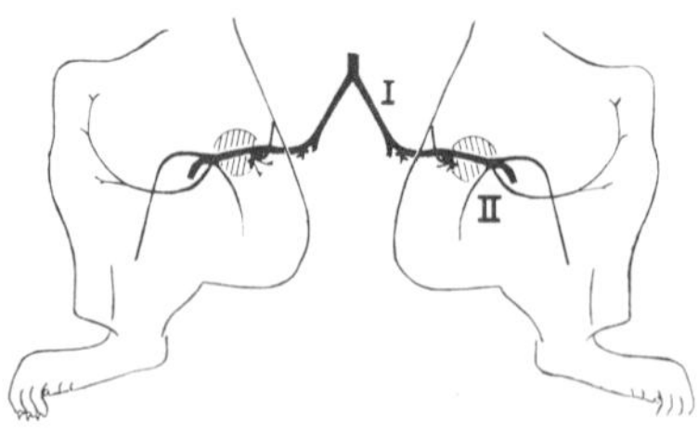

Figure 1. Schematic representation of the hindlimbs of a rat illustrating the two experimental models (I and II) that were used. In I, an 0.3 mm coarctation was applied to the left iliac artery and the iliolumbar artery was ligated (poststenotic model). In II, several femoral artery side branches, including the saphenous and deep femoral artery, were ligated leaving only the small epigastric branch patent (prestenotic branch). The shaded area highlights the vessel segment that was used for in vitro experimentation.

diameter curves were fitted with a polynomial equation to determine D_o, i.e. the diameter at which AWT was maximal. Furthermore, the intercept between the passive extension curve and the isobaric line calculated from Laplace's law at 100 mmHg was determined as an estimate of resting vessel diameter at a transmural pressure of 100 mmHg (D_{100}, [14, 17]). In addition, the ratio of responses to 30 mM K^+ and 125 mM K^+ was determined as an estimate of the sensitivity of the smooth muscle for stimulation. At the end of these functional experiments, vessels were set at D_o and fixed.

Structural analysis was performed on paraffin cross sections stained with Lawson's solution. Media cross sectional area (CSA), defined as the area enclosed by the internal and external elastic lamina, was measured by planimetry.

The imposed diameters (D) and the measurements of WT and CSA were used to calculate media thickness (Mt), media to lumen ratio (M/L), and circumferential wall stress. In all experiments a post– or prestenotic vessels was studied in parallel with a contralateral control. Measurements of diameters, CSA, Mt, M/L, maximal active wall tension and maximal active wall stress were compared between experimental and contralateral side with Student's t–test for paired observations. Comparison of relations of tension – diameter and stress – strain was performed using a univariate repeated measures analysis of variance.

RESULTS

Four weeks after surgery mean intra–arterial pressure poststenosis averaged 22 ± 3 mmHg compared to 76 ± 6 mmHg on the contralateral side and pulse pressure was virtually absent. In the prestenosis experimental model, femoral artery flow averaged 0.27 ± 0.05 ml/min vs 1.15 ± 0.1 ml/min.

Structural and functional properties of prestenotic femoral arteries did not differ from those in contralateral control vessels. Findings in poststenotic and control femoral arteries are summarized in Table 1. They are shown for three conditions: (i) no–distension zero–stress, (ii) distending conditions at which stimulation resulted in optimal force development (D_o) and (iii) at 100 mmHg. Under all conditions CSA was significantly smaller poststenosis (−30% at D_o). Internal diameter was larger at 100 mmHg than at the mechanical optimum. It was smaller in poststenotic vessels (−12% vs control) at the optimum, but not at 100 mmHg. This results from two observations (see Fig. 2): (i) passive tension – diameter curves did not differ between both experimental groups (the stiffness factor ß averaged 6.0 ± 0.3 and 5.6 ± 0.2 mm^{-1} for experimental and control vessels) and (ii) active tension – diameter curves were shifted to smaller diameters in poststenotic vessels compared to controls.

Findings with respect to media thickness (Mt) follow from the measurements of CSA and D. Under all conditions Mt was significantly smaller in poststenotic than control vessels (Fig. 2). At D_o it averaged 31.7 ± 1.0 and 38.9 ± 1.4 µm, respectively. The combination of reduced media mass and unaltered passive tension – diameter curves results in a paradoxical leftward shift of the stress – strain curves of poststenotic vessels. Disproportionate changes of the mass of distensible and non–distensible components in the vessel wall may be responsible for this [12].

DNA content in poststenotic vessels was 560 ± 40 ng per mm vessel length, compared to 540 ± 20 ng/mm in controls. Furthermore the density of nuclear profiles in the media was 388 ± 15 and 298 ± 10 per 4 µm cross section of poststenotic and control vessels, respectively. This indicates that poststenosis, arterial smooth muscle cell number was not affected but arterial smooth muscle cell size reduced, leading to increased cellular density.

Table 1. Structural and functional properties of poststenotic and contralateral femoral arteries. Effects of distending conditions.

	Distension		
	100 mmHg	Optimum	None
CSA	√	√	√
D	=	=	=
Mt	√	√	√
M/L	√	=	√
AWT	√	√	?
AWS	√	=	?
ED½	√	=	?

Multiple comparisons between properties of isolated poststenotic and contralateral femoral arteries of the rat studied 4 weeks after the surgical intervention at three different levels of distension (corresponding to a transmural pressure of 100 mmHg, at the mechanical optimum and in the absence of external distending forces). CSA, media cross sectional area; D, internal diameter; Mt, mean media thickness; M/L, media to lumen ratio; AWT, maximal active wall tension; AWS, active wall stress; ED½, sensitivity for contractile responses to a depolarizing stimulus. Corresponding values in contralateral control vessels at optimal distension (D_0) were: 93 ± 3 10^3 μm², 728 ± 8 μm, 39 ± 1 μm, 10.8 ± 0.5%, 9.8 ± 1.0 N/m and 224 ± 37 N/m². ? – For obvious reasons functional recordings were not performed in undistended vessel segments; √, observations in poststenotic vessels were significantly smaller than in control; =, comparable between both experimental groups.

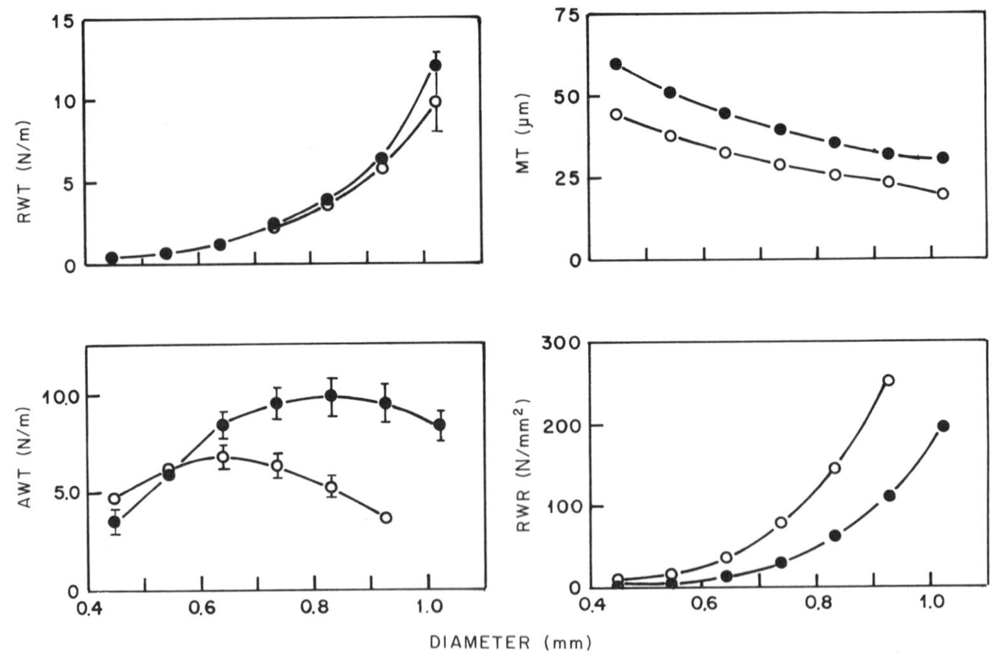

Figure 2. Relationships of resting wall tension (RWT), media thickness (Mt), active wall tension (AWT) and resting wall stress (RWS) versus imposed diameter. Data are shown as mean ± SEM (n = 10) for poststenotic (open circles) and contralateral control femoral arteries (closed circles).

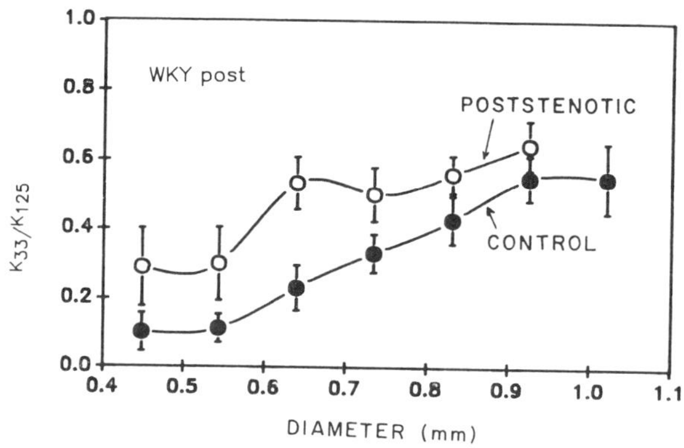

Figure 3. Relationship of vessel sensitivity to imposed diameter. The ratio of force responses to 30 mM and 125 mM K+ is shown as means ± SEM (n = 10) for poststenotic (open circles) and contralateral control femoral arteries (closed circles).

Indices of sensitivity and maximal responsiveness to contractile stimuli were determined to gain more insight in potential selective remodeling of arterial smooth muscle cells. Maximal active wall tension was obtained at a smaller diameter in poststenotic vessels and its amplitude was significantly smaller (6.8 ± 0.6 N/m vs 9.8 ± 1.0 N/m). Maximal active wall stress was, however, comparable in both groups (189 ± 26 and 224 ± 37 N/m^2). Figure 3 summarizes the relationship between sensitivity of arterial smooth muscle to contractile stimuli and imposed diameter. Sensitivity increased in all vessels with increasing distension. The relationship was shifted to smaller diameters in poststenotic vessels compared to controls.

DISCUSSION

Combining these findings indicates that chronic pressure reduction primarily modifies arterial smooth muscle cell (ASMC) volume leading to (i) a reduction of arterial wall mass, arterial diameter, and contractile reactivity, (ii) paradoxical elevation of stiffness and (iii) resetting of length sensitive elements.

It has long been recognized that pressure elevation may increase arterial wall mass [1, 18, 19]. In large arteries this involves primarily an increase of ASMC size [20]. ASMC hypertrophy can be reversed by pressure reduction although it should be realized that in the case of antihypertensive drugs this may be offset by reflex activation of neurohumoral mechanisms [9, 11].

Especially in essential and genetic hypertension, not all types of arteries display hypertrophy [3, 5, 20]. Therefore, the possibility that arterial structural diameter may be altered has gained interest in recent years. Baumbach and Heistad [21] were among the first to elaborate on this hypothesis of remodeling. They observed that the external diameter was reduced in cerebral arterioles of SHRSP, despite significant media hypertrophy. It had been suggested earlier that while arterial wall mass may be determined by wall stress, arterial diameter may be primarily influenced by shear stress [18, 19, 22].

Several techniques can be used to measure the arterial diameter. Yet, there is in principal not a single diameter but rather a set of pressure–volume relationships. Evaluation of radial dimensions at controlled axial length under activated and inactivated conditions is, however, not always practical. This is, for instance, the case for small vessels isolated from skin biopsies of human volunteers [23, 24]. We have used recordings of isometric force vs imposed circumference introduced by Mulvany and Halpern [14]. Our approach differs, however, in that we consider the vascular wall not only as an elastic element but along the lines described by Johnson [25]. We consider the wall as being composed of contractile elements coupled in series and in parallel to elastic structures. Furthermore, a third length- (or load-) sensitive component is taken into account representing the excitation–contraction coupling process.

Using this approach we found that in poststentoic arteries: (i) passive tension – diameter curves were not altered; (ii) passive circumferential stress – strain curves were steeper as a result of reduced media thickness; (iii) active tension – diameter curves were shifted to smaller diameters and peak force, but not maximal active wall stress, was reduced; (iv) sensitivity – diameter relationship was shifted to the same extent as the active tension – diameter curve. Combined with morphometric measurements this suggests that the size of the contractile elements was reduced without marked alteration of the poorly distensible components and that this was accompanied with resetting of length sensitive elements in excitation–contraction coupling. Stereologic measurements of the volume density of collagen and elastin are being performed to substantiate this hypothesis. We propose that disproportionate mass changes of vessel wall components play a pivotal role in remodeling [12] and that this is accompanied by changes in vascular wall function.

Using an approach of arterial diameter that is presently popular in isolated vessel research, our observations differed both quantitatively and qualitatively. Several groups estimate and compare diameters at a fixed and preset transmural pressure (eg 100 mmHg). Under this condition we note that (i) diameter of poststenotic vessels is comparable to control (i.e. no remodeling), (ii) the decrease in media thickness is exaggerated, (iii) media to lumen ratio is reduced, (iv) the reduction of AWT is exaggerated and a difference in AWS ensues; controls and poststenotic vessels are on a different point on the descending limb of the AWT–D curve, and (vi) poststenotic vessels are hypersensitive to contractile stimuli. The conclusion is that chronic pressure plus flow reduction reduce mass of the media without affecting diameter, resulting in reduced contractility and enhanced excitability.

Changes in post- but not in prestenotic vessels indicate that reduction of pressure is primarily responsible for the structural and functional remodeling. The relative contributions of mean pressure and pulse pressure can not be inferred from our present findings. Unlike Langille and O'Donnel [22], we did not observe a reduction of diameter following chronic flow reduction, attributed to species and especially age differences. Flow may modify the production and organization of elastic components during morphogenesis of blood vessels, while the established extracellular matrix may be rather refractory to endothelial influences triggered by changes in shear stress [19, 22].

In conclusion the arterial remodeling observed following chronic stress reduction is both structural and functional in nature and may involve primarily a reduction of arterial smooth muscle cell volume.

Acknowledgement

This work was supported by the Royal Dutch Academy of Sciences (KNAW) and by the Dutch Heart Foundation (NHS).

DISCUSSION

Dr. Gotsman: What was the time course of the changes that you observed?

Dr. J. De Mey: Similar experiments were also performed 4 hrs after the ligation. It will not surprise you that at that point in time we did not observe any mass changes. All the data that I discussed were acquired after 4 weeks.

Dr. J. Spaan: If you have a stenosis, you reduce the pulse pressure as well. How much is that compared to mean pressure and what are the effects of this particular variable?

Dr. J. De Mey: Not only was the mean pressure dramatically reduced, but pulse pressure was virtually absent. This experimental approach does not allow to speculate about the role of mean vs pulse pressure. However, if we take the literature and other observations from our laboratory, I would guess that pulse pressure rather than mean pressure, is of prime importance for arterial smooth cell mass.

Dr. J. Spaan: This consideration may be important for post–stenotic vessels within the heart where pressure will always be pulsatile, because of the contraction of the heart itself. You would not expect to find this in the heart. Is that true?

Dr. J. De Mey: Obviously this kind of experiment is hard to perform in the heart. Your comments call for specific pulse pressure reducing experiments, which we hope to perform.

Dr. N. Westerhof: Do your vessels develop spontaneous tone if you wait long enough?

Dr. J. De Mey: They develop spontaneous tone, and they definitely develop tone in response to stretch. That was one of the reasons to keep them in calcium free solution in between stimulations during *in vitro* mechanical recordings.

Dr. N. Westerhof: But your segment length is not maintained. Your mean stretch is in the radial direction and not in the longitudinal direction because you put the segment in your apparatus and then it sits at the length it happens to sit. Is that right?

Dr. J. De Mey: The distensions and the length changes that were imposed and those I was referring to in answer to your question are all in the radial direction. Axial length is maintained constant throughout the experiment.

Dr. J.K. Li: It is known that arterial compliance decreases in hypertension. Since you do not have a positive change in pressure. Do you have a positive change in volume so that you can give an estimate of the compliance changes?

Dr. J. De Mey: No. Since pulse pressure was absent we were not able to measure any index of compliance in the intact animal.

REFERENCES

1. Folkow B. Physiological aspects of primary hypertension. *Physiol Rev* 1982; 62: 347–504.
2. Cox RH. Mechanical properties of arteries in hypertension. In: Lee RMKW (eds), *Blood Vessel Changes in Hypertension: Structure and Function*. Boca Raton, FL: CRC Press, 1989, pp 65–98.
3. Mulvany MJ. Structure and function of small arteries in hypertension. *J Hypertension* 1990; 8: S225–S232.

4. Lever AF. Slow pressor mechanisms in hypertension: a role for hypertrophy of resistance vessels? *J Hypertension* 1986; 4: 515–524.
5. Bund SJ, West KP, Heagerty AM. Effects of protection from pressure on resistance artery morphology and reactivity in spontaneously hypertensive and Wistar–Kyoto rats. *Circ Res* 1991; 68: 1230–1240.
6. Lever A, Harrap SB. Essential hypertension: a disorder of growth with origins in childhood? *J Hypertension* 1992; 10: 101–120.
7. Folkow B, Gurevich M, Hallback M, Lundgren Y, Weiss L. The hemodynamic consequences of regional hypotension in spontaneously hypertensive and normotensive rats. *Acta Physiol Scand* 1971; 83: 532–541.
8. Tsoporis J, Fields N, Lee RMKW, Leenen FHH. Arterial vasodilation and cardiovascular structural changes in normotensive rats. *Am J Physiol* 1991; 260: H1944–H1952.
9. Struijker Boudier HAJ, Van Bortel LMAB, De Mey JGR. Remodeling of the vascular tree in hypertension: drug effects. *TIPS* 1990; 11: 240–245.
10. Hajdu MA, Heistad DD, Baumbach GL. Effects of antihypertensive therapy on mechanics of cerebral arterioles in rats. *Hypertension* 1991; 17: 308–316.
11. Tsoporis J, Leenen FHH. Effects of arterial vasodilators on cardiac hypertrophy and sympathetic activity in rats. *Hypertension* 1988; 11: 376–386.
12. Hajdu MA, Heistad DD, Ghonheim S, Baumbach GL. Effects of antihypertensive treatment on composition of cerebral arterioles. *Hypertension* 1991; 18 (suppl II): II15–II21.
13. Labarca C, Paigen K. A simple, rapid and sensitive DNA assay procedure. *Anal Biochem* 1980; 102: 344–352.
14. Mulvany MJ, Halpern W. Contractile properties of small arterial resistance vessels in spontaneously hypertensive and normotensive rats. *Circ Res* 1977; 41: 19–26.
15. Boonen HCM, De Mey JGR. Increased calcium sensitivity in isolated resistance arteries from spontaneously hypertensive rats: effects of dihydropyridines. *Eur J Pharmacol* 1990; 179: 403–412.
16. Freslon JL, Guidicelli JF. Vascular effects of captopril and dihydralazine in spontaneously hypertensive rats. *Prog Appl Microcirc* 1985; 8: 142–151.
17. Mulvany MJ, Warshaw DM. The active tension–length curve of vascular smooth muscle related to its cellular components. *J Gen Physiol* 1979; 74: 85–104.
18. Thoma R. *Untersuchungen uber die histogenese und histomechanik des gefasssystems*. Stuttgart: Verlag von Ferdinand Enke. 1893.
19. Glagov S, Vito R, Giddens DP, Zarins CK. Micro-architecture and composition of artery walls: relationship to location, diameter and the distribution of mechanical stress. *J Hypertension* 1992; 10 (suppl 6): S101–S104.
20. Owens GK. Control of hypertrophic versus hyperplastic growth of vascular smooth muscle cells. *Am J Physiol* 1989; 257: H1755–H1765.
21. Baunbach GL, Heistad DD. Remodeling of cerebral arterioles in chronic hypertension. *Hypertension* 1989; 13: 968–972.
22. Langille BL, O'Donnel F. Reductions in arterial diameter produced by chronic decreases in blood flow are endothelium dependent. *Science* 1986; 231: 405–407.
23. Aalkjaer C, Heagerty AM, Petersen KK, Swales JD, Mulvany MJ. Evidence for increased media thickness, increased neuronal uptake, and depressed excitation–contraction coupling in isolated resistance vessels from essential hypertensives. *Circ Res* 1987; 61: 181–186.
24. Heagerty AM, Aalkjaer C, Bund SJ. Effects of drug treatment on human resistance arteriole morphology in essential hypertension: direct evidence for structural remodelling of resistance vessels. *Lancet* 1988; 26: 1209–1212.
25. Johnson PC. The myogenic response. In: *The Cardiovascular System, Vol II: Vascular Smooth Muscle*. Bethesda, MD: Am Physiol Soc, 1980, pp 409–442.

CHAPTER 28

MYOCARDIAL COLLAGEN AND ITS FUNCTIONAL ROLE

Joseph S. Janicki[1], Beatriz B. Matsubara[2], and Ameer Kabour[1]

ABSTRACT

Even though normally present in relatively small amounts, myocardial collagen strongly influences ventricular diastolic function. Removal of less than half of the normal amount results in a dilated ventricle with increased compliance. In contrast, an abnormal increase in collagen concentration results in a stiffer myocardium and ventricular diastolic dysfunction.

INTRODUCTION

In the myocardium, the interstitial collagen matrix surrounds and supports cardiac myocytes and the coronary microcirculation [1]. It also: 1) serves as an important determinant of ventricular diastolic function [2] and size [3]; 2) coordinates the transmittal of force generated by myocytes to the ventricular chamber [4]; 3) prevents ventricular aneurysm and rupture [5]; and 4) opposes myocardial edema [6]. In view of these many functional roles, it is not unexpected to find that an alteration in the myocardial mechanical properties and ventricular structure and function will result from either a degradation of collagen or an abnormal increase in interstitial collagen concentration. Our current understanding of collagen matrix remodeling, which results in either inadequate or excessive amounts of collagen, and its functional consequences will be the focus of this communication.

MECHANICAL PROPERTIES AND ORGANIZATION OF MYOCARDIAL COLLAGEN

Cardiac connective tissue consists predominantly of collagen; a stiff material with a high tensile strength. The mechanical behavior of a composite material such as the

---

[1]Dalton Research Center and Department of Internal Medicine, University of Missouri, Columbia, MO 65212, USA and [2]Universidade Estadual Paulista–Botucatu, Brasil.

Interactive Phenomena in the Cardiac System, Edited by
S. Sideman and R. Beyar, Plenum Press, New York, 1993

myocardium, will depend not only on the concentration of collagen but also its fibril and fiber diameter, degree of crosslinking, spacial alignment, crimp properties, and collagen types [2]. In general, areas of tissue which require a high tensile strength will have an elevated collagen content and larger diameter collagen fibers that have a greater percentage of covalent crosslinks. Collagen fibers that are oriented parallel to the direction of stress will contribute significantly to the elasticity of the composite material as opposed to fibers aligned perpendicular to the stress direction. The crimp property of collagen refers to the amount to which a collagen fiber is coiled. Once uncoiled, the stress required for further elongation increases exponentially. Tissue containing predominantly type I collagen (e.g. tendons) has a higher modulus of elasticity than tissue with mostly type III collagen (e.g. uterus). Nonhuman primate cardiac tissue contains 80 to 90% type I and 10 to 15% type III collagen [7].

The collagen network consists of three major components, the epimysium, perimysium and endomysium. The epimysium is a sheath of collagenous connective tissue which, in the case of papillary muscle, surrounds the entire muscle. Included in the perimysial component are tendinous extensions of the epimysium which branches to form weaves of collagen around groups of myocytes. Adjacent weaves are joined by collagen fibers, referred to as strands. There are also coiled perimysial fibers which form an array in parallel with muscle fibers. Portions of the perimysial weave and the larger–diameter, coiled perimysial fibers are usually quite evident between rows of muscle fibers when viewed with the light microscope. The endomysium represents the ultrastructural component of the collagen network. It consists of a network of fibers that surround individual myocytes and of fibers or struts that connect myocytes to neighboring myocytes and capillaries.

INADEQUATE COLLAGEN MATRIX

In the myocardium, a latent collagenase system coexists with the collagen matrix [8]. Hence there exists the potential for a rapid degradation of collagen. In the arrested heart with rigor, O'Brien and Moore [9] observed the pressure–volume curve of the left ventricle (LV) to significantly shift to the right following a 90 minute incubation in a solution of collagenase, indicating that the ventricle had become more distensible following collagen degradation. Others [3, 6] have obtained similar results using an *in vivo* model of presumed myocardial collagenase activation [10]. As a consequence of this model there is a 35% decrease in collagen concentration due to disappearance of perimysial coiled fibers and strands and of endomysial collagen surrounding myocytes as well as struts. At any level of end diastolic pressure, left ventricular volume was increased by at least 70% following collagen degradation and the ventricle was more distensible particularly at larger filling volumes. Regional ultrastructural collagen degradation is also evident after transient episodes of ischemia [11] which is thought to be responsible for the subsequent regional dilation, increased compliance and paradoxic expansion and thinning (i.e. "stunned" myocardium). Postmortem examination of human myocardium from dilated cardiomyopathic hearts revealed the absence of thick coiled perimysial fibers, disruption of lateral connections of collagen between muscle fibers, and numerous widened interstitial spaces [12]. As shown above, an inadequate collagen matrix leads to ventricular dilation, increased compliance and possibly sphericalization of the ventricle. Thus, it is likely that collagen disruption and degradation are responsible for the increase in size and compliance, and the change in shape of the dilated cardiomyopathic heart.

MYOCARDIAL FIBROSIS

Myocardial collagen concentration is increased in renovascular [7, 13–15] and genetic [16–18] hypertension, and with chronic elevations in plasma aldosterone [19]. This remodeling of the collagen matrix occurs at both the micro– and ultrastructural levels and includes: new collagen fibers and thickening of existing fibers and tendons; increased density of the weave and network surrounding myocytes; expanded areas of perivascular collagen; and microscopic scars [13, 20, 21]. Accompanying this fibrosis is an increase in myocardial and LV diastolic stiffness. Bing et al. [22] and Holubarsch et al. [23] maintained that the 30 to 60% elevation in myocardial collagen secondary to various forms of left ventricular pressure overload in the rat explained the greater (i.e. 40 to 50%) passive papillary muscle stiffness. More recent studies have clearly demonstrated a relation between increased myocardial and ventricular stiffness and collagen concentration in: the non-human primate with experimental hypertension [7]; in rats with renovascular [15]; perinephritic [24], or genetic [17, 18] hypertension; and in rats with myocardial fibrosis secondary to perinephritis and/or isoproterenol [24], renovascular hypertension and isoproterenol [24] or coronary embolization [25]. Finally, Brilla and colleagues [18], using an angiotensin converting enzyme inhibitor, reported a return to normal passive stiffness in SHR following a complete regression of collagen concentration and LV mass to levels found in WKY.

In these various models of LV pressure overload, there was also significant myocyte hypertrophy which accompanied the fibrosis and one could argue that myocyte enlargement, not fibrosis, was responsible for the diastolic dysfunction. Several recent studies, however, discount this possibility. Bing et al. [26] prevented the increase in collagen content associated with chronic aortic constriction with ß–amino proprionitrile and concluded that elevations in resting tension depend upon an increase in collagen content but not hypertrophy. Others [17] were able to prevent myocyte hypertrophy with hydralazine but not the abnormal accumulation of collagen in spontaneously hypertensive rats (SHR). The consequences of this fibrosis was an abnormally elevated passive myocardial stiffness which was similar to that measured in the untreated SHR with fibrosis and hypertrophy but significantly greater than the stiffness obtained in the genetic control (WKY). Finally, Gelpi and his colleagues [27] found LV diastolic chamber compliance to be normal in dogs with normal collagen concentration and significant hypertrophy secondary to perinephritic hypertension.

As presented above, an experimentally–induced, abnormal accumulation of myocardial collagen results in an increase in diastolic LV stiffness. Thus, a disproportionate increase in this structural protein relative to myocyte enlargement could be considered a pathologic remodeling process. This also appears to be the case clinically. In the athlete with a significant increase in LV mass which presumably represents physiologic hypertrophy, diastolic function is normal at rest and even enhanced during exercise [28, 29]. In contrast, hypertensive patients with less hypertrophy than that in the athlete are found to have significant diastolic dysfunction [30] which is not related to the increase in LV mass [31, 32].

Combining these clinical observations with experimental results and the finding that collagen concentration is increased in humans with systemic hypertension [16], it is reasonable to conclude that diastolic dysfunction in hypertensive patients is the result of excessive myocardial collagen.

CONCLUSIONS

The myocardial collagen matrix is intimately related to the myocyte, myofibril and muscle fiber as well as the coronary vasculature and is an active participant in determining ventricular architecture and diastolic function, and myocardial structural integrity and mechanical properties. Removal of less than half of the normal amount of collagen, results in myocardial edema and a dilated ventricle with increased compliance. Remodeling of the collagen matrix, which results in an abnormal increase in collagen concentration, consists of a thickening of existing fibrillar collagen and the addition of new collagen at all structural levels of the matrix. The consequences of this remodeling process are an adverse increase in passive elasticity of the myocardium and LV diastolic dysfunction. This pathophysiologic aspect of the hypertrophic process is independent of the concomitant remodeling of the myocyte. Thus an alteration in the extracellular matrix which results in an abnormal accumulation of interstitial collagen is a major distinguishing factor between physiologic and pathologic hypertrophy.

Acknowledgement

This work was supported in part by NHLBI Grant Nos. RO1–HL–31701 and RO1–HL–46461 and American Heart Assoc. Grant–In–Aid No. 901397.

DISCUSSION

Dr. F. Prinzen: You compared photomicrographs of collagen from the scanning electron microscope with magnifications of 5000x and light microscope pictures with decreased magnification. Was your quantification usually based on the light microscopic pictures?

Dr. J.S. Janicki: The values for collagen concentration were determined using light microscopy and a magnification of 80x. There is no valid way of morphometrically quantifying the amount of collagen at the ultrastructural levels. The other way to quantify collagen concentration would be to measure hydroxyproline, which is a biochemical determination. The results of Caulfield and Wolkwicz [10], which were similar to ours, were in terms of hydroxyproline, so the two methods correlate reasonably well.

Dr. F. Prinzen: The reason for my question is that you showed different types of collagen with different orientations to the fibers struts and tendons and weaves. What then is the function of these various components which determine the compliance of the heart muscle.

Dr. J.S. Janicki: I did not have time to go into all of those results. One of our conclusions, based on our studies which utilized the model described by Caulfield and Wolkowicz [10], was that it is the ultrastructural collagen which is most important in determining ventricular size, and compliance. I based this conclusion on the fact that when we gave saline alone we saw the same reduction in collagen as with oxidized glutathione but ventricular size and compliance were normal. The only difference between rats receiving saline and oxidized glutathione was at the ultrastructural level. In the hearts that received oxidize glutathione the ultrastructural collagen was abnormal while in hearts receiving saline it was normal. Based on this observation, we concluded that the ultrastructural collagen which surrounds the myocytes and joins one myocyte to the other is the most important.

Dr. R. Chadwick: Do you see any difference in twisting during filling?

Dr. J.S. Janicki: We have not studied this phenomenon.

Dr. R. Chadwick: The fetal heart and the newborn heart are evidently very stiff, yet have very little collagen. Do you have any comments about that?

Dr. J.S. Janicki: Borg and Caulfield *[Collagen in the heart. Texas Reports on Biol and Med 39:321–333, 1979]* determined that there was no collagen in the newborn heart, but that it rapidly increases with age. I am not aware of any study that shows the newborn heart to be stiffer than expected.

Dr. W.M. Chilian: What influence does oxidized glutathione have on systemic hemodynamics?

Dr. J.S. Janicki: Oxidized glutathione doesn't appear to have an effect. You have to remember that the model described by Caulfield and Wolkowicz [10] included the infusion of 20 ml of saline. Accordingly, this is a volume overload to the heart with an acute increase in systemic blood pressure, that is not due to oxidized glutathione. The rats receiving oxidized glutathione are healthy and they gain weight as normally expected. We have kept them for periods of four months with no adverse affects.

Dr. W.M. Chilian: You have concluded that collagen is responsible for impaired diastolic dysfunction. How can you really distinguish between cause and effect? Couldn't diastolic dysfunction and overstretch of the myocardium be the factors which lay down more collagen?

Dr. J.S. Janicki: We are further investigating the stimulus for abnormal collagen deposition. However, the athlete, who has tremendous hypertrophy and dilated ventricle does not have diastolic dysfunction. In contrast, patients with systemic hypertension who have less hypertrophy than the athletes have diastolic dysfunction. In addition, we measured in post–mortem hearts from such patients an increased collagen [16]. Thus, pathologic hypertrophy is associated with an increase in collagen concentration.

Dr. E. Yellin: Comparing the normal vs the hypertrophied failing heart, do you know the ages of the normal group? Are they comparable to the ages of those with heart failure?

Dr. J.S. Janicki: There were no differences in ages. We realized that there is an increase in myocardial collagen with ageing and tried to avoid this complication by using normal post–mortem hearts from patients of similar age.

Dr. Y. Kresh: It seems to me that even with a loss of collagen, the structural integrity of the myocardium is maintained. In part because there is also a fluid–matrix, not only a collagen matrix. Is it this fluid–matrix gel that maintains the structure? I wonder why in the acute state, when we did a DTNB infusion, known to activate the latent collagenase, the heart initially dilated? After some time the pressure–volume relation flips to the other side and becomes stiffer. The heart developed tissue edema after the collagen matrix was lost (dissolved); something else must have replaced it. You did not discuss this effect.

Dr. J.S. Janicki: I did not discuss the acute results because of time constraints. We have looked at these hearts 3 hours after infusion and it did not matter if they were given saline alone or saline with oxidized glutathione [6]. The ventricles in both groups were dilated and they were stiffer. They were stiffer because they had myocardial edema as measured by wet/dry weight ratio. Edema will quickly increase myocardial stiffness and offset any decreases in compliance.

Dr. Y. Lanir: Was the treated heart zero volume point shifted?

Dr. J.S. Janicki: I did that artificially to try and show that there was indeed an increase in compliance in this group. This was merely an attempt to remove the dilatation aspects so as to visually compare compliance.

Dr. Y. Lanir: The pressure–volume relations are non–linear so one would expect that a shift in the zero volume point would give rise to lower compliance, just by virtue of the non–linearity.

Dr. J.S. Janicki: Compliance was rigorously compared using non–linear statistical techniques. It took a significantly greater amount of volume to go from 0 to 25 mmHg filling pressure in the groups with increased compliance when compared to normal ventricles.

Dr. G. Hasenfuss: How does collagen change during regression of hypertrophy?

Dr. J.S. Janicki: We did one regression study with spontaneous hypertensive rats where we treated them with an angiotensin converting enzyme (ACE) inhibitor; the treatment period was 16 weeks. We picked 16 weeks because the synthesis and presumably degradation rates of collagen in the myocardium are very slow; 0.6% of the total collagen per day. If there is equilibrium then one can expect the same sort of degradation rate and, according to our calculations it would take at least 90 days for one–half of the collagen to degrade if there was no synthesis. Thus, we designed our regression studies to be greater than 90 days and we were successful in regressing the collagen with an ACE inhibitor [18].

Dr. D. Kass: Have you ever plotted individual correlations between estimates of chamber stiffness from one of your rat studies and measures of collagen, not just the mean? Did they both go up? On an individual basis is there a reasonably tight correlation in interanimal variability between those two variables?

Dr. J.S. Janicki: There is definitely a good correlation between the collagen we measure and diastolic stiffness in each individual heart.

Dr. D. Kass: With the glutathione effect, abnormal amounts of collagen will reverse. Have you investigated the outcome when that reverses and the collagen comes back?

Dr. J.S. Janicki: We did not use glutathione in animals with various abnormal accumulations of collagen. We only gave glutathione to normal rats. However, I have to emphasize again: I do not think it is the glutathione that caused the degradation in collagen. Caulfield and Wolkowicz [10] reported hydroxycholine to return to normal after 6 months. At 4 months we observed an incomplete return to normal.

Dr. D. Kass: Does chamber stiffness come back again?

Dr. J.S. Janicki: Yes. In fact, at the ultrastructural level it was back to normal even in the hearts that received oxidized glutathione, even though the collagen we normally measure was still below normal [6]. Thus, while oxidized glutathione did not appear to cause the initial degradation in collagen, it somehow retarded the reparative process so that it took longer to restore the ultrastructural collagen.

Dr. T. Arts: You compare the athletes who generally have a volume load, with patients with pressure load. These types of hypertrophy might be different in these groups.

Dr. J.S. Janicki: Yes, it is physiologic hypertrophy in the athlete, and pathologic hypertrophy in the patient with systemic hypertension.

Dr. T. Arts: Another point may be, there are athletes with pressure overload. Maybe you should look into the weight lifters.

Dr. J.S. Janicki: Weightlifting will result in a combination of the two types of overload. They do get ventricular dilatation and increased ventricular mass. However, the percentages due to volume and to pressure overload are not known.

Dr. T. Arts: Do they get more collagen?

Dr. J.S. Janicki: This is not known.

REFERENCES

1. Borg TK, Caulfield JB. The collagen matrix of the heart. *Fed Proceedings* 1981; 40: 2037–2041.
2. Janicki JS, Matsubara BB. Myocardial collagen and left ventricular diastolic function. In: Gaasch WH, LeWinter MM (eds), *Left Ventricular Diastolic Dysfunction*. Philadelphia: Lea & Febiger, 1993 (in press).
3. Matsubara BB, Henegar JR, Janicki JS. Role of normal fibrillar collagen matrix in determining size and function of rat left ventricle. *Am J Physiol* 1993; in press.
4. Robinson TF, Factor SM, Sonnenblick EH. The heart as a suction pump. *Sci Am* 1986; 254: 84–91.
5. Factor SM, Robinson TF, Dominitz R, Cho S. Alterations of the myocardial skeletal framework in acute myocardial infarction with and without ventricular rupture. *Am J Cardiovas Pathol* 1986; 1: 91–97.
6. Matsubara BB, Henegar JR, Janicki JS. Functional and morphological consequences of induced myocardial collagen damage. *Circulation* 1992; 86: I–171.
7. Weber KT, Janicki JS, Shroff SG, Pick R, Chen RM, Bashey RI. Collagen remodeling of the pressure–overloaded, hypertrophied nonhuman primate myocardium. *Circ Res* 1988; 62: 757–765.
8. Montfort I, Perez–Tamayo R. The distribution of collagenase in normal rat tissues. *J Histochem Cytochem* 1975; 23: 910–920.
9. O'Brien LJ, Moore CM. Connective tissue degradation and distensibility characteristics of the non–living heart. *Experientia* 1966; 22: 845–847.
10. Caulfield JB, Wolkowicz PE. Mechanisms for cardiac dilatation. *Heart Failure J* 1990; 6: 138–150.
11. Zhao M, Zhang H, Robinson TF, Factor SM, Sonnenblick EH, Eng C. Profound structural alterations of the extracellular collagen matrix in postischemic dysfunctional ("stunned") but viable myocardium. *J Am Coll Cardiol* 1987; 10: 1322–1334.
12. Weber KT, Pick R, Janicki JS, Gadodia G, Lakier JB. Inadequate type I collagen fibers in dilated cardiopathy. *Am Heart J* 1988; 116: 1641–1646.
13. Abrahams C, Janicki JS, Weber KT. Myocardial hypertrophy in the macaque fascicularis: Structural remodeling of the collagen matrix. *Lab Invest* 1987; 56: 676–683.
14. Contard F, Koteliansky V, Marotte F, Dubus I, Rappaport L, Samuel J. Specific alterations in the distribution of extracellular matrix components within rat myocardium during the development of pressure overload. *Lab Invest* 1991; 64: 65–75.
15. Doering CW, Jalil JE, Janicki JS, Pick R, Aghili S, Abrahams C, Weber KT. Collagen network remodeling and diastolic stiffness of the rat left ventricle with pressure overload hypertrophy. *Cardiovasc Res* 1988; 22: 686–695 .
16. Pearlman ES, Weber KT, Janicki JS, Pietra G, Fishman AP. Muscle fiber orientation and connective tissue content in the hypertrophied human heart. *Lab Invest* 1982; 46: 158–164.
17. Narayan S, Janicki JS, Shroff SG, Pick R, Weber KT. Myocardial collagen and mechanics after preventing hypertrophy in hypertensive rats. *Am J Hypertens* 1988; 2: 675–682.
18. Brilla CG, Janicki JS, Weber KT. Cardioreparative effects of lisinopril in rats with genetic hypertension and left ventricular hypertrophy. *Circulation* 1991; 83: 1771–1779.
19. Brilla CG, Pick R, Tan LB, Janicki JS, Weber KT. Remodeling of the rat right and left ventricles in experimental hypertension. *Circ Res* 1990; 67: 1355–1364.
20. Caulfield JB. Alterations in cardiac collagen with hypertrophy. *Perspect Cardiovasc Res* 1983; 8: 49–57.
21. Pick R, Janicki JS, Weber KT. Myocardial fibrosis in nonhuman primate with pressure overload hypertrophy. *Am J Pathol* 1989; 135: 771–781.

22. Bing OHL, Matsushita S, Fanburg BL, Levine HJ. Mechanical properties of rat cardiac muscle during experimental hypertrophy. *Circ Res* 1971; 28: 234–245.
23. Holubarsch CH, Holubarsch T, Jacob R, Medugorac I, Thiedemann K. Passive elastic properties of myocardium in different models and stages of hypertrophy: A study comparing mechanical, chemical, and morphometric parameters. *Perspect Cardiovasc Res* 1983; 7: 323–336.
24. Jalil JE, Doering CW, Janicki JS, Pick R, Shroff S, Weber KT. Fibrillar collagen and myocardial stiffness in the intact hypertrophied rat left ventricle. *Circ Res* 1989; 64: 1041–1050.
25. Carroll EP, Janicki JS, Pick R, Weber KT. Myocardial stiffness and reparative fibrosis following coronary embolization in the rat. *Cardiovasc Res* 1989; 23: 655–661.
26. Bing OHL, Fanburg BL, Brooks WW, Matsushita S. The effect of the lathyrogen ß–amino proprionitrile (BAPN) on the mechanical properties of experimentally hypertrophied rat cardiac muscle. *Circ Res* 1978; 43: 632–637.
27. Gelpi RJ, Pasipoularides A, Lader AS, Patrick TA, Chase N, Hittinger L, Shannon RP, Bishop SP, Vatner SF. Changes in diastolic cardiac function in developing and stable perinephritic hypertension in conscious dogs. *Circ Res* 1991; 68: 555–567.
28. MacFarlane N, Northridge DB, Wright AR, Grant S, Dargie HJ. A comparative study of left ventricular structure and function in elite athletes. *Brit J Sports Med* 1991; 25: 45–48.
29. Nixon JV, Wright AR, Porter TR, Roy V, Arrowood JA. Effects of exercise on left ventricular diastolic performance in trained athletes. *Am J Cardiol* 1991; 68: 945–949.
30. Shapiro LM, McKenna WJ. Left ventricular hypertrophy: relation of structure to diastolic function in hypertension. *Brit Heart J* 1984; 51: 637–642.
31. Shahi M, Thom S, Poulter N, Sever PS, Foale RA. Regression of hypertensive left ventricular hypertrophy and left ventricular diastolic function. *Lancet* 1990; 336: 458–461.
32. Szlachcic J, Tubau JF, O'Kelly B, Massie BM. Correlates of diastolic filling abnormalities in hypertension: A Doppler echocardiographic study. *Am Heart J* 1990; 120: 386–391.

Cardiac Function and Circulation

CHAPTER 29

VENTRICULAR–ARTERIAL INTERACTION: CARDIAC EFFECTS OF MEAN VERSUS PULSATILE ARTERIAL LOAD

David A. Kass[1]

ABSTRACT

The influence of the two principal components of vascular loading, mean resistance and pulsatile load, on the contractile and energetic performance of the left ventricle are discussed. The data suggest that while large changes in mean resistance leading to varying ejection fraction can influence both cardiac systolic mechanics and energetic efficiency, substantial changes in pulsatile loading do not. They provide an explanation for why pulsatile loading does *not* necessarily result in a coronary supply/demand imbalance. By not significantly altering chamber systolic performance of elastance (i.e. stiffness), the pulsatile load results in parallel increases in coronary systolic pressure and flow, allowing adequate perfusion despite the reduced mean diastolic perfusion pressure. Future studies are required to better determine how cardiac disease alters the interplay between vascular load and cardiac performance.

INTRODUCTION

Unlike the simplified loads generally employed in isolated muscle and cell studies, the intact cardiac chamber must pump its contents into a branched vascular network, imposing far more complex dynamics. A complete evaluation of cardiovascular interaction must therefore consider both mean and pulsatile components of arterial load, and their influences on chamber contractile performance and energetics [1, 2]. Since it is generally difficult to selectively vary these components *in vivo*, most data has derived from isolated heart studies. In such preparations, the ventricle "ejects" into a servo-controlled volume

[1]Associate Professor of Medicine, The Johns Hopkins Medical Institutions, Div. of Cardiology, Carnegie 565A, 600 N. Wolfe Street, Baltimore, MD 21205, USA.

Interactive Phenomena in the Cardiac System, Edited by
S. Sideman and R. Beyar, Plenum Press, New York, 1993

influences on chamber contractile performance and energetics [1, 2]. Since it is generally difficult to selectively vary these components *in vivo*, most data has derived from isolated heart studies. In such preparations, the ventricle "ejects" into a servo-controlled volume pump, either by a direct volume command signal, or as a consequence of computed interactions between the real heart and a simulated vascular system (usually 3-element Windkessel) [3]. Either approach represents a simplification of real coupling, and underplays the potential role of pulsatile components and wave reflections. However, human studies increasingly demonstrate the prominence of these components with normal aging [4, 5]. Furthermore, recent data suggests that systolic hypertension is an independent risk factor for cardiovascular morbidity and mortality, heightening interest in the effects of such load on cardiac contractile performance and energetics [6].

In this report, I discuss the influence of the two major aspects of vascular loading, namely mean resistance and pulsatile load (primarily determined by compliance and wave reflections), on the contractile and energetic performance of the left ventricle. The question asked is whether either aspect significantly alters systolic performance and energetic efficiency of the heart. Such data are clearly important in order to understand how vasoactive therapies, commonly used to treat hypertension and heart failure, interact with the heart.

DEFINITIONS

In order to approach the question of how arterial loading influences cardiac contractile function and energetics, one first must settle on definitions for both properties. Over the past two decades, numerous methods have been proposed for characterizing chamber systolic function. These include the end-systolic pressure-volume relations (ESPVR) [7], stroke-work or dP/dt_{max} - end-diastolic volume relation [8, 9], and circumferential fraction shortening - wall stress relation [10], to name a few. Each reflects different aspects of systolic function, and all were initially purported to provide "load independent" measures of contractility. However, none really do this, and recent studies suggest that no such entity probably exists [11]. Nevertheless, we need some way of defining "systolic properties", and for the purpose of this discussion, I have chosen the ESPVR for several reasons. It represents an outer boundary of cardiac performance for the heart, and thus determines the effective work space (pressure-volume area) within which the heart operates [12]. As it lies near end-ejection, it also easily links with ejection parameters such as stroke work and ejection fraction [13].

As for energetic efficiency, there are equally many definitions from which to choose. The most common would be external work divided by total oxygen consumption (SW/MVO_2). However, this definition is clearly load dependent, since with increased resistance, SW declines, while MVO_2 increases. The ratio of force-time integral to MVO_2 has also been used by many investigators to index efficiency [14], however, this too is load dependent [15]. Suga et al. proposed the relation between total pressure-volume area and MVO_2 to be minimally "load-dependent" [16]. Pressure-volume area is defined by the sum of external work, and a potential work bounded by the ESPVR and EDPVR, between end-systolic volume and the zero-pressure volume intercept (V_o). In numerous studies, Suga and colleagues have explored this relation, showing it to be linear and minimally altered (in their preparation) by a myriad of varied ejection patterns [15, 17]. The inverse slope of this relation is a measure of chemomechanical transduction efficiency, and the intercept the sum of MVO_2 costs of basal metabolism and E-C coupling. For the purpose of this discussion, the MVO_2-PVA relation will be used to define cardiac efficiency.

EFFECTS OF MEAN RESISTANCE

In 1983, Maughan et al. reported data from isolated canine ventricles "ejecting" into a simulated arterial loading system [18]. The computer vascular model was the 3–element Windkessel, containing a peripheral resistor, proximal series resistor (characteristic impedance), and lumped capacitor. Varying resistance over a 2 fold range (increase and decrease) resulted in minimal ESPVR change, with a small parallel shift to the left with increasing resistance. Interestingly, a similar shift was reported by Freeman et al. several years later in studies in intact dogs [19, 20]. In this instance, resistance was changed either pharmacologically or mechanically, and both resulted in little change in ESPVR slope, and a slight leftward shift at higher resistances. It should be remembered that for the *in situ* studies, resistance is not the only thing altered, since compliance and wave velocity (and thus wave reflections) of the arterial system vary with mean pressure. However, the results spotlighted the notion that very large changes in arterial resistance could alter the ESPVR, and thus enhance or reduce the total pressure–volume working space for the heart.

Further evidence that mean arterial resistance could alter cardiac systolic function by effecting the extent of ejection was provided by Hunter [21]. In this study, comparisons were made between isovolumic contractions and ejecting beats, both achieving similar end–systolic volumes (V_{es}). Traditional concepts predicted that the ejecting beat would always generate a lower end–systolic pressure (P_{es}) at this same V_{es}, due to deactivation processes associated with shortening [22]. However, the opposite was found, particularly at low to normal range ejection fractions. The ejecting beats started at a larger end–diastolic volume in order to arrive at the same V_{es}. A positive effect of this larger initial volume on length–dependence of myofilament activation was proposed to counter negative shortening effects, resulting in the net observed behavior.

From the perspective of myocardial energetics, Suga and colleagues have reported that the MVO_2–PVA relation was minimally altered by the pattern or extent of ejection. However, these investigators have also found negligible ESPVR change with varying resistance. Differences in experimental methodology may play a role. For example, isolated heart studies performed by Suga have utilized a direct volume–command servo system [23]. This typically produces pressure–volume loops with sharp corners – reflecting a sudden onset and termination of ejection, with small high frequency oscillations observed during ejection [24]. In contrast, the isolated model used by Maughan, Hunter, Sunagawa, and others, utilized a computer–simulated arterial system, with the volume signal generated as a consequence of the heart's interaction with this simulated vasculature. Since none of the earlier studies performed with the computer simulated arterial loading system had evaluated simultaneous mechanics and *energetics*, we recently undertook experiments to further explore this issue [25].

As with the earlier studies, isolated blood–perfused canine left ventricles were connected to the servo–controlled pump system and allowed to contract either isovolumically or against a 3–element Windkessel loading model. The right ventricle was vented (zero load), and blood drained through a flow probe and oxygen content analyzer to determine MVO_2. A range of 6 resistances were selected at random, and the hearts allowed to contract against this load at four–five randomly chosen preload volumes. Before and after each set of ejection contractions, hearts were set to beat isovolumically, and similar measurements at varying preloads obtained. Sufficient time was provided at each EDV (3–5 minutes) to allow mechanical and energetic responses to stabilize. At each afterload, multiple beats at varying preloads were used to define both the ESPVR and the MVO_2–PVA relation.

Results of this study are summarized in Fig. 1. Values for the end–systolic pressure–volume relation slope, and inverse slope of the MVO_2–PVA relation are shown at varying afterloads. The data are grouped by the ejection fraction that resulted with each arterial load, with EF referenced to V_o (i.e. EF = SV/(EDV–V_o)). Figure 1A shows slope and intercept results for ESPVR, with data normalized to isovolumic contraction results (i.e. EF = 0, R = ∞). There was an increase in ESPVR slope with rising EF, suggesting that chamber systolic performance actually improved with greater ejection. The volume intercept also had small negative shifts at higher EFs, further increasing the PV work space. This runs counter to muscle results in which shortening deactivation always results in a reduction in contractile force. However, in the intact heart, it is in part the fact that blood is ejected into a hydraulic circuit (not a fixed stress) that may play a critical role. Specifically, to achieve a similar range of end–systolic pressures and volumes at larger EFs, ejecting beats must start at larger end–diastolic volumes. This could enhance the contractile response. It is worth noting that these results differ somewhat from those of Maughan et al. [18], specifically in that ESPVR slope change was observed, and that the positive effect

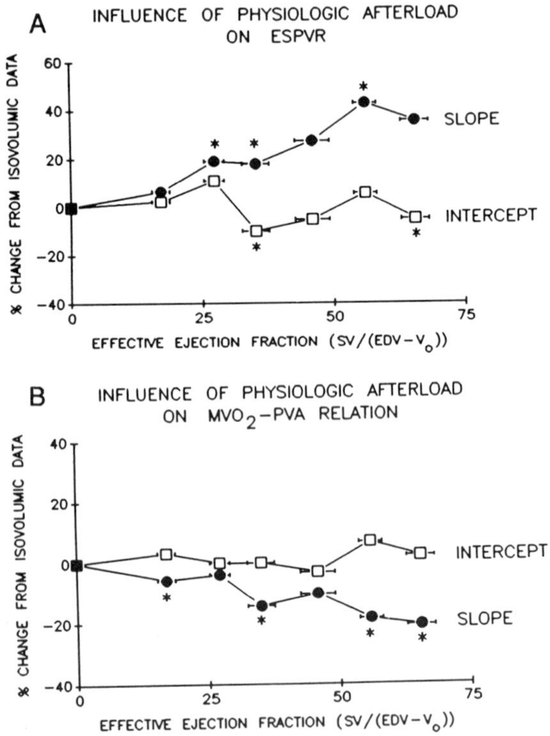

Figure 1. Influence of mean resistance on left ventricular contractile performance and energetics. **Panel A** shows influence on the end–systolic pressure–volume relation (ESPVR). Changes in resistance (R) loading resulted in changes in the effective ejection fraction of the heart, defined by the ratio SV/(EDV–V_o), where V_o is the volume axis intercept of the ESPVR. Slope and intercept data for the ESPVR are shown normalized to values for isovolumic contractions (i.e. EF = 0, R = ∞. There was an increase in ESPVR slope and slight leftward shift with increasing ejection fraction (reduced R). **Panel B** shows similar data for the myocardial oxygen consumption – pressure–volume area relation (MVO_2–PVA). In this instance, only the slope varied, and it fell (enhanced efficiency) at reduced resistive load.

was greatest at physiologic EFs. A potentially important difference lies in methodology. For the earlier study, a given EDV was established, and then arterial loading rapidly varied. In our study, resistance was altered, and then EDV varied – often requiring several minutes to achieve a steady state. This was essential to perform the simultaneous measurements of chamber energetics, however, it may well have influenced the results [25].

Figure 1B shows the results for the slope and intercept of the MVO_2–PVA relation for these same experiments. There was a reduction of this slope at the higher ejection fractions (reduced resistance) that had increased contractile performance. A fall in the MVO_2–PVA slope translates to an improvement in chemomechanical transduction efficiency. The intercept, reflecting basal metabolism and E–C coupling costs, did not change. Thus, not only did mean resistance have an effect on the total systolic pressure/volume generating capacity of the heart, but it altered its energetic efficiency. Ongoing studies combining direct measurements of calcium transients with whole heart mechanics are currently exploring the mechanisms underlying these load–dependent changes. The data suggest that vasodilator therapy in humans with high peripheral resistance (essential hypertension or heart failure) may effect more than just cardiac unloading by also improving cardiac systolic performance and energetic efficiency.

EFFECTS OF PULSATILE LOADING

While disparities between isovolumic and ejecting beat data at varying arterial resistances are important, their relation to physiologic loading changes that occur more commonly in man is less obvious. Rarely are alterations in resistance as marked as that between a low or normal value and an infinite one. However, a more common vascular change is one that accompanies normal human aging, namely the increase in pulsatile load due to stiffening of the vasculature. In this instance, mean pressure and flow are little changed, however the pattern of ventricular stresses attained during ejection are markedly different. A number of prior investigators have attempted to study how pulsatile loading alters cardiac function and energetics. These studies relied on preparations in which the descending thoracic aorta was stiffened or bypassed by a stiffer tube [26–28]. Interestingly, none of these studies had found a significant increase in MVO_2 nor clear evidence of a contractile effect when hearts ejected into the stiffer load. In the previously cited isolated heart study of Maughan et al. [18], compliance and characteristic impedance (of the simulated arterial model) were also varied over a two fold range, and virtually no effect on the ESPVR was found. However, this variation in compliance falls short of magnitude of change that can occur with aging. Despite the paucity of supporting data, many investigators believed that pulsatile load was disadvantageous to cardiac systolic performance and energetic efficiency.

To better assess this interaction, we undertook a set of experiments in which virtually the entire thoracic aorta was surgically bypassed *in situ* by a plastic tube [29]. A short length of 1 cm diameter dacron graft was sutured to the ascending thoracic aorta and attached to a 40 cm long 1 cm i.d. plastic tube (Tygon). This tube was reinserted into the abdominal aorta just above the level of the iliac bifurcation. By placement of vascular clamps occluding the native aorta at the diaphragm and ascending limb, blood flow could be redirected to pass via the plastic conduit, eliminating the major portion of vascular compliance. Pressure–volume data were recorded using a conductance catheter/micromanometer, vascular pressure–flow data by ultrasonic meter and manometer, and myocardial oxygen consumption by continuous total drainage of coronary sinus blood via a flow probe and oxygen content analyzer. Blood was also diverted into a reservoir, and by changing the fluid level in the reservoir, steady state variations in circulating blood volume were obtained. Data were measured at each steady state volume, to yield both ESPVR and MVO_2–PVA relations. An example of pressure, volume, and flow data for native aorta versus stiff (plastic) aorta is displayed in Fig. 2. As can be seen, the switch to the stiff aorta markedly increased end–systolic pressure (by a mean of 52 mmHg or 47% with very little change in mean pressure (+11.9%) (Table 1). Estimated arterial compliance fell by an average of 60–80% by the bypass technique. Both MVO_2 and PVA were increased by 32.3 and 38%, respectively, from the switch to the stiffer vasculature.

ESPVR and MVO_2–PVA relations for an example dog is shown in Fig. 3. Absolute volume was not calibrated in these experiments, but shown relative to the V_0 obtained for the native aorta data. The left panel displays pressure–volume loops with ejection into the native aorta, and the right panels similar data with ejection into the stiff (tygon) aorta. There was very little difference in the slopes of these two sets of relations despite the marked change in vascular loading. There was a slight volume axis shift in the ESPVR in this example. The lower panel displays the MVO_2–PVA relation for both data sets. The results were virtually superimposable. Mean data are provided in Table 2, revealing no significant change in contractile function (ESPVR slope or intercept) or energetic efficiency (MVO_2–PVA relation slope and intercept) due to the marked change in pulsatile loading. These data contrast to the results described earlier in response to marked changes in mean arterial resistance. However, with varied mean resistance, the extent of ejection (EF) changed markedly, whereas the marked pulsatile loading change generated in the present study did not significantly alter EF (Table 2).

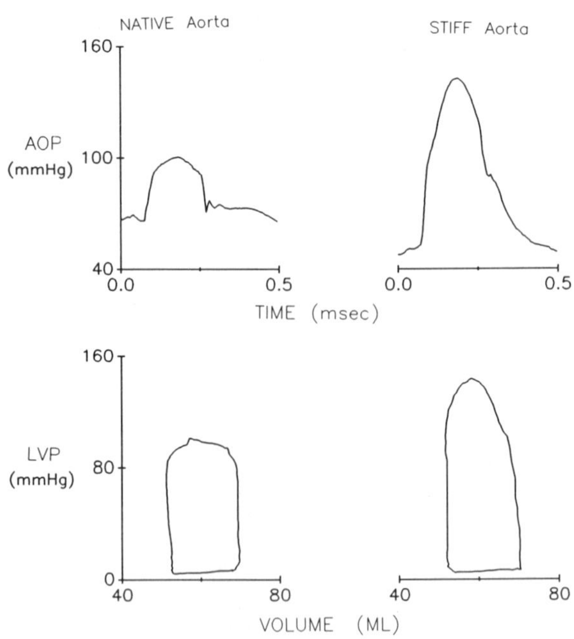

Figure 2. Alteration in aortic pressure and pressure–volume loop shape with reduced arterial compliance model. Upper panels show data for flow in the native aorta versus a stiff plastic bypass tube (see text for details). There is a marked increase in pulse pressure about a very similar mean pressure. Corresponding lower panels display the pressure–volume loops, showing the late systolic peaking present with the greater pulsatile load due to reduced compliance.

Table 1. Hemodynamic, vascular, and energetic consequences of switch to increased pulsatile load (stiff aorta).

Parameter	Native Aorta	Stiff Aorta	p
Systolic Arterial Pressure	109.8 ± 18.6	161.6 ± 34.9	<0.001
Diastolic Arterial Pressure	75.7 ± 18.1	62.7 ± 17.9	<0.01
Mean Arterial Pressure	91.7 ± 20.5	102.6 ± 22.5	<0.05
Mean Arterial Resistance	3.0 ± 1.5	3.6 ± 1.1	<0.05
Arterial Compliance	1.1 ± 0.5*	0.15 ± 0.07*	<0.01
Ejection Fraction	50.4 ± 12.5	42.1 ± 13.4	NS
Cardiac Output	1.9 ± 0.55	1.7 ± 0.44	NS
MVO_2	0.102 ± 0.03	0.135 ± 0.05	<0.01
PVA	2499 ± 864	3450 ± 1547	<0.05

Pressures are in mmHg, Resistance in mmHg/ml/sec, Compliance in ml/mmHg. (*) denotes that numbers are average of upper and lower range estimates for compliance. Cardiac output is L/min. MVO_2, the myocardial oxygen consumption, is in ml $O_2 \cdot 100g^{-1} \cdot beat^{-1}$. PVA, the pressure–volume area, is in mmHg·ml/100 gm.

Table 2. Influence of increased pulsatile load on end–systolic pressure–volume relation (contractile function) and MVO_2–PVA relation (energetics). Mean values for slope and intercept are provided. For ESPVR, the intercept includes a positive offset due to lack of absolute volume calibration of the volume–conductance catheter used to measure *in vivo* volume.

		Native Aorta	Stiff Aorta	p
ESPVR				
Slope	(mmHg/ml)	6.74 ± 2.82	7.14 ± 3.81	NS
Intercept	(ml)	48.5 ± 26.1	46.7 ± 30.9	NS
MVO_2–PVA				
Slope	(ml O_2/mmHg·ml·10^{-5})	2.03 ± 0.57	2.06 ± 0.54	NS
Intercept	(ml O_2/100g/beat)	0.02 ± 0.007	0.02 ± 0.012	NS

NS – not significant.

The data suggest that it is the absolute extent of ejection rather than the systolic stress pattern which influences net contractility and energetic efficiency.

Another important difference between the present study of pulsatile loading effects and prior isolated heart studies is the presence of closed–loop coronary perfusion *in situ* as opposed to open–loop (fixed) coronary perfusion used in the isolated hearts. One might expect that with reduced peripheral arterial compliance, diastolic coronary perfusion is compromised due to a fall in perfusion, despite simultaneous increased systolic load. To test this, we have recently initiated studies in which a second flow probe is placed about the proximal left anterior descending coronary artery to measure phasic flow. An example of the flow patterns with native and plastic aorta is shown in Fig. 4. Onset and end of systole are noted by vertical lines. With flow via the native aorta, there is a characteristic phasic coronary flow pattern with nearly 76% of flow occurring during diastole, and 24%

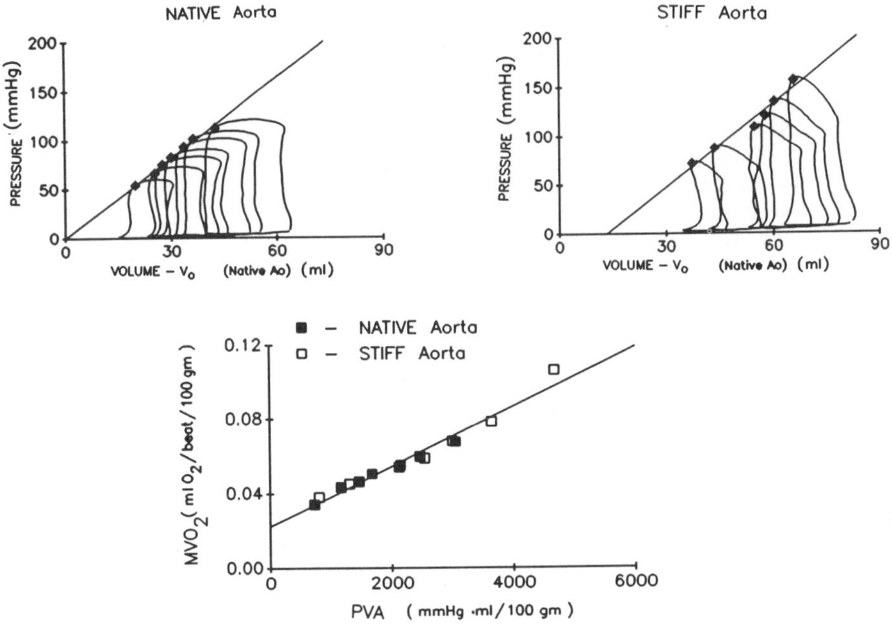

Figure 3. Pressure–volume relations obtained by combining varying preload contractions are shown to obtain ESPVR (upper panels) and MVO_2–PVA relations. There is very little change in the slope of the ESPVR due to the switch from native to stiff plastic (low compliance) aorta. A small rightward shift is observed in this example, although this was not significant for the data overall (see Table 2). The MVO_2–PVA relations were superimposable, demonstrating no change in myocardial efficiency.

during systole. Interestingly, when flow was routed via the stiff tygon aorta, the magnitude of diastolic flow was maintained, but there was nearly a doubling of the extent of systolic flow.

This result is *inconsistent* with the concept that increased systolic wall stress during ejection into the stiff aorta initially limits systolic flow and compromises diastolic flow. The results are intriguingly consistent with a novel model of coronary pressure–flow relations proposed by Krams et al., based on a time–varying elastance [30]. In this model, the relation between coronary artery pressure and flow is not dependent upon the magnitude of wall stress, but rather on the contractility or stiffness of the myocardium – determined by the ventricular time–varying elastance. This has been recently confirmed in isolated septal studies of Resar et al. [31]. As we have demonstrated above, switching from native to stiff aorta did not significantly alter the slope of the ESPVR and thus chamber stiffness. However, since systolic pressures rose markedly at a similar chamber stiffness, this model predicts a similar rise in systolic flow – which is precisely what was observed. What is most intriguing about the results is that they provide an explanation for why pulsatile loading does *not* necessarily result in a coronary supply/demand imbalance. By not significantly altering chamber systolic performance of elastance (i.e. stiffness), the pulsatile load results in parallel increases in coronary systolic pressure and flow – allowing adequate perfusion despite the reduced mean diastolic perfusion pressure.

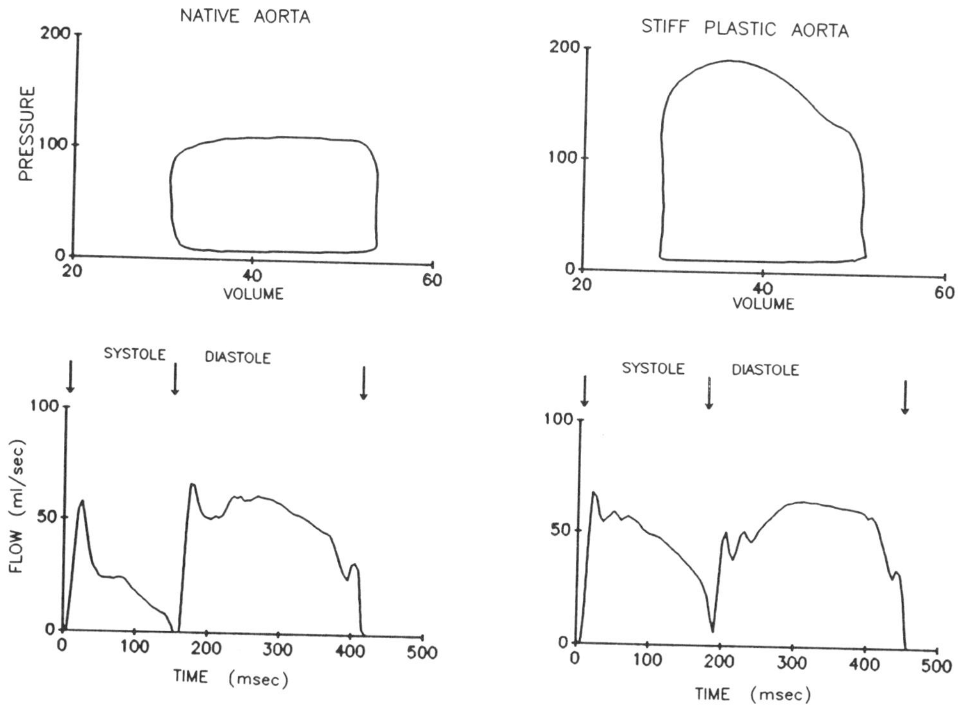

Figure 4. Influence of aortic stiffening on coronary phasic flow profiles. Upper panels display pressure–volume loops for native versus stiff plastic aortas. Lower panels show coronary flow patterns. For native aorta, coronary flow is predominately diastolic, with only 24% of flow during systole. In contrast, with the stiffened aorta and marked rise in pulsatile load, there is a substantial rise in systolic flow, and little change in diastolic flow.

CONCLUSIONS

This brief report describes several recent studies to test whether mean and pulsatile arterial loading can influence cardiac systolic mechanics and energetic efficiency. The data suggest that while large changes in mean resistance leading to varying ejection fraction can influence both parameters, that substantial changes in pulsatile loading do not. Furthermore, recent data suggest that systolic coronary perfusion is enhanced in the setting of a widened pulse pressure and systolic hypertension, consistent with a recent theory of coronary flow based on a time–varying elastance model. Future studies are required to better determine how cardiac disease alters the interplay between vascular load and cardiac performance, and what circumstances must exist for coronary supply to become inadequate in the closed–loop perfusion setting.

Acknowledgements

The author gratefully acknowledges the collaboration and major contributions of Drs. Daniel Burkhoff, Raymond Kelly and Pieter de Tombe, and the superb technical assistance of Richard Tunin in conducting these studies.

DISCUSSION

Dr. L.E. Ford: Are your figures representative of all your data?

Dr. D. Kass: This is an example of the data, and there were some differences between individual dog results. However, the mean results clearly demonstrate no significant differences.

Dr. L.E. Ford: It seems that the duration of systole was substantially longer in the hearts that had the stiffer ventricles; the time from the onset of systole to the onset of diastole is longer.

Dr. D. Kass : We defined systole from the time at which aortic flow starts and when it stops. End–systole fails just short of where the coronary flow drops. Thus, it is not as long as it might appear. There is some prolongation, that is true.

Dr. E. Yellin: Have you or the adherents of the end–systolic pressure–volume relation, tried to reconcile Mark Noble's concepts that the later part of the aortic outflow is due to the momentum that is carrying the blood out of the ventricle and really is not related to the active state of the ventricle. Physically, this makes sense and he has shown it. How does that influence your thinking, since systole may end long before aortic valve closure, i.e. end ejection.

Dr. D. Kass: Demonstration that there are effects of both the magnitude of ejection and the rate of ejection goes back to an early study Dr. Suga did in which inertial elements as well as internal resistors were added to try and explain disparities between isovolumic and ejecting beats. Dan Burkhoff has done a recent study in the isolated heart trying to look at this, where these factors have also been added in. What we can not explain are what appear to be the fundamental effects of ejection on lengthening contractile force generation, the duration of systolic pressure development, and changing the nature of early relaxation in the ejecting beats. Dr. Burkhoff is trying to describe it by a model that examines calcium binding kinetics. It basically is a myofilament interaction calcium kinetics model which he has been able to use to explain both the efficiency changes as well as the contractile state changes.

Dr. N. Westerhof: A lengthening of systole seems logical because of the larger swing in aortic pressure, and it would be logical if you found that. Your elastance E_{max} is considerably changed from your graph; it seems that the intercept differs from the pressure–volume relation, so it is difficult to say what happens.

Dr. D. Kass: The intercept of those relationships must be regarded cautiously, because this study was not done where the absolute volume position was accurately calibrated. I am confident of the slope because that was calibrated to a gain from a flow probe, whereas it is difficult to calibrate the absolute position of those relationships with the conductance catheter. On average, there was no significant volume shift, but I would take this with a grain of salt.

Dr. G. Mitchell: You stated that this theory of stiffening of the aorta would increase load and diminish perfusion and then you seem to refute that, where you show nice diastolic perfusion. Your diastolic pressure was one half the diastolic pressure of the controls. Isn't that a little misleading?

Dr. D. Kass: I do not think it is that misleading. The mean diastolic pressure change is not that great due to the late systolic pressure rise. Once aortic flow stops, you operate at a relatively high systolic pressure. It is true that it falls off fairly rapidly, but during the early phase of diastolic coronary perfusion mean perfusion pressures remain fairly high. Coronary resistance may also have fallen. The intriguing thing is that these effects balance out and that we do not see more diastolic perfusion. We do not see less either. What is observed is that the increase in required flow to compensate for the elevation in work load and oxygen consumption is made up for in systole. This is what is intriguing.

REFERENCES

1. Yin FCP (editor). *Ventricular/Vascular Coupling: Clinical, physiological, and engineering aspects*, New York: Springer–Verlag, 1987.
2. Kass DA, Kelly RP. Ventriculo–arterial coupling: Concepts, assumptions, and applications. *Annals Biomed Eng* 1992; 20: 41–62.
3. Sunagawa K, Burkhoff D, Lim KO, Sagawa K. Impedance loading servo pump system for excised canine ventricle. *Am J Phys* 1982; 243: H346–H350.
4. Avolio AP, Deng FQ, Li WQ, Luo YF, Huang ZD, Xing LF, O'Rourke MF. Effects of aging on arterial distensibility in populations with high and low prevalence of hypertension: comparison between urban and rural communities in China. *Circulation* 1985; 71: 202–210.
5. Nichols WW, O'Rourke MF, Avolio AP, Yaginuma T, Murgo JP, Pepine CJ, Conti CR. Effects of age on ventricular–vascular coupling. *Am J Cardiol* 1985; 55: 1179–1184.
6. Rutan GH, Kuller LH, Neaton JD, Wentworth D,N., McDonald RH, McFate Smith W. Mortality associated with diastolic hypertension and isolated systolic hypertension among men screened for Multiple Risk Factor Intervention Trial. *Circulation* 1988; 77: 504–514.
7. Suga H, Sagawa K, Shoukas AA. Load independence of the instantaneous pressure–volume ratio of the canine left ventricle and effects of epinephrine and heart rate on the ratio. *Circ Res* 1973; 32: 314.
8. Glower DD, Spratt JA, Snow ND, Kabas JS, Davis JW, Olsen CO, Tyson GS, Sabiston DC, Rankin JS. Linearity of the Frank–Starling relationship in the intact heart: the concept of preload recruitable stroke work. *Circulation* 1985; 71: 994–1009.
9. Little WC. The left ventricular dP/dT max –end diastolic volume relation in closed–chest dogs. *Circ Res* 1985; 56: 808–815.
10. Mirsky I, Aoyagi T, Crocker VM, Fujii AM. Preload dependence of fiber shortening rate in conscious dogs with left ventricular hypertrophy. *J Am Coll Cardiol* 1990; 15: 899.
11. Kentish JC, ter Keurs HEDJ, Ricciardi L, Bucx JJJ, Nobel NIM. Comparison between sarcomere length–force relations of intact and skinned trabeculae from rat right ventricle. *Circ Res* 1986; 58: 755–768.
12. Kass DA, Maughan WL. From "Emax" to pressure–volume relations: A broader view. *Circulation* 1988; 77: 1203–1212.
13. Kass DA, Grayson R, Marino P. Pressure–volume analysis as a method for quantifying simultaneous drug (amrinone) effects on arterial load and contractile state. *J Am Coll Cardiol* 1990; 16: 726–732.
14. Hasenfuss G, Holubarsch C, Heiss W, Meinertz T, Bonzel T, Wais U, Lehmann M, Just H. Myocardial energetics in patients with dilated cardiomyopathy. *Circulation* 1989; 80: 51–64.
15. Suga H, Goto Y, Nazawa T, Yasumara Y, Futaki S, Tanaka N. Force–time integral decreases with ejection despite constant oxygen consumption and pressure–volume area in dog left ventricle. *Circ Res* 1987; 60: 797–803.
16. Suga H. Ventricular Energetics. *Phys Rev* 1990; 70: 247–277.
17. Suga H, Hayashi T, Sueheiro S, Hisano R, Shirahata M, Ninomiya I. Equal oxygen consumption rates of isovolumic and ejecting contractions with equal systolic pressure volume areas in canine left ventricle. *Circ Res* 1981; 49: 1082–1091.
18. Maughan WL, Sunagawa K, Burkhoff D, Sagawa K. Effect of arterial impedance changes on the end–systolic pressure–volume relation. *Circ Res* 1984; 54: 595–602.
19. Freeman GL, Little WC, O'Rourke RA. The effect of vasoactive agents on the left ventricular end–systolic pressure–volume relation in closed–chest dogs. *Circulation* 1986; 74: 1107–1113.

20. Freeman GL. Effects of increased afterload on left ventricular function in closed–chest dogs. *Am J Physiol* 1990; 259: H619–H625.
21. Hunter WC. End–systolic pressure as a balance between opposing effects of ejection. *Circ Res* 1989; 64: 265–275.
22. Schroff SG, Janicki JS, Weber KT. Evidence and quantification of left ventricular systolic resistance. *Am J Physiol* 1985; 249: H353–H370.
23. Goto Y, Igarashi Y, Yasumura Y, Nozawa T, Futaki S, Hiramori K, Suga H. Integrated regional work equals total left ventricular work in regionally ischemic canine heart. *Am J Physiol* 1988; 254: H894–H904.
24. Suga H, Goto Y, Yasumura Y, Nozawa T, Futaki S, Tanaka N, Uenishi M. O2 consumption of dog heart under decreased coronary perfusion and propranolol. *Am J Physiol* 1988; 254: H292–H303.
25. Burkhoff D, de Tombe PP, Hunter WC, Kass DA. Contractile strength and mechanical efficiency of left ventricle are enhanced by physiological afterload. *Am J Phys* 1991; 260 (29): H569–H578.
26. Urschel CW, Covell JW, Sonnenblick EH, Ross J,Jr., Braunwald E. Effects of decreased aortic compliance on performance of the left ventricle. *Am J Physiol* 1968; 214: 298–304.
27. O'Rourke MF. Steady and pulsatile energy losses in the systemic circulation under normal conditions and in simulated arterial disease. *Cardiovasc Res* 1967; 1: 313–326.
28. Randall OS, Van Den Bos GC, Westerhof N. Systemic compliance: does it play a role in the genesis of essential hypertension? *Cardiovasc Res* 1984; 18: 455–462.
29. Kelly RP, Tunin R, Kass DA. Effect of reduced aortic compliance on cardiac efficiency and contractile function of *in situ* canine left ventricle. *Circ Res* 1992; 71: 490–502.
30. Krams R, Sipkema P, Zegers J, Westerhof N. Contractility is the main determinant of coronary systolic flow impediment. *Am J Phys* 1989; 257: H1936–H1944.
31. Resar JR, Livingston JZ, Yin FCP. In–plane myocardial wall stress is not the primary determinant of coronary systolic flow impediment. *Circ Res* 1992; 70: 583–592.

CHAPTER 30

THE VEINS AND VENTRICULAR PRELOAD

John V. Tyberg, Nairne W. Scott-Douglas, Yudi Wang, and Dante E. Manyari[1]

ABSTRACT

A pressure-volume model of the peripheral circulation is presented with a discussion of the effects of congestive heart failure on the venous capacitance bed.

INTRODUCTION

The venous system remains the most poorly understood element in the circulation, much more being known about the heart, the arterial system, and the microcirculation. Furthermore, some of what is thought to be understood may be, if not incorrect, subject to serious misinterpretation. In the latter category may be the concept of "venous return". There can be no doubt that venous return is a very useful concept when analyzing the beat-to-beat circulatory changes that accompany standing up or a rapid deep inspiration; the difficulty comes when "an increase in venous return" is used to denote the steady-state condition caused by the venoconstriction-induced translocation of blood from the peripheral to the central circulations. In congestive heart failure when cardiac output is known to be depressed, steady-state venous return *cannot* be increased [1].

Also, the analogy of the emptying lung [2] has led to an emphasis on right atrial (RA) pressure and venous resistance as the principal determinants of venous return. In this formulation, it is the reduction in RA "back pressure" which allows venous return to increase. However, this inverse relationship between RA pressure and venous return (cardiac output) has been interpreted alternatively by Levy, who suggested that it is the increase in cardiac output that *causes* the decrease in RA pressure (i.e. increasing cardiac output depletes the venous reservoir) [3]. While this "chicken-and-egg" problem cannot be resolved conclusively because both interpretations are internally consistent, the objective of a recently proposed model [4] was to support Levy's interpretation of the inverse relation

[1]Departments of Medicine and Medical Physiology, The University of Calgary, Calgary, Alberta T2N 4N1, Canada.

Interactive Phenomena in the Cardiac System, Edited by
S. Sideman and R. Beyar, Plenum Press, New York, 1993

between RA pressure and cardiac output and to interpret recent data in the context of that model.

AN ALTERNATIVE MODEL OF THE PERIPHERAL CIRCULATION

The fact that an increase in cardiac output causes a decrease in venous and RA pressures becomes clear from an examination of Fig. 1. In this figure, the idealized human circulatory values chosen by Levy [3] are used and, for simplicity, systemic vascular resistance has been assumed to be constant (20 mmHg/L/min). The horizontal scale is defined only in relative units and is based on the observation that approximately 70% of the blood is contained within the venous system at normal cardiac outputs and pressures [5]. When cardiac output is zero, the pressures in the idealized venous and arterial compartments are equal and are assumed to be 7 mmHg. This pressure is defined as mean circulatory pressure (P_{mc}) [5], sometimes termed mean circulatory filling pressure or mean systemic filling pressure. Mean circulatory pressure is the value of pressure everywhere in the circulation after the heart has stopped beating (if flow is zero, there can be no pressure gradients in a resistive circuit and all pressures must be equal). (In practice, it is not simple to determine this value experimentally [6].) Mean circulatory pressure is also a measure of "the fullness of the circulation" [6], a measure of the circulating blood volume relative to the "tone" of the vasculature. As shown presently, mean circulatory pressure is the value from which arterial pressure increases and venous pressure decreases, as cardiac output increases.

When cardiac output increases from 0 to 1 L/min, a new steady state is reached as the heart pumps an incremental volume of blood (ΔV_1) from the venous reservoir and transfers it to the arterial reservoir (Fig. 1). Because of the values of the compliances which

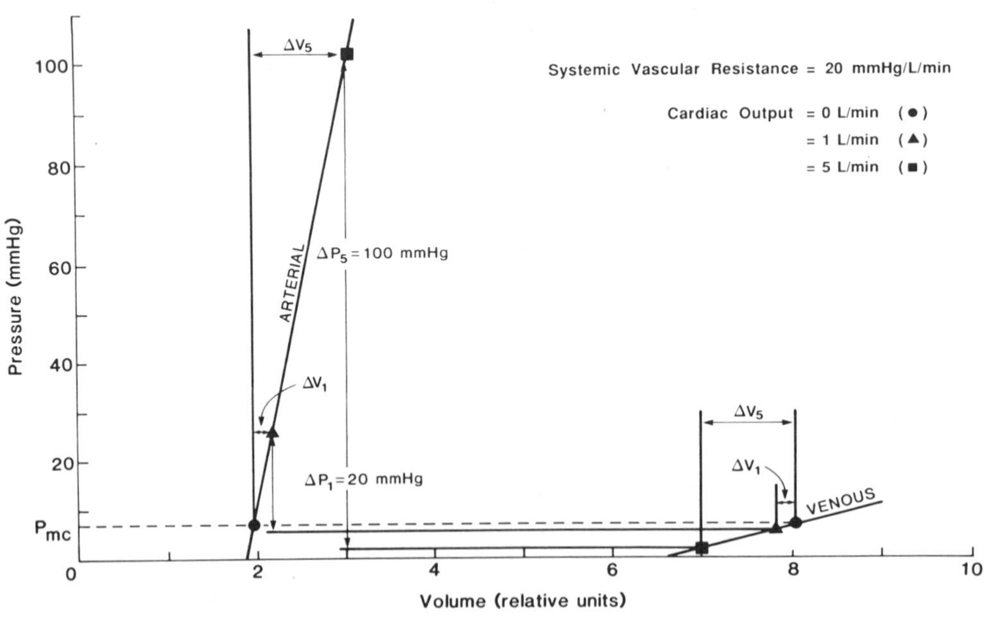

Figure 1. Relative arterial and venous pressure–volume relations. (Modified from Tyberg [4] and published with permission of Mosby–Yearbook, Inc.)

have been assumed, this transfer of blood lowers venous pressure by 1 mmHg (to 6 mmHg) and raises arterial pressure by 19 mmHg (to 26 mmHg). The resulting arterial–to–venous gradient (20 mmHg) is just sufficient to drive a flow of 1 L/min through the systemic vascular resistance back into the venous compartment, consistent with the establishment of a new steady state. When the cardiac output increases to a normal value (5 L/min), a larger volume of blood must be transferred (ΔV_5) from the veins to the arteries. This transfer of blood effects normal mean values of venous and arterial pressures (2 and 102 mmHg, respectively). The gradient thereby established (100 mmHg) drives a flow equal to the cardiac output back through the systemic vascular resistance (100 mmHg = 5 L/min x 20 mmHg/L/min).

Changes in venous capacitance tend to be dominated by changes in so–called unstressed volume (unstressed volume is the volume that would exist at a venous pressure of zero if the quasi–linear portion of the venous pressure–volume relation were extrapolated to the zero–pressure axis) [5]. It does not really exist in that all direct studies of vascular pressure–volume relations indicate that the relation is curvilinear and tends to parallel the volume axis near zero pressure [7]. Nonetheless, it has proved to be a useful parameter with which to characterize the position of the pressure–volume relation. True changes in venous compliance (i.e. the reciprocal of the slope of the pressure–volume relation) can be demonstrated [8] but are small, relative to the changes in unstressed volume and to previous expectations based on models which assumed that the pressure–volume relation of the vasculature, like the voltage–charge relation of an electrical capacitance, passes through the origin [9, 10].

The small changes in compliance that have been demonstrated do not appear to be larger than those to be expected from a priori geometric considerations (i.e. if one assumes that the relative change in volume is constant for a given pressure change, the slope of the pressure–volume relation [the reciprocal of compliance] must decrease in proportion to the increase in unstressed volume). Although the small slope changes in the directly measured intravascular pressure–diameter relation are unequivocal [8], the slopes of pressure–volume relations described by other techniques may be less physiologically significant in that they are model–dependent and sometimes involve a lumped capacitance in which the contribution of a given vascular element (e.g. venules) might be less at lower outlet pressures than at higher pressures. Finally, from a teleologic viewpoint Greenway has suggested that a change in unstressed volume is preferable to a change in compliance in that the effect of a change in compliance would tend to diminish at low venous pressures and in circumstances under which translocation of volume might be most beneficial [11].

THE VEINS IN CONGESTIVE HEART FAILURE

As implied at the outset, it has been widely assumed that an important component of the pathophysiology of congestive heart failure is venoconstriction. However, direct experimental evidence has been lacking until recently. Using the increasingly accepted pacing–induced canine model of chronic congestive heart failure [12, 13] and classic indicator–dilution methods, Ogilivie and Zborowska–Sluis demonstrated that heart failure results in a profound leftward shift in the relation between mean circulatory filling pressure and total blood volume [14]. The decrease in unstressed volume was almost 50% and the changes in compliance were of no statistical or physiologic significance. This strongly suggests that chronic congestive heart failure involves profound constriction of the venous–capacitance vasculature.

We have used the model of acute heart failure developed by Smiseth and Mjøs in which the canine left coronary artery is incrementally embolized by 50 μm microspheres until LV end–diastolic pressure reaches 20 mmHg (at that time, cardiac output is usually reduced by about 50%) [15]. We studied the effects of 3 different vasoactive agents, nitroglycerin, enalaprilat (a parenteral angiotensin–converting enzyme inhibitor), and hydralazine. In order to distinguish effects on venous capacitance from arteriolar effects, we used a modification of ^{99m}Tc–blood pool scintigraphy [16] to measure changes in total vascular volume and administered each drug in equihypotensive dosages (i.e. in each case, mean arterial blood pressure was reduced by 20%). We reasoned that this procedure would result in equal effects on the arteriolar circulation, which largely determines vascular resistance, and that changes in total vascular volume could, for the most part, be ascribed to changes in venous capacitance, since approximately 70% of the blood is contained in the venous vasculature [5]. Relative to our control observations, this model of heart failure produced a 15% reduction in total vascular (primarily venous) unstressed volume.

Nitroglycerin, enalaprilat, and hydralazine were then given in three different groups of dogs. Relative to the unstressed volume during heart failure, nitroglycerin increased unstressed volume by 30%, enalaprilat by 11%, and hydralazine by 0% [17]. These observations showed that vasodilators, administered in a dosage to produce equal arteriolar effects, can have vastly different effects on the venous capacitance bed. As widely recognized, nitroglycerin has a relatively large effect on venous capacitance, enalaprilat clearly dilates the veins but is only 1/3 as effective as nitroglycerin, and, consistent with textbook teaching, hydralazine has no effect on venous capacitance even though its effects on the arteriolar bed were equal. Effects on LV end–diastolic pressure were consistent with the venous effects: nitroglycerin lowered pressure the most, enalaprilat was intermediate, and there was no significant effect with hydralazine. Thus, for equal effects on the arteriolar bed, therapeutic vasodilators may have very disparate effects on venous capacitance and it is the venous effects which determine changes in cardiac filling pressure.

DISCUSSION

Dr. Y. Kresh: What you are saying is quite intriguing. It takes courage to go against the established sacred view of cardiac output regulation. The cardiac output is self–limiting. The limit is set, in–part, by the circulating volume (mostly venous). That may explain why the only way kids, after a Fontan operation, can compensate for not having a right heart is by simply having to volume load the venous side of the system (increase in CVP, to overcome the pulmonary circulation resistance). Once the loading of the left side is exhausted, that limits the cardiac output that can be recruited. In fact, years ago we proposed to replace the whole heart with a single mechanical artificial chamber (simulating the Fontan–like circuit), it became evident that it does not matter how much power (energy) is generated by the native heart or to the mechanical (artificial) heart, it is not going to increase the cardiac output unless it can translocate additional volume to the venous side by splenic–circulation recruitment etc. Is that what you are really saying?

Dr. J.V. Tyberg: Yes, and I certainly do not want to argue with the view that the heart pumps out what it gets back. However, I am arguing for the importance of *displacement of volume* and of concentrating on a change in a pressure–volume relationship rather than in a pressure–flow relationship, which seems to be a less fundamental way to look at capacitance.

Dr. E.L. Yellin: I do not understand why, in hemorrhage for example, when the tone of the vessels is not changing, it does not go up and down the same pressure–volume curve.

Dr. J.V. Tyberg: I do not really understand why either, but I believe our data and I believe Art Shoukas' data [8], which is less equivocal methodologically than ours. I think that a large part of it is an α–adrenergic effect. Some of it may be related to angiotensin itself. Also, Dr. Chilian has some interesting data about flow–related effects but, regardless how they are hormonally mediated, the changes that you suggest do occur: the slope does not change very much but the unstressed volume does.

Dr. E.L. Yellin: You are saying that there is a great deal of reflex activity during these maneuvers.

Dr. J.V. Tyberg: Yes. With nitroglycerin, for instance, I envision that the patient in heart failure with a great deal of stress has a great deal of α–adrenergic tone which shifts the venous pressure–volume relationship to the left, i.e. toward the pressure axis. That shift can be overcome by nitroglycerin, which perhaps shifts it back to a maximum volume at that pressure. The magnitude of the nitroglycerin–induced rightward shift depends on your starting point.

Dr. E.L. Yellin: I understand the effect of the drug. But, without the drug, why does the slope not change if an organ bed becomes stiffer, i.e. with more tone?

Dr. J.V. Tyberg: We have been using these terms, stiffness and compliance, badly for a long time in cardiology. The interesting thing to me is that, to a remarkable degree, the veins do change their volume at the same pressure.

REFERENCES

1. Packer M. Editorial: Abnormalities of diastolic function as a potential cause of exercise intolerance in chronic heart failure. *Circulation* (Suppl III). 1990; 81: III–78–III–86.
2. Permutt S, Caldini P. Regulation of cardiac output by the circuit: venous return. In: Baan J, Noordergraaf A, Raines J, eds. Cardiovascular System Dynamics. Mass Institute of Technology; 1975: 465–479.
3. Levy MN. The cardiac and vascular factors that determine systemic blood flow. *Circ Res* 1979; 44: 739–747.
4. Tyberg JV. Venous modulation of ventricular preload. *Am Heart J* 1992; 123: 1098–1104.
5. Rothe CF. Reflex controls of veins and vascular capacitance. *Physiol Rev* 1983; 63: 1281–1341.
6. Rothe CF. Mean circulatory pressure: its meaning and measurement. *J Appl Physiol* 1993; 74: 499–509.
7. Katz AI, Chen Y, Moreno AH. Flow through a collapsible tube: Experimental analysis and mathematical model. *Biophys J* 1969; 9: 1261–1279.
8. Shoukas AA, Bohlen HG. Rat venular pressure–diameter relationships are regulated by sympathetic activity. *Am J Physiol* 1990; 259: H674–H680.
9. Guyton AC, Coleman TG, Granger HJ. Circulation: overall regulation. *Ann Rev Physiol* 1972; 34: 13–46.
10. Greenway CV. Simple model of the circulation. *Physiologist* 1981; 24: 63–67.
11. Greenway CV, Seaman KL, Innes IR. Norepinephrine on venous compliance and unstressed volume in cat liver. *Am J Physiol* 1985; 284: H468–H476.
12. Whipple GH, Shefield LT, Woodman EG, Theophilis C, Friedman S. Reversible congestive heart failure due to rapid stimulation of the normal heart. *Proc N Engl Cardiovasc Soc* 1962; 20: 39.
13. Coleman HN, Taylor RR, Pool PE, Whipple GH, Covell JW, Ross J Jr, Braunwald E. Congestive heart failure following chronic tachycardia. *Am Heart J* 1971; 81: 790–798.
14. Ogilvie RI, Zborowska–Sluis D. Effect of chronic rapid ventricular pacing on total vascular capacitance. *Circulation* 1992; 85: 1524–1530.
15. Smiseth OA, Mjos OD. A reproducible and stable model of acute ischaemic left ventricular failure in dogs. *Clin Physiol* 1982; 2: 225–239.
16. Robinson VJB, Smiseth OA, Scott–Douglas NW, Smith ER, Tyberg JV, Manyari DE. Assessment of the splanchnic vascular capacity and capacitance: a new application of equilibrium blood–pool scintigraphy. *J Nucl Med* 1990; 131: 154–159.
17. Wang Y, Scott–Douglas NW, Manyari DE, Tyberg JV. Different effects of vasoactive agents on vascular capacitance in dogs with experimental heart failure (abstract). *FASEB J* 1991; 5: A776.

CHAPTER 31

WHY SMALLER ANIMALS HAVE HIGHER HEART RATES

Nicolaas Westerhof and Gijs Elzinga[1]

ABSTRACT

Diastolic blood pressure is the main driving pressure for coronary perfusion. Diastolic pressure depends on mean pressure and the ratio of the decay time of aortic pressure in diastole (τ) and the duration of diastole (T_d). The ratio of τ, a morphological, arterial parameter, and T_d, a functional, cardiac parameter, is the same in all mammals. This could mean that smaller animals have higher heart rates i.e. shorter duration of diastole to match the shorter time constant of the diastolic pressure decay and to guarantee adequate coronary perfusion.

INTRODUCTION

In most mammals mean arterial blood pressure is about 100 mmHg. The systolic and diastolic aortic pressures are about 120 and 80 mmHg, in spite of a considerable variation in heart rate. It is supposed that the constancy of mean pressure is beneficial for organ perfusion (mainly brain) and renal (glomerular) filtration. The heart is a special organ: as a result of its contraction blood flow through the myocardium during systole is small if not negligible. Myocardial blood flow thus mainly depends on the pressure in the diastolic phase and the duration of diastole.

Diastolic pressure decreases with a characteristic time, the decay time. This decay time (τ) is determined by the product of total arterial compliance (C), i.e. the storage capacity of the arteries, and the peripheral resistance (R_p) through which blood leaves the arterial system. The decay time is therefore entirely determined by arterial and arteriolar properties. In small mammals the decay time is shorter than in large mammals. To prevent diastolic pressure from decaying to very small values a shorter duration of the diastolic

[1]Laboratory for Physiology and Institute for Cardiovascular Research, Free University of Amsterdam, 1081 BT, Amsterdam, The Netherlands.

Interactive Phenomena in the Cardiac System, Edited by
S. Sideman and R. Beyar, Plenum Press, New York, 1993

period in small mammals seems essential. We therefore studied the relation between the decay time (τ) and the duration of diastole (T_d) in a large range of mammals.

METHODS

The peripheral resistance (R_p, in $mmHg \cdot s \cdot ml^{-1}$) is the ratio of mean pressure and mean flow (F, cardiac output), and was determined from our own experiments on cat, dog, baboon and man and from data in the literature on rat, guinea pig and rabbit where this parameter was given directly or where pressure and flow were reported.

There are a number of methods to measure total arterial compliance (C, in $ml \cdot mmHg^{-1}$): from the decay time of pressure in diastole and peripheral resistance [4], from the input impedance of the entire arterial system [2], from a fit of the aortic flow calculated using a three-element Windkessel model with measured pressure as input [3] and via areas under the diastolic pressure decay [4]. Using these data and taking the average value per species total arterial compliance was also determined for these animals [5]. The time constant (τ, in seconds) was derived from the product of peripheral resistance and arterial compliance. For details see Westerhof and Elzinga [5].

For many mammalian species heart rate (inverse of the heart period, T) and information on the electrocardiogram (ECG) are given by Altman and Dittmer [6]. We determined the duration of ejection (T_s) by subtracting from the QT–time the duration of the QRS–complex using Altman and Dittmer's tables [6]. The duration of diastole (T_d) is the difference of T and T_s. The duration of the entire cardiac cycle, diastole and ejection were determined for the range from rat to elephant.

All parameters were related to body mass (M, in kg). The allometric equation applied to the data is $X = X_0 M^b$ with X the parameter of interest and b the exponent. By relating the logarithm of the parameter with the logarithm of body mass and applying linear regression the exponent can be determined. It was tested if exponents were different from zero (independence of slopes, $p<0.05$). It was also tested if slopes were different (comparison of slopes, 5% significance level).

RESULTS

For peripheral resistance we find:

$$R_p\,(M) = R_{p,o}\, M^{-0.93} \quad . \tag{1}$$

The exponent for arterial compliance is +1.23 and for decay time a value of +0.29 is found. All slopes of are significantly different from zero ($p<0.05$).

The exponents for the times are T: 0.27, T_d: 0.30 and T_s: 0.20, and are all different from zero ($p<0.05$). The exponents of these three times are not different from each other. The exponents of the heart period and the duration of diastole are not different from the arterial decay time.

DISCUSSION

We found that heart period (inverse of heart rate) and arterial decay time are similarly related to body size.

The dependence of the decay time on body mass can be understood from the following findings. The stress in the wall of arteries is given by Laplace's law [7], it depends on pressure and the ratio of wall thickness (h) and radius (r). This ratio (h/r) is similar (about 10%, [3]) in large arteries, independent of the species, so that wall stress is also similar. Pulse wave velocity (c) is about 5 m/s in all mammals [7]. Since pulse wave velocity can be written as

$$c^2 = Eh/2\rho r \tag{2}$$

with E and ρ the modulus of elasticity of the arterial wall and blood density, respectively [7]. These material properties, in view of the same wave velocity, appear to be the same in mammals. This has been reported to be indeed the case [3]. The velocity of the pulse wave can also be given by:

$$c^2 = (dP/dA)\ (A/\rho) \tag{3}$$

with P pressure and A (aortic) area (the Moens–Korteweg equation, [7]). Finally, the velocity of blood (v = F/A, with F flow) in the aorta is similar [7].

The decay time can now be written as $\tau = R_p\, C$, with $R_p = P/F$ and $C = L\ dA/dP$, with aortic length L. Thus

$$\tau = (P/F)\ (A/A)\ L\ (dA/dP) = L\ (P/v)\ (h/r)\ (E/2)\quad . \tag{4}$$

With mean blood pressure, blood velocity, h/r (and thus wall stress) and E (material constant) the same in mammals, the decay time depends on length only. Aortic length was found to depend on body mass with an exponent of 0.33 [3] and the time constant is thus predicted to vary with this exponent as well. The exponent of the decay time (0.29 ± 0.07 (SE)) could not be shown to differ from 0.33.

Apparently pressure, stress, blood velocity and material properties of the arterial wall and blood density (E, ρ) were kept constant during evolution, with the result that the time constant of the arterial system became dependent on body size (length).

The slope of the relation between heart period and body mass was found to be 0.27. Milnor [7] reported 0.32 and Schmidt–Nielsen [8] found 0.25. From the data of Holt et al. [9] a value of 0.27 can be derived. These values are close to our results.

The ratio of the duration of diastole and the decay time (T_d/τ) and the ratio of the heart period and the decay time (T/τ) are found to be independent of body mass. It can be reasoned that with the same mean pressure the diastolic pressure is similar when the ratio T_d/τ is the same. Thus the body not only keeps mean pressure constant but diastolic (and systolic) pressure as well.

Because cardiac metabolism increases with heart rate it seems desirable in evolutionary terms that the heart rate is kept low. However, pressure in diastole would then decrease to very low values, an undesirable condition for coronary perfusion. Since the ratio of the duration of diastole to heart period (T_d/T) is the same, coronary perfusion takes place in the same fraction of time in all mammals. Adequate coronary perfusion is, with similar diastolic pressure and similar fractional duration of perfusion, guaranteed.

Acknowledgement

The critical reading of the manuscript by Hans van Beek is greatly appreciated. In part supported by grant #890902 from NATO Scientific Affairs Division.

DISCUSSION

Dr. R. Chadwick: Extremely fascinating. We should do more of this kind of scaling. Surely you must have thought about animal longevity. Small animals with higher heart rates do not live as long as big animals with lower heart rates. It is tempting to think that there might be approximately the same total number of heart beats on average for all of these animals. Have you looked at that?

Dr. N. Westerhof: I have not looked at it, but it is known as a good approximation that the number of heart beats is a given quantity so the rat will have about the same number of heart beats as the elephant over his life–time. Man does not fit so well.

Dr. D. Allen: I liked your analysis. But animals obviously exercise and then they increase their heart rate rather substantially and I wonder whether some of the deviations from the line might be because some animals spend more of their time exercising and therefore they have optimized heart rates, somewhere between the resting and the exercising level, whereas other more sedentary animals will have heart rates near the resting level most of the time.

Dr. N. Westerhof: There are several problems with all of these figures. As stated, I am not looking to exercise, but some of the animals have been anesthetized and some may have had more training. There are lot of complications that give noise on the figures; some of the very small animals, like the guinea pig, are very sensitive in heart rate to anesthesia, so there is some doubt here about the accuracy. It would be nice to have all the information on the conscious animal as it is sitting quietly.

Dr. J–K. Li: Regarding the cardiac period, in your allometric equation the exponent is very close to 0.33, which means that it is related to the length of the aorta or the effective length of the arterial system. Can you comment on that?

Dr. N. Westerhof: I have tried to indicate that if you look at decay time of arterial pressure in diastole, it is related, in a good approximation, to body length because all of the other parameters like pulse wave velocity and blood velocity are very similar in mammals.

Dr. J–K. Li: We looked at the propagation constant as well as the reflection coefficient and we found them very similar in mammals. Another philosophical comment is that some time ago people have found that total number of heart beats in a mammal's life span is fixed, so that a smaller mammal, even though its heart beats faster, lives a much shorter life.

Dr. L.E. Ford: Were the pressure vs flow measurements made at a constant volume? Were the measurements of power averaged over the cardiac cycle, or was it the peak power, or power at a constant volume or a particular time in the cardiac cycle?

Dr. N. Westerhof: I did not go into this. That is a point in itself. The pump function is taken under one fixed condition. That means constant contractile state, constant filling, constant heart volume.

Dr. L.E. Ford: But are the measurements instantaneous values or are they average?

Dr. N. Westerhof: That is average flow and average pressure and power is calculated by instantaneous multiplication and integration over time (mean power).

Dr. L.E. Ford: A number of things which you have pointed out in this very nice study were anticipated by A.V. Hill in a much rougher form, about 45 years ago. In a lecture to the Royal Institution, he pointed out these differences in the time periods in animals. He expected that the cardiac output of the animal would vary, roughly with the length of the animal. His calculation was based on the notion that the blood would have to be accelerated a lot more rapidly in a larger animal. He concluded that the animal heart could not generate sufficient power to provide the necessary acceleration of the blood. He also pointed out that the power and efficiency points on the curve were different; the maximum efficiency occurrs at a higher pressure (or force) and lower velocity. He related this observation to the way bicycle racers chose their pedaling frequency. In a short race they optimize the power output by pedaling at a somewhat higher rate whereas in a long race they optimize the efficiency by pedaling at a lower rate.

Dr. T. Arts: If you look at the human or any other animal as a function of age, the stiffness of the arteries change very much. Is this optimization criterion valid during a whole life or not?

Dr. N. Westerhof: We have not studied age. It is more complex because not only compliance changes but also peripheral resistance. I do not know what happens with age. We do not have enough data to do this. I would be more interested in situations like hibernation where output is very low but mean pressure is also very low and therefore compliance is very large. It may well be, just an hypothesis, that the heart rate and decay time are low, i.e. there could still be a relation between them.

Dr. E. Ritman: Hibernation is of course very interesting, but there are also diving mammals that cut off the blood supply temporarily. For instance, with the diaphragm they cut off the aorta. So this type of relationship may still be valid for the mass that is perfused at the time. Do you know if anybody has looked at that?

Dr. N. Westerhof: I know very little about this. I have looked in the literature to whales because I wanted to have large animals with large body mass, but I could only find two references. While most of these points are averaged over a number of animals, for the whale, we have only two whales, one by N.T. Smith in 1963 and one recently in *Circulation*, or *JACC* (1992), so we have limited data.

Dr. E. Ritman: Were those the whales that were harpooned with electrocardiograms?

Dr. N. Westerhof: Yes, so we do not know how accurate the heart rate is; they may have been a little excited.

REFERENCES

1. Randall OS, van den Bos GC, Westerhof N. Systemic compliance: does it play a role in the genesis of essential hypertension? *Cardiovasc Res* 1984; 18: 455–465.
2. van den Bos GC, Westerhof N, Randall OS. Pulse wave reflection: can it explain the differences between systemic and pulmonary pressure and flow waves? *Circ Res* 1982; 51: 479–485.
3. Toorop GP, Westerhof N, Elzinga G. Beat-to-beat estimation of peripheral resistance and arterial compliance during pressure transients. *Am J Physiol* 1987; 252: H1275–H1283.
4. Yin FCP, Liu Z. Estimating arterial resistance and compliance during transient conditions in humans. *Am J Physiol* 1989; 257: H190–H197.
5. Westerhof N, Elzinga G. Normalized input impedance and arterial decay time over heart period are independent of animal size. *Am J Physiol* 1991; 261: R126–R1336.
6. Altman PL, Dittmer DS (eds). Biological Handbook. *Fed Am Soc Exptl Biol*, Bethesda, 1971; pp 278; 320: 336–341.
7. Milnor WR. Hemodynamics. *Williams and Wilkins*, Baltimore, 1989; pp 165–167.
8. Schmidt-Nielsen K. Scaling. *Cambridge Univ Press*, New York/Melbourne, 1984; pp 126–128..
9. Holt JP, Rhode EA, Kines H. Ventricular volumes and body weight in mammals. *Am J Physiol* 1968; 215: 704–714.

CHAPTER 32

FEEDBACK EFFECTS IN HEART–ARTERIAL SYSTEM INTERACTION

John K–J. Li[1]

ABSTRACT

Dynamic arterio–ventricular interaction in terms of left ventricle elastance and nonlinear arterial system compliance, pulse wave reflections and coronary blood flow was investigated, combining the use of analog models of the circulation with data from animal experiments. Results show that dynamic factors, as well as "feedback" effects are important.

INTRODUCTION

Blood pressure and flow pulses generated with each heartbeat encompass the effects of the ventricular contractile performance and the viscoelastic loading behavior of the arterial tree. This signifies the importance of understanding the interaction between the contracting left ventricle (LV) and the distributing arterial system (AS). Furthermore, the coronary vasculature within the myocardium is dependent on aortic blood pressure for its perfusion. Coronary blood flow occurs mostly in diastole when the aortic valve is closed. We investigated the role of pulse wave reflections and coronary flow in the dynamic interaction of the LV and the arterial system and concluded that their inclusion is important in the dynamic interaction study and that their role resembles that of functional feedback.

METHODS, MATERIALS AND PROCEDURES

Theoretical Analysis

We have previously developed a nonlinear arterial system model to include the pressure–dependent characteristics of arterial compliance [1] in the form of

[1]Cardiovascular Research Laboratory, Department of Biomedical Engineering, Rutgers University, Piscataway, NJ 08855–0909, USA.

Interactive Phenomena in the Cardiac System, Edited by S. Sideman and R. Beyar, Plenum Press, New York, 1993

$$C(P) = a \cdot \exp(bP) \tag{1}$$

where a and b are empirical constants derived from pressure–diameter measurements. This nonlinear model is coupled to the resistance (R_v)–elastance (E(t)) model of the LV [2, 3] (Fig. 1).

From simultaneous measurement of aortic pressure (P) and flow (Q), the flow through the compliance branch is

$$Q_c(t) = Q(t) - P(t)/R_s \tag{2}$$

It is dependent on the pressure–dependent compliance and the rate of change of pressure,

$$Q_c(t) = C(P)\ dP(t)/dt \tag{3}$$

Equating (2) and (3), results in

$$dP(t)/dt = (Q(t) - P(t)/R_s)\ /\ C(P) \tag{4}$$

This equation defines the relationship between aortic pressure and flow for the nonlinear compliance. The equation can be solved numerically.

The lumped interaction model does not afford pulse transmission characteristics. Pulse wave propagation and reflections can be examined separately [4]. Measured pressure and flow can be considered as the sum of the forward (f) and the reflected (r) components [5, 6], given by

$$P = P_f + P_r \tag{5}$$

$$Q = Q_f + Q_r \tag{6}$$

By estimating Z_o in the early ejection phase as the instantaneous ratio of aortic pressure to flow above the end–diastolic level,

$$Z_o = (P - P_d)/Q \tag{7}$$

forward and reflected waves can be obtained [5],

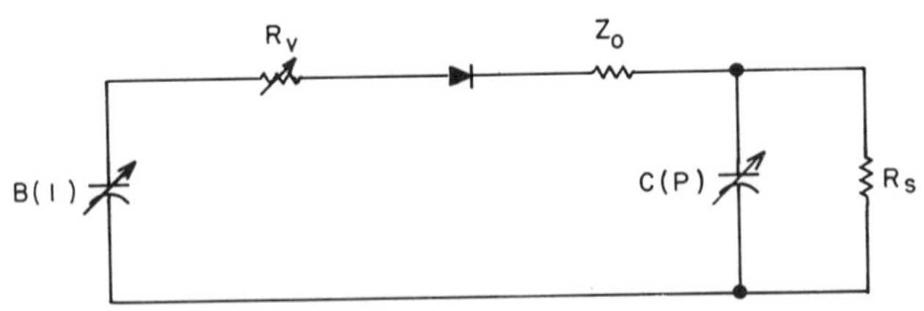

Figure 1. Model of the left ventricle (LV) and the arterial system (AS) with LV represented by a time–varying compliance and a resistance R_v, and with the AS represented by a modified Windkessel model with a pressure dependent compliance C(P), characteristic impedance Z_o and resistance R_s.

$$P_f = (P + QZ_o) / 2 \tag{8}$$

$$P_r = (P - QZ_o) / 2 \tag{9}$$

The reflection coefficient is given by

$$R_f = P_r/P_f \tag{10}$$

which can also be defined in terms of impedances,

$$R_f = (Z - Z_o) / (Z + Z_o) \tag{11}$$

Input impedance has been used to characterize the behavior of systemic, pulmonary and the coronary arterial systems.

For the LV, elastance E(t) is defined from pressure (P_v) and volume (V),

$$P_v(t) = E(t)\,[V(t) - V_d)] - R_vQ(t) \tag{12}$$

and

$$V(t) = EDV - \int Q(t)dt \tag{13}$$

where V_d is the dead volume, and EDV is the end–diastolic volume. This last expression assumes the flow to the coronary arteries is small during ejection. E(t) is readily computed by assuming values for the ejection fraction and V_d [7].

The external work (W) performed by the LV is the sum of a steady component (W_s) and a pulsatile component (W_p),

$$W = W_s + W_p \tag{14}$$

and

$$W_s = \bar{P} \cdot SV \tag{15}$$

where SV is the stroke volume. The pulsatile work is dependent on the forward and reflected waves. For this reason, a pulsatile energy transmission efficiency is introduced to account for the net amount of pulsatile energy that is transmitted to the periphery.

Animal Experiments

Experiments were performed on adult mongrel dogs of either sex, weighing between 20–25 kg each. Each animal was anesthetized with intravenous Nembutal (30 mg/kg) and placed on a respirator. A left lateral thoracotomy was performed to expose the heart and the great vessels. A segment of the ascending aorta as well as the left coronary artery were isolated for placement of cuff–type electromagnetic flow probes for measurement of aortic and coronary flows. A catheter–tip pressure transducer advanced from an exposed femoral artery provided simultaneous measurement of aortic pressure. Another transducer inserted through the apex measured LV pressure. A standard lead electrocardiogram (ECG) were also recorded. Data were taken at control, arterial load alterations by intravenous infusions of methoxamine (MTX) and nitroprusside (NTP), and during brief counterpulsation experiment.

Simultaneous recordings were made on an eight channel FM tape recorder, and on a paper recorder. The data were digitized at 100 Hz and appropriately filtered for analysis.

RESULTS

Figure 2 illustrates the temporal relationship of aortic pressure to the pressure–dependent compliance. It is clear that compliance varies continuously throughout the cardiac cycle and reaches its maximum, not at peak systolic pressure, but at end–systole. This arterial compliance is related to the time–varying compliance of the LV shown in Fig. 3, plotted as elastance.

Increased arterial load through increased blood pressure (MTX infusion) increased wave reflections, but decreased arterial compliance. The reverse was observed for the unloading conditions by nitroprusside infusion. The progressive alterations in pressure–dependent compliance in response to blood pressure changes are seen in Fig. 4. The pulsatile energy transmission efficiency is also altered accordingly (Fig. 5).

Since aortic pressure is a main determinant of coronary perfusion, particularly in diastole, the brief counterpulsation, or increased wave reflections, applied at selected diastolic intervals can significantly alter coronary blood flow. This is illustrated in Fig. 6.

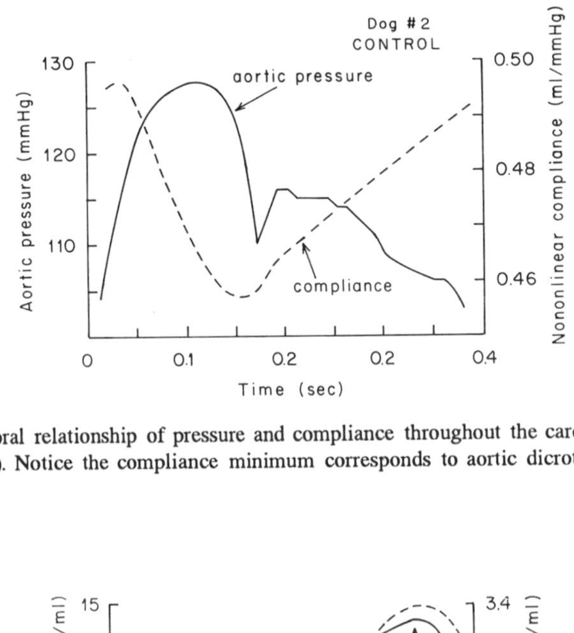

Figure 2. The temporal relationship of pressure and compliance throughout the cardiac cycle (CONTROL condition of Dog #2). Notice the compliance minimum corresponds to aortic dicrotic notch [14].

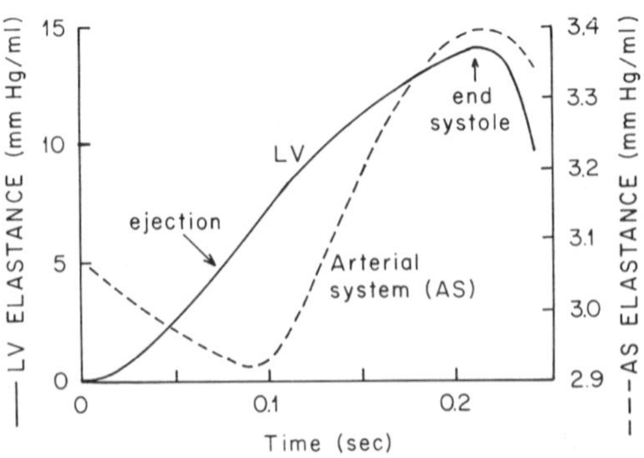

Figure 3. Left ventricular (LV) and arterial system (AS) elastance throughout systole.

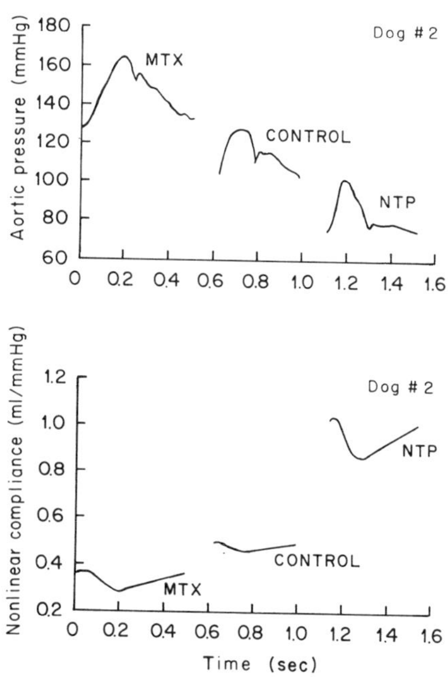

Figure 4. Aortic pressure and nonlinear compliance from CONTROL, MTX and NTP conditions of experiment Dog #2 [14, 15].

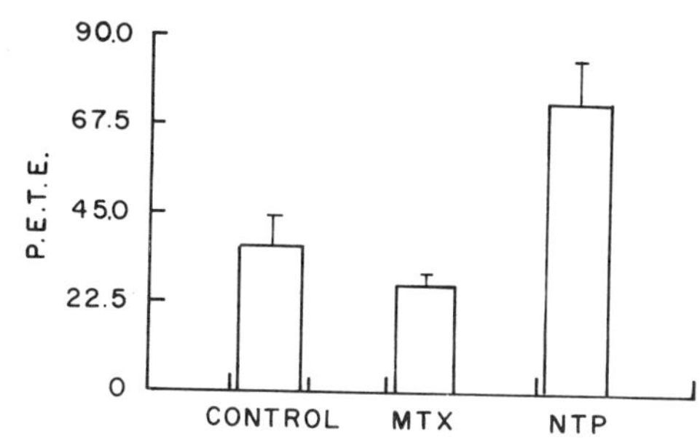

Figure 5. Summary of pulsatile energy transmission efficiency for CONTROL, MTX and NTP conditions.

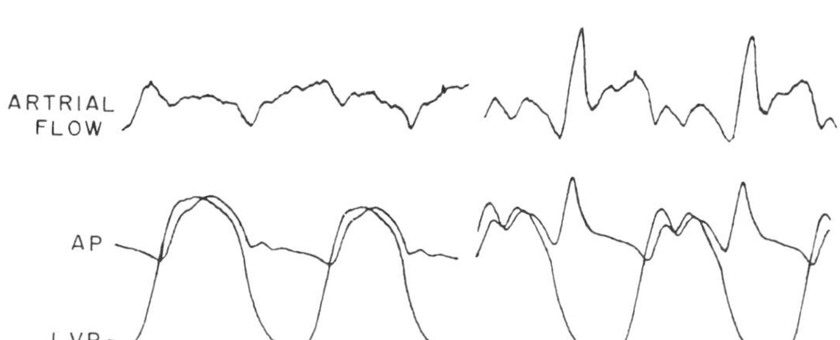

Figure 6. Coronary artery flow, left ventricular pressure (LVP) and aortic pressure (AP) measured during control (left) and brief diastolic counterpulsation (right).

DISCUSSION

Although the heart and arterial system may be each isolated for study and modeled as separate entities, they exist in a coupled state in the living animal. It is therefore important to understand the dynamic relationship between the two. Identifying such relationships is often done through the use of computer modeling so that complicated, multi-variable systems can be manipulated with relative ease and the responses analyzed. Animal experiments are necessary however, to update and evaluate the model predictions.

Many previous interaction studies considered only mean or steady-state values. They are limited therefore by the fact that the consequence of the dynamic LV-AS interaction cannot be obtained [8, 9]. Most interaction studies have also focused on systolic events; diastolic events were little studied.

Diastolic aortic pressure serves as the coronary perfusion pressure which governs, to some extent, the entrance flow. Thus, coronary flow during diastole is largely determined by the arterial system, particularly its compliance. Since the value of the compliance determines the amount of blood available for coronary flow, as well as the amount of wave reflections, the state of the arterial system feedbacks upon the heart, through coronary flow, and placing an effect on ventricular performance. This aspect of arterio-ventricular interaction has received little attention. Pulse wave reflections arriving in diastole can augment aortic pressure, thus increase the perfusion of the coronary arteries. This is important when flow is compromised as in the case of myocardial ischemia [10, 11]. The counterpulsation experiment demonstrated this. Properly timed reflected waves can therefore enhance the ventricular performance. Under differential loading conditions in the natural cardiovascular system, however, the pulsatile energy transmission efficiency is proportionally dependent on the amount of reflected waves [12, 13] which, like the pressure-dependent compliance [14, 15], serve as "feedback" effects on the heart.

CONCLUSION

Analysis of the heart-arterial system interaction needs to be dynamic in nature. Pressure-dependent arterial compliance and pulse wave reflections have feedback effects on the performance of the left ventricle.

Acknowledgment

I would like to thank my graduate students Pamela Geipel, David Berger and especially Ying Zhu.

DISCUSSION

Dr. E. Ritman: The reflected waves travel in one direction at any one time. Is that right?

Dr. J.K-J. Li: No. We have studied repeated reflections. These forward and reflected waves are actually the summation of individual forward and reflected waves which occur in different times throughout the cardiac cycle.

Dr. E. Ritman: I understand it is different in the different parts of the cardiac cycle but at any one time can the blood in your model flow in different directions?

Dr. J.K–J. Li: Yes.

Dr. E. Ritman: You are assuming that the heart is fixed in space, whereas in fact it may be moving around the blood. Yet the root of the aorta, perhaps not as much as the pulmonary artery or trunk, seems to move at times in the cardiac cycle as a sleeve over an arm so that the blood itself does not have to move as much as the actual heart or vessel wall around it. Can that be accounted for in this model in some fashion?

Dr. J.K–J. Li: No, we do not show any motion of the heart. We only look at pressure and flow.

Dr. D. Kass: Would you consider late systolic wave reflections to be detrimental?

Dr. J.K–J. Li: Wave reflection is necessary for normal cardiovascular function. We have shown it in a study we have just completed. We have shown that with preload and cardiac properties constant, the pressure generated by the heart is lower compared to without reflections. The systolic wave reflection is necessary for the proper function of the heart under normal conditions.

Dr. D. Kass: I am confused because late systolic wave reflections are usually shown to add a late bump to the end–systolic pressure. I am not sure what kind of systolic wave reflection this is. Most people have said that increase of late systolic load does not necessarily improve coronary perfusion. However, our data suggests otherwise.

Dr. J.K–J. Li: Late systolic reflection is actually detrimental to the failing heart during ejection. If one removes the reflection, under normal conditions the heart does not work as well.

Dr. D. Kass: Methoxamine is a systemic vasoconstrictor and it is presumably significantly effecting peripheral arterial resistance and, for that matter, coronary resistance and so it is a little more difficult to interpret. In the studies where we are bypassing the aorta, mean flow is identical. In some ways that is more analogous to what happens as systolic reflections occur since people's cardiac outputs do not fall because they have late systolic wave reflections. At least, I am not aware of data that there is a reduction.

Dr. J.K–J. Li: Late systolic reflection is necessary for the normal heart. But if you look at a heart that is not in normal conditions, either pressure overload or volume overload conditions, or even if the peripheral arterial system has changed, reflection is actually detrimental.

Dr. W. Welkowitz: One can produce the same effect as a reflected wave with assisted circulation by varying the timing. One can do that easily by using a balloon pump. One finds that the effect is very much dependent on the timing. In other words, one can maximize coronary flow with a certain timing. Incidentally, this is not the same timing that best unloads the heart. Thus, one has the choice of unloading the heart or maximizing coronary flow, but all reflected wave situations give you improved coronary flow. There is a certain narrow range that will.

Dr. D. Kass: With the counterpulsation balloon blowing up during systole, I would expect that you would acutely afterload the ventricle, and the net outflow for that beat would be less, so the effects are complicated by changes in instantaneous outflow. If you could somehow produce and time a wave reflection without changing outflow from the ventricle, so that you are only looking at the effect of a pressure wave coming back at various times in the cardiac cycle, then my prediction would be that it really will not matter when it comes back – with respect to the coronary flow change vs work load.

Dr. W. Welkowitz: It does. That is the interesting observation. Lets say the normal way of inflating is during diastole. One can then vary both the inflate time and deflate time so that you get a shifting of the waves in time due to the adjusting. One then finds that coronary flow changes radically, but only for certain timing arrangements. In other words, there is no uniformity. The system is very sensitive to the on–time and the off–time, or if you like, to the phase of the wave coming back to the ascending aorta.

Dr. L.E. Ford: The answer to the question of whether it was beneficial or detrimental might have to do with the operating conditions being considered. At rest it may be detrimental, but during exercise it might be beneficial. If the duration of systole shortens and the reflected wave comes back against a closed valve, it will not increase the load on the ventricle but it might increase coronary filling, in the same way that reflective waves are said to promote the backward flow of blood into the renal arteries. So it might not be a detriment to the ventricle when cardiac output has to be optimized, that is during exercise.

Dr. J. Spaan: How did you calculate the work of the forward wave and the backward wave?

Dr. J.K–J. Li: We have calculated the power associated with the forward wave and the reflected wave to demonstrate that pulsatile energy transmission efficiency is altered by reflections.

Dr. J. Spaan: Do you multiply the forward pressure and the forward flow waves for the forward wave, and the backward pressure wave and the backward flow wave for the backward wave?

Dr. J.K–J. Li: That is correct.

Dr. J. Spaan: That should not be allowed, because the work is pressure times flow and if you have the integral of that to measure average during a cycle, so then you have (P1 + P2) · (Q1 + Q2). If you are going to split that up to a P1·Q1 and a P2·Q2, you are left over with a double product.

Dr. J.K–J. Li: That works out because cross terms cancel out. They are instantaneously resolved forward and reflected pressure and forward and reflected flow and the power is product so you have instantaneous pressure times instantaneous flow.

Dr. J. Spaan: I do not think that what you are doing is appropriate but it is difficult to work that out. To have a product is always a little difficult.

Dr. J. Janicki: Concerning future work. The trend here is to try and make these models more and more realistic. I was wondering if you foresee the need to eventually add the effects of respiratory variations. For example, variations in intrathoracic pressure will affect both the preload and afterload to the left ventricle. I wonder what your thoughts are on this issue.

Dr. J.K–J. Li: We are working on the effects of pulsus paradoxus.

Dr. J. Janicki: But do you think this is something important to think about in these kind of models?

Dr. J.K–J. Li: Yes, perhaps.

Dr. N. Westerhof: You have to realize that forward and backward separation of pressure and flow is interesting to look at; but whether wave shapes means much in a quantitative sense is another matter. It is like input impedance and pressure–flow wave shape; it would appear as incorrect realization of the arterial system. So is the reflection coefficient a correct realization of the arterial system? Pressure and flow are a result of the interaction of heart and arterial system. That is a dangerous thing. Secondly, I do not know what separation of power means in all sorts of components. I will give another example. If you calculate power from LV pressure and cardiac output waveshapes, or from aortic pressure and cardiac output, you get exactly the same overall answer. However, if you separate it in an oscillatory and a mean component you get completely different answers. What does that mean? Therefore, I have a little hesitation to see what happens if you separate forward and backward power and what do we learn from it?

Dr. J.K–J. Li: If you look at pulsatile energy transmission, the net amount of this energy which is transmitted to the peripheral–vascular beds depends on wave reflections.

Dr. N. Westerhof: But what do you think happens to the reflected power?

Dr. J.K–J. Li: The reflected power is dissipated as the reflected wave has to go through the arterial system, encountering damping due to the viscous property of the walls as well as geometry changes.

REFERENCES

1. Li JK–J, Cui T, Drzewiecki G. A nonlinear model of the arterial system incorporating a pressure–dependent compliance. *IEEE Trans Biomed Eng* 1990; 37: 673–678.
2. Shroff SG, Janicki JS, Weber KT. Evidence and quantitation of left ventricular systolic resistance. *Am J Physiol* 1985; 249: H358–370.
3. Little WC, Freeman GL. Description of LV pressure–volume relations by time–varying elastance and source resistance. *Am J Physiol* 1987; 253: H83–90.
4. Li JK–J. *Arterial System Dynamics*. New York University Press, 1987.
5. Li JK–J. Time domain resolution of forward and reflected waves in the aorta. *IEEE Trans Biomed Eng* 1986; BME–33: 783–785.
6. Berger DS, Li JK–J, Laskey WK, Noordergraaf A. Repeated reflection of waves in the systemic arterial system. *Am J Physiol* 1993; 264: H269–H281.
7. Berger DS, Li JK–J Temporal relationship between left ventricular and arterial system elastances. *IEEE Trans Biomed Eng* 1992; 39: 404–410.
8. Van Huis GA, Sipkema P, Westerhof N. Coronary input impedance during cardiac cycle as determined by impulse response method. *Am J Physiol* 1987; 253: H317–324.
9. Toorop GP, Van den Horn GJ, Elzinga G, Westerhof N. Matching between feline left ventricle and arterial load. Optimal power or efficiency. *Am J Physiol* 1988; 254: 279–285.
10. Li JK–J, Welkowitz W, Zelano J, Molony DA, Kostis KB, Mackenzie JW. Effects of balloon inflation and deflation rates on global and regional ventricular performance. *Progr Artif Organs* 1983; pp 137–140.
11. Li JK–J. Regional left ventricular mechanics during myocardial ischemia. In: Sideman S and Beyar R (eds) *Simulation and Modeling of the Cardiac System*, NY: Martinus Nijhoff, 1986, pp 501–507.
12. Li JK–J. Increased pulse wave reflections and pulsatile energy loss in acute hypertension. *Angiol J Vasc Disease* 1989; 40: 730–735.
13. Zhu Y, Li JK–J, Drzewiecki G. Arterial compliance variation throughout the cardiac cycle. *Proc 14th IEEE Eng Med Biol Conf* 1992; pp 758–759.
14. Zhu Y. Hemodynamic Basis and Nonlinear Model Analysis of Hypertension and Aging. *MSc Thesis*, Rutgers University, NJ, 1993.
15. Li JK–J, Zhu Y. Arterial compliance and its pressure dependence in hypertension and vasodilation. *Angiology, J Vasc Dis* 1993; in press.

INTEGRATED ANALYSIS

CHAPTER 33

THE RELATIONSHIP BETWEEN ALTERED LOAD AND IMPAIRED DIASTOLIC FUNCTION IN CONSCIOUS DOGS WITH PACING INDUCED HEART FAILURE

Richard P. Shannon[1]

ABSTRACT

The complexities of diastolic dysfunction are being recognized with increasing frequency. Prior studies of diastolic dysfunction in both clinical disease states and experimental models have overlooked the major role which altered loading conditions may play in the evolution of diastolic dysfunction. In order to determine the relative importance of the multiple determinants of diastolic dysfunction in disease states requires a large animal model, suitable for chronic study in which the determinants can be controlled independently. This manuscript reviews recent work from our laboratory in which we investigated the mechanisms of diastolic dysfunction in conscious dogs with dilated cardiomyopathy induced by rapid ventricular pacing.

INTRODUCTION

The effects of altered load and contractile state on commonly employed indices of left ventricular (LV) function has been studied extensively in the normal myocardium [1–6]. However, when these very same indices are applied to the study of diastolic abnormalities in cardiovascular disease states, the influences of load and impaired contractility are often overlooked in favor of the assumption that intrinsic myocardial abnormalities, not altered load, are the dominant determinants of diastolic dysfunction. Such conclusions are based on the fact that the preponderance of data regarding diastolic dysfunction are derived from *in vitro* studies of isolated myocytes, trabeculae, or isolated heart preparations in which loading conditions can be controlled. However, when the intrinsic abnormalities in

---

[1]Cardiovascular Division, Beth Israel Hospital and the New England Regional Primate Research Center, One Pine Hill Drive, P.O. Box 9102, Southborough, MA 01772–9102, USA.

Interactive Phenomena in the Cardiac System, Edited by
S. Sideman and R. Beyar, Plenum Press, New York, 1993

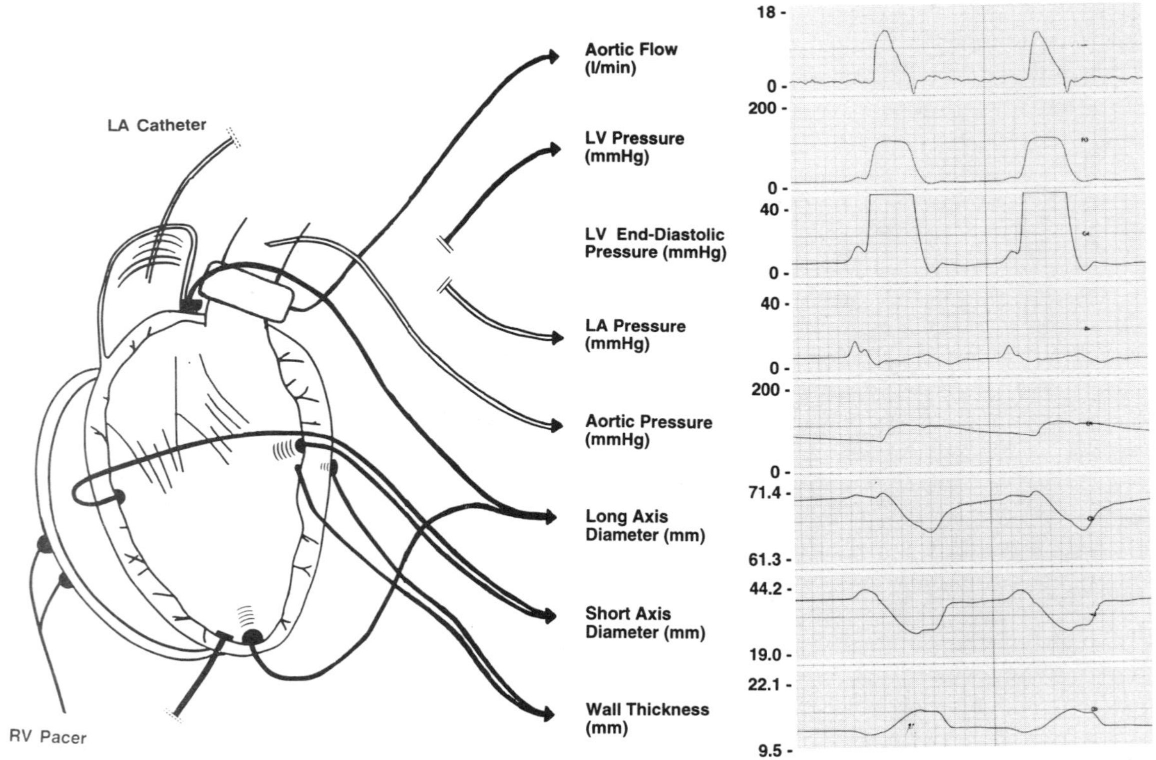

Figure 1. Schematic illustration and representative hemodynamic recordings from a dog studied at control.

myocardial calcium handling, which have been observed *in vitro* preparations, and alterations in the extracellular matrix are cast in the context of the intact, whole animal model, it is not intuitively clear whether abnormalities in calcium handling or altered loading conditions are the dominant influence.

Pacing induced heart failure in conscious dogs provides an experimental model suitable for chronic study with the additional advantage that myocardial tissues can be harvested at the time of sacrifice to assess intrinsic alterations in myocardial diastolic properties. In the present review, we discuss our findings relating to abnormalities in diastolic function and examine the contribution of the following major determinants of diastolic function: a) intracellular calcium handling, b) altered loading conditions, c) alterations in the extracellular matrix d) altered coronary blood flow.

METHODS

The findings reviewed here have been reported previously from our laboratory [7–9]. The observations were made essentially in 13 mongrel dogs who were instrumented as has been described previously [7, 8]. Figure 1 is a representative illustration of the instrumentation employed. All animals used in these studies were maintained according to the guidelines for the "Care and Use of Laboratory Animals" of the Institute of Laboratory Animal Resources, National Council (DHHS Publication No. [NIH] 85–23, revised 1985) and the Standing Committee on Animal Care of Harvard Medical School. The methods for measuring hemodynamics and data analysis as well as the methods for assessing the extracellular matrix have been described in detail previously [8]. Specifically, end diastolic and end systolic wall stress were measured and used as indices of LV loading conditions. After 3–4 weeks of rapid ventricular pacing when the animals had developed severe congestive heart failure, the elevated end systolic and end diastolic wall stresses were reduced to levels observed in the control state by rapid controlled hemorrhage (30–50 ml/min), under conditions in which heart rate was held constant by left atrial pacing [8].

Assessment of regional myocardial blood flow was made using radioactive microspheres in six sham operated controls and nine dogs studied as part of the diastolic dysfunction protocol. The technique has been described elsewhere [8].

Assessment of Intracellular Calcium Homeostasis [9]

Following the completion of the studies in the conscious state, six sham operated controls and nine dogs with pacing induced heart failure were sacrificed using pentobarbital anesthesia. Right ventricular trabeculae were harvested from each animal and prepared for *in vitro* organ bath studies. A subset of trabeculae were loaded with the bioluminescent indicator, aequorin, as previously described. The *in vitro* experiments were conducted with muscle stretched to L_{max} at 30°C and a pacing frequency of 0.33 mHz. Resting intracellular calcium levels were determined by the technique of fractional luminescence.

RESULTS

Intracellular Calcium Handling

Figure 2 reveals the prolongation in tension and aequorin light signals in sham operated control dogs and dogs with heart failure following 3–4 weeks of rapid ventricular pacing. However, the impairment in relaxation was not associated with a difference in

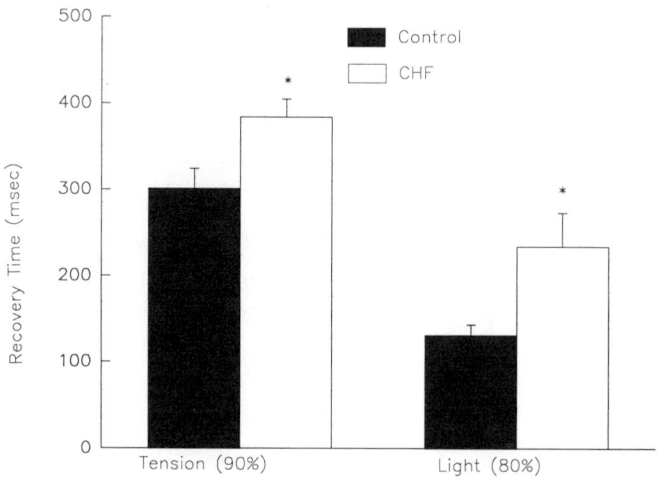

Figure 2. Prolongation in the tension and light signals in dogs with advanced heart failure compared to sham controls.

resting systolic calcium levels (control: 0.29 ± 0.05μM; CHF: 0.31 ± 0.05μM), as assessed by the method of fractional luminescence.

Relationship to Load

Figure 3 reveals the alterations in indices of diastolic function at control and then at 3–4 weeks following rapid ventricular pacing when severe symptomatic heart failure was manifest. Of note, there were significant prolongations in the time constant of isovolumic relaxation, determined by using three distinct mathematical models for assessing isovolumic relaxation. There was a similar marked increase in radial myocardial stiffness, but no significant difference in the coefficient of chamber stiffness normalized for wall volume. However, these impairments in both active and passive phases of diastole occurred in the setting of marked increases in end systolic and end diastolic wall stress as well as a significant decrease in LV dP/dt (control: 2865 ± 155 mmHg/s; CHF: 1539 ± 103 mmHg/s) and ejection fraction (control: 50 ± 3%; CHF: 28 ± 2%).

In order to ascertain the potential contribution of altered load to the impairment in diastolic function, we normalized the elevated loading conditions observed in dogs with advanced heart failure using rapid, controlled hemorrhage. Figure 4 reveals the effect of such normalization on diastolic function. With heart rate held constant, both the isovolumic relaxation time constant and radial myocardial stiffness constant returned to control levels in the dogs with CHF. Notably, the marked impairment in LV systolic function persisted. Thus the marked alterations in LV loading conditions observed during advanced heart failure contributed prominently to the observed impairment in diastolic function.

Importantly, there was no difference in the hydroxyproline or volume percent of myocardium occupied by collagen, nor in the ratio of type I to type III collagen. Thus, there were no significant differences in the type or content of collagen at this stage in the heart failure process.

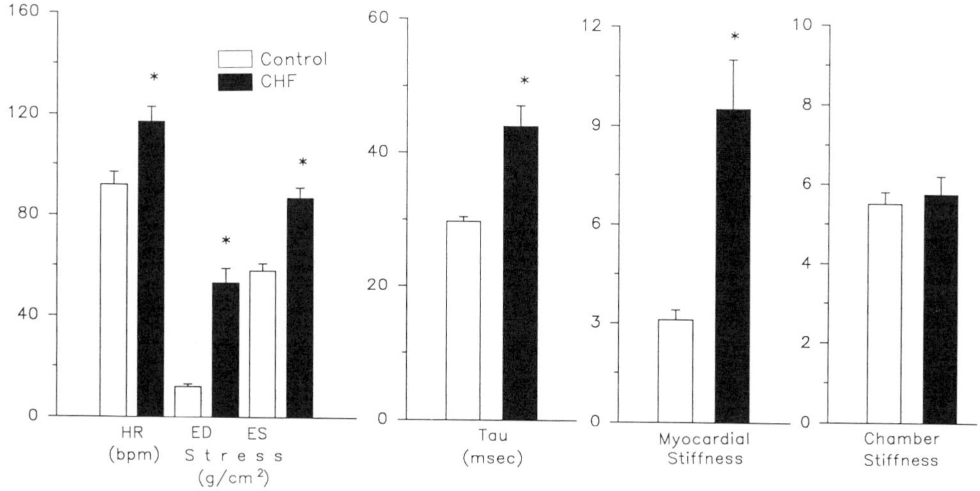

Figure 3. Changes in LV diastolic function at control and following three weeks of rapid pacing. There was significant prolongation of the isovolumic relaxation time constant and the radial myocardial stiffness constant.

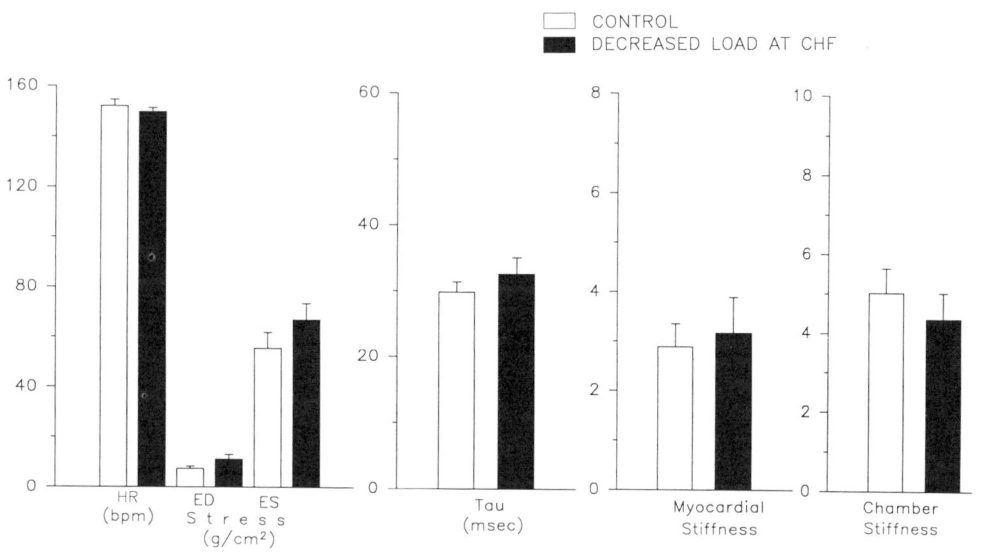

Figure 4. Changes in LV diastolic function at control and following three weeks of rapid pacing. With heart rate held constant, when the markedly elevated loading conditions observed in heart failure were reduced to levels observed in controls, there was no difference in the indices of diastolic function.

Alterations in Coronary Blood Flow

Figure 5 revels the relationship between altered myocardial loading conditions, myocardial perfusion, and abnormalities in diastolic function. At baseline, transmural coronary blood flow was significantly less in dogs with advanced heart failure (1.18 ± 0.11

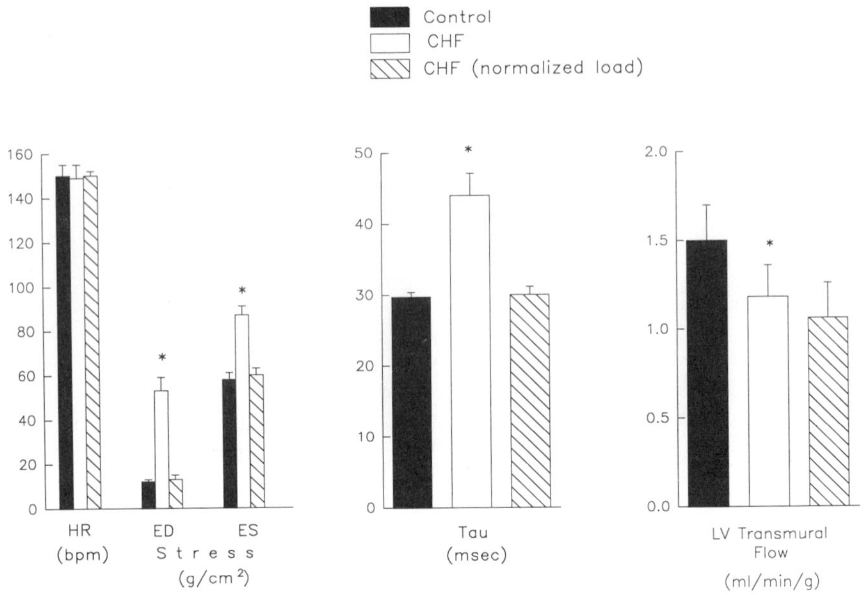

Figure 5. The relationship between the improvement in indices of diastolic function during normalization of load in heart failure and the changes in transmural myocardial blood flow. The improvement in diastolic function was associated with a further reduction in blood flow suggesting that myocardial ischemia was unlikely to explain the impaired diastolic function evident in heart failure.

ml/mm/g) compared to sham operated controls (1.50 ± 0.10 ml/mm/g). However, the endocardial/epicardial blood flow ratio (endocardial/epicardial) was not significantly different between the two groups (control: 1.31 ± 0.08; CHF: 1.15 ± 0.09). Thus, it was unlikely that the baseline reductions in coronary blood flow observed in dogs with heart failure represented myocardial ischemia as balanced transmural myocardial perfusion, as reflected by the endo/epi ratio, was maintained. Furthermore, when LV end diastolic wall stress was reduced to normal levels in the dogs with heart failure, average transmural myocardial blood flow was reduced further, suggesting that the improvement in diastolic function was not likely due to resolution of myocardial ischemia.

DISCUSSION

This manuscript summarizes the findings from our laboratory on the nature and extent of diastolic impairments in the canine model of dilated cardiomyopathy induced by rapid right ventricular pacing. We focus on the findings following 3–4 weeks of rapid pacing, which is a stage characterized by symptomatic heart failure and severe contractile dysfunction. The major findings include: 1) there are distinct abnormalities in intracellular calcium homeostasis which result in prolongation of the tension and light signals in trabecular strips harvested from dogs with severe symptomatic congestive heart failure after 3–4 weeks of pacing. The abnormalities are strikingly reminiscent of findings from trabeculae strips obtained from humans with end-stage cardiomyopathy. However, the prolongation in the dissipation of tension and light occurred despite the absence of significant differences in resting intracellular calcium. 2) Despite these significant abnormalities evident *in vitro* studies, the marked abnormalities in active and passive indices of diastolic function were reversible by normalizing the increases in end systolic and end diastolic stresses which accompanied advanced heart failure. Furthermore, the diastolic abnormalities appeared independent of changes in collagen type or content. 3) The abnormalities in diastolic function appeared to be independent of altered myocardial perfusion as coronary blood flow was reduced further during experiments in which load was normalized and diastolic function ameliorated.

The ability to make multiple measurements of diastolic function and ventricular geometry during the evolution of the heart failure process together with measurements of intracellular calcium handling *in vitro* are critical to establishing the relevance and contribution of the multiple abnormalities in the determinants of diastolic function observed in this model. Although the contribution of altered load and impaired contractility to abnormalities in diastolic function has been noted previously in normal myocardium, these data demonstrate that load is a major determinant of diastolic abnormalities in advanced symptomatic stages of heart failure in conscious dogs. These findings give rise to an interesting experimental paradigm in which the determinants of diastolic disfunction in heart failure are dynamic. We suggest that the mechanism of impaired diastolic function in early and advanced heart failure is increased ventricular load, which results in significant but importantly reversible forms of diastolic dysfunction. However, later in the heart failure process, myocardial ischemia may supervene perhaps related to impaired subendocardial flow reserve, which is itself a consequence of increased diastolic pressures and stresses. Once myocardial ischemia supervenes, there are associated changes in the extracellular matrix including myocyte necrosis and reparative fibrosis as well as potential further impairment in intracellular calcium regulation which may lead to irreversible, load independent, diastolic abnormalities.

The observation of the reversible nature of the diastolic abnormalities noted at this stage in the heart failure process raises questions as to the role of altered *in vitro* intracellular calcium handling, evident in the trabeculae harvested from these same dogs. One potential explanation is that the prolongation of tension and calcium signals is important in the maintenance of active tension for longer periods, required in the face of increased wall stress. Alternatively, these abnormalities may reflect early changes in calcium sequestration which may be accentuated later in the heart failure process and, at that point, serve a more dominant role in the diastolic abnormalities. Further studies will be required to reconcile these complex interactions. In addition, the findings reviewed in this manuscript underscore the importance of an integrative approach to the understanding of the role of diastolic abnormalities in disease states characterized by primary contractile abnormalities and ventricular dilatation.

Acknowledgements

The author wishes to thank Stephen F. Vatner, M.D. for his review of the manuscript. The work reviewed in this manuscript was supported in part by US Public Health Service grants HL 38070 and RR 00168.

DISCUSSION

Dr. F. Prinzen: The functional and structural abnormalities in your model of rapid ventricular pacing could be due to a combination of two factors, the high heart rate and ventricular pacing. You will not be amazed that I focus on the asynchronous activation of the ventricles, because of our experimental findings (Chapter 24). It was nice to see ultrastructure changes, especially at the sarcomere level. You see this fiber disarray type, which is also known to be caused by ventricular pacing at the normal heart rate *[Kaipawich et al., Am Heart J 1991;121:827–828]*.

Dr. R. Shannon: We do not know what the specific inciting events are. They occur very early. They are reversible early, but if one takes the animals out to 5–6 weeks, we find that it is not easily reversible. There is this reversible injury early, but ultimately there are changes which occur that are no longer reversible. Whether those ultrastructural changes reverse, I do not know.

Dr. F. Prinzen: Dr. Janicki has made (see Chapter 28) a distinction between physiological and pathological collagen development hypertrophy, whether or not collagen content is increased. You show a pathological change, without increase in collagen or in muscle mass.

Dr. R. Shannon: Correct. At this stage we see neither increase in mass nor increase in the extracellular matrix. But there are rather dramatic ultrastructural changes. In Dr. Janicki's and Dr. Weber's experience, if one waits 5–6 weeks, one actually sees changes at the light microscopic level. It may be just a different, more advanced, point in the evolution. I do not think they see increases in mass at that point, which is a very peculiar feature and may well relate to the nature of the insult.

Dr. J. Janicki: The group in South Carolina reported significant myocardial edema in this model *[Spinale et al. Am J Physiol 1991; 261: H308–H318]*. I wonder if you saw similar increases in water. That itself could explain a lot of the diastolic functional changes.

Dr. R. Shannon: We did not look at it specifically. However, I do not think, if that were the case, that edema would be so readily reversible with normalization of the load.

Dr. J. Janicki: I was surprised at the amount of excess water they obtained. With regard to collagen, your results agree well with what we saw when we removed myocardial collagen; we both observed ventricular dilatation. Perhaps at a later time with, for example, activation of the renin–angiotensin system, you would get an abnormal accumulation of collagen and diastolic dysfunction.

Dr. E.L. Yellin: This is a very nice comprehensive study dealing with many aspects of the failure model. If you walked into a physician's office with a heart rate of 150 you would most probably be considered to have some kind of a dysfunction. But if you walked into physician's office with a heart rate of 150 immediately after you were exercising, you would be functioning fine. The idea of saying you improve or correct diastolic dysfunction by unloading the dog is fallacious. The reason the dog was operating at a high pressure and a high volume was because that was the only way the cardiac output could be maintained, so it really was not dysfunctional, it was functional, and when you unloaded, you probably were not getting the cardiac output that was required, but you were getting normal stresses.

Dr. R. Shannon: That is correct. You see a dramatic fall in cardiac output if one normalizes the load. It has something to do with the nature of pacing the right ventricle, although it can be reproduced by atrial pacing, as well as the fact that it is chronic. We never exercised the dogs for 24 hours and all the changes occurred by one day of rapid pacing, so it is peculiar, and I do not know that I understand it.

Dr. E.L. Yellin: Saying that you correct dysfunction by unloading the ventricle leads to an incorrect approach. You did not correct anything. You just forced the animal to function at a lower load; the diastolic function looked normal, but the cardiac output was low. Therefore it was not normal.

Dr. R. Shannon: I do not disagree. It is for precisely that reason that *in vitro* studies like the work we have done with Dr. J. Morgan do not provide the entire picture. If one can reproduce the same diastolic prolongation and radial–myocardial stiffness by simply loading a ventricle, does that imply an intrinsic abnormality in that ventricle, or is that simply a phenomenon of the load that is required to maintain cardiac output at that state. That is the point we are trying to make. I do not disagree with you. If you take a normal heart, you can make the indices abnormal by applying a similar load.

Dr. D. Allen: Regarding the intriguing calcium transient with the strange bump at the end: You said that the bump was sensitive to calcium channel blockers, but of course so is the peak under normal conditions. Are you saying that the bump is *selectively* sensitive to calcium channel blockers?

Dr. R. Shannon: Yes. The bump, or second component, persists in the presence of ryandine. One can eliminate the peak impressive early calcium transient with ryandine, but it does not eliminate the second component which is eliminated by verapamil. That is the basis of this statement.

Dr. T. Arts: You are working at a very high heart rate. Generally, at higher heart rates the valves are less efficient. Do you have an idea about aortic valve function? Maybe your overloading is partly caused by the fact that the heart is pumping more than you can see from the measured cardiac output.

Dr. R. Shannon: I do not have information on valve competence or flow during rapid right ventricular pacing. It is no small feat, using these very sophisticated crystals, to actually make very precise measurements at that rapid rate. But it could be done.

REFERENCES

1. Karliner JS, LeWinter MM, Mahler F, Engler R, O'Rourke RA. Pharmacologic and hemodynamic influences on the rate of isovolumic left ventricular relaxation in the normal conscious dog. *J Clin Invest* 1977; 60: 511–521
2. Gaasch WH, Blaustein AS, Andrias CW, Donahue RP, Avitall B. Myocardial relaxation. II. Hemodynamic determinants of rate of left ventricular isovolumic pressure decline. *Am J Physiol* 1980; (*Heart Circ Physiol* 8) 239: H1–H6.
3. Gaasch WH, Carroll JD, Blaustein AS, Bing OHL. Myocardial relaxation: effects of preload on the time course of isovolumetric relaxation. *Circulation* 1986; 73(5): 1037–1041.
4. Bahler RC, Martin P. Effects of loading conditions and inotropic state on rapid filling phase of left ventricle. *Am J Physiol* 1985; 248: H523–H533.
5. Cheng C–P, Freeman GL, Santamore WP, Constantinescu MS, Little WC. Effect of loading conditions, contractile state, and heart rate on early diastolic left ventricular filling in conscious dogs. *Circ Res* 1990; 66: 814–823.
6. Blaustein AS, Gaasch WH. Myocardial relaxation. VI. Effects of β–adrenergic tone and asynchrony on LV relaxation rate. *Am J Physiol* 1983; (*Heart Circ Physiol* 13) 244: H417–H422.
7. Shannon RP, Komamura K, Stambler BS, Manders WT, Vatner SF. Alterations in myocardial contractility in conscious dogs with dilated cardiomyopathy. *Am J Physiol* 1991; 260: H1903–H1911.
8. Komamura K, Shannon RP, Pasipoularides A, Ihara T, Lader AS, Patrick TA, Bishop SP, Vatner SF. Alterations in left ventricular diastolic function in conscious dogs with pacing–induced heart failure, *J Clin Invest* 1992; 89: 1825–1838.
9. Perreault CL, Shannon RP, Komamura K, Vatner SF, Morgan JP. Abnormalities in intracellular calcium regulation and contractile function in myocardium from dogs with pacing–induced heart failure. *J Clin Invest* 1992; 89: 932–938.

CHAPTER 34

INTERACTIONS: THE INTEGRATED FUNCTIONING OF HEART AND LUNGS

Eric A. Hoffman[1]

ABSTRACT

The heart and lungs are two dynamic organ systems functioning in a highly integrated inter–relationship within the unique negative pressure environment of the intact thorax. Noninvasive imaging techniques have afforded us the opportunity to study the interdependence of these two organ structures with evaluation focused both on intra and inter organ relationships. It is through a recognition of these interdependent phenomena that one begins to appreciate their importance to the prediction of the total mechanical response of the cardiopulmonary system when piecing together individual response characteristics determined with components of the system held in isolation. Highlights of a number of measurements made from what has been termed dynamic and electron beam x–ray CT as well as recent work utilizing magnetic resonance imaging (MRI) are presented. Our earlier work related to the intracardiac interrelationships serving to maintain the heart at a near constant volume throughout the cardiac cycle. Here we will expand to include heart–lung and lung–heart interactions as they affect both cardiac and pulmonary function. The overall theme is systems integration serving to dictate function and functional efficiency.

BACKGROUND: INTRACARDIAC EFFECTS

The Total Heart Volume

Within the intrathoracic, fetal milieu, whereby the lungs and the uterus are fluid filled, the fetal heart must develop so as to circulate blood through the systemic vascular bed while surrounded by the noncompressible pulmonary structures. This marks the beginning of heart–lung and lung–heart interactions. To investigate how this early environment might affect global cardiac mechanics after birth, perhaps by dictating

---

[1]Department of Radiology, University of Iowa College of Medicine, Iowa City, IA 52242, USA.

myocardial fiber organization, we have evaluated what we have termed the total heart volume. This is defined as the contents of the pericardial sac. Using anesthetized dogs scanned in the Dynamic Spatial Reconstructor [1], we have demonstrated that the total heart volume throughout the cardiac cycle remains within 5% of the end–diastolic (ED) value [2]. This relationship can be seen in Fig. 1, whereby a volume drop between end–diastole and end–systole is consistently limited to 5% or less of the total ED volume of the heart. Although our measurements have been validated to be accurate to ±5%, the repeatability of the volume drop across animals and species along with the smooth transition between diastole and systole and back has lead us to believe that this small variation is real and not simply noise in the measurement. This relationship was also found in awake normal human volunteers scanned via MRI. Here [3], 3 mm thick contiguous (interleaved acquisition) spin echo images were gathered to measure the total heart volume. The gated scan sequence took approximately 2.5 hours total scanning time. As in the dogs, there was a consistent drop in total heart volume through systole, but the total volume stayed within 4% of the ED heart volume throughout the cycle. The constant heart volume relationship is maintained largely through a reciprocal emptying and filling of the atria and ventricles with the epicardial apex remaining fixed in space as the atrio–ventricular valve plane moves in as a piston, descending towards the apex in systole.

To understand the regional wall motion associated with the maintenance of heart volume constancy, we employed a magnetic resonance tagging technique referred to as SPAMM [4]. The protons are double flipped in planes, realigning them with the primary magnetic field. Thus, in these planes, the myocardium reconstructs as black (no signal). With panes established in two orthogonal directions, simultaneously, the reconstructed images of the heart appear to have a mesh of black stripes. Since this striping is due to the local proton characteristics of the myocardium, as the myocardium contracts, the stripes distort. By tracking the stripe intersections, we can map myocardial motion [5]. Through this process, we have found that the basal myocardium twists, untwists, and then moves inwards in systole. Contrarily, apical myocardium shows a twisting and inwards motion throughout systole. It is the untwisting at the base of the heart in systole without a concomitant untwisting at the apex which presumably contributes to the pulling down of the valve plane.

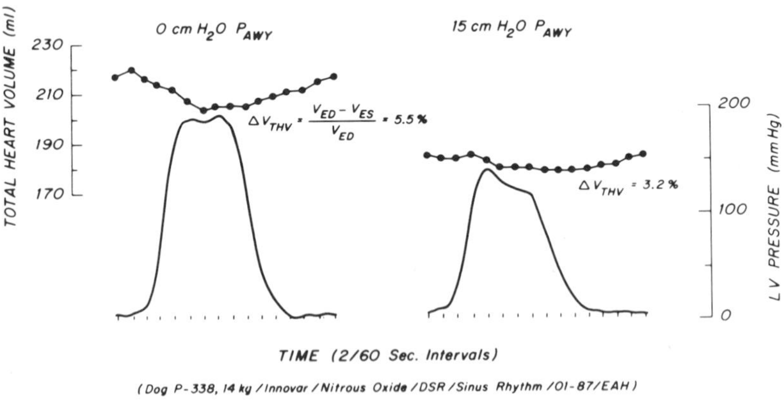

Figure 1. Intracardiac integration. Variation in total heart volume (cardiac cycle dependence): Total heart volume plotted as a function of intracardiac cycle phase. Lungs were held at 0 and 15 cm H_2O airway pressure. (Dog P–338, 14 kg/Innovar/Nitrous Oxide/DSR/Sinus Rhythm/01–87/EAH.)

It is clear that when one scans a short axis plane of the heart, with the scanning plane fixed in the universe, the original myocardial plane of interest moves in systole out of the scanning plane towards the apex. We adapted a scanning protocol, first discussed by Rogers et al. [6], and added the SPAMM scanning sequence. We added two selective pre–saturation regions 20 msec prior to the standard SPAMM sequence. These two 4 cm wide regions were parallel, and their edges were approximately 8 mm apart. Because the longi–tudinal magnetization of these regions were set to zero before tagging, tags were only present in the 8 mm unaffected region. Following tagging and broad band presaturations, 8 mm thick images were acquired at the short axis spatial location of the unaffected region. This experiment was repeated, moving the selected slice, 4 mm at a time, from the base towards the apex. Because the slice was being moved into an untagged region, the tags gradually disappeared from the initial slice level. If the tagged plane appeared at a later point in time at a more apical short axis level, they originated from the initial 8 mm region, and underwent displacement into the initially saturated region. In this manner, we were able to piece together, albeit laboriously, a representative short axis temporal sequence which depicted the motion of the basal myocardium through its apical descent through systole, assuming cycle to cycle repeatability of cardiac motion. The difference in motion of the myocardium as assessed via a fixed location in space versus the motion seen following the actual descent of the short axis slice is depicted in Fig. 2. In each of the two panels, the septal wall of the left ventricle (LV) is to the left and the free wall is to the right. Motion is tracked by forming non–overlapping triangles [7] from sets of three tag intersection points and triangle centroid motion is depicted with the ED point shown as a dot with the

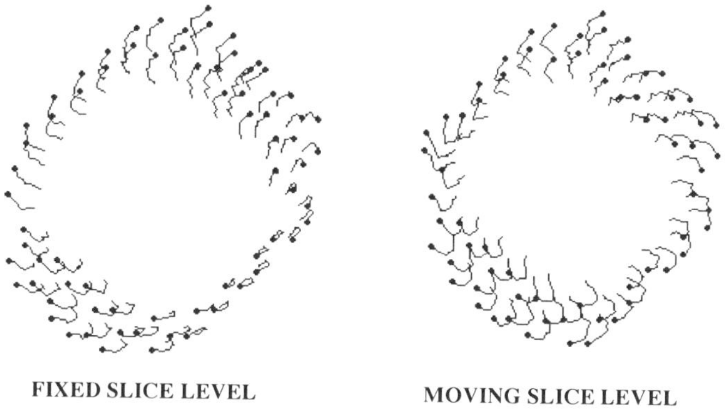

Figure 2. Interaction of muscle fiber orientation and electrical activation sequencing. SPAMM was used to lay down two orthogonal sets of stripes within a basal short axis section of myocardium. The stripes distort as the heart moves with systolic events. Stripe intersections are located, and a delaunay triangulation is used to form a set of non–overlapping triangles. The centroids of the triangles are tracked throughout systole and displayed with solid circles representing a triangle's ED centroid location, and the tail of each circle represents the motion of that circle location as it moves through systole. We track a basal slice through its descent towards the apex in systole **(right panel)**: this tracked or "moving" short axis slice is compared short axis location tracked at a fixed point in the universe through systole **(left panel)**. Panels represent the septal myocardium on the left and the LV free wall on the right. When the muscle is followed throughout its apical descent (right panel), the motion is fairly uniform around the wall. Note the two phases of motion at this level: the myocardium twists (approximately 5–7 degrees) in one direction in early systole and untwists in late systole. This twisting and untwisting can be seen in both images, but it is more pronounced when one correctly follows the myocardium through its apical descent.

tail representing motion in systole. Note that the LV freewall, as viewed at a fixed level in space, appears to be akinetic while motion is fairly uniform around the wall when the true myocardial motion is followed in three dimensions. Furthermore, note that the twisting and untwisting which we had previously [3] noted to occur at the base is not only present when following true 3D motion, but in fact the magnitude of untwisting is more pronounced. Total twist is on the order of 5–7 degrees, and the apical descent of the short axis is on the order of 1.5–2.0 cm. It is the untwisting which we believe to be important in atrio–ventricular interactions. Greenbaum et al. [8] have demonstrated three distinct layers of fibers, based upon orientation angle, at the base of the heart and two at the apex. This may or may not be coincident to the three versus two phases of motion that we find at the base and apex, respectively.

Atrial Stiffness and Ventricular Afterload

In a second series of dog studies, when anesthetized with inovar and nitrous oxide, the dogs were in atrial fibrillation for the first hour or so of anesthesia and then either spontaneously converted to sinus rhythm or were convertible, surprisingly, via xylocain. In sinus rhythm with lungs held at 0 cm H_2O airway pressure during DSR scanning, the mean change in total heart volume between end–diastole and end–systole was 3% while in atrial fibrillation, the mean change was 9%.

We have previously shown that a feature of the normal functioning of the heart in sinus rhythm in both dogs [2] and humans [3] is the phenomena of the epicardial apex remaining fixed in space while the atrio–ventricular (A–V) valve plane moves in a piston like motion towards the apex in systole. In Fig. 3, we demonstrate how the A–V valve plane motion is altered in atrial fibrillation. Mid–long axis sections through the LV are

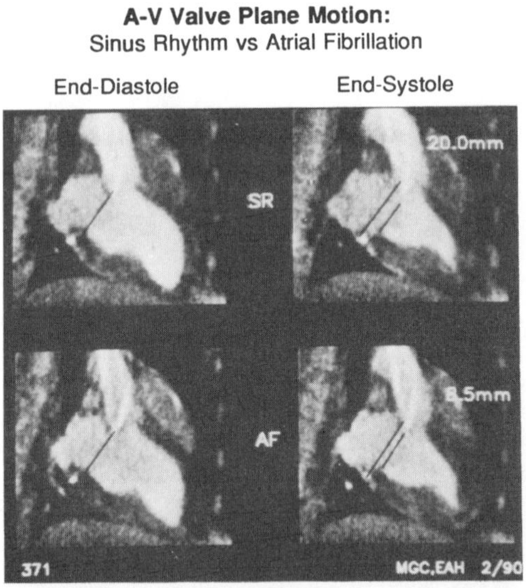

Figure 3. Atrio–ventricular interaction. AV–V valve plane motion: sinus rhythm vs atrial fibrillation: Mid sagittal sections calculated from a volumetric dynamic spatial reconstructor scan of a dog in (AF) and out (SR) of atrial fibrillation. Heart rate was maintained constant between the two conditions by pacing using a bipolar coronary sinus pacing catheter. A line is drawn in space at the mitral valve plane in the ED images and then transferred to the associated end–systolic (ES) picture. In the ES images, a second, more apical line denotes the ES position of the mitral valve plane. Note that the valve plane moves only 8.5 mm towards the apex in systole during atrial fibrillation while it moves 20.0 mm without atrial fibrillation.

depicted at ED (left column) and ES (right column) in sinus rhythm (upper row) and atrial fibrillation (bottom row). In the left column we have drawn a line in space at the level of the A–V valve plane. In the right column we have drawn the same line at the same point in space and than have added a second line at the new location of the valve plane. Note that in the case of SR, the valve plane moved 20 mm while in the same dog in AF the valve plane moves only 8.5 mm. This valve plane motion reduction was a consistent finding in dogs with atrial fibrillation, suggesting that atrial stiffness may play a significant role in ventricular afterload by resisting the LV "wringing" based long axis shortening.

Suga and colleagues [9, 11] have shown, using an isolated LV preparation as a model of LV contraction, that the P–V relationship along with an estimate of ventricular volume at zero pressure can be used to calculate the total work of the LV. They have described this work as the time–varying elastance model. Later work [10] has shown that a strong linear correlation exists between total work and MVO_2 as well as myocardial blood flow (MBF). The model has been useful in studying cardiac performance under a number of conditions and is well–validated through a number of techniques including dynamic CT [12]. Since MBF and MVO_2 correlate with the work of the heart, then abnormal circumstances (i.e. increased atrial stiffness where the P–V derived relationships no longer serve to reflect total work of the heart), will be reflected in an alteration of the slope of the total work vs. MBF (or MVO_2) relationship.

To test this hypothesis, we studied seven dogs [13] with the goal being to measure myocardial blood flow using a contrast dilution technique [14] and total work estimated using the pressure–volume relationship derived from the volumetric images. These dogs were scanned in the Dynamic Spatial Reconstructor while in atrial fibrillation and after conversion, with heart rate maintained constant across conditions via pacing with a bipolar pacing catheter placed in the coronary sinus. The goal was not to study true sinus rhythm, but rather to understand the potential role atrial stiffness might play in ventricular afterload. As Murphy's law would have it, three out of the four dogs reverted to sinus rhythm before we could begin scanning and never converted back into atrial fibrillation. Of the four that were in atrial fibrillation during scanning, one dog had a significantly different filling pressure in sinus rhythm versus atrial fibrillation. Of the remaining three dogs, we were able to make a very interesting, albeit small, set of observations. From the predicted total work using the pressure–volume loops in atrial fibrillation as compared with sinus rhythm for volumetric measurements of both the LV and the right ventricle (RV), total work was consistently less, on the order of 20%, in atrial fibrillation as compared with paced sinus rhythm. On the other hand, as total work was found to be less in atrial fibrillation, myocardial blood flow estimated from time intensity curves in the LV free wall was found to be greater in atrial fibrillation as compared to paced sinus rhythm by an average of 16%. This suggests a dissociation between calculated total work and myocardial blood flow. These data serve to highlight the importance of considering atrial–ventricular interactions when evaluating ventricular afterload. Under pathologic states, atrial stiffness in addition to aortic pressure may serve to impede ventricular emptying and to contribute to ventricular myocardial work of contraction.

Atrial Baffles: An Added Ventricular Afterload?

With the notion that a constant total heart volume (±5%) is an index of the normal, integrated functioning of the heart in the intact thorax, coupled with the findings that in dogs atrial fibrillation disrupts the constant total heart volume (THV) relationship, we have turned our attention to congenital heart disease where repairs entail placement of a non–compliant baffle into the atria. We have selected hypoplastic left heart syndrome (HLHS)

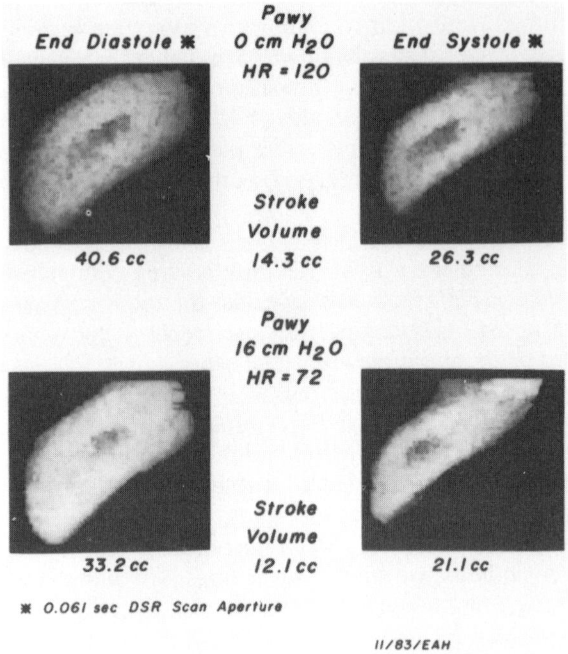

Figure 4. Heart–lung interaction—geometry of LV with lung inflation (dog 11.4 kg, supijne, anesthetized): Shaded surface displays of the LV cavity at ED and ES of an intact anesthetized dog with the heart scanned via the DSR while lungs were held at an airway pressure (Pawy) of 0 and 16 cm H_2O. Note that the LV volume is reduced with lung inflation at both ED and ES. This was accompanied by a consistent reduction in overall heart volume and RV volume.

with staged repair leading to the Fontan procedure, and transposition of the great arteries with a mustard or senning procedure. These two abnormalities complement each other in that the final surgical repairs result in either a single ventricle (Post Fontan) or a ventricular pair (Post Mustard or Senning) connected to an atrial system tethered by the presence of interposed baffling.The state of the art in the field of imaging has clearly developed to a point whereby we can now begin to assess not only the "plumbing", but we can now begin to evaluate the mechanical functioning of the heart. Perhaps the disruption of the constant THV relationship is an index of inefficiency; it is certainly an index of an abnormal integration of the cardiac components.

Fogel et al. have to date [15] prospectively studied 28 single ventricle patients with a mean age of 41 months; 23 had morphologic functional single RVs and five had morphologic functional single LVs. Subjects were studied to evaluate changes in cardiac mechanics as assessed via SPAMM tagging of three short axis levels spanning base to apex to test the hypothesis that mechanics will significantly change through the steps of a staged fontan procedure. Findings have lead to the demonstration that indeed significant changes in regional wall mechanics take place throughout the staged repair [15]. With increased attention to the mechanical properties of the heart throughout staged surgical procedures, we now have the tools to better understand the mechanisms behind our successes and failures and we may be able to influence the long term viability of the single ventricle.

Effects of the Lung on the Heart

Early studies of the DSR were designed to show the effect of lung inflation on the heart and we showed that lung inflation served to decrease the total heart volume at all phases of the cardiac cycle as seen in the right panel of Fig. 1. Both the RV and the LV ED volumes were reduced. Although LV stroke volume was reduced with lung inflation, as depicted in Fig. 4, ejection fraction was preserved. It was concluded that the drop in cardiac output, in the case of static lung inflation maneuvers, was due to decreased ED volume. With lung inflation, at the smaller heart volume, the percent change in total heart volume through the cardiac cycle was reduced. Although the ejection fraction was low at both lung volumes in this study, the ejection fraction remained the same with and without lung inflation indicating that the fall in stroke volume was primarily due to the loss of pre-load (ED volume). The study lead us to the notion that lung inflation gated to systole and lung exhalation during diastole might serve as a LV assist device, using the naturally occurring interaction between heart and lungs.

In theory, cardiac-cycle specific changes in intra-thoracic pressure should have effects on both ventricular preload and afterload, and potentially improve cardiac performance. Some current theories of the mechanism of closed-chest "cardiac massage" rely on such an explanation. Such changes have in fact been studied and documented by Pinsky and his colleagues [16, 17]. They studied the effect of cardiac cycle-specific jet ventilation in a dog model of acute ventricular failure. Success of cardiac gated respiration was not obtainable in the normal heart in Pinsky's studies. To study this phenomena using a non-invasive imaging technique, we have developed a respirator whereby a single board computer is programmed by macros to control a bank of high frequency needle valves and gated to external signals allowing for the creation of any respiratory wave form desired. We were able to use electron beam x-ray CT (Imatron 20) to evaluate the ventricular stroke volume and cardiac mechanics. Two representative images are shown in Fig. 5 demonstrating a fixed diaphragm during apnea for comparison with diaphragm descent timed to systole. Through physical slewing of the animal in the scanner, we were able to scan with the imaging plane along the true LV short axis and thus we were able to accurately identify the division of the atria and ventricles for ventricular volume measurements.

We measured stroke volumes, ejection fraction, wall motion, and myocardial blood flow with the electron beam CT scanner [18]. Carotid blood flow was monitored with an ultrasonic probe. In 6 mongrel dogs, inspiration gated to cardiac contraction significantly increased ejection fraction (13.4% ± 6.5%, $p<0.001$), stroke volume (3.7 ± 2.7 cc/stroke, $p<0.001$) and cardiac output (37% ± 28%, $p<0.001$) over standard ventilation. Neither carotid blood flow nor heart rate changed significantly. Presumably carotid flow remained constant through an autoregulation mechanism. The cardiac chambers were contrast enhanced, and stroke volumes under the two conditions were calculated from the multislice imaging studies without the need for invasive procedures. Note that even in the normal, healthy (anesthetized) heart cardiac gated respiration can serve as an effective LV assist device through heart lung interaction.

In this particular example, an understanding of the interactions of heart and lung brought about through non-invasive detection techniques such as ultrafast volumetric imaging may yield important new patient management approaches. A recurrent problem in the medical and surgical intensive care population is the patient with co-existent respiratory and cardiac failure. These patients are supported with positive pressure ventilation (usually standard volume cycled ventilation), inotropic infusions, and not infrequently with mechanical cardiac assist devices such as the intra-aortic balloon pump or the ventricular assist device. Inotropic infusions have inherent risks and benefits. While they may improve

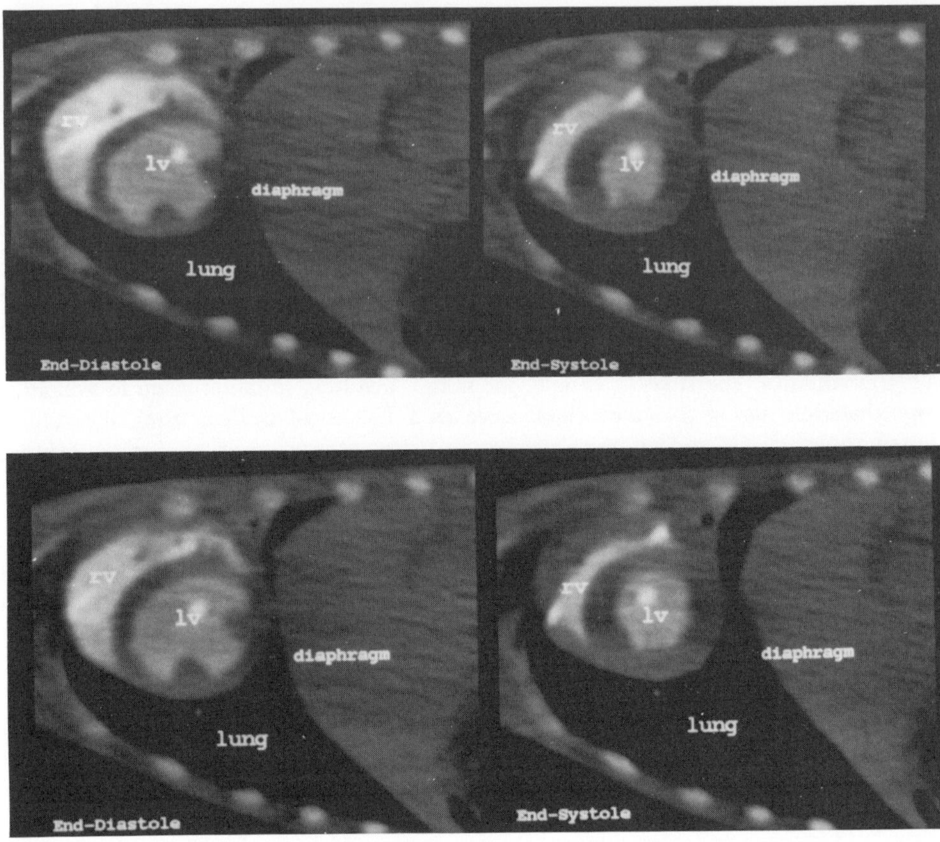

Figure 5. Heart–Lung Interaction: These images depict an electron beam CT based image data set where the short axis of the heart was directly scanned by slewing the dog in the scanner and dynamically scanning during apnea **(top)** and again during cardiac gated respiration with lung inflation gated to systole **(bottom)**. Note the constant location of the diaphragm in apnea and the caudal shift of the diaphragm during systole with systolic gated respiration.

perfusion to the cardiac and cerebral circulation, there may be detrimental effects in the pulmonary or splanchnic circulations. Devices such as the IABP or VAD necessitate intra–vascular placement of a foreign body with the attendant risk of infection or vascular injury. An alternative may be the naturally occurring interaction between the lungs and the heart.

EFFECT OF THE HEART ON THE LUNGS

Pulmonary Blood Flow

On the pulmonary side of the heart lung interactions, a number of studies of our own and others have lead us to the belief that gravity and the intrathoracic position of the heart are determinants of regional lung expansion (and ventilation) while gravity and vascular conductance are determinants of regional perfusion. Because of the non–

overlapping parameters between ventilation and perfusion (heart position and vascular conductance) it may be possible to modify one of the two parameters without modifying the other and thus cause a mismatch in the ventilation/ perfusion relationship. To study regional distribution of pulmonary blood flow, we have again used electron beam CT. Blood flow and its parameters can be calculated by applying an appropriate blood flow model to samples of regional lung density changes and changes in the feeding vessel caused by contrast passage [19]. Assuming a sharp enough bolus, such that the amount of contrast enhanced blood leaving a region is minimal prior to the full bolus arrival, blood flow can be calculated using equations derived from conventional microsphere approaches to blood flow analysis [19], as described by Wolfkeil et al. [27].

To express blood flow per gram of parenchyma, we assume the region of interest (ROI) to be composed of air and "water" (i.e. blood + parenchyma) [22, 23]. Because of the disparate densities of these two components, we can use the CT gray scale values (Hounsfield number) of the images to calculate the fraction of each component in the ROI.

The water fraction, for example, can be calculated by subtracting the CT value of pure air from the mean CT value of a ROI to give a number relating to the amount (density) of parenchyma + blood present in the selected region. Because of the linear relationship between Hounsfield number and density, comparing this value to the continuum ranging from pure water (Hounsfield number = 0) to pure air (Hounsfield number = −1024) yields the percentage of the ROI which is water (parenchyma + blood). The air fraction of an ROI, then, is simply 1.0 − "water" fraction. Furthermore, the amount of blood present within the ROI can be computed by comparing the area under the "time–intensity" curve of the ROI to the area under the curve in the feeding vessel. To the extent that the area under the ROI curve is less than the curve in pure blood, the ratio of the curves gives the percentage blood volume in the region of interest. Subtracting this result from the water fraction leaves the percentage of the ROI which is lung parenchyma. Multiplying the percentage of parenchyma, the number of voxels in the ROI, and the voxel dimension finally yields the volume of parenchyma in cm^3 (grams).

As demonstrated in Fig. 6, our findings have shown that, in the right lung, there is a significant ventral–dorsal gradient in regional blood flow in the supine body posture and the gradient is reduced or eliminated in the prone body posture [24]. Of note in these two panels is the fact that the significant relationship between parenchymal blood flow and lung height (slope of −1.71 and r = −0.73) is not simply reversed with shift in body posture from supine to prone (slope of −0.54 and r = −0.49). While 73 percent of the variability in parenchymal blood flow in the supine posture is explained by lung height, only 49% is explained in the prone posture. In both postures, the coefficient of variation in the data was 31. These findings were typical of all dogs studied and data suggest that a direct gravitational effect on the lung is not the sole, or even primary, explanation for non uniform distribution of blood flow to the lungs. This finding is consistent with our original hypothesis: In the dog, as shown in Fig. 7 through the maximum intensity projections of a volumetric electron beam CT scan of the thorax, the arterial branching pattern is such that the major pulmonary vessel is the one traveling from the hilum to the dorsal–basal lung region of the lower lobe. (see figure legend for description of anatomic orientation of images) Thus, when the dog is supine, conductance might be expected to drive blood to the dependent lung region [25] while gravity also drives blood down. This combines to produce a significantly larger flow in the dependent than the non–dependent lung region. In the prone body posture, gravity drives blood down while conductance drives blood up, and the combined effect is a more uniform ventral–dorsal distribution of flow. The surprising finding from our studies to date is that the significant prone versus supine blood flow difference seems to hold true only for the right lung. In the left lung, the slope of the regression describing

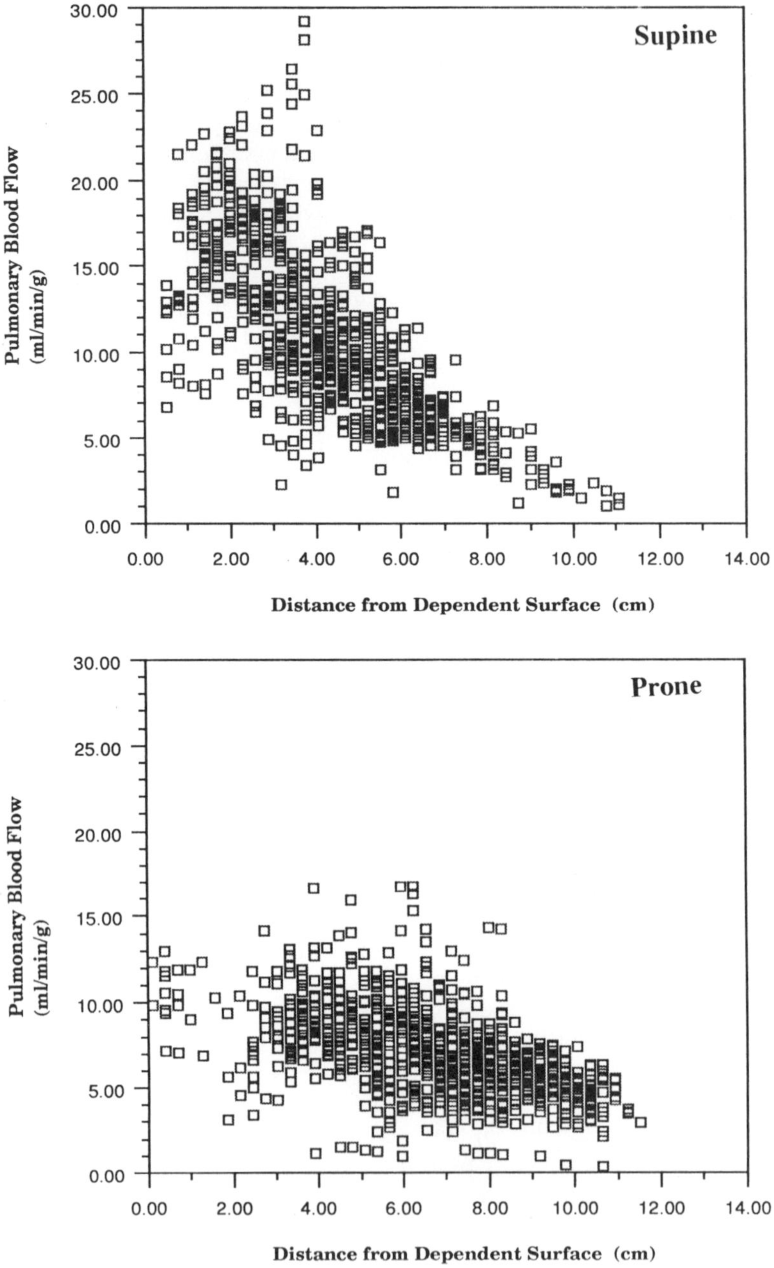

Figure 6. Distribution of pulmonary blood flow was sampled via electron beam CT scanning during passage of contrast material through the lungs. Data is representative of anesthetized dogs studied supine **(top)** and prone **(bottom)**. Blood flow data from 3x3 voxel (0.008 ml) samples are plotted as a function of lung height.

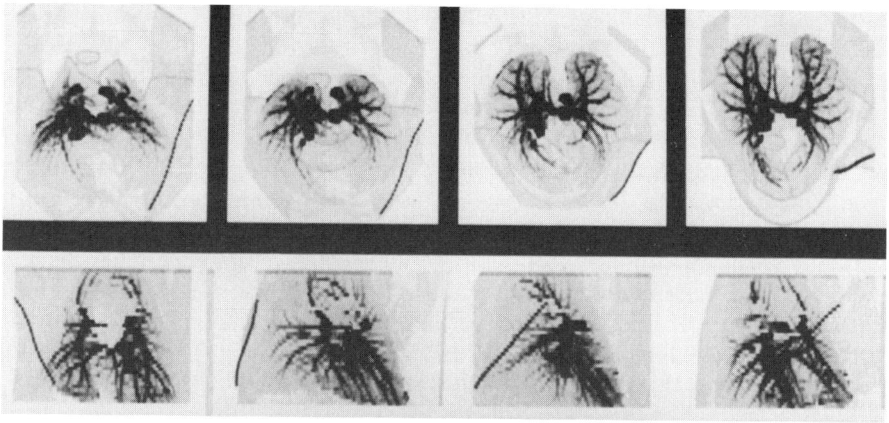

Figure 7. Interaction between gravity and vascular conductance. Maximum intensity volume renderings (brightness inverted) of a volumetric scan of the lung. An electron beam CT scanner was used to image the thorax of a supine anesthetized dog during a continuous drip of IV contrast agent. The top panels demonstrate multiple angles of view of the rendering rotated about the right to left body axis. The bottom panels demonstrate multiple angles of view with the rotation occurring about the cephalo–caudal body axis. Note, for instance, the lower panel third from the left. Here the spine is to the right and the caudal lung surface is towards the bottom of the picture. Note the clear direction of vascular conductance focused towards the dorsal lung regions.

a ventral to dorsal perfusion gradient in the supine body posture was reduced and less significant. The left lung in the supine body posture appears to have a much stronger zone 4 condition which reduces the supine ventral to dorsal blood flow gradient. Of note is the branching pattern of the pulmonary arterial tree in the dog. A monopodial branching structure is characteristic of many vertebrates other than humans whereby small side branches fork off of a large main pulmonary artery which traverses from the carina to the dorsal–basal portion of the lower lobes.

We have used the volumetric imaging capabilities of the electron beam scanner to reconstruct the pulmonary vascular anatomy of the supine and prone dog to further evaluate the relationship between anatomical and functional parameters, such as shown in Fig. 7. From such images we have shown the compression of the dorsal/ basal portion of the vascular tree in the supine posture. The compression was found to be greater in the left lung, and may be due to the weight of the heart in the left side of the chest cavity along with a rotation of the lung lobes caused by the change in shape of the rib cage and diaphragm which is responsible for this altered vascular geometry. This altered vascular geometry may explain the enhanced zone 4 condition found in the left lung. Vascular compression, due to the weight of the heart, could counteract both the gravitational and vascular conductance effects which combine to cause a steep gradient in blood flow in the right lung in the supine body posture. In the prone body posture, the heart is supported by the sternum, and the right and left lungs show less of a difference. In preliminary studies, we have lifted the heart into a "prone" position with the dog in a supine body posture. We opened the chest, exteriorized sutures placed around the pericardial sac, reapproximated the chest wall, and evacuated the pneumothorax. We used electron beam CT scanning to evaluate pulmonary blood flow before surgery, after surgery, and after heart lift. At the onset of the studies, we hypothesized that the lifting of the heart would allow for expansion of the dependent alveoli at FRC and thus create a more homogeneous lung density serving to facilitate a more homogeneous distribution of the inspired gas. To our surprise, the gradient in lung density increased slightly with heart lift. From blood flow studies in these initial experiments at multiple lung volumes, and from observations made in the above described studies, we hypothesize that as the dependent lung is unburdened of the weight of the heart, pulmonary blood flow and blood volume increase in the dependent lung regions. This increased blood volume counteracts the potential for alveolar expansion when the alveoli are relieved of the heart weight, and regional air content at FRC in the dependent regions may remain unchanged or is reduced. This has been a particularly difficult study when coupling the complexity of the electron beam CT studies themselves with the difficulty of opening the chest, suturing the pericardial sac bilaterally, and then needing to re-close the chest, to fully evacuate the thorax, and accomplish all of this without leaving residual atelectasis. It does, however, help to further emphasize the importance of studying the system in its integrated, interactive state.

Pulmonary Ventilation

Studies of regional lung air content distribution have lead to the conclusion that the intrathoracic position of the heart is a major determinant of the regional distribution of ventilation, and the presence of lobar fissures allow the lobes of the lungs to slip [26] and accommodate shape changes of the diaphragm and rib cage without altering the volumes of the alveoli. Studies of dogs on the DSR, depicted in Fig. 8, show that there is a significant gradient in lung air content at FRC with the dependent (lower) lung regions having less air than the non-dependent (top) regions suggesting that the alveoli are more expanded in the non-dependent lung region. With inflation steps, a greater portion of the bolus of air goes to the dependent lung regions as the non-dependent lung regions reach their non-compliant limits earlier. With the dog in the prone posture, the situation is not simply reversed but rather the lung in more uniformly expanded at FRC and thus inspired air is more uniformly distributed throughout the inflation steps. Figure 8 demonstrates that there is a significant ventral-dorsal gradient in regional lung expansion in the supine body posture which disappears when the dog is shifted into the prone body posture [22, 27]. Interestingly, this ventral-dorsal gradient in regional lung expansion re-appears in the non-dependent lung with the dogs in the left or right lateral decubitus body postures, suggesting that gravity directly acting on the lung is not the only factor in determining regional variation in lung expansion. There are numerous factors at work including altered chest wall shape as well as inherent regional variations unrelated to any well defined cartesian coordinate system [28].

With the observation that the dog manages to match ventilation and perfusion in the prone body posture without large gradients leaving the non-dependent lung exposed to high, continuous strain, and with the thought that, since humans in the upright posture have significant, continuous exposure of the non-dependent (apical) lung region to large strains, it was hypothesized that perhaps humans have not evolved to walk uprights in relationship to the cardiopulmonary system. An animal was sought that lived in the opposite body posture to the dog, and a sloth was selected. Contrary to the initial hypothesis, the sloth showed the same lung density gradient supine and lack of gradient prone as was found in the dog [27]. However, whereas the dog rib cage and diaphragm changed shape considerably prone vs. supine, the sloth has a very rigid chest wall (22 rib pairs) and showed no significant change in chest wall geometry with change in body posture. The similarity between dog and sloth was the shift in the intrathoracic position of the heart, and we believe that it is the sternal support of the heart in the prone posture versus the lung support of the heart supine which in part alters regional lung expansion differences.

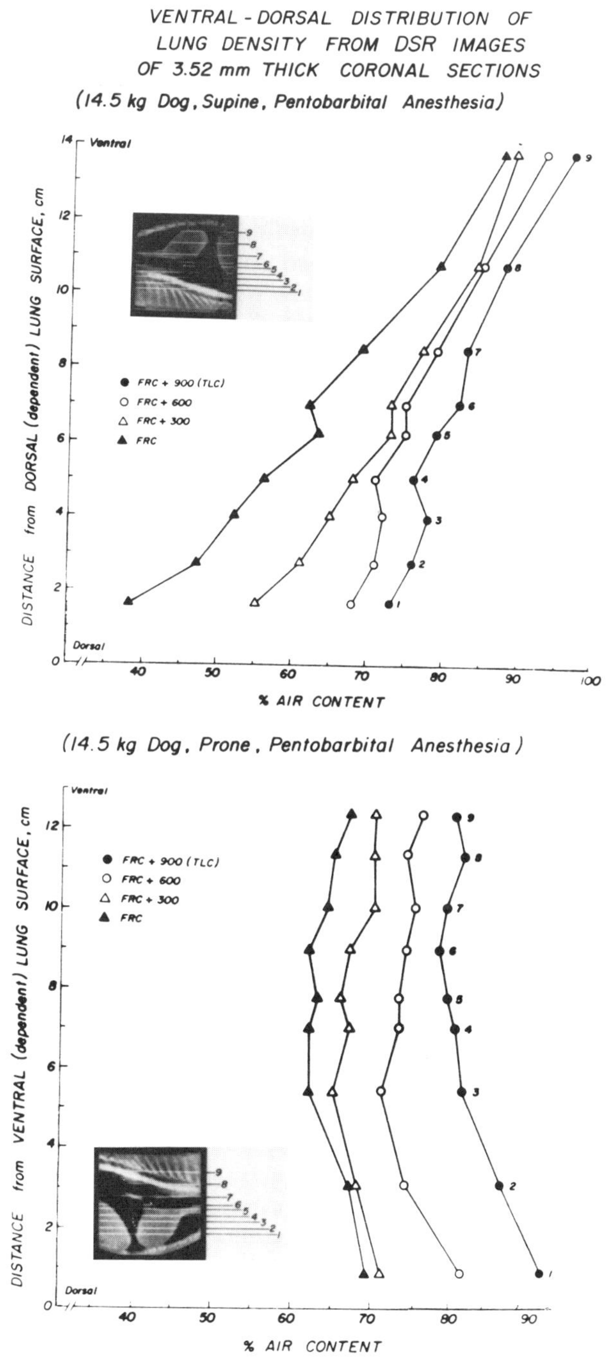

Figure 8. Heart–lung interactions: Distribution of regional lung air content was sampled in isogravimetric (coronal) planes through the volumetric image data sets of an anesthetized dog studied supine **(Top)** and prone **(Bottom)** at multiple 300 ml steps from functional residual capacity (FRC) to total lung capacity (TLC). Lung air content is plotted as a function of lung height.

Presumably, in the dog, lobar slippage is able to minimize the effects of chest wall shape changes on regional variation in lung expansion while lobar slippage may not accommodate the altered support requirements of the heart. It is interesting to note that the sloth is born with lobar fissures, but these fissures reportedly fibrose over shortly after birth, perhaps from disuse since the rib cage does not change shape with changes in body posture. Shaded surface displays of the in vivo lungs of the dog and sloth demonstrate the altered ventral lung geometry determined by the shifts of the intrathoracic position of the heart with change in body posture. An animal which has essentially no functional lobar fissures is the horse. Olson and Lai–Fook [29] have shown that in ponies there is a very sharp pleural pressure gradient supine, which again is eliminated prone. The pleural pressure gradient was so steep, that there is a suggestion that nearly 1/3 to 1/2 of the dorsal lung is collapsed.

A particularly interesting finding to date has been that, despite the dramatic difference in blood flow supine versus prone (Fig. 6) and the accompanying difference in regional lung air content supine versus prone (Fig. 8), the relationship between the regional

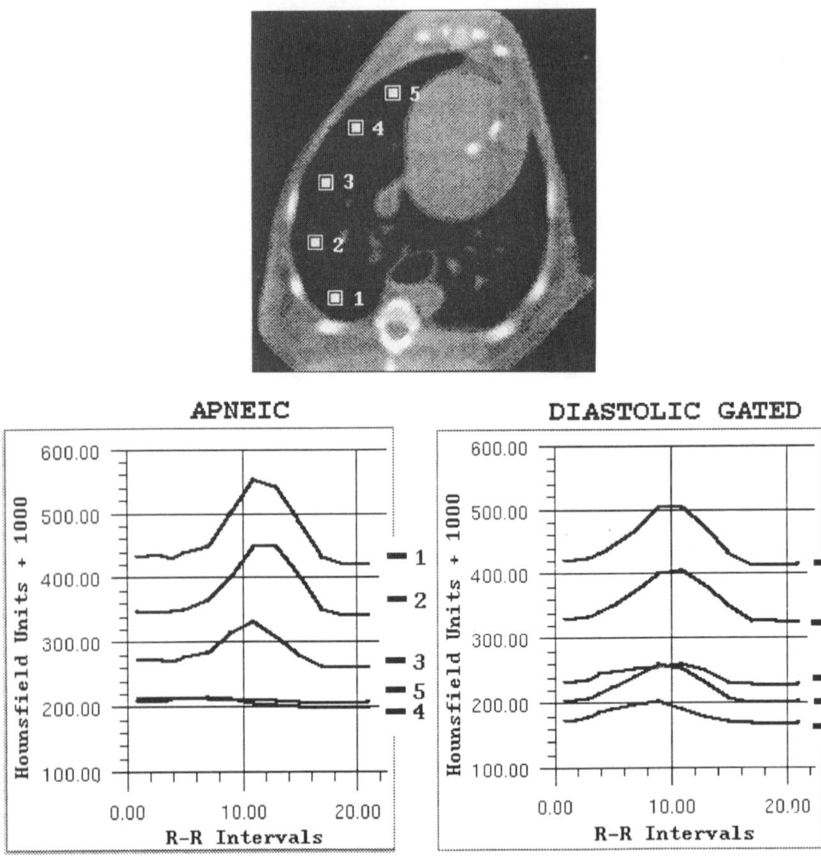

Figure 9. Respiratory–cardiac cycle interactions: The lower panels represent intensity changes measured within the lung regions defined in the upper panel with data representing the passage of x–ray contrast agent through the lungs during electron beam CT scanning. The higher the peak of the curve relative to the baseline of the curve, the greater the blood flow in that region. The two conditions depicted are pulmonary blood flow during apnea and pulmonary blood flow during diastolic gated ventilation (inspiration occurrs at each heart beat during diastole and expiration occurrs in systole).

parenchymal volume versus regional lung air content appears to remain strong across dogs and across body postures within a given dog. This suggests that regional alveolar expansion may serve to compress local vascular (capillary) beds serving to reduce regional blood volume. We have discussed above that the weight of the heart on the left lung in the supine body posture serves to bring about zone 4 conditions whereby blood flow is reduced by external compression on the extra alveolar vessels. Thus, heart support and alveolar expansion appear to compete for control of regional lung blood volume under certain conditions.

Cardiac and Pulmonary Phase Interrelationships

Finally, we return to the example of respiratory gated ventilation. An example of cardiac cycle and respiratory cycle interactions is demonstrated graphically in Fig. 9. The heights of the regional time intensity curves in a dynamic electron beam CT sequence following contrast agent through the lung field are directly related to blood flow. As seen by the increased rise in curves 4 and 5, blood flow to the non–dependent lung regions are significantly increased when the lung is deflating or at FRC during the time when the heart is pumping blood into the pulmonary vascular bed. There are distinct gravitationally based blood flow gradients in both the apneic and diastolic gated conditions, with the greater flow going to the dependent lung regions and in the apneic state shown on the left; there is essentially no measurable flow to the upper most regions of the lung in this particular dog. However, when the lung and cardiac cycles are synchronized such that the lung is either deflating, or at rest as the heart is pumping blood into the pulmonary arteries, blood flow is significantly enhanced in the non–dependent lung regions as evidenced by the increased height of the curves in this region.

CONCLUSION

Our studies show an integration of function of the four chambers of the heart to maintain a constant heart volume relationship, which in turn may be influenced by the in utero, intrathoracic fetal milieu. At birth, the constant heart volume may serve to minimize work of the heart. Atrial stiffness can pose an important afterload on the LVs as a consequence of the constant volume pump configuration, and the lung can impinge on the cardiac fossa at inspiration and this interaction can be harnessed to improve cardiac output and myocardial blood flow through cardiac gated respiration. On the other side of the relationship, pulmonary blood flow distribution can be altered by altering the phase relationship between the cardiac and respiratory cycle, and support of the heart by the lung can serve to alter both regional ventilation and regional pulmonary blood flow. The heart and lungs work in an integrated environment and care must be taken in the final analysis to come back to the integrated whole at times to understand the implications of measurements made in isolation.

DISCUSSION

Dr. E. Yellin: Considering the popularity these days of the pacing induced failure model with a dilated heart, do you think that the mechanical heart–lung, or heart–diaphragm interaction, would increase and be a significant part of the whole process?

Dr. E. Hoffman: I am not sure because under normal respiration you do not really have much of a coupling between breathing and heart beats. On average, you are breathing in sometimes during systole and breathing out sometimes during systole, and I am not sure that this would play an important role. However, if you could gate respirations so that you are always breathing in during systole so that you are assisting the heart, this may actually allow the heart to recover. In some ways it may serve partly as an assist device.

Dr. E. Yellin: When you were gating your tidal volume must be very small then similar to synchronous jet ventilation.

Dr. E. Hoffman: It is a little bit more than jet ventilation because we need some tidal volume in order to squeeze down on the heart. I believe that it is a mechanical effect of lungs squeezing down on the heart; we reduce tidal volume to about 1/3 of the normal tidal volume. If we were to reduce it all the way down to the equivalent of jet ventilation, we would most likely not get improvement of cardiac output.

Dr. G.F. Mitchell: You showed that inflation, whether during systole or diastole, would improve ejection. My experience in patients with heart failure who require positive pressure ventilation has generally been that they do not necessarily do too well. Standard clinical teaching is that positive pressure ventilation, if anything, will diminish cardiac output. How do you reconcile these observations? Moreover, most of these patients have heart rates of 120–140 bpm rather than 60 bpm. I wonder how you would do your gating in that situation.

Dr. E. Hoffman: You could gate up to 120–140 bpm. However, if you maintain your tidal volume at 30% normal, you may hyperventilate the patient, in which case you may have to start adjusting for CO_2 and so forth. With the heart gated to the cardiac cycle, vs just normal peak ventilation, cardiac output increases, whereas PEEP ventilation causes output to decrease. In fact, the first study on the DSR in the Mayo Clinic, where we looked at the change in chamber volume with static lung inflation, was designed to start looking at the question "why does the cardiac output fall during PEEP ventilation." The leading hypothesis at the time had been that as you increase resistance to the pulmonary vascular bed, you back blood up in the RV ventricle and push the septum over and decrease the volume available to the LV. At least in the static inflation we have shown that you just decrease the volume of both chambers and it is an effect of the lung compressing the heart. It may be that when you gate to the cardiac cycle you are getting enough of an improvement by the lung on the heart, so that you are overcoming detrimental changes in the pulmonary vascular resistance. Whereas when you are using PEEP ventilation, then the two are not tied together; you are not getting the improvement through timed compression on the heart, while you are getting the decrement in cardiac output because of the possible increases in the pulmonary vascular resistance and compression on the heart in both diastole and systole.

Dr. R. Beyar: The effect that you may have with gated respiration may be similar or analogous to what we have shown with our vest–type cardiac assist. We can assist the heart and get 20% increase in cardiac output in severe heart failure by getting intrathoracic pressure of about 10–20 mmHg. I wonder what kind of pressure cycling and variation you get with your respiration.

Dr. E. Hoffman: With a normal tidal volume ventilation you would expect pleural pressure to change by probably 10–15 cm water. Here we are getting maybe 7 cm water change in pleural pressure. I would guess that this is similar to your measurements. But here we are doing two things at once: respirating the lungs and improving cardiac output. As I remember, you also compressed the abdomen at Johns Hopkins.

Dr. R. Beyar: No. At Johns Hopkins we compressed only the chest. But we have shown at the Technion that with compression of the abdomen you can have further benefit.

REFERENCES

1. Ritman EL, Robb RA, Harris LD. *Imaging Physiological Function: Experience with the Dynamic Spatial Reconstructor*. Praeger:New York 1985.
2. Hoffman E, Ritman E. Invariant total heart volume in the intact thorax. *Am J Physiol* 1985; 249: H883-890.
3. Hoffman EA, Rumberger J, Dougherty L, Reichek N, Axel L. A geometric view of cardiac "efficiency". *JACC* 1989; 13(2): 86A.
4. Axel L, Dougherty L. MR Imaging of Motion with Spatial Modulation of Magnetization. *Radiology* 1989; 171: 841–845.
5. Clark NR, Reichek N, Bergey P, Hoffman EA, Brownson D, Palmon L, Axel L. Circumferential myocardial shortening in the normal human left ventricle: Assessment by magnetic resonance imaging using spatial modulation of magnetization. *Circulation* 1991; 84: 67–74.
6. Rogers NJ, Shapiro EP, Weiss JL, Buchalter MB, Rademakers FE, Weisfeldt ML, Zerhouni EA: Quantification of and correction for left ventricular systolic long axis shortening by magnetic resonance tissue tagging and slice selection. *Circulation* 1991; 84: 721–731.
7. Delaunay B. Sur la sphere vide. *Bul Acad Sci USSR VII: Class Sci Mat Nat* 1934; 793–800.
8. Greenbaum RA, Ho SY, Gibson DG, Becker AE, Anderson RH. Left ventricular fibre architecture in man. *Brit Heart J* 1981; 45(3): 248–263.
9. Khalafbegui F, Suga H, Sagawa K. Left ventricular systolic pressure–volume area correlates with oxygen consumption. *Am J Physiol* 1979; 237(5): H566–H569.
10. Nozawa T, Yasumara Y, Futaki S, Taneka A, Igarashi Y, Goto Y, Suga H: Relation between oxygen consumption and pressure–volume area of in situ dog heart. *Am J Physiol* 1987; 253(22): H31–H40.
11. Suga H. Total mechanical energy of a ventricle model and cardiac oxygen consumption. *Am J Physiol* 1979; 236(5): H498–H505.
12. Chung N, Wu X, Bailey KR, Ritman EL. LV pressure–volume area and oxygen consumption: evaluation in intact dog by fast CT. *Am J Physiol* 1990; 27: H1208–H1215.
13. Cristescu MG, Ritman EL, Hoffman EA. Mechanics, Energetics and Constant Heart Volume: Atrial Fibrillation vs. Sinus Rhythm. *FASEB J* 1990; 4: A433.
14. Wong T, Wu L, Chung N, Ritman EL. Myocardial blood flow estimated by synchronous, multislice, high speed tomography. *IEEE Trans Med Imag* 1989; 8: 70–77.
15. Fogel MA, Gupta KB, Weinberg PM, Hoffman EA. Strain and wall motion analysis of single ventricles throughout staged fontan reconstruction using magnetic resonance tagging (Young Investigator Award). *JACC* 1993; 21: 2A.
16. Pinsky MR, Matuschak GM, Klain M. Determinants of cardiac augmentation by elevations in intrathoracic pressure. *J Appl Physiol* 1985; 58(4): 1189–1198.
17. Pinsky MR, Matuschak GM, Bernardi L, Klain M. Hemodynamic effects of cardiac cycle–specific increases in intrathoracic pressure. *J Appl Physiol* 1986; 60(2): 604–612.
18. Hanson CW, Haywood MT, Hoffman EA. Cardiopulmonary dynamics with EKG gated ventilation. *JACC* 1992; 19: 189A.
19. Tajik JK, Kugelmass SD, Hoffman EA. An automated method for relating regional pulmonary structure and function: Integration of dynamic multislice CT and thin–slice high–resolution CT. *SPIE Proc* 1905. 1992; in press.
20. Boyd DP, Lipton MJ. Cardiac computed tomography. *Proc IEEE* 1983; 71: 298–307.
21. Wolfkiel CJ, Ferguson JL, Chomka EV, Law WR, Labin IN, Tenzer ML, Booker M, Brundage BH. Measurement of myocardial blood flow by ultrafast CT. *Circulation* 1987; 76: 1262–1273.
22. Hoffman EA. Effect of body orientation on regional lung expansion: A computed tomographic approach. *J Appl Physiol* 1985; 59: 468–480.
23. Hoffman EA, Ritman EL. Heart–lung interaction: Effect on regional lung air content and total heart volume. *Annals Biomed Eng* 1987; 15(3&4): 241–257.
24. Larsen RL, Bridges CR, Beck KC, Hoffman EA. Regional pulmonary blood flow via Cine X–ray computed tomography. *FASEB J* 1990; 4(3): A1074.
25. Beck KC, Rehder K. Differences in regional vascular conductance in isolated dog lungs. *J Appl Physiol* 1986; 61: 530–538.
26. Rodarte JR, Hubmyer RD, Stamenovic D, Walters BJ. Regional lung strain in dogs during deflation from total lung capacity. *J Appl Physiol* 1985; 58: 164–172.

27. Hoffman EA, Ritman EL. Effect of body orientation on regional lung expansion in dog and sloth. *J Appl Physiol* 1985; 59: 481–491.
28. Hoffman EA, Acharya RS, Wollins JA. Computer–aided analysis of regional lung air content using three–dimensional computed tomographic images and multinomial models. *Int J Math Modeling* 1986; 7: 1099–1116.
29. Olson LE, Lai–Fook SJ. Pleural liquid pressure measured with rib capsules in anesthetized ponies. *J Appl Physiol* 1988; 64: 102–107.

CHAPTER 35

CAROTID–CARDIAC INTERACTION: HEART RATE VARIABILITY DURING THE UNBLOCKING OF THE CAROTID ARTERY

Metin Akay,[1] Giora Landesberg,[2] Walter Welkowitz,[1] Yasemin M. Akay,[1] and Dan Sapoznikov[2]

ABSTRACT

Multiresolution representations of the heart rate variability (HRV) using the wavelet transforms are proposed to characterize the autonomic nervous system regulation of cardio–vascular activity during carotid surgery. Results suggest that the power in all frequency bands was low during the surgery and increased after the declamping of the carotid artery.

INTRODUCTION

The cardiovascular system and in particular the heart, interacts with the central nervous system to produce heart rate controls, ventricle elastance controls, and arterial resistance controls [1, 2]. Much of this control comes from sensing the carotid sinus pressure with stretch receptors. It has been demonstrated that in situations such as assisted circulation all of these controls come into play to produce the desired assistance to the failing heart [3].

When there is a blockage of the carotid artery we can expect the controls to be effected due to both restricted blood flow to the brain and to mechanically induced pressure changes in the carotid sinus. The interaction of the heart with this complex control system can be studied by analyzing the variations of heart rate in such cases before, during, and after carotid endarterectomy.

The heart rate variability can also be used to study the autonomic nervous system (ANS) [4]. The autonomic nervous system modulates the cardiovascular control during the

[1]Department of Biomedical Engineering, Rutgers University, Piscataway, NJ 08855, USA, and [2]Department of Anesthesiology and Cardiology, Hadassah University Hospital, Jerusalem, Israel.

Interactive Phenomena in the Cardiac System, Edited by
S. Sideman and R. Beyar, Plenum Press, New York, 1993

traumatic preoperative procedure. The status of the autonomic nervous system is reflected in the electrical activity of the heart since it provides beat–by–beat regulation of the cardiovascular system.

The application of spectral analysis techniques to beat–to–beat heart rate and blood pressure variations has provided an important tool for noninvasively understanding tonic cardiovascular regulation [5]. Results using spectral analysis techniques showed that there are three major spectral regions. The high frequency region (HF, above 0.25 Hz) represents shifts in respiratory rate. The mid–frequency region (approximately 0.15 Hz) is linked to the response of the baroreceptor reflex, and the low frequency region (approximately 0.08 Hz) is related to thermoregulation fluctuation and vasomotor tone (renin–angiotensin system) [5].

These spectral components of the heart rate variability data (HRV) and blood pressure can be used clinically to assess the ANS, with separate measures of the sympathetic and parasympathetic systems. The high frequency component in HR variability appears to be mediated solely by the vagal tone since it disappears completely with vagal or muscarinic blockade. The mid–band frequency component is an indicator of the sympathetic tone but is also modulated by vagal activity [5].

Power spectral analysis of HR and blood pressure variability which represents the activity of the ANS could provide an important noninvasive prediction of high risk patients who may develop cardiovascular complications during vascular surgery [6].

Little is known about the characteristics of heart rate fluctuations during cardiovascular surgery both in the time and frequency domains. The purpose of this study is to characterize the heart rate fluctuations during surgery by determining how the signal changes in the frequency domain during the surgery. Here we introduce the wavelet transform method to analyze the heart rate fluctuations. The wavelet transform method based on multiresolution signal decompositions is free of assumptions regarding the characteristics of the signal and is able to localize the non–stationary signal more accurately (both in the time and frequency domains) than the methods of Wigner–Ville (WV) and the short term Fourier transform [7–9]. This time and frequency localization can be achieved by the wavelet transform since it uses short windows at higher frequencies and long windows at low frequencies.

METHODS

Wavelet Transform

The wavelet orthonormal bases provide an important tool in signal analysis [7–9]. The difference information between the approximation of heart rate fluctuations at resolutions 2^{j+1} and 2^j can be extracted by decomposing the signal on a wavelet ortho–normal basis of $L^2(R)$ [7]. $L^2(R)$ denotes the vector space of measurable, square–integrable one–dimensional functions $f(x)$. In $L^2(R)$, a wavelet orthonormal basis in the vector space V_{2_j} can be given as a family of functions $[2^{j/2}\phi(x - 2^j x - n)]_{j,n \in Z}$ which can be built by dilating the unique function $\phi(x)$ called a scaling function. The scaiing function $\phi(x)$ can characterize the multiresolution approximation of the vector space V_{2_j}. The projection of the signal $f(x)$ onto the orthonormal bases of $L^2(R)$ can be estimated as follows [7]:

$$A_{2^j} = 2^{-j} \sum_{n=-\infty}^{\infty} < f(u), \phi_{2^j}(u - 2^{-j}n) > \phi_{2^j}(x - 2^{-j}n) \tag{1}$$

$n, j \in Z$.

The discrete approximation of $f(x)$ can be estimated by using the inner products at the resolution 2^j, which can be estimated as follows [7]:

$$A_{2^j}^d f = \langle f(u), \phi_{2^j}(u - 2^{-j}n) \rangle \tag{2}$$

The consecutive $A_{2^j}^d f$ can be explained as a low–pass filtering of $f(x)$ followed by a uniform sampling at a rate 2^j. For each scale change, the higher frequencies of the signal will be eliminated. $A_{2^{j-1}}^d f$ can be calculated by using a recurrence algorithm as follows [7]:

$$\langle f(u), \phi_{2^j}(u - 2^{-j}n) \rangle = \sum_{k=-\infty}^{\infty} \bar{h}(2n - k) \langle f(u), \phi_{2^{j+1}}(u - 2^{-j-1}k) \rangle \tag{3}$$

where $\bar{h} = h(-n)$ represents the mirror filter of $h(n)$

$$h(n) = \langle \phi_{2^{-1}}(u), \phi(u - n) \rangle \tag{4}$$

where $h(n)$ represents the low–pass filter. $A_{2^j}^d f$ can be estimated by convolving $A_{2^{j+1}}^d f$ with $h(n)$ and storing every other sample of the output [7].

The wavelet function, $\psi(x)$, called the orthogonal wavelet can be estimated at resolution 2^j as follows [7]:

$$\psi_{2^j} = 2^j \psi(2^j x) \tag{5}$$

The functions of $\psi(x)$, $\psi_{2^j}(x - 2^{-j}n)$, which are an orthonormal bases of the vector space O_{2^j} have good localization properties in the time and frequency domains [7].

The orthogonal projection of a signal $f(x)$ on the vector space O_{2^j} can be estimated as follows [7]:

$$D_{2^j}^d f = \langle f(u), \psi_{2^j}(u - 2^{-j}n) \rangle \tag{6}$$

where $D_{2^j} f$ represents the discrete detailed signal. The inner product can be estimated from the higher resolution discrete approximation as follows [7]:

$$\langle f(u), \psi_{2^j}(u - 2^{-j}n) \rangle = \sum_{k=-\infty}^{\infty} \bar{g}(2n - k) A_{2^{j+1}}^d(k) \tag{7}$$

where $\bar{g}(n) = g(-n)$ represents the mirror filter of $g(n)$ [7].

$$g(n) = \langle \psi_{2^{-1}}(u), \ \phi(u - n) \rangle \tag{8}$$

where $g(n)$ represents the high–pass filter. Since filters $g(n)$ and $h(n)$ are quadrature filters, the high–pass filter $g(n)$ can be estimated as follows [7].

$$g(n) = (-1)^{1-n} h(1 - n) \tag{9}$$

The vector space O_{2^j} is orthonormal to the vector space V_{2^j}. As a summary, A_{2^j} and D_{2^j} can be estimated from $A_{2^{j+1}}$ by convolving with the filters $h(n)$ and $g(n)$, respectively. The details of the wavelet transforms are described elsewhere [7].

Kolmogorov–Smirnov (K–S) Test

The K–S test was successfully applied to the detection of stimulus–related (evoked response) activity in the electroencephalogram [11] and to the distributions of the transition states of the ion channel activity [12]. The value of the K–S test has also been demonstrated in acoustical signal detection associated with coronary artery disease [13].

The K–S test compares the cumulative distribution of sample data sets with that of a known or reference data set. Since the K–S test makes no assumption regarding the type of data distribution, it is applicable to any distribution of data. In our case, the K–S test was an attractive method for statistical analysis of the detailed signal, $|D_j f|^2|$, of the heart rate fluctuations at different frequency bandwidths. Different distribution functions (or data sets) yielded different cumulative distribution function estimates using the K–S test.

The behavior of the distribution functions between the largest and smallest values characterizes the distributions. The K–S distance, D, represents the maximum absolute difference between two cumulative distribution function as follows [11–13]:

$$D = \max_{0<x<\infty} |F_N(x) - R(x)| \tag{10}$$

where $F_N(x)$ and $R(x)$ represent the cumulative distribution functions of the sample (unknown) and the reference functions, respectively.

In our case the reference distribution is provided by the one hour time segment after the declamping time and the sample cumulative distribution functions are all the other one hour segment for each detailed signal at the different frequency bandwidths.

In our case of two unknown cumulative distribution functions, the maximum distance D_i can be calculated as follows [11–13]:

$$D_i = \max_{0<x<\infty} |F_{1a} - F_i| \tag{11}$$

where F_{1a} represents the cumulative distribution function of the detailed signal within an hour period after the declamping, and F_i represents the cumulative distribution function of the detailed other signals each with a one hour period (non–adjacent segments).

RESULTS AND DISCUSSION

Files of 24–hour R–R intervals were recorded from a Holter Marquette series 8000 analysis system. Files of R–R intervals with their annotations (normal beats, premature ventricular beats, ectopic beats) were transferred to an IBM–386 compatible computer disk. The R–R intervals between two consecutive normal QRS complexes were calculated by noting any irregular beats. Then, the irregular beats were replaced by the values obtained by linear interpolation from the normal beats. The irregular beats were determined by using a threshold obtained by updated averages and standard deviations of the R–R intervals. The details of the recording and interpolation procedures have been described elsewhere [10]. Then, the 24 –hour R–R intervals were transferred as a function of time after the interpolation procedure to a Sun 4.0 System for wavelet analysis. We performed multiresolution decomposition for three sets of parameters D_{2^j} where $-1 < j < -3$. The wavelet transform method was applied to the heart rate fluctuations obtained from five patients for 5 h before and 3 h after declamping in patients undergoing carotid endarterectomy. The three wavelet transforms represent the following signal bandwidths: 1) 0.250–0.500 Hz, 2) 0.125–0.250 Hz, 3) 0.062–0.125 Hz.

All the patients ended the surgery with no cardiac or neurological damage. Figure 1A shows the heart rate in msec for 5 h before and 3 h after the declamping in one of those patients undergoing carotid endarterectomy. Figures 1B to 1D show the corresponding power of the three wavelet decompositions which define the power at each time sample,

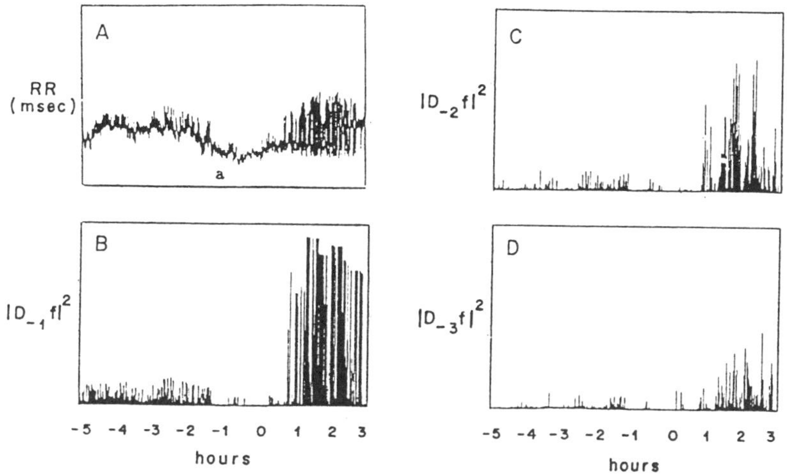

Figure 1. The resolution decomposition of the 8 h R–R intervals obtained from patient 1 who underwent carotid surgery. **A:** R–R intervals. **B, C, D:** The corresponding three frequency bandwidths (discrete detail signals, D_{2^j}) as a function time. From top to bottom the resolution decreases by a power of 2.

respectively. This patient was a 64 year old male who underwent left carotid endarterectomy with cervical block anesthesia without the need of any additional systemic drug. The blood pressure of this patient fell from 188/74 to 157/66 within 30 minutes after declamping. The heart rate and the corresponding power of the three wavelet decompositions which define the power were calculated at each time sample in 1 h segments from 5 h before to 3 h after the declamping. The results show that the power of the heart rate fluctuations in all three wavelet bands was low during surgery and increased after carotid declamping. For this reason, we statistically analyzed the 1 h segment of RR intervals in msec and all three wavelet bands before declamping as well as for the 3 hours after declamping to establish the significance of the 1 h segment after declamping. For each 1 h segment, the cumulative distribution function (CDF) values were estimated for these three wavelet bands. Then, the CDFs of 1 h segments before and after declamping were compared with the CDF of the 1 h segment that immediately follows the declamping.

The standard for comparison is the K–S distance D which can have a maximum of one for extremely contrasting functions and a minimum of zero for functions that are essentially the same. The K–S distances between the cumulative distribution functions of the five segments before declamping and the two segments after declamping versus the segment following the declamping are shown in Fig. 2 for the R–R intervals and each of the three wavelet bands. The figure shows that the R–R interval and the first wavelet bands followed the same statistical patterns, which implies that the probabilistic distributions of the 5, 4 and 3 hours before and 2 and 3 hours after declamping were approximately the same. In other words, the power in the first wavelet was higher during 5,4, and 3 hours before and 2 and 3 hours after declamping time compared with those of 2 and 1 h before and 1 after declamping. However, the power in the second and third wavelet bands was very low during all the 1 h segments before and 1 h after declamping.

Since the value of S, the K–S test significance, in each case is smaller than 0.001, the results are statistically significant [11–13].

Reinstitution of blood flow after cleaning the atheroma from inside the artery at the area of the baroreceptors could be responsible for the increase of the power in all frequency ranges. It should be noted that the blood pressures of these patients fell drastically within 30 minutes after declamping. All patients ended the surgery with no cardiac or neurological damage.

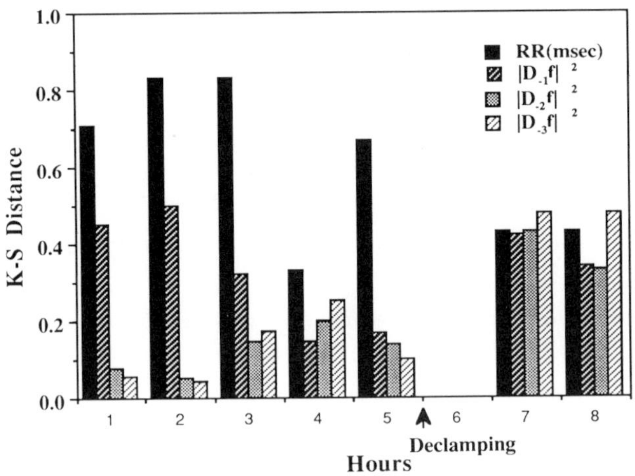

Figure 2. The K–S distance between 1 h segments for the RR and the three wavelet bands following declamping.

CONCLUSIONS

The wavelet transform method was utilized in this study to characterize autonomic nervous system regulation of cardiovascular activity in order to better understand short–term cardiovascular regulation. The wavelet transform was chosen since it has the ability to localize the change in the characteristics of the non–stationary heart fluctuations during surgery without loosing the time and frequency information.

A strong relationship between all three wavelet bands before and after declamping has been established using the statistical analysis technique known as the Kolmogorov–Smirnov (K–S) test, which does not make any assumption regarding the statistical distribution of the data. Results showed a highly significant relationship between all the wavelet bands and the declamping time. Results also showed that 1 h segments of each wavelet band immediately following declamping is statistically unique, that is, distinguishable from all other segments considered. This implies that the increased power in each wavelet band after surgery is caused by the declamping.

However, the mechanisms responsible for the hemodynamic alterations and even for myocardial ischemic events occurring during carotid clamping and declamping [10] in carotid endarterectomy are not completely understood. Since the behavior of the ANS during major surgery and cardiac ischemic events can be tracked carefully and accurately using wavelet transforms, we believe that this technique will further improve our understanding of the interactions of the control systems with the cardiovascular system.

DISCUSSION

Dr. E. Ritman: It is well known that pulsatility of the carotid sensing organ is very important. Have you looked, for instance with echo, at pulsatility after surgery.

Dr. W. Welkowitz: No, we have not. But it certainly is a good idea because it is an easy region to look at since it is right near the surface. We have not looked at whether anatomically these blockages impinge on the carotid sensor. One thing that has bothered us is that it is hard to distinguish the effects of brain blood flow from mechanical effects on the sensors. We may be able to get at some of these questions by looking at the blood pressure, since it is very sensitive to the characteristics.

Dr. R. Mates: How does the post–operative variability compare with normal patients who do not have chronic blockages?

Dr. W. Welkowitz: We are monitoring normals now for 24 hrs and it takes some time to analyze these records. The records show quite a bit of variability, especially at night during sleep. We would like to compare the K–S patterns of a normal with a K–S pattern before and after surgery.

Dr. J. Bassingthwaighte: You have used the wavelet transform as an alternative to the Fourier transform. Would you comment on its virtues?

Dr. W. Welkowitz: If you perform a fast Fourier Transform (FFT) on the heart rate variability, which we have done, you do not get the information that you are looking for. You get only frequency information. From the FFT it is not easy to pick out particular frequencies of interest and to follow them in a time course. What some people have done is to take short time Fourier Transforms, but the shorter the time over which you take the Fourier Transform, the poorer is the resultant Fourier Transform. The wavelet transform method does not have these problems. The technique allows you to look at frequency domains over periods of time. Since in most cases we are interested in the effects over a long time, you can use this technique to follow the frequency characteristics over time. The closest approach to this method is to use analog comb filters. The problem with using analog systems was that the output signals were very sensitive to the particular filter characteristics. The wavelet transforms seem to be free of such limitations.

Dr. J. Bassingthwaighte: How do you go about choosing the orthogonal basis function?

Dr. W. Welkowitz: We picked the frequency bands in powers of two. In the approach we use, the frequency bands must have this characteristic. We picked the highest one to give us a range covering the effect of the parasympathetic system. Then we divided the ranges by two and then two again.

Dr. T. Arts: Fourier analysis can generally be used quite well, especially if you make a comb filter with octaves in a row. Then you can calculate the power of the signal as a function of time. Thus you get an idea about power variability in spectral windows and that is about what you showed here. I think that is not the strong point of wavelets. The strongest point of wavelets is at phase differences. Follow a wave in time, and observe how it changes because the phase information is still in it. I did not see this aspect in your plans.

Dr. W. Welkowitz: The time information in our results can give you the phase information. I do not quite agree with you on the short term Fourier Transforms since we did some. Depending upon how short a period you use, you get a lot of erroneous information. You can get the phase information from Fourier Transforms, however this information is not too accurate unless your data is very good. We seem to get much more consistent results with the wavelet transform. If you use a short window, you will get good time resolution at the expense of poor frequency resolution.

Dr. L.E. Ford: How did you deal with the extra systoles? Also, how did you deal with changes of pressure? I did not notice that you had changes in pressure, but if you did, you would have expected changes in heart rate going along with it.

Dr. W. Welkowitz: Some pressure data were obtained. We are going to analyze the data in the same time–frame as the other data. I agree with you that there is an effect of pressure. We have not completed this work as yet. As far as the extra systoles are concerned, the data was actually edited first, extrasystoles were dropped out and interpolation was carried out to add in the missing beats.

Dr. L.E. Ford: Did you take out the beats following the extra systole for a certain period as well?

Dr. W. Welkowitz: Yes. The data we analyzed was edited in that fashion.

REFERENCES

1. Blombery PA, Ferguson IA, Rosengarten DS, Stuchbery KE, Miles CR, Black AJ, Pitt A, Anderson ST, Harper RW, Federman J. The role of coronary artery disease in complications of abdominal aortic aneurysm surgery. *Surgery* 1987; 101: 150–5.
2. Gouny P, Bertrand M, Coriat P, Kieffer E. Perioperative cardiac complications of surgical repair of infrarenal aortic aneurysms. *Ann Vasc Surg* 1989; 3: 328–34.
3. Roger VL, Ballard DJ, Hallett Jr JW, Osmundson PJ, Puetz PA, Gersh BJ. Influence of coronary artery disease on morbidity and mortality after abdominal aortic aneurysmectomy: a population–based study. *J Am Coll Cardiol* 1989; 14: 1245–52.
4. Eagle KA, Coley CM, Newell JB. Combining clinical and Thallium data optimizes prospective assessment of cardiac risk before major vascular surgery. *Ann Int Med* 1989; 110: 859–866.
5. Akselrod S, Gordon D, Ubel FA,. Shannon DC, Barger AC, Cohen RJ. Power spectrum analysis of heart rate fluctuations: a quantitative probe of beat to beat cardiovascular control. *Science* 1981; 213: 220–222.
6. Zbilut JP, Lawson L. Decreased heart rate variability in significant cardiac events. *Crit Care Med* 1988; 16: 64–6.
7. Mallat SG. A theory for multiresolution signal decomposition: the wavelet representation. *IEEE Trans on PAMI* 1989; 7: 674–693.
8. Akay YM, Akay M, Welkowitz W, Lefkowicz S, Palti Y. Time–frequency analysis of the turbulent sounds produced by femoral artery stenosis in dogs using wavelet transform. *Proc IEEE EMBS*, Paris, 1992.
9. Healy DM Jr and Weaver JB. Two applications of wavelet transforms in magnetic resonance imaging. *IEEE Trans on Information Theory* 1991; 2: 840–860
10. Landesberg G, Erel J, Anner H, Eidelman LA, Weinmann E, Luria MH, Sapoznikov D, Berlatzky Y and Cotev S. Perioperative myocardial ischemia in carotid endarterectomy under cervical block anesthesia and prophylactic nitroglycerin infusion. *J Cardiothor Vasc Anesthesia* 1992; in press.
11. Bachen NI. Detection of Stimulus–Related (Evoked Response) Activity in the Electroencephalogram (EEG). *IEEE BME* 1986; 6: 245–251.
12. Akay M, Welkowitz W, Semmlow JL, Kostis J. Application of the ARMA method to acoustical detection of coronary artery disease. *Med Biol Eng Comput* 1991; 29: 365–372.
13. Akay M and Craelius W. Mechanoelectric feedback in cardiac myocytes from stretch–activated ion channels. *IEEE Trans on BME* 1992; in press.

CHAPTER 36

Right and Left Ventricle Interaction and Remodeling in Congenital Heart Disease

Richard S. Chadwick[1], Annabelle Azancot–Benisty[2], Jacques Ohayon[3], and Yuho Ito[4]

ABSTRACT

A biomechanical model of the left ventricle (LV) using loading conditions and short–axis echocardiographic shape information predicts significant differences in fiber disorganization and contractility among normals and patients with congenital heart disease characterized by right ventricular (RV) pressure or volume overload.

INTRODUCTION

The LV and RV are intimately linked both functionally and anatomically [1]. In a previous echocardiographic study we investigated ventricular interdependence in normal fetuses, newborns, infants and in congenital heart disease with RV pressure or volume overload using a quantitative computerized geometric method [2, 3]. LV short–axis echocardiographic shapes were described and quantified by a shape factor (SF) that changed monotonically with increasing LV distortion. A significant positive correlation was found between SF and RV and LV pressure ratios [3]. However, a geometric approach cannot assess the influence of mechanical and functional factors such as wall thickness, muscle fiber organization, interstitial collagen, and contractility on RV and LV interaction; consequently we applied a biomechanical model and validated this model in children with RV volume and pressure overload [4,5]. This present work extends that model to include variable fiber disorganization, and uses the model in an inverse mode to make predictions

[1]Theoretical Biomechanics Group, Biomedical Engineering and Instrumentation Program, National Center for Research Resources, National Institutes of Health, Bethesda, MD 20892, USA; [2]Laboratoire d'Explorations Fonctionelles, Hôpital Robert Debré, 75019, Paris, France; [3]Laboratoire de Mécanique Physique, Université Paris Val de Marne, 94010 Créteil Cedex, France; [4]Hiroshima University of Medicine, 2nd Department of Internal Medicine, 1–2–3 Kasumi Minami–Ku, 734 Japan.

Interactive Phenomena in the Cardiac System, Edited by
S. Sideman and R. Beyar, Plenum Press, New York, 1993

concerning contractility, and muscle fiber remodeling, given the loading conditions and the deformed geometry of the LV.

EXPERIMENTAL METHODS

Patient Groups

Group 1 (G1) consisted of a control population (n=16) aged one day to six months in which the physical and echocardiographic examinations revealed the absence of cardiac abnormalities. This group was subdivided according to age into G1a < 1 month and G1b ≥ 1 month. Group 2 (G2) consisted of atrial septal defects (n = 8) aged 9 days to 48 months presenting RV volume overload with normal pulmonary artery pressures. Only five required cardiac catheterization; in the others RV pressure was estimated by continuous wave Doppler, and LV systolic pressure was evaluated by systemic cuff arterial blood pressure. The pulmonary to systemic shunt ratio was equal to 2.7 ± 0.5. Group 3 (G3) comprised of patients with RV pressure overload and RV hypertrophy (n = 14) aged 1 day to 13 years. Seven patients presented D Transposition of the great vessels (TGV) with intact septum, four of which had a Senning procedure. TGV patients are separately analyzed as G3a. The other patients (G3b) included pulmonary atresia (PA) with ventricular septal defect (n = 2), tetralogy of Fallot (TOF) (n = 1), atrioventricular canal (n = 1), ductus arteriosus (n = 1), truncus arteriosus (n = 1), and idiopathic pulmonary hypertension (n = 1). The ratio of LV peak systolic pressure to RV peak systolic pressure was 1.22 ± 0.49. All patients underwent cardiac catheterization with fluid-filled catheters allowing RV and LV pressure measurements. All patients were in sinus rhythm without evidence of bundle block at the time of the study, and none presented a pericardial effusion.

Echocardiographic and Doppler Methods

Cross-sectional echocardiograms were performed with a Toshiba 160 SSH phased array using a 3 MHz or 5 MHz transducer. Complete examinations were performed, although only LV short axis parasternal views were considered in the study. For consistency between patients and further quantification, the anatomic landmarks required were the tips of the anterior and posterior mitral leaflets centered in the frame of view. The entire LV was visualized and special care was taken to obtain the septal portion and clear definition of its attachments to the RV. Analysis was performed at end-systole (the frame just before mitral valve opening) and end-diastole (the frame just after mitral valve closure). Real time videotape recordings were analyzed frame by frame in slow motion allowing selection of the best single frames. These frames were printed for subsequent geometric quantification. Continuous wave Doppler ruled out pulmonary hypertension in Group 2 using the simplified Bernoulli equation on peak tricuspid regurgitation jet velocity.

Geometric Quantification

The following methodology was utilized to obtain the LV and RV geometric parameters (Fig. 1) required as input data for modeling. End-diastolic and end-systolic epicardial and endocardial contours of the RV and LV were traced. The LV endocardial contours were subsequently used for calculation of cavity area and SF. A line (Oy) was constructed perpendicular to and bisecting the center of the line (Ox) connecting the mitral valve attachments. We measured the inner and outer radii R_i and R_0 along the positive

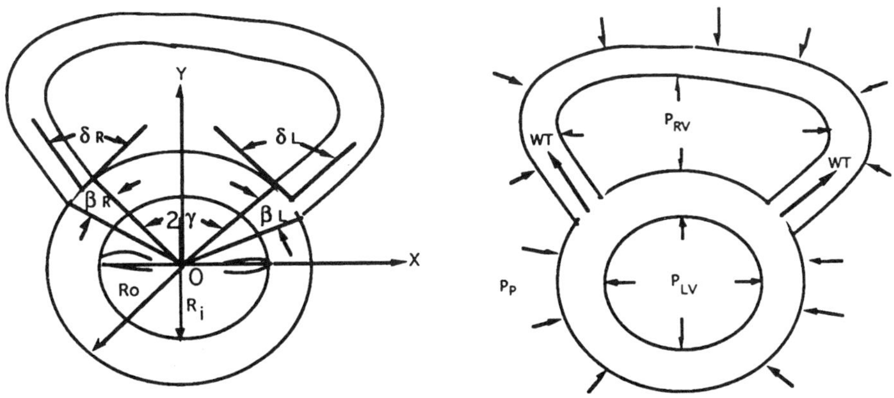

Figure 1. Left: Measured LV and RV geometrical parameters. **Right:** loading conditions. P_{LV} – LV cavity pressure; P_p – pericardial pressure; P_{RV} – right ventricular cavity pressure; WT – RV wall tension.

y–axis, and calculated their ratio $\alpha_m = R_o/R_i$. The septal arc length, $(2R_o\gamma)$ was determined by the angular aperture (2γ) between the inner septal attachments. Rays were drawn from the center O to the borders of the left and right septal attachments to obtain the angles β_R and β_L. Intersections of the tangents to the LV outer contour and to the midwall direction of the septal attachments define the angles δ_R and δ_L.

MATHEMATICAL PROCEDURE

The Shape Factor (SF)

The methodology used here for obtaining SF evolved from a previous study [2]. The LV endocardial boundaries of the end–diastolic and end–systolic frames for each patient were digitized on a Wacom SD–42 digitizing table. Computer programs were written to: (a) determine the center of gravity (c.g.) of the digitized boundary points; (b) obtain a cubic spline representation of the radius, with origin at the c.g., as a function of arc length; (c) twice differentiate the radius as a function of arc length to obtain the curvature as a function of arc length; (d) obtain a Fourier representation of this curvature function. Fourier coefficients were also directly computed for the curvature obtained as output of the biome–chanical model described below, which generated the shapes shown in Fig. 2. These shapes serve as templates for an arbitrarily assigned shape factor scale. A shape factor could then be assigned to a patient's endocardial boundary by linear interpolation between the Fourier coefficients of the template shapes and the Fourier coefficients computed in step (d).

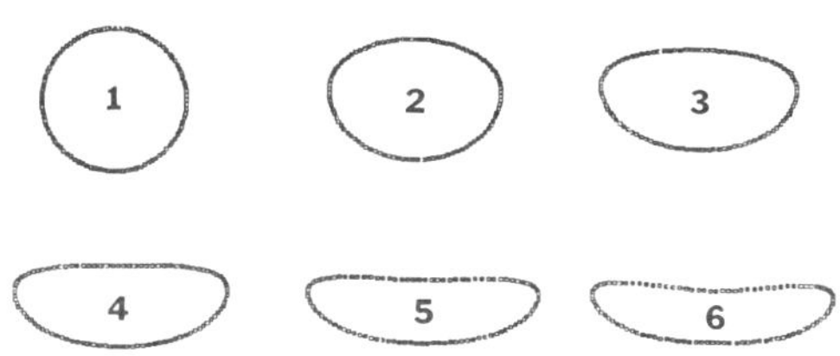

Figure 2. Computed LV endocardial boundary shapes and their corresponding shape factors.

The Biomechanical Model

A 2D biomechanical model is used to analyze end–diastolic and end–systolic short axis echocardiograms of the LV. End–diastole and end–systole are considered as mechanical equilibrium configurations corresponding to minimal and maximal states of activation. Both of these states are derived from a common geometrical reference, the hypothetical unloaded passive state. We approximate this reference state as a circular annulus with end–diastolic values of the geometric parameters shown in Fig. 1. The LV is loaded by its cavity pressure (P_{LV}), the RV cavity pressure (P_{RV}), pericardial pressure (P_P), and RV wall tension (WT) which must be computed from P_{RV}, P_P, and the geometry.

The myocardial tissue is represented as a homogeneous, incompressible, fluid–fiber–collagen continuum. The linearized equations of equilibrium of the model and their solution have been previously given [5]. However, in the present study we modified the constitutive law to include fiber disorganization:

$$\sigma_{ij} = -(P - \beta'\kappa T_o)\delta_{ij} + (1-\kappa)\ \tau_i\tau_j\ T_f + 2\{\mu + (1/3)\kappa E_f\}\,\varepsilon_{ij} \qquad (1)$$

where κ is the fiber disorganization parameter, $0 \le \kappa \le 1$. Note that when $\kappa = 0$, the stress tensor σ_{ij} reduces to that of a fluid–fiber–collagen continuum having only circumferential muscle fibers, while $\kappa = 1$ corresponds to a completely random or isotropically oriented set of muscle fibers. For intermediate values of κ, Eq. (1) represents a mixture of the two extremes. Others quantities in Eq. (1) are: the myocardial tissue pressure P; the activation parameter β' (0 at end–diastole and 1 at end–systole); the contractility parameter T_o (dyne/cm^2) represents the maximal active tension of muscle fibers; the Kronecker delta symbol δ_{ij}; the direction field of the circumferential muscle fibers $\tau = \mathbf{e}_\theta$; the effective elastic modulus of the isotropic collagen matrix μ (dyne/cm^2); the effective elastic modulus of the muscle fibers $E_f = (1-\beta')E + E^*\beta'$ where E (dyne/cm^2) is the passive elastic modulus and E* (dyne/cm^2) is the maximally active elastic modulus (also a contractility parameter); and the fiber tension $T_f = \beta' T_o + E_f\ \tau_i\varepsilon_{ij}\ \tau_j$ where ε_{ij} is the tissue strain tensor.

Algorithm for Solving the Inverse Problem

The inverse problem of finding biomechanical parameters that result in computed shapes within specified error bounds for given geometrical reference values and loading conditions is not unique. The best that can be achieved is a range of "acceptable values" for each parameter. The definition of "acceptable values" will be given in the following explanation. Computations are carried out on a Macintosh II FX, using a scheme that iterates between end–diastolic and end–systolic states. (1) First, computations at end–diastole are performed. The measured end–diastolic geometric parameters α_m, β (the mean of β_L and β_R), 2γ, and δ (the mean of δ_L and δ_R) are used to approximate the reference geometry for each patient. Utilizing end–diastolic RV, LV and pericardial pressures, the end–diastolic SF and α are computed in a 3D grid of points in diastolic rheological parameter space (E, μ, κ). A set of preliminary acceptable values of (E, μ, κ) were defined as those for which the magnitude of the difference between the computed SF and α and their values determined from the traced contours were less than specified error bounds, e. For SF < 3, we used $e_\alpha = 0.1$ and $e_{SF} = 0.2$, while for SF > 3, we used $e_\alpha = 0.2$ and $e_{SF} = 0.3$. The unknown reference α was sometimes adjusted so that these conditions could be satiSFied. (2) Next, the process is repeated for a 3D grid of points in systolic rheological parameter space (E*, T_o, κ) using the same geometrical reference quantities, the end–systolic RV, LV and pericardial pressures, and the measured systolic/diastolic LV cavity area ratio AR (± 15% measurement error) as input. A theoretical relationship exists between AR, loading conditions, and the parameters α, μ, E ,E*, T_0, κ, which can be explicitly solved for T_0 to reduce the systolic grid to a search in (E*, κ) space. Since systolic shapes are not very sensitive to E and μ, their mean values could be used in the systolic calculations. Acceptable values of (E*, T_0, κ) were similarly defined as those for which the above conditions between computed and measured SF and α were satiSFied. In addition, the (E*, T_0, κ) space was constrained to satiSFy the inequality: $3 \leq (E^* - E)/T_0 \leq 4$. This constraint follows from a theoretical relationship between $(E^* - E)/T_0$ and the sarcomere length/effective actin length ratio [6]. This algorithm produced a narrow range of acceptable κ's. Another cycle of diastolic and systolic computations using the narrower range of κ refines the ranges of all the parameters.

RESULTS AND DISCUSSION

Intergroup comparisons of the averaged means ± the averaged half–ranges of the computed fiber disorganization parameter (κ) and contractility (T_0), are respectively plotted in Figs. 3 and 4. The lowest κ was found for G1 regardless of age. G3 was characterized by the highest degree of fiber disorganization and the narrowest ranges, with marked increase in κ for G3a (TGV). G2 fiber disorganization was at an intermediate level. Contractility T_0 was severely decreased in G3 with narrow ranges, especially for G3a (TGV). G2 demonstrated an increased contractility compared to G1 and G3.

The biomechanical model provided information on fiber disorganization and intrinsic contractility based on shape analysis of 2D echocardiographic images and hemodynamic loading conditions that were either measured during catheterization or estimated by Doppler. Such information is otherwise currently impossible or very difficult to obtain *in vivo*. Studies on fiber disorganization currently require *in vitro* morphometry, while *in vivo* contractility assessment is confounded by functional abnormalities such as paradoxical septal wall motion evaluated by M–mode.

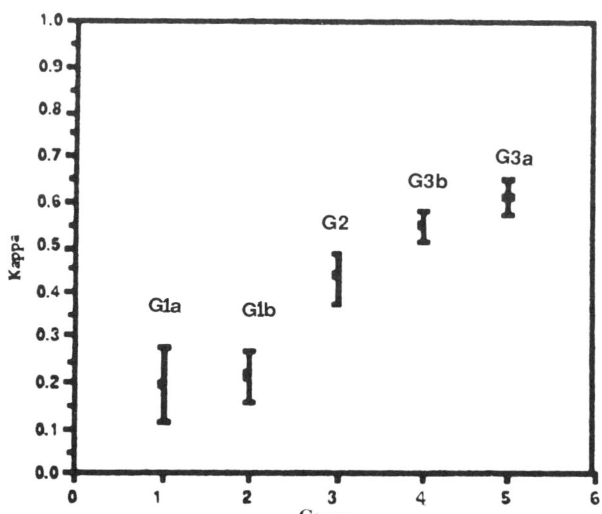

Figure 3. Intergroup comparison of computed fiber disorganization parameter κ.

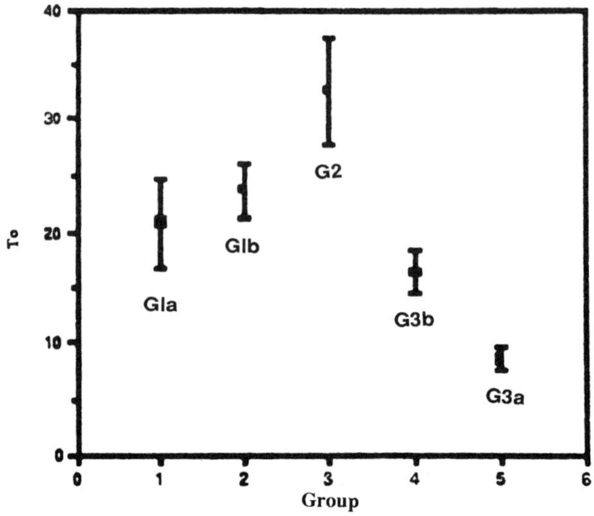

Figure 4. Intergroup comparison of computed fiber contractility parameter T_o (units of 10^5 dyne/cm^2).

Our model predicts some degree of fiber disorganization in all patients, including normals. The model parameter κ indicates disorganization on a macroscopic fiber level rather than disarray at the local myocyte level. Fiber disorganization in normals has been found in gross dissections and histological sections, particularly at the subaortic septal region, and the junctional areas of the ventricular septum with the ventricular free walls [7, 8]. We found that fiber disorganization was lowest in the youngest group (G1a), which is consistent with the belief that the septum equally shares RV and LV fibers in the fetus and newborn [9]. Apparently, LV fiber disorganization increases with RV hypertrophy. This process may be initiated by the large number of RV fibers encircling and "choking" the LV [9]. In our model major LV fiber disorganization is predicted in patients with RV hypertrophy (G3) irrespective of the type of heart disease, although it was most marked with TGV (G3a). Extensive fiber disorganization concomitant with RV pressure overload is in concurrence with morphometric observations from hearts having PA with intact septum and TOF [10].

Our model predicts that intrinsic LV contractility, which is characterized in the model by the isometric tension parameter T_0, is depressed in patients with RV pressure overload (G3). This seems to be in general agreement with the clinical and experimental findings of others. It has been suggested that associated myocardial ischemia is responsible for the depressed contractility in TGV [11]. Cytoskeletal interference with contractile proteins by stress–induced polymerization of microtubules has also recently been demonstrated experimentally with RV pressure overload [12]. Our finding that LV contractility is enhanced in patients with RV volume overload (G2) was not anticipated since previous clinical and experimental evidence has not been consistent [1, 13].

CONCLUSION

In vivo morphometric confirmation of our quantitative predictions of fiber disorganization is still required. Nevertheless, we propose that fiber disorganization is an adaptation of the LV to prevent the occurrence of even greater LV distortions in the presence of abnormal loading conditions resulting from structural anomalies that evolve in utero. The biomechanical model shows that fiber disorganization increases the effective shear modulus, a material property that resists distortions of the LV. This strategy is particularly effective during systole when active fiber stiffness and disorganization cooperatively act to resist distortion. This may explain why patients with RV volume overload (G2) have circular LV cavities at end–systole, but distorted LV cavities at end–diastole. Apparently, the strategy fails in patients with RV pressure overload (G3), since reduced contractility reduces the mechanical advantage of fiber disorganization in resisting LV distortion.

Acknowledgments

This work was partially supported by a grant from La Fondation de France.

DISCUSSION

Dr. R. Beyar: Does the right ventricular pressure overload depress contractility of the LV? The other question: what does it mean when we have a heart with a fiber disorientation of say 0.5? What does it mean in terms of how the fibers are arranged there and what do you get for a normal heart?

Dr. R. Chadwick: The first question is whether or not right ventricle pressure overload depresses contractility of the left ventricle. I believe that the literature is fairly consistent in saying that it does. We did not have any trouble finding papers that supported that. There are two hypotheses. One is that associated septal hypertrophy induces ischemia, which depresses contractility. Another hypothesis was presented at the AHA meeting in New Orleans [12]. In an experimental study on pulmonary artery banded cats, it was demonstrated that individual myocytes had an associated proliferation of cytoskeletal microtubules. They felt that these microtubules might be interfering with the normal contractile protein cycle. As to the question of fiber disorganization and the meaning of the parameter κ. When κ is zero, all the fibers are oriented in a well–defined manner. When κ is one, all of the fibers are oriented at random, or isotropically. When κ is 0.5, half the fibers are oriented and half are directed randomly. There is some fiber disorganization even in the normal heart. Some years ago our NIH Director, Dr. Healy (then Dr. Bulkley) and Dr. Weisfeldt showed that about 10% of the fibers are disorganized in a normal heart. Our model predicts about 15% of the fibers are disorganized in normals.

Dr. T. Arts: You discussed remodelling, which I see as adaptation of shape to mechanical load. In that case, if you say that shear is a sensor for growth, I have a problem in the sense that the cell does not know inside which directions it has. As you know, shear in one direction is just stress in another direction. It depends on what coordinate system you take. The cell does not really have a coordinate system. I have a problem: what might be the feedback mechanism for the kind of adaptation you are thinking of?

Dr. R. Chadwick: There are two ways to think about this. Dr. Art's view is that each cell is very selfish, and just wants to make sure that its own conditions are as good as possible. One can take another point of view where signals might be fed back over a larger scale, and that maybe there is some "social responsibility" where a population of cells are seeking to preserve the function of the ventricle. It is interesting to speculate that there may be both local and regional feedback. I do not think it is important that a cell should know the direction of shear. Shear is not present in a ventricle of circular cross–section. Not worrying about whether shear is positive or negative, when you have a distorted ventricle, you get a significant shear component one way or another throughout the ventricle. Perhaps not knowing the sign might explain why a cell does not know which way to orient itself. It just goes in some direction.

Dr. Y. Lanir: You took a constant shear parameter and considered an isotopic structure. I believe that some of your results of disorganization result from the fact that in large deformation, the network reorganizes itself reversibly by the large strain. So at least some of this disorganization is not an adaptation, but simply a matter of passive change of the fibers architecture compatible with the strain field that is applied on the tissue.

Dr. R. Chadwick: That is a very good question. In fact our model is currently based on a linearized analysis so there will be some error in accounting for large deformations. Furthermore, we assume the same κ in systole and diastole, i.e. we do not have fiber orientation changing from directed to undirected within a beat. However, I seriously doubt that finite deformation effects can account for such a large scale change in κ from 0.2 to 0.6, which is what we have found. These are huge changes and if you look at the morphology, you would see the existence of gross fiber disarray for some diseases. Our model seems to be consistent with these morphometric studies.

Dr. E. Hoffman: In some of the studies that we have been doing with MRI tagging. The unique feature of being able to lay down this mesh is that we have been able to get the distribution of strain and a measure of the heterogeneity of strain. You are showing this heterogeneity of fiber orientation to correlate with increased heterogeneity of strain relative to the normals. Now we have interpreted heterogeneity of strain to be bad: the loss of normal endocardial, epicardial differences in strain and so forth. I gather that you are saying that heterogeneity of strain may actually be good.

Dr. R. Chadwick: I do not know whether strain heterogeneity is ultimately good or bad, but I am suggesting that fiber disorganization is an adaptation that helps to preserve the normal geometry of the ventricle in the presence of abnormal loading conditions.

Dr. D. Allen: As I understand it, you have contractile elements in your model and they can change their length. I wonder how realistic the tension–length curve is that you have given to these elements?

Dr. R. Chadwick: We think it is quite realistic. We have used the same local time–varying elastance model that we have used before, as have many other cardiac modelers.

Dr. D. Allen: Can you tell us what length–tension relation you used for the contractile elements?

Dr. R. Chadwick: We used a linear length–tension relationship at end–systole. The parameters of the line, T_0 and E^*, were found by solving the inverse problem. The values obtained for these parameters were consistent with values measured on papillary muscles.

Dr. Tsujioka: Your calculation is based on echo imaging. Usually an echo image is very noisy, so I have two questions. How did you digitize echo image and how stable was the digitized result?

Dr. R. Chadwick: Dr. Azancot–Bensity, who is an echocardiologist, established the location of the boundaries [4]. She drew the boundary contours, which were then digitized with about 100 points each. It was stable as long as we used enough points.

Dr. Tsujioka: Did you use any smoothing method?

Dr. R. Chadwick: Cubic splines were fit to the digitized points, so that derivatives required some smoothing. Dr. Ohayon worked very hard to overcome some initial difficulties.

REFERENCES

1. Janicki JS, Weber KT. Altered left ventricular function in pulmonary hypertension. In: ***The Diagnosis and Treatment of Pulmonary Hypertension***, Weir EK, Archer SL, Reeves JT (eds), 1992 Futura Publishing Inc., Mount Kisco, NY, pp 61–78.
2. Azancot A, Caudell TP, Allen HD, Horowitz S, Sahn DJ, Stoll C, Theis C, Valdes-Cruz LM, Goldberg SJ. Analysis of ventricular shape by echocardiography in normal fetuses, newborns and infants. *Circ* 1983; 68: 1201–1211.
3. Azancot A, Caudell TP, Allen HD, Toscani G, Debrux JL, Lamberti A, Sahn DJ, Goldberg SJ. Echocardiographic ventricular shape analysis in congenital heart disease with right ventricular volume or pressure overload. *Am J Cardiol* 1985; 56: 520–526.
4. Azancot-Benisty A. *Interaction du Ventricle Droit et du Ventricule Gauche: Mecanique du Ventricule Gauche*. 1990 These de Doctorat de l'Universite Paris XII.
5. Chadwick RS, Lewkowicz M, Ohayon J. An analytical approach to the biomechanics of some cardiac diseases. In: *Imaging, Measurements and Analysis of the Heart*, Sideman S, Beyar R (eds), 1991 Hemisphere Publishing Corp., Mount Kisco, NY, pp 99–112.
6. Chadwick RS, Ohayon J. A theory for local myocardial energetics and O_2 demand based on an active rheological law. In: Cardiovascular Dynamics and Models, Brun P, Chadwick RS, and Levy BI (eds), 1988 Colloque INSERM vol. 138, Paris, pp 151–159.
7. Becker AE, Caruso G. Myocardial disarray, a critical review. *Br Heart J* 1982; 47: 527–538.
8. Bulkley BH, WeiSFeldt ML, Hutchins GM. Asymmetric septal hypertrophy and myocardial fiber disarray. Features of normal, developing, and malformed hearts. *Circ* 1977; 56: 299–298.
9. Becker AE, Caruso G. Congenitial heart disease: a morphologist's view on myocardial dysfunction. In: *Pediatric Cardiaology,* Becker AE, Losekoot G, Maicelette C, Anderson, RH (eds), 1981 Churchill Livingstone Inc. vol. 8, Edinburgh, Scotland, pp 307–323.
10. Bulkley BH, D'Amico B, Taylor AL. Extensive myocardial fiber disarray in aortic and pulmonary atresia. Relevance to hypertrophic cardiomyopathy. *Circ* 1983; 67: 191–198.
11. Hausdorf G, Grävinghoff L, Keck EW. Incoordinate contraction and relaxation in d-transposition of the great arteries with intact septum-Analysis of pressure-dimension relations. *Basic Res Cardiol* 1986; 81:134–141.
12. Tsutsui H, Kent RL, Ishihara K, Nagatsu, M, Cooper IV, G. Cytoskeletal role in the contractile dysfunction of pressure overload cardiac hypertrophy. *Circ* 1992; 86: I 860 (abs).
13. Ferlinz J. Left ventricular function in atrial septal defect: are interventricular interactions too complex to permit definitive analysis? *JACC* 1988; 12: 1237–1240.

CHAPTER 37

Macroscopic Three-Dimensional Motion Patterns of the Left Ventricle

Theo Arts[1], William C. Hunter[2], Andrew S. Douglas[2], Arno M.M. Muijtjens[1], Jan W. Corsel[1], and Robert S. Reneman[1]

ABSTRACT

The pattern of displacements in the left ventricle (LV) can be described by 13 modes of motion and deformation. Three functional modes of deformation are essential for ejection: a decrease in cavity volume, torsion, and ellipticalization. Four additional modes are used to describe asymmetric deformation. Six modes of rigid body motion describe rotation and translation. In the LV 14–20 radiopaque markers were inserted in the wall of the LV. They were distributed more or less evenly from base to apex and around the circumference. Torsion and volume changes require the definition of a cardiac coordinate system. The point at which ejection focusses is used as the origin, and the torsion axis is used as the z–axis. In the present study the coordinate system was positioned objectively by a least squares fit of the kinematic model to the measured motion of markers. In five dogs in the control state the kinematic parameters were determined as a function of time for all 13 modes. The torsion axis was displaced 4 ± 2 mm (mean±sd) from the center of the cross–section of the LV towards the lateral free wall. The direction of the torsion axis closely coincided with anatomical landmarks at the apex and base. During systole, a unique relation was found between the ratio of cavity volume to wall volume and torsion. This relation was universal to all LVs, the cylinder–symmetric mathematical model of cardiac mechanics inclusive. In diastole the patterns of deformation seem less universal and reproducible.

INTRODUCTION

The complicated motion pattern of the left ventricle (LV) may be simplified considerably by describing it as a sequence of appropriately chosen major modes of

---

[1]Cardiovascular Research Institute Maastricht, University of Limburg, Maastricht, The Netherlands and [2]Department of Biomedical Engineering, Johns Hopkins University, Baltimore, MD 21205, USA.

Interactive Phenomena in the Cardiac System, Edited by
S. Sideman and R. Beyar, Plenum Press, New York, 1993

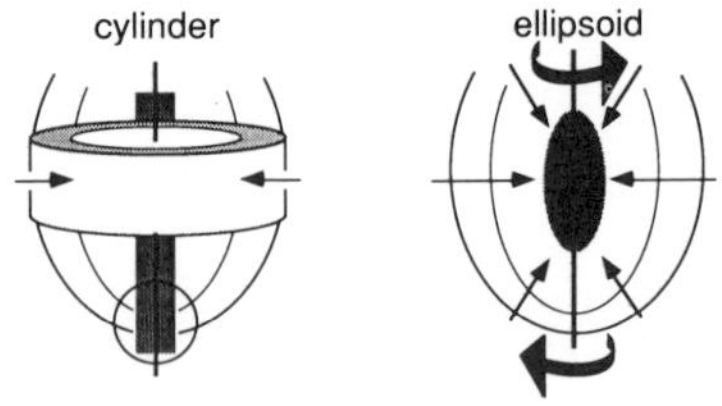

Figure 1. Left: In a cylindrical model, the ejected (shaded) region crosses the LV wall at the apex. **Right:** Using an ellipsoidal model for ejection, the ejected region is separated from the wall. The functional modes of deformation are ejection, torsion as indicated by the arrows, and base to apex ellipticalization.

deformation, rotation and translation. The simplest mode of deformation is a spherically symmetric radial displacement of the wall, which is related to a decrease in cavity volume and an increase in wall thickness during the ejection phase [1–3]. In the field of displacement of the wall as extrapolated to the cavity, ejected volume is disappearing in a mathematically singular point located at the center of the cavity.

Left ventricular kinematics are described much more accurately when considering additional modes of deformation. One mode of this kind is torsion of the LV around the base to apex axis [4–7], which is quantified by axial–circumferential shear in the wall. Another mode is circumferential contraction in combination with longitudinal extension, often referred to as ellipticalization [8–11]. The combination of the three modes was described in detail in a cylindrical symmetric model of the LV [7, 12, 13]. When describing the kinematics of the left ventricular ejection for the whole LV, the cylindrical model cannot be used, because the axis of the cylinder crosses the LV wall at the apex. The volume near the cylinder axis will be ejected, and this volume cannot be part of the wall (Fig. 1). Obviously, the shape of the LV is neither spherical nor cylindrical, but more that of a prolate ellipsoid with a distinct base to apex axis.

To describe stresses and strains in the fibers of the wall during the ejection phase, three functional modes of deformation can be recognized. The mode of ejecting volume from the cavity is needed for pumping. The modes of torsion and ellipticalization are related to equilibria of forces, and play an important role in transmural evening of fiber stress and strain.

For the torsion and ellipticalization modes, the mechanical equilibrium is described by the state of minimum energy. A deformation mode with amplitude k of the kinematic parameter describes a pattern of displacement $\vec{u}$ as a function of the position $\vec{x}$ in the wall. Then for a small change in stored mechanical energy ΔE in the fibers it holds:

$$\Delta E = \int_{wall} \sigma_f \Delta e_f dV \quad ; \qquad e_f = k\, f(\vec{u}(\vec{x})) \tag{1}$$

where σ_f and e_f indicate fiber stress and fiber strain, respectively. The energy changes as a function of kinematic parameter k. At equilibrium:

$$\frac{\partial E}{\partial k} = \int_{wall} \sigma_f \frac{\partial e_f}{\partial k} dV = 0 \tag{2}$$

The angle β between fiber direction and circumference at location $\vec{x}$ determines the relation between displacement and fiber strain (right part Eq. (1)). For the equilibria of torsion and ellipticalization it holds:

$$\int_{wall} \sigma_d \sin\beta \cos\beta \, dV = 0 \qquad\qquad \int_{wall} \sigma_f \, (1 - 3\sin^2\beta) \, dV = 0 \qquad (3)$$

In the present study, the functional modes of deformation are reconstructed by following the motion of radiopaque markers, inserted in the wall of the LV [14, 15].

To follow the motion of the wall of the LV, six modes of motion have to be added, in addition to the functional modes of deformation, to describe rotation and translation of the whole LV in the three–dimensional (3D) space [16]. Besides, due to gravitational forces, the LV deforms asymmetrically during diastole. The related pattern of deformation has been described by four asymmetric modes, related to deformation of a sphere to an ellipsoid: e_{xx}, e_{yy}, e_{xy}, e_{yz} and e_{zy}, where the z–axis coincides with the long axis of the LV [17]. The three functional motion modes are distinct from the ten other modes, the latter of which are not functionally related to the ejection of blood.

EXPERIMENTS

In five anesthetized open chest dogs, 14–20 radiopaque markers were implanted in the wall of the LV. Stainless steel markers (1.5 mm OD) were inserted at three equally spaced parallel short axis cross–sections in the anterior, lateral and posterior part of the free wall of the LV. The markers were inserted in pairs, one just below and the other 7 mm below the epicardial surface. One or two markers were positioned in the septal wall through the right ventricle. For identification of the anatomical base to apex axis, two ring–shaped markers were attached to the apical dimple and to the invagination between the aortic root and the left atrium. The positions of the markers were recorded by biplane cineangiography with 90 frames per second. In each projection the position of the markers was detected by computerized image analysis. The 3D location of the markers was obtained by pairing the marker images in both projections [14, 15]. Using a least squares method, the kinematic model was fitted to the measured motion of the markers [16].

Given the LV in the reference state, the location of the kinematic center and the direction of the torsion axis are defined by five parameters. To start the motion analysis, the configuration of the LV at approximately mid–ejection is used as the state of reference. The center and the direction of the axis are estimated on the basis of anatomical landmarks. The 13 kinematic parameters were calculated using a least square method for each frame in time. The total residual sum of the squared distances between the model and the measured marker positions were further minimized by varying the location of the center and the orientation of the torsion axis in the reference state. Experimental results on patterns of deformation were compared with the simulated deformation of the LV in a cylindrically symmetric model of left ventricular mechanics [7].

RESULTS

Generally, a good and stable numerical convergence was obtained in the experiments, resulting in a standard deviation of ±0.3 mm between measured and calculated marker positions. Stable estimates were obtained of the 13 parameters for each frame and the location and orientation of the coordinate system in the reference configuration. In the control state, the torsion axis was found to be close to the anatomical base to apex axis. The center of the torsion axis crosses the equatorial plane of the LV at a distance of 4 ± 2 mm (mean ± sd), displaced towards the lateral aspect of the free wall.

Figure 2 shows a control beat example of the time course of the seven kinematic parameters which are related to deformation. During the ejection phase, LV cavity volume decreased by a 0.14 fraction of wall volume. Torsion, as expressed by axial–circumferential shear deformation in the wall (k_2), increased by 0.113 radians. Axial shortening was a fraction of 0.04 less than circumferential shortening, resulting in ellipticalization of the LV during the ejection phase. Interestingly, the parameters k_4–k_7 were practically constant during the ejection phase, indicating a minor asymmetric deformation. These latter four parameters vary significantly in diastole, indicating the effect of gravity on the shape of the diastolic ventricle in the open chest.

Figure 3 represents the control beats in five experiments. Left ventricular pressure is plotted as a function of the ratio of cavity volume to wall volume. Furthermore, one loop has been added, describing the pressure–volume plot as generated by a mathematical model of LV mechanics. The bold parts of the curves reflect the relation during the ejection phase. In the control situation in the various experiments, the loading states appeared to be quite different. The end–diastolic ratio of cavity volume to wall volume ranged from 0.22 to 0.49, and the end–systolic ratio ranged from 0.12 to 0.29.

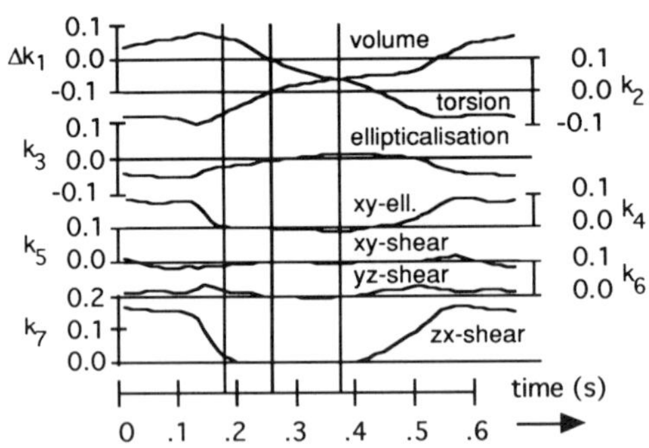

Figure 2. The time course of kinematic parameters related to deformation of the LV during the cardiac cycle. The vertical lines indicate the beginning of ejection, the reference frame of deformation, and the end ejection, respectively. The parameter Δk_1 is associated with changes in ventricular cavity volume, k_2 with torsion, k_3 with the ratio of axial length to diameter, k_4–k_7 with asymmetric linear (shear) deformation. The positive x–,y– and z–directions point to the right, the posterior side, and the apex, respectively.

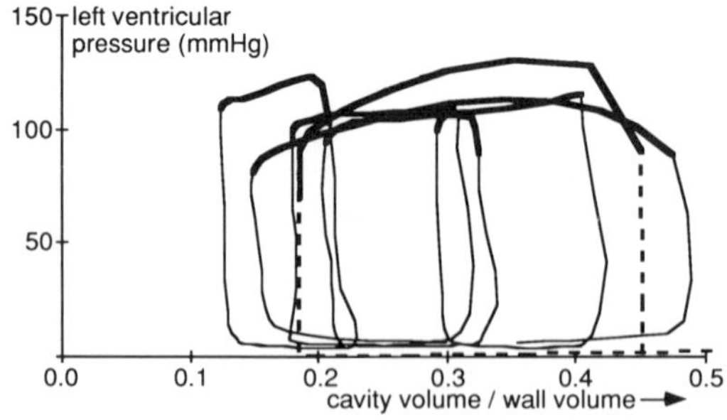

Figure 3. Left ventricular pressure as a function of normalized LV volume. The bold parts of the curves indicate the ejection phase. The dashed line refers to the results of a computer simulation.

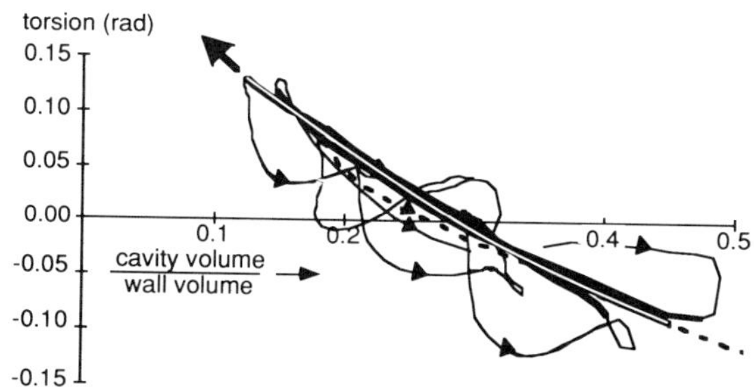

Figure 4. Torsion as a function of normalized LV volume. The bold parts of the curves indicate the ejection phase. The dashed, and partly white line refers to the results of a computer simulation.

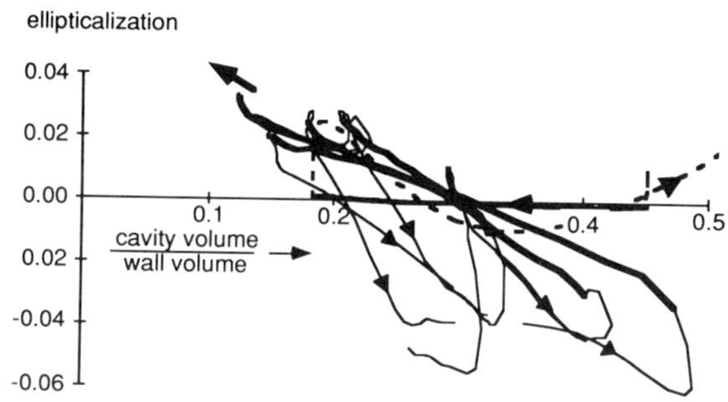

Figure 5. Ellipticalization as a function of normalized LV volume. The bold parts of the curves indicate the ejection phase. The dashed line refers to the results of a computer simulation.

In Figs. 4 and 5, representing the control beats in five experiments, the torsion and ellipticalization are plotted as a function of the ratio of cavity volume to wall volume, respectively. Included in each figure is a curve generated by computer simulation of LV wall mechanics. The bold parts of the curves reflect the relation during the ejection phase. All systolic curves were forced to cross the normalized volume axis at 0.3 by appropriate vertical shift of the individual curve. Strikingly, all systolic torsion–volume curves appear to coincide in one unique curve, which appears to be identical with the curve generated by the simulation. The systolic ellipticalization–volume curves are more different from one experiment to another. During diastolic filling, both the torsion and ellipticalization curves are individually very different.

DISCUSSION

Normal motion of the wall of the LV can be described quite accurately by the 13 motion modes. Three deformation modes are needed for the ejection of blood during systole. Four additional modes reflect asymmetric deformation, which are predominantly important during the diastolic phase. The six rigid body motion modes are not evaluated. When comparing different hearts, the pattern of systolic deformation appears to be quantitatively similar in all experiments after proper normalization. All motion modes are evaluated as a function of the dimensionless ratio of cavity volume to wall volume.

Normally, the axis of the LV is determined on the basis of anatomical landmarks. The anatomical landmarks used in the present study are only an initial estimate of this axis. The final location and direction of the torsion axis is calculated on the basis of the motion of the markers by numerical iteration. The torsion axis appears to be close to the anatomical axis, albeit displaced approximately 4 mm towards the lateral free wall of the LV.

Torsion is expressed by the axial–circumferential shear in the wall. In this definition the circumferential–axial shear is supposed to be zero because of rotational symmetry of the pattern of deformation as related to torsion. In order to obtain the symmetric shear component as related to the deformation of the myocardial material, torsion should be halved. Torsion appears to have a unique quantitative relationship with normalized volume. Moreover, this relation is identical to the relation predicted by an earlier theoretical model of the LV mechanics [7]. The theoretical model was based on the equilibrium of torsion and axial force; torsion was indicated to be a means to even out transmural differences in the strain of the myocardial fibers. Because the model and all control experiments have the same relation between the torsion and the normalized volume, we believe that the basics of the mechanics of the LV are now quite well understood.

The mode of ellipticalization does not relate to the normalized volume as uniquely as the torsion, and the differences between experiments are larger. Furthermore, the ellipticalization–volume curve predicted by the model [7] does not fit the experiments as well as in the case of torsion. Thus, the role of ellipticalization of the LV is not well understood. According to previous model studies, ellipticalization is related to the equilibrium of axial force, which is partly determined by the forces in the mitral valve papillary muscle system [18, 19].

In the present study, general relations are found between dimensionless quantities such as the ratio of cavity volume to wall volume, torsion and ellipticalization. The amplitude of changes in these parameters during the ejection phase depends on the hemodynamic state, which, as shown in Fig. 2, vary considerably with the large variations in the normalized cavity volume in the control state. During ejection, changes in these parameters occur simultaneously. The ratio of changes in these parameters during ejection appears to reflect the pattern of motion, and is much less dependent on hemodynamic load than on the changes in these quantities themselves. Recognition of the motion pattern is important in characterizing the mechanical function of the LV. That means that measuring a change in one parameter such as torsion is not as valuable as the measurement of the ratio of torsion to a change in the normalized volume. It would seem that for clinical applications it would be more useful to stress the search for a ratio of changes of the parameters than to analyze the change of one individual parameter.

In diastole, the relation between the various motion modes is variable. Evidently, the analysis of diastolic motion is much more complicated than systolic motion. No general patterns in diastolic motion could be recognized so far. Because of the large variations in diastolic motion patterns, normal and abnormal diastolic motion cannot be differentiated as easily as in systolic motion. It is to be expected that recognition of aberrant ventricular motion can be based best on data obtained in systole.

CONCLUSIONS

The motion pattern of the LV in the normal open chest canine preparation can be measured by using radiopaque markers inserted in the wall of the LV. Evaluation of systolic motion requires three functional modes: the ratio of cavity volume to wall volume, torsion and ellipticalization. Four additional modes are related to asymmetric deformation of the ventricle, which mainly occurs during diastole. Finally, six rigid body motion mode are needed. The location of the center of ejection and the orientation of the torsion axis are determined on the basis of the motion of the markers in the wall independent of anatomical landmarks. A unique relation is found during systole between the normalized cavity volume and torsion. This relation is universal to all LVs, and is identical with the prediction of our mathematical model [7]. The patterns of deformation in diastole seem less universal and much less reproducible.

DISCUSSION

Dr. E. Ritman: How was this work done?

Dr. T. Arts: An open chest canine dog in the supine position in a bi–plane x–ray set–up.

Dr. E. Ritman: That bothers me somewhat; within the closed chest with the lung and no pneumothorax, the epicardial surface of the heart is constrained to the extent that it can not move as much as it can in the open chest and that may alter the motion of your heart quite a bit.

Dr. T. Arts: I agree. Especially in the diastolic phase, because then the heart is very deformable. It is lying there in the open air, so it flattens with gravity. I believe that in the closed thorax the shape will not change that much. At the beginning of systole it jumps very quickly into some systolic state. Then the heart feels very stiff, and shape is determined by the internal forces.

Dr. E. Ritman: I think it is sort of chicken and egg problem here. I wonder if all the muscle does is to contract with a certain strain and then the heart twists. It has no option. It is not as though there is somebody in there saying "Let's twist" so that the strains are equal. It may be just the opposite way around.

Dr. T. Arts: According to our models, the distribution of strain is a result related to the basic physics of mechanics. I would not say it is proven, but there is some evidence that it is correct.

Dr. R. Beyar: You suggest that diastolic deformation is variable and I disagree with that. It may be variable in your experiments, but isovolumic relaxation has been clearly shown by a lot of methods to be very consistent. These include the multiple markers method, human data with MRI, dog data with MRI and our recent apical twistometer. All consistently show a pattern of rapid untwisting during isovolumic relaxation.

Dr. T. Arts: As far as I can see, it is the jump from the systolic to the diastolic torsion curve as a function of cavity volume. This jump is indeed always downward, that is right. But if you look more carefully, the distance over which it jumps is not really well defined. I am not so sure about it. In systole you should think of a variance in the order of a few percent and in diastole the recoil may be on the order of 20–30%, and with a much larger variance.

Dr. R. Beyar: You have a spread of the load, which may explain it in these dogs.

Dr. L.E. Ford: Your model is intended to account for the possibility that all of the fibers shorten by the same amount. The available data on this point are a little less than ideal in that they have been obtained in microscopic studies of muscle taken out of a relaxed ventricle. These kinds of marker studies would enable you to see how much shortening actually occurs during ejection in the muscles at various layers of the heart. Have you analyzed the data to see if in fact the strain is equal through the heart wall.

Dr. T. Arts: This is our largest problem. In trying to relate endocardial and epicardial shortening, you should compare it with the diastolic heart. In diastole there is nearly no torsion. At least, the torsion is completely different from what you find during systole. You can not use the studies that are done *in vitro*. There have been several studies which looked into deformation in the systolic phase. Hunter and Douglas have recently found *[Rodriguez E, Hunter W, Royce M, Leppo M, Douglas A, Weisman H. A method to reconstruct myocardial sarcomere lengths and orientations at transmural sites in beating canine hearts. Am J Physiol 1992; 263: H293–H306]* that shortening is indeed quite homogeneously distributed from the endocardial to the epicardial layers, if you consider the interval of the ejection phase. You should not start at the end of diastole but immediately after the jump at the beginning of systole.

Dr. L.E. Ford: Could you analyze your data to see whether in fact the markers were moving towards each other by the same amount in the epicardium and endocardium?

Dr. T. Arts: They probably do, along the fiber orientation probably they do. The problem is that I do not know the fiber orientation.

Dr. E. Yellin: Did your model predict that there would be no base to apex shortening?

Dr. T. Arts: No. The model says that axial shortening and midwall shortening should be similar. That means that no change in shape is expected. Experimentally, a little change was found so the shape factor does not fit our model. I think it is fair to show this.

Dr. Y. Kresh: I am convinced that sarcomere length changes are not sufficient to account for the global chamber ejection fraction. There must be another mechanism to facilitate an ejection fraction of 60–70%. I am not saying your explanation of regional shortening does not account for it; there must be additional components that will dislocate or remove volume from the chamber other than straight sarcomere length changes.

Dr. T. Arts: No. Sarcomere shortening is of the order of 10% over the whole ejection phase. Then the ejection fraction is 50–70%.

Dr. Y. Kresh: It will not work if there is no torsion.

Dr. T. Arts: Even then I would also get it, but the distribution of sarcomere shortening from the endocardial to epicardial layers would not be even. The average of sarcomere shortening would not be affected.

Dr. J.K-J. Li: Can you indicate where the maximum velocity of shortening is?

Dr. T. Arts: The velocity of shortening is maximum close to where the aortic flow is maximum. This point also closely matches the point where the rate of torsion is maximum.

Dr. E. Yellin: The whole model is predicated on shortening. Shortening takes place everywhere and that is what ejects volume. There is lots of experimental evidence, and certainly there is evidence conceptually, that blood has to leave the ventricle on its own momentum; late in systole some of the blood is leaving the ventricle on its own momentum. Therefore there could be a volume change in the ventricle without shortening, due to shape change. In other words, shortening could completely stop and blood could still leave the heart because it has inertia.

Dr. T. Arts: Our data do not show that. If you look at the change in volume, it stops where flow crosses zero and then it looks more or less stable until the end of ejection. Then the aortic valve closes.

Dr. E. Yellin: If blood leaves, the volume has to decrease. My point is that some of the decrease in volume late in systole is not due to sarcomere shortening, but to a shape change due to blood leaving on its own inertia; it is being sucked out.

Dr. T. Arts: It might be, but we did not measure a shape change. It is part of the pump function and that means that the sarcomeres are shortening. The inertia effect seems not to be related to a change of shape.

Dr. E. Yellin: During the ejection phase the sarcomeres stop shortening, blood leaves the heart, and whatever you see after that point is a shape change, because the sarcomeres have stopped shortening.

Dr. T. Arts: We did not measure a shape change at the end of the ejection phase. In other experiments we have measured epicardial shortening with a video technique. Then you see that the length of the fibers follows very well the pattern of volume change. The sarcomeres stop shortening at the moment of closure of the aortic valve.

Dr. E. Yellin: Let me put it in another way. Suppose the sarcomeres stop shortening, and we have a little Maxwell demon who sits at the aortic valve and prevents the valve from closing, and sucks blood out of the ventricle. What would happen?

Dr. T. Arts: You create a vacuum and the fibers will shorten anyway.

Dr. E. Yellin: Yes, you will create a vacuum! And that is why ventricular pressure is less than aortic pressure sometime in mid-systole.

Dr. T. Arts: Yes, but fibers shorten anyway. You do not know if this is active force generation by the fibers, or whether they are shortened by their environment.

Dr. E. Yellin: Interesting point; they could stop shortening, blood could still leave and the ventricle could distort. We can not prove it, but it is worth thinking about.

REFERENCES

1. Ingels NB, Daughters GT, Stinson EB, Alderman EL. Evaluation of methods for quantitating left ventricular segmental wall motion in man using myocardial markers as a standard. *Circulation* 1980; 61: 966–972.
2. Kresh JY, Brockman SK. A model-based system for assessing ventricular chamber pressure-volume-dimension relationship: regional and global deformation. *Ann Biomed Eng* 1986; 14: 15–33.
3. Slinker BK, Glantz SA. The accuracy of inferring left ventricular volume from dimension depends on the frequency of information needed to answer a given question. *Circ Res* 1985; 56: 161–174.
4. Hansen DE, Daughters GT, Alderman EL, Ingels NB, Stinson EB, Miller DC. Effect of volume loading, pressure loading, and inotropic stimulation on left ventricular torsion in humans. *Circulation* 1991; 83: 1315–1326.
5. Ingels NB, Daughters GT, Stinson EB, Alderman EL. Measurement of midwall myocardial dynamics in intact man by radiography of surgically implanted markers. *Circulation* 1975; 52: 859–867.
6. Arts T, Veenstra PC, Reneman RS. A model of the mechanics of the left ventricle. *Ann Biomed Eng* 1979; 7: 299–318.
7. Arts T, Reneman RS. Dynamics of left ventricular wall and mitral valve mechanics: a model study. *J Biomech* 1989; 22: 261–271.
8. Potel MJ, MacKay SA, Rubin JM, Aisen AM, Sayre RE. Three-dimensional left ventricular wall motion in man. Coordinate systems for representing wall movement direction. *Invest Radiol* 1984; 19: 499–509.
9. Rankin JS, McHale P, Arentzen CE, Ling D, Greenfield JC, Anderson RW. The three-dimensional dynamic geometry of the left ventricle in the conscious dog. *Circ Res* 1976; 39: 304–313.

10. Olsen CO, Rankin JS, Arentzen CE, Ring WS, McHale PA, Anderson RW. The deformational characteristics of the left ventricle in the conscious dog. *Circ Res* 1981; 49: 843–855.
11. Hunter WC, Sugiura S, Douglas AS. Systolic changes in local shape of left ventricular wall. *Ann Conf Eng Med Biol* 1986; p 124.
12. Chadwick RS. Mechanics of the left ventricle. *Biophys J* 1982; 39: 279–288.
13. Reneman RS, van der Vusse GJ, Arts T. Cardiac microcirculation, a general introduction. *Bibl Anat* 1981; 20: 477–483.
14. Garrison JB, Ebert WL, Jenkins RE, Vionoulis SM, Malcom H, Heyler GA. Measurement of three-dimensional biplane cine- angiograms. *Comp Biomed Res* 1982; 15: 76–96.
15. Hunter WC, Zerhouni EA. Imaging distinct points in left ventricular myocardium to study regional wall deformation. In: *Innovations in Diagnostic Radiology*, Anderson JA (ed), Springer–Verlag: New York. 1989; 169–190.
16. Arts T, Hunter WC, Douglas A, Muijtiens AMM, Reneman RS. Description of the deformation of the left ventricle by a kinematic model. *J Biomech* 1992; 25: 1119–1128.
17. Walley KR, Grover M, Raff GL, Benge W, Hannaford B, Glantz SA. Left ventricular dynamic geometry in the intact and open chest dog. *Circ Res* 1982; 50: 573–589.
18. Yellin EL, Nikolic S, Frater WM. Left ventricular filling dynamics and diastolic function. *Prog Cardiovasc Dis* 1990; 32: 247–271.
19. Arts T, Meerboum S, Reneman RS, Corday E. Stresses in the closed mitral valve, a model study. *J Biomech* 1983; 7: 539–547.

CHAPTER 38

Cardiovascular Flow Velocity Measurements by 2D Doppler Imaging for Assessment of Vascular Function

Dan R. Adam[1,2], Kenneth M. Kempner[2], Mark A. Vivino[2], Eben E. Tucker[3] and Michael Jones[4]

ABSTRACT

Clinical two-dimensional (2D) Doppler ultrasound flow velocity measurement is important for determination of arterial wall shear stress, blood-tissue exchange, myocardial and valvular function. Such 2D Doppler flow velocity images are usually displayed in color, superimposed on the gray-scale, cross-section structural images of the tissue. There are several limitations to this technique of flow measurement, some due to the instrumentation and some to the way the measurement is made. In this report we concentrate on the latter, identifying the main causes of errors and distortion, and outlining the methodology for minimizing them. The suggested method takes into account the spatial location and orientation of both the ultrasound transducer and the blood vessel. It allows quantification of vascular flow patterns, thus enhancing the usefulness of this important non-invasive diagnostic tool.

INTRODUCTION

The flow of blood and its velocity distribution across the artery have significant effects on the processes within the arterial wall. Transport of metabolic constituents and exchange of substances from blood to the endothelial cells depend on blood volume and its velocity in the artery [1]. Similarly, the damage caused to the endothelial layer, a

[1]Heart System Research Center, Department of Biomedical Engineering, Technion-IIT, Haifa, [2]Division of Computer Resources and Technology, [3]Cardiology Branch, NHLBI, [4]SLAMS, NHLBI, NIH, Bethesda, MD 20892, USA.

Interactive Phenomena in the Cardiac System, Edited by S. Sideman and R. Beyar, Plenum Press, New York, 1993

mandatory stage in the pathological development of coronary artery disease and arterial stenosis, also depends on flow velocity [2]. The high velocities, which occur in areas of bifurcation and bending, and the large shear stresses associated with them, affect shear-induced platelet aggregation [3]. In order to estimate the intensity of these normal and pathological processes near and at the walls, the blood flow velocity must be determined. Yet, the non–invasive measurement of blood flow velocity in a specific location of the cardiovascular system is a challenge. Some of the imaging modalities have been modified to allow flow measurements. The imaging systems (MRI, CT, ultrasound) usually produce images of cross–sections, sequences of such cross–sections or projections (X–ray angiography). Unless the image plane coincides with the vascular central longitudinal cross–section, the measurement of flow velocity from these images may produce erroneous values. Errors may also be introduced when the flow direction is not accounted for in the data analysis.

There is clearly a clinical demand for measurement of the flow velocity pattern across the flow field. In the study and development of artificial cardiac valves, quantitative assessment of the 3D flow jets through and around the valve is required. The studies of vessel stenosis development, blood clot formation and effective flow volume, require quantitative estimation of the 3D flow profile in the arterial lumen. Until new probes are configured to acquire flow information directly in 3D, there is a need for development and improvement of measurement, processing and display techniques. These techniques use temporal and spatial sequential sets of 2D images, and with additional information from either the measurement itself or from the acquired images, would better enable quantification of 3D flow profiles.

The concept of reconstructing a 3D image from 2D cross–sectional images has been applied to the cardiovascular system. Several groups have attempted to reconstruct in 3D the contour of the entire heart (or the left ventricle) from 2D echo ultrasound images. Multiple images of structural cross–sections of the heart have been taken at various orientations in order to reconstruct its shape [4–8]. Since the introduction of esophageal probes, the better image quality and the nearly fixed location of the echo ultrasound transducer within the body have made these systems better suited for 3D reconstruction [9]. The accuracy for volume measurements has been demonstrated [10, 11]. The further development of miniaturized probes has allowed intravascular generation of 2D images and therefore, the 3D reconstruction and visualization of arterial structures [11–14], including coronary arteries [15].

These methods have not yet been well adapted for flow measurements. Both external and esophageal echo ultrasound scanning transducers are available with Doppler flow imaging capability. While both allow 2D images of intra–ventricular flow, the accuracy of the measurements is too low for quantitative evaluation and 3D reconstruction. Intravascular probes may produce superior images, but the position of the probe within the vessel affects and distorts the 3D pattern of flow substantially.

The determination of 3D flow patterns may be also achieved by a different modality, magnetic resonance imaging (MRI). Various approaches have been taken [16–18] to allow flow velocity mapping. Validations of this measurement versus flow phantoms [19] and ultrasound [20] demonstrate good results. But the spatial resolution of MRI flow velocity measurement is too low, the acquisition time is much more than the cardiac cycle, and the price is extremely prohibitive.

Doppler echo ultrasound imaging has the many advantages of being non–invasive, nearly real–time and relatively inexpensive, but its flow measurement is inaccurate. Our effort is directed towards identifying the main causes which reduce the accuracy, and limit the ability to quantify the flow measurement. This effort includes reducing the errors generated by the varying angles between the transducer and the flow. This is achieved by measuring the orientation of the former and taking into account the direction of the latter. We try also to address the problem of limited information, since currently the clinician is provided with cross–sectional data only, by measuring and displaying the data in 3D.

METHODS

The selection of equipment was limited to include only off–the–shelf instruments, and of proven, long–used technology. Though a few ultrasound scanners have recently been offered with limited digital output (optical disk or digital link to a personal computer), the majority of manufacturers offer only video output. Our measured data is recorded on an analog tape and requires, therefore, the equipment for controlling both the tape recorder movement and the video sampling board.

Equipment

Doppler Echo Ultrasound Imaging System selected for this study is a system (Acuson Computer Sonography System 128XP–10, Acuson Co.) which produces excellent images from its 7.5 MHz Linear Array probe (Acuson Probe L7384) and, thus, is well suited for studies of superficial vessels. The system allows either continuous scanning and recording, or acquisition into internal RAM and then recording (by Panasonic Video Recorder AG–7350). The system is set for imaging the carotid arteries (common and external) with a constant zoom to allow a window of 2 cm depth by 2.8 cm length, with a dynamic range of +/– 8 cm/sec or +40 cm/sec. An electromagnetic receiver antenna is mounted on the linear array ultrasound probe, for measurement of spatial location and orientation.

Spatial Location and Orientation Measurement System is based upon an electromagnetic position and orientation measurement system (standalone 'A Flock of Birds,' by Ascension Technology Corp.), with a transmitter antenna mounted on an extension from the wall and the receiver antenna mounted on the linear array ultrasound transducer. The antennas are mounted close to each other, to obtain the specified accuracy (translational 0.1" RMS, Angular 0.5° RMS) and resolution (translational 0.03" RMS, Angular 0.1° RMS). The system is controlled by a PC, which serves also as a digital recorder, capturing the readings transmitted by the system at a rate of 30 times per sec.

Tape Recorder, Time Code Generator and Sampling Controller are used for recording and playback. During the experiments, the data is recorded concurrently with a time code (SMPTE Time Code reader/generator TRG–50PC, Horita Co.) which is recorded on one of the audio channels in the recorder. During playback, (by Panasonic Video Player AG–7650), the different data sections are selected by reading this time code (BCD–5000 Video Controller) and triggering the frame grabber system in the computer when the selected time is reached. The frame grabber system is a two board system (Media Master 2000, Scion Co., and 64Mb RAM Powercard), installed in a Macintosh Quadra 950.

The video tape recorder is also used to record the analog signals of the ECG, Respiration and flow (the latter in animal experiments only). These analog signals are preconditioned and multiplexed (FM Recording Adaptor model 3, Vetter Co.) into one of the audio channels in the recorder. These signals must be de–multiplexed utilizing the same device, before being sampled by an A/D converter.

Data Recording

The hardware described above allows for continuous sampling of more than 8 sec of 520x480 interlaced frames at 30 frames/sec, directly into RAM mounted on the sampling board which is installed in our computer. This constraint suggests that the length of the data recordings be about 1 min. for each sequence under stationary conditions.

We decided upon recording sequences at two longitudinal (parallel to the long axis) cross–sections at 90° to each other and at 12 transverse cross–sections as nearly parallel as possible. This decision was made so as to minimize the number of sequences to be recorded, while allowing collection of sufficient data to describe the arterial lumen and the flow profile in this particular artery, The hand–held ultrasound transducer is manipulated at each location over the vessel until a 'good' image is obtained. There are no constraints on the location or orientation of the transducer, except that while the recordings are made the transducer should not be moved. A set of such 14 sequences would produce, after data analysis, the flow profile in 3D during one cardiac cycle.

The video tape recorder is used to record concurrently on one of its audio channels the physiological signals of interest – ECG and respiration. These signals are sampled by a 12 bit A/D converter at 120 samples/sec. The second audio channel is used to record the time code from the time code generator. This time code allows exact registration of each video frame recorded, and comparison between the data recorded on the video tape and the spatial location and orientation data recorded on disk. The spatial location and orientation data are recorded 30 times per sec, with time information provided by the same time code generator.

Data Analysis

The Doppler echo ultrasound image sequences are processed and analyzed somewhat differently for the longitudinal vs. the transverse cross–sections. The longitudinal cross–sections serve two purposes:

a) The determination of the direction of flow in the 3D space, relative to the orientation of the transducer. We assume the flow to be laminar (which is usually the case, at least during the diastolic period). The direction of flow is taken along the center of geometry of the arterial lumen. Thus, the direction of flow is calculated at each point from the structural information within the image, and not from the flow information. Since the direction of the ultrasonic beam is known (set by the operator to be 0°, +60° or −60°, all in the image plane), the values of flow obtained in this mode are recalculated, taking into account the angle between these two directions.

b) The recalculated values of flow in the longitudinal cross–sectional images serve as the gold standard for the recalculated values of flow in the transverse cross–sections.

The flow values in the transverse cross–sections are processed by taking into account the known direction of flow in the 3D space, and the measured spatial location and orientation of the ultrasound transducer. Since the flow value at each point must be modified according to the cosine of the angle between the two vectors, the values changes quite significantly.

The recalculated flow values in the transverse cross–sections are used to adjust flow velocity values in the longitudinal cross–sections: In the vicinity of the border between the tissue and the arterial lumen (or cavity), at the proximal (towards the transducer) portions of the flow images, flow velocity values are often displayed superimposed on tissue structure. Similarly, adjustment should be made in the more distal portions of the images, where 'no–flow' is shown in areas of flow (due to the wall–motion filters cutoff).

RESULTS

The data required for the processing procedures include sequences of images of longitudinal and transverse cross–sections of the carotid arterial lumen, with the color Doppler flow information. The resultant image sequences will differ in two ways: 1. The color–encoded flow values will be much more accurate, and 2. since the flow values will be calculated for the entire volume of the lumen, orthogonal cross–sections will be presented, though the values can be presented for any desirable oblique cross–section.

Since the flow velocity patterns are four dimensional, with the velocity value depending on the three spatial dimensions and time, it is beneficial to display the results as a sequence of images of the 3D volume of blood flowing in the arterial lumen. It is possible to look closely at any specific cross–section, thus avoiding misinterpretation due to partial information.

DISCUSSION

This report outlines a new way of measuring and processing of Doppler echo ultrasound images. There have been several demonstrations of using measurements of the 3D spatial orientation of the ultrasonic probe for calculating the orientation of the ultrasound beam and thus reconstructing the myocardial walls in 3D space [4–8]. Here, we use this method not only for reconstruction of the 3D shape of the arterial lumen and the flow velocity distribution, but also for recalculation of the velocity values with a significant reduction of errors and distortions.

Several modifications must still be made in the instrumentation to reduce measurement errors, e.g. errors due to diffraction of the ultrasonic beam when it crosses layers of different acoustical impedances. Also, there is currently no reasonable solution for the problem of estimating the localized flow direction during turbulent flow, and therefore the calculation of turbulent flow velocity is inherently incorrect.

In spite of these limitations, non–invasive flow velocity measurements become increasingly important as clinical tools for diagnosis and for evaluating physiological function. Pre operative studies allow assessment of severity of obstruction in arteries, and an evaluation of flow volume. The recalculation of flow velocity values, as outlined in this report, is expected to yield significantly smaller errors than those produced by the currently available commercial equipment.

CONCLUSIONS

We have outlined here a method for measuring the 3D spatial orientation of the ultrasonic probe, thus allowing calculation of the orientation of the ultrasound beam, as well as the direction of flow, in the spatial coordinates of the image. Since Doppler echo ultrasound imaging includes superposition of flow data with structural information, it is possible to estimate the general direction of flow in the image coordinates, specifically in a vessel. It is therefore possible to increase the accuracy of the calculations of flow velocity values by taking into account the angle between the ultrasound beam and the flow direction.

The increased accuracy of the calculated flow velocity values allow readjustment of flow values in areas of ambiguity, and may reduce distortions near the blood–wall interface. It also allows the computation of flow velocity values at different viewing angles and the construction of a 3D description of flow patterns in a vessel.

DISCUSSION

Dr. E. Yellin: Can you go from a color coding to velocity vectors and do a velocity map using vectors rather than color?

Dr. D. Adam: Since flow velocity vectorial values are calculated in our approach, it is possible to do that. The problem is that the users, the clinicians, are not used to look at the vectors. They are more used to look at the colors, and therefore we calculate the velocity vectorial values, but display their amplitude in color coded maps.

Dr. E. Yellin: You would have to do it off line.

Dr. D. Adam: Currently we do all the calculations off line, and the process is labor intensive. Once the procedure is verified, and accepted, it can be implemented on line, since the whole procedure is not computationally intensive and does not require delays.

Dr. E. Ritman: Since you are still struggling with the technique itself, obviously you did not have time to think about the display problem. It seems to me though, that your study of quantifying the flow velocity measurement is very much related to the sort of questions that we are interested in, such as the shear at the endothelium (which can be deduced from the gradient and velocities near the wall). How are you going to handle the display of your results with the sort of data sets that you get? To project it in 3D is going to be confusing.

Dr. D. Adam: There are two steps here. First, there is the problem of the correct calculation of the velocity values in 3D. The flow "velocity" values obtained in the longitudinal cross–sections are really distorted by the blood–wall interface and filtration, so estimating the velocities along the wall from these measurements is quite inaccurate. Our approach is to obtain the values near the wall from the transverse cross–sections, once they are recalculated correctly, by taking into account the transducer orientation versus the flow orientation. Those who currently study flow can obtain measurements from the transverse cross–sections, but the measurements of the orientation of the transducer vs the flow are far from being accurate. Therefore, the correct calculation is the first important issue. The display is the second step. Once all of the corrected data is available in the 3D volume, one can cut different cross–sections in any direction and show the vectors of the flow at the various locations. Showing the flow velocity values within the "artery," but with a "transparent tissue" around it, may also be a useful way of display.

REFERENCES

1. Bassingthwaighte JB, Wang CW, Chan IS. Blood–tissue exchange via transport and transformation by endothelial cells. *Circ Res* 1989; 65: 997–1020.
2. Dewey CF, Davies PF, Gimbrone MA. Turbulence, disturbed flow and vascular endothelium. In: Yoshida Y, Yamaguchi T, Caro CG, Glagov S, Nerem RM (eds) *Role of Blood Flow in Atherogenesis*. Springer–Verlag: Tokyo, pp 201–204, 1988.
3. O'Brien JR. Shear–induced platelet aggregation. *Lancet* 1990; 335: 711–713.
4. Moritz WE, Pearlman AS, McCabe DH, Medema DK, Ainsworth ME, Boles MS. An ultrasound technique for imaging the ventricle in three–dimensions and calculating its volume. *IEEE Trans Biomed Eng* 1983; 30: 482–492.
5. Geiser EA, Ariet M, Conetta DA, Lupkiewicz SM, Christie LG, Conti CR. Dynamic three–dimensional echocardiographic reconstruction of the intact human left ventricle: Technique and initial observations in patients. *Am Heart J* 1982; 103: 1056–1065.
6. Sawada H, Fujii J, Kato K, Onoe M, Kuno K. Three–dimensional reconstruction of the left ventricle from multiple cross sectional echocardiograms: Value for measuring left ventricular volume. *Br Heart J* 1983; 50: 438–442.

7. McCann HA, Chandrasekaran K, Hoffman EA, Sinak LJ, Kinter TM, Greenleaf JF. A method for three-dimensional ultrasonic imaging of the heart in vivo. *Dynamic Cardiovasc Imaging* 1987; 1:97–109.
8. Levine RA, Handschumacher MD, Sanfilippo AJ, Hagege AA, Harrigan P, Marshall JE, Weyman AE. Three-dimensional echocardiographic reconstruction of the mitral valve, with implication for the diagnosis of mitral valve prolapse. *Circulation* 1989; 80: 589–598.
9. Martin RW, Bashein G. Measurement of stroke volume with three-dimensional transesophageal ultrasonic scanning: Comparison with thermodilution measurement. *Anesthesiology* 1989; 70: 470–476.
10. Martin RW Bashein G, Detmer PR, Moritz WE. Ventricular volume measurement from a multiplanar transesophageal ultrasonic imaging system: An in vitro study. *IEEE Trans Biomed Eng* 1990; 37: 442–449.
11. Kuroda T, Kinter TM, Seward JB, Yanagi H, Greenleaf JF. Accuracy of three-dimensional volume measurement using biplane transesophageal echocardiographic probe: In vitro experiment. *J Am Soc Echocardiogr* 1991; 4: 475–484.
12. Kitney RI, Moura L, Straughan K. 3-D visualization of arterial structures using ultrasound and voxel modeling. *Int J Card Imaging* 1989; 4: 135–143.
13. Potkin BN, Bartorelli AL, Gessert JM, Neville RF, Almagor Y, Roberts WC, Leon MB. Coronary artery imaging with intravascular high-frequency ultrasound. *Circulation* 1990; 81: 1575–1585.
14. Nissen SE, Grines CL, Gurley JC, Sublett K, Haynie D, Diaz C, Booth DC, DeMaria AN. Application of a new phased-array ultrasound imaging catheter in the assessment of vascular dimensions. *Circulation* 1990; 81: 660–666.
15. Rosenfield K, Losordo DW, Ramaswamy K, Pastore JO, Langevin RE, Razvi S, Kosowsky BD, Isner JM. Three-dimensional reconstruction of human coronary and peripheral arteries from images recorded during two-dimensional intravascular ultrasound examination. *Circulation* 1991; 84: 1938–1956.
16. Van Dijk P. Direct cardiac NMR imaging of heart wall and blood flow velocity. *J Comput Assist Tomogr* 1984; 8: 429–436.
17. Bryant DJ, Payne JA, Firmin DN, Longmore DB. Measurement of flow with NMR imaging using a gradient pulse and phase difference technique. *J Comput Assist Tomogr* 1984; 8: 588–593.
18. Mohiaddin RH, Amanuma MA, Kilner PJ, Pennel DJ, Manzara C, Longmore DB. MR phase-shift velocity mapping of mitral and pulmonary venous flow. *J Comput Assist Tomogr* 1991; 15: 237–243.
19. Van Rossum A, Sprenger KH, Peels FC, et al. In vivo validation of quantitative flow imaging in arteries and veins using magnetic resonance phase shift techniques. *Soc of Magnetic Resonance in Medicine*, Amsterdam, 1989; 205.
20. Kilner PJ, Firmin DN, Rees RSO, et al. Magnetic resonance jet velocity mapping for assessment of valve and great vessel stenosis. *Radiology* 1991; 178: 229–235.

CLOSING DISCUSSION: *A View into the Future*

Dr. S. Sideman: Nine years ago, in the first Henry Goldberg Workshop, there was a debate between the clinicians and cardiac scientists on the role of modelling as a tool to explain and predict what we do not know. I believe we have passed this phase and experience has shown that while a model is not a substitute for reality, it is a tool, calibrated by available experimental/clinical data, by which we can learn specific unmeasurable elements of reality under very well controlled conditions. This is its strength and this is its function. When we started our research into cardiac function some 10 years ago or so, I believed that by combining information and putting it in equations, we could simulate the whole heart and that it would be easy to do it.... Well it is not easy, and it could probably not be done, because whatever we do, we can not recreate reality. We can at best simulate parts of it. Should we combine the different models? Yes, provided that we want to get specific answers to specific questions. I do not foresee today an overall model describing ***all*** the functions of the heart. That is a tremendous, and perhaps unrealistic, goal. What we can do and should do is relate the different disciplines and the different parameters and try to learn more and more about the characteristics of more and more parameters under different conditions. A model is a tool to approach reality as close as we can. In 10 years I will probably be more optimistic, but after 10 years of a lot of modeling, I feel we are still working with a very broad brush and the fine brush, if you allow me to say so, is in the hands of God. We can only hope to approach it! To my students I convey a very humble message: all you have to do is touch one hair of the tail of the donkey on which the Messiah is riding! I don't ask for anything more!

I believe we all share the excitement of learning new things from different points of view and seeing the progress of cardiac science. I would like to initiate a short and hopefully useful discussion, trying to look into the crystal ball and anticipate potential future research work. It may be useful, or it may be pipe-dreams. Nevertheless, I do not see anybody better qualified to do it than the people sitting here.

Dr. J. Bassingthwaighte: I have learned a great deal here about a whole variety of different aspects. Let's start with calcium. Dr. Marban discussed calcium explicitly. Dr. Strauss's presentation related ATP and adenosine to calcium and calcium currents and activation. I tend to translate everything that is electrical–mechanical into something metabolic, which is how Dr. Hasenfuss ended when he talked about heat. The question is, how do we relate the generated force to the chemical supply? In each situation, such as ischemia described by Dr. Allen, we ask, "what happened to the supply of nutrient, and therefore what would happen to the electromechanical force development?" It is one thing to show that the immediate precursors of activation, let's say by a drop in PCr or rise in phosphate, are involved. But what happens to the substrates in between? Is it just oxygen insufficiency? Does the electron transport system fail? What are the interactions between the different cell types? What are the storage mechanisms for substrates, oxygen as well as fatty acid, glycogen and so on. Each of these topics merited and received, attention.

Dr. Somlyo, in talking about the morphology in explicit ways, gave hint to a major event, namely the interactions between different cell types, the endothelial cell, the myocyte, the smooth muscle cells and so on. That brings back the relationship between the ATP and intracellular calcium in vasoregulation and the to–and–fro which occurs between force development at the myocyte and what is happening in the intact organ. Clearly the intact organ and the intact cell behave differently from the isolated or skinned cell. Drs. Sys and Ford went back to energetics. Dr. Sys and Dr. Brutsaert brought out the ideas of endothelial cell/myocyte interaction, although I have to admit that I do not understand how endocardial endothelium affects ventricular contraction. But there is clearly some observation there that demands understanding. The next two presentations, of Drs. Landesberg and Sideman and of Rudy, were overt cases of trying to be the physiologist, physician, bioengineer or, if you want to call it so, the integrators of the system. These were both successful in different ways. What was interesting too is that they both gave well integrated synthetic approaches to figuring out how the system works and yet the topics were not overlapping. Such approaches will inevitably be brought together before long, and later associated with metabolism. The integrated system synthesis will eventually bring it all back together.

The questions to be asked are: What can we learn from this exciting session to do next? What are the particular problems, what are the conflicts that we see exposed today? Can we identify those fairly clearly? Which new types of approaches should we use in the future? What should be the next effort to bring the system into workable order? Not that it is in disarray, but it certainly needs more tight ordering.

Dr. R. Chadwick: I would like to see more cross–fertilization between models dealing with either mechanical, electrical, or chemical questions. If one is studying arrhythmias, for example, how does that affect pumping efficiency? People have not really studied the effects of electrical abnormalities on mechanical performance and that should be done.

Dr. R. Beyar: We deal with a global heart. We take a nose–dive into the cellular mechanism, stay there for a while and, like pilots, we should be able to pull the stick up each time and go back to the whole cardiac system. We should be able to relate the cellular mechanisms that we are studying in very fine details to the global ventricular performance and to patient health and well being. I would like to give an example. There have been a whole class of studies on ventricular elastance from an experimental mechanical point of view. We have now learned how it all stems from calcium kinetics and contractile mechanics. We should be able to go back and forth between the cellular mechanism of calcium kinetics and global ventricular elastance and try to explain global mechanical features of cardiac function in terms of cellular mechanism. Models are very important in helping us to understand this interaction.

Dr. Y. Rudy: It is important to remember that even at the microscopic level of the cell, isolated components do not do the same thing as they do when they are in the cell or when the cell is in an ensemble of cells. I can give many examples, but Dr. Marban gave one, the skinned cell preparation vs the intact cell. We have talked about calcium transients. I have discussed EADs (early after depolarization) that result from spontaneous release of calcium from the SR during calcium overload. But calcium overload also uncouples cells at the gap junctions, therefore affecting not only the generation of the action potential by the single cell but also its propagation between cells. It is important to study component processes in isolation, but it is also important to remember that when they are part of a bigger system (cell, tissue), they are not exactly the same as they were in isolation.

Dr. J. Bassingthwaighte: We have seen some very nice modelling presented; models were demonstrated in one way and another here. There is lots of quantitative thinking in this room. My overt suggestion would be, should we not put together models for excitation–contraction (EC) coupling, including all of the force–development, all of the crossbridge interactions, the ATP generating part of this sequence, the substrate utilization to form ATP, and then put that into multi–cellular models, myocyte models, which have endothelial cells appropriately positioned, and try to master such a model. Is that a worthwhile effort to bring about the response to Dr. Beyar, namely, to have something that can be utilized and expressed toward a clinical end. How else might you do this? These are approaches that will allow you to take the basic cellular physiology and put it together so that one can understand the working organ.

Dr. A. Landesberg: The importance of a model is its ability to test the influence of different events. We can not put in the model all of the biochemical end events that happen in the cell. We cannot put into the model also the ATP and all the biochemical processes, as we would get a huge model with a lot of parameters. We would never be able to measure all of the processes in the cell, the calcium transient, the amount of calcium bound to troponin, the amount of ATP, the hydrolysis. The advantage of a model is the ability to test the importance of different events that occur in the cell. The most important event in testing the model is the time constant. For example, calcium kinetics is very important to demonstrate the kinetics of one beat. But when you are talking on force length, frequency relation or the kinetic of ATP is more important. One of the important things in a model is to determine what process we are going to model, what is the time interval and what is the main biochemical process that determines the characteristics of the cardiac muscle. For example, our model that couples calcium kinetics with crossbridge cycling can also calculate, since we can calculate the number of crossbridges in the strong state, the energy and heat produced. Dr. Hasenfuss has shown us that tension depends on heat. When he checked the force and the tension dependent heat he got a straight line and this demonstrated to him that in the depleted cardiac muscle the contractile element is not working normally. Only a model can test the main problems in different cardiac mechanisms.

Dr. E. Ritman: There are two issues we need to think about as far as the future is concerned. One concerns modeling. One should always ask, why are you modeling? What is the question you are trying to get a handle on and how will the model help there? In addition, how should you modify the model, or some aspect of the model, in response to new real information that becomes available. We have heard here the results of modeling what you might call more real data. How are we going to link the two and respond to each other? Hopefully the models will stimulate experiments that need to be done.

The second issue is a very striking absence of molecular and perhaps genetic aspects from this series of presentations. I realize this is a buzz word and we should not get onto the band–wagon just because it is popular. Nonetheless, we are limited in the sort of questions we are able to ask and address with the methodology used. I suspect that in future workshops, the molecular aspect needs to be incorporated in some fashion.

Dr. S. Sideman: The genetic field is one we should definately enter. We can contribute in system analysis and in dynamic studies. I do not feel that we presently have the handle to do the things that we can really contribute to, but it will come, within a short time. The rational to deal with genetic engineering and molecular biology in this forum is that we can contribute our own strength to it, once we find the tools and the means to do it. But I have no doubt that we are headed there, because we are hungry for excitement, knowledge and challenges and this is the place to find it.

Dr. E. Ritman: There are a lot of people working with molecular medical techniques. I am told that in principal it is quite a simple technique and it may, in fact be rather boring for some people, but it brings up some interesting new information. I am afraid that many molecular people working with molecular techniques are sort of like Mickey Mouse as the Sorcerer's apprentice chopping up the broomstick, conjuring up little broom sticks running around out of hand. They do not know how to put all their data together in terms of the integrated body, and this is perhaps where integrated physiology can have some impact.

Dr. M. Gotsman: I would like to relate for a moment to our large scale studies. One thing that worries me is that we have "modelers" and we have "datists." Some have data and some can create models. The trouble is that the models may sometimes get out of hand and sometimes do not necessarily take the data into hand. We are trying to fit together the way in which the ventricle contracts, the way in which the ventricle is oriented. We look at a very big model, the model of the total ventricle, and one way we can study it is by putting markers inside and seeing how it contracts. But we have not asked many questions: if you have a given mass of sarcomere, what determines how much is synthesized to create this mass? what induces its alignment and normalizes stress? what turns it on? what turns it off? We have not asked what is the transducer which orientates it. If it becomes hypertrophic and gets out of hand, why does it get out of hand? All of these things should be amenable to modeling. The next stage maybe is to move beyond just the fiber orientation and look at the transducers which cause the fiber orientation and the kinds of myosin, and actin, and the speed with which all of these reactions occur.

Dr. Janicki has talked about collagen. What turns the collagen on? What turns it off? Why do we synthesize the collagen? Why is it degraded? What orientates the collagen? How does it attach itself to the surrounding muscle cells? Does it attach to blood vessels or does it wrap around the blood vessels? What makes it do these things? What determines these shape changes in the LV in terms of collagen? Does it take weeks, months or years? I think we are moving into the next phase, examining new tools, not new ideas. We are going to be taking the same modeling techniques but we are going to ask the questions at a molecular level.

I also have a question about restenosis: why does restenosis occurs at a particular sight? What are the flow characteristics which turn it on as opposed to the chemical characteristics which turn it on and off? We have not answered a lot of questions at the macro scale level, so lets talk about the subcellular level as a modification or as a future extension of what we have been talking about today.

The paper on flow in the carotid artery imparts a message that atheroma occurs at the carotid bifurcations. Once the flow alterations are induced, how does the secondary changes in flow remodel the artery? We have to ask the correct questions! The molecular biologists can explain how the cells stick together or not, how they interact, how they cross membranes or emerge from them, so that we have an extension of our previous basic ideas.

Dr. N. Westerhof: There was a lot of sophisticated high level modeling reported here, and most used models to interpret data. However, models have a limit. A model is necessary to organize your thoughts, help with future experiments, and that has always a limit. Take for example, Poiseuille's Law. It is very nice to think of molecules, even maybe nuclei of atoms, etc., but at that level you can not model laws like Poiseuille's. So you make a big jump and you forget all about the details and about statistical mechanics etc., and you go to another set of equations and you model the Poiseuille's Law. There is always a trade-off between how complex a model should be and what you gain from it. My personal opinion is to favor models that can be more or less comprehended. You need a computer to calculate the details in a nonlinear system, as is most often the case in biological science. But every model has its limitation, and to go on, you have to start from a different level of assumptions and go to a higher level of system.

Dr. E. Yellin: A comment can be made that we are dinosaurs doomed to extinction. But dinosaurs were destroyed by a large meteorite or comet and we are going to be destroyed by a molecule, and I do not think we should be destroyed! I am not sure that we have to move toward molecular biology. We have to raise new questions. How are these things done? Let the molecular biologist do it. But if we are not here to look at the functional correlates of what they are doing, then all of their little broomsticks will be meaningless. A message has to come from this meeting to NIH: mechanics and systems and organs have to remain a viable area of study so that the molecular people can have some meaning placed on their results. Someone has to discuss these things. Someone has to talk about shear and transport and so on, so that the molecular people will know where to go.

Dr. L.E. Ford: I want to respond to the statement on what we should make known to the NIH. If we take one of the questions raised here, "why is there an abnormal hypertrophy in the septum and what are the things that contribute to it," and we call the NIH's attention to it, we might obtain a rude response from the highest level. The current director of the NIH, Dr. B. Healey (whose name was Buckley, about 10 years ago), published a paper about the development of myofibrilla disarray and abnormal hypertrophy in the centroid shapes of the LV. Centroid shapes are those in which there is no change in the stress with changes in their orientations. To my knowledge, her findings were never followed up. The point is, there is a lot of data out there, and a lot of models, and they should be incorporated together.

Dr. S. Sideman: On the global scale, we are trying to do the impossible, which makes it fun, because if it was possible it would be boring. We are trying to understand things that are quite complicated and unclear and sometimes unreasonable, or at least they look so. We are trying to decipher how the herat works. Molecular engineering, molecular biology and genetics are a very important part in making it work. That is where we can and should get involved and I have no doubt that this will happen soon. Whoever will be the first to come up with a good model relating molecules and genes to function will do an important work. Today, we work on the ionic-calcium-control of the activation-contraction system, which is already at the subcellular level. It is just another step into the molecular dimension. I hope it will come soon enough to have it on the agenda of the future Henry Goldberg Workshops.

Dr. J. Bassingthwaighte: It is kind of a semantic issue. There is a philosophical issue embedded in this conversation. The way we need to look at a model is that it is an hypothesis; it is the clean quantitative description of the hypothesis that we pose. In posing an hypothesis, you ask the question how do I disprove it, because you can never prove it. So this is in a sense the basis of the scientific method and it is one of the things that is a major strength in this group. Let me add another thing that was brought to our attention by Platt. Dr. J.R. Platt, in a wonderful article in *Science [#3966, 1964; 146: 347–355]* titled "Strong Inference," emphasizes that one has not only an hypothesis that one wishes to test, but the essential corollary to having an hypothesis which you want to disprove is to have an alternative hypothesis. That then strengthens your ability to design experiments in the sense that you then try to design your experiment so as to distinguish between your first hypothesis and your alternative hypothesis. If you can distinguish between these two you can disprove one of the hypothesis. So you can extrapolate this strategy for the scientific development deeper and deeper. What are our hypotheses? These days we have had several different hypotheses in several different areas. We have had several different hypotheses in any one area. Some are contradictory to others. We have not really gotten to the issue, in the mechanical modeling of the myocardium, of what are the contradictory aspects between these different models and how do we design an experiment to distinguish between them which results in disproof of at least one of the hypotheses and maybe both. I think that we are not really getting to the heart of this issue of examining each other's model hypotheses so carefully that we can distinguish among them from these various experiments.

Our simulation resource facility in Seattle is sponsored by the National Center for Research Resources, a sponsor of this Workshop. Over the door is written: *No Simulation without Experimentation*. Those of you from outside of the US might recognize this as a distortion of a slogan from the time of the founding our country, "No taxation without representation." Hypothesis and test go hand in glove. You develop the hypotheses, you develop the experiment to disprove the hypotheses and you go from there. There has to be a very close relationship between the experimentalist and the analyst. My own belief is that almost need to be the same person and if the analyst is not a part of the experimental team, you do not see all of the nuances, the things that help to disprove the hypothesis.

Dr. S. Sideman: If science is the quest for understanding the unknown, then modeling is a vehicle we must use in this voyage. The secret of understanding the complicated system that we deal with, the cardiac system, requires to decipher the interactions that make the heart work. There is not one point of view, or one discipline, that can give a complete satisfactory explanation to the phenomena that occur. The term "integration" represents the level which combines the interactions under some circumstances. To take a philosophical outlook, I would say that this is how we should proceed in the future: cooperation of spirits, interaction of ideas and integration of data.

As we come to the end of this exciting meeting, I would like to thank the people who helped make this meeting possible: The Advisory Committee which is chaired by Mike Weisfeldt, and the Organizing Committee: Dr. Beyar my co–Chairman, Jim Bassingthwaighte, Robert Reneman, Eric Ritman, and last but definitely not least, Walter Welkowitz. Special thanks go to the people of the NIH who helped us to get organized, here in Washington, particularly Richard Chadwick and Dan Adam, who is at the NIH on sabbatical, proving that you can do something worthwhile while you are on sabbatical...

Finally, my most hearty and sincere thanks to all the participants for their cooperation in this exciting voyage to unknown horizons.

THE EDITORS

Samuel Sideman, D.Sc., R.J. Matas/Winnipeg Professor of Biomedical Engineering, is Chairman of the Department of Biomedical Engineering, Director of the Julius Silver Institute of Biomedical Engineering, and Head of the Cardiac System Research Center of the Technion–Israel Institute of Technology.

Born in Israel (1929), he received his B.Sc. and D.Sc. from the Technion and his M.Ch.E. from the Polytechnical Institute of Brooklyn. On the faculty of the Technion since 1957, he served as Dean of Faculty, Dean of Students, and Chairman of the Department of Chemical Engineering, was a Visiting Professor at the University of Houston and CCNY, a Distinguished Visiting Professor at Rutgers University, NJ, and is a Visiting Professor of Surgery (Bioengineering) at the University of Medicine and Dentistry, New Jersey (UMDNJ), USA.

His interests include transport phenomena, with particular emphasis on the analysis and simulation of the cardiac system. He has authored and co–authored over 250 scientific publications and co–edited 12 books. A recipient of a number of professional awards and citations, President of the Assembly for International Heat Transfer Conferences, on the editorial board of some major scientific journals, he is a Senior Member of a number of professional societies, Fellow of the American Institute of Chemical Engineering and the New York Academy of Science.

Rafael Beyar, M.D., D.Sc., is an Associate Professor in the Department of Biomedical Engineering and is Associate Head of the Cardiac Research Center at the Technion.

Born in Israel (1952), he received his M.D. from Tel Aviv University and obtained his D.Sc. in Biomedical Engineering from the Technion–Israel Institute of Technology. In the Julius Silver Institute, Department of Biomedical Engineering, Technion–IIT since 1984, he was (1985 to 1987) at the Division of Cardiology, Johns Hopkins University Hospital, Baltimore. He was a Visiting Professor of Medicine and a Visiting Scientist to Alberta at the University of Calgary (1991–1992).

His interests include modeling, simulation of the cardiovascular system, 3D analysis of ventricular function, MRI, coronary flow, CPR and cardiac assist. He is a member of medical and engineering societies, and a recipient of a number of institutional and national excellence awards. He has authored and co–authored over 100 scientific publications and is co–editor (with Prof. Sideman) of 9 volumes dealing with imaging, analysis, simulation and control of the cardiac system.

CONTRIBUTORS

Mark Abovsky, Department of Biomedical Engineering, Technion–Israel Institute of Technology, Haifa, 32000, Israel

Dan R. Adam, D.Sc., Heart System Research Center, The Julius Silver Institute, Department of Biomedical Engineering, Technion–IIT, Haifa, Israel, and Division of Computer Resources and Technology, NIH, Bethesda, MD, USA

Metin Akay, Ph.D., Department of Biomedical Engineering, Rutgers University, Piscataway, NJ 08855, USA

Yasemin M. Akay, M.Sc., Department of Biomedical Engineering, Rutgers University, Piscataway, NJ 08855, USA

David G. Allen, MB.BS, Ph.D., Department of Physiology, University of Sydney, NSW 2006, Australia

Norman R. Alpert, Ph.D., Departments of Physiology and Biophysics, University of Vermont, Burlington, VT, USA

Luc J. Andries, Ph.D., Department of Physiology and Medicine, University of Antwerp, Groenenborgerlaan 171, 2020 Antwerp, Belgium

Theo Arts, Ph.D., Departments of Physiology and Biophysics, Cardiovascular Research Institute Maastricht, University of Limburg, P.O. Box 616, 6200 MD Maastricht, The Netherlands

Michelle D. Azan–Backx, V.M.D., Postdoctoral Fellow, Division of Cardiology, Department of Medicine, The Johns Hopkins University, 844 Ross Building, Baltimore, MD 21205, USA

Annabelle Azancot–Benisty, M.D., Ph.D., Laboratoire d'Explorations Fonctionelles, Hôpital Robert Debré, 75019, Paris, France

Peter H. Backx, V.M.D., Ph.D., Assistant Professor, Division of Cardiology, Department of Medicine, The Johns Hopkins University, 844 Ross Building, Baltimore, MD 21205, USA

James B. Bassingthwaighte, M.D., Ph.D., Center for Bioengineering, University of Washington, WD–12, Seattle, WA 98195, USA

Rafael Beyar, M.D., D.Sc., Heart System Research Center, The Julius Silver Institute, Department of Biomedical Engineering, Technion–IIT, Haifa, 32000, Israel

Dirk L. Brutsaert, M.D., Ph.D., Department of Physiology and Medicine, University of Antwerp, Groenenborgerlaan 171, 2020 Antwerp, Belgium

Rolf Bünger, M.D., Ph.D., Department of Physiology, Uniformed Services University of the Health Sciences, Bethesda, MD 20814–4799, USA

Simeon P. Cairns, Ph.D., Department of Physiology, University of Sydney, NSW 2006, Australia

Donald L. Campbell, Ph.D., Department of Pharmacology, Duke University Medical Center, Durham, NC 27710, USA

Richard S. Chadwick, Ph.D., Theoretical Biomecanics Group, Biomedical Engineering and Instrumentation Program, National Center for Research Resources, National Institutes of Health, Bethesda, MD, USA

William M. Chilian, Ph.D., Texas A&M University, Health Science Center, College Station, TX 77843, USA

Jan W. Corsel, Cardiovascular Research Institute Maastricht, University of Limburg, Maastricht, The Netherlands

Jenny Dankelman, Laboratory for Measurement and Control, Delft University of Technology, Mekelweg 2, 2628 CD Delft, The Netherlands

Tammo Delhaas, M.D., Departments of Physiology and Biophysics, Cardiovascular Research Institute Maastricht, University of Limburg, P.O. Box 616, 6200 MD Maastricht, The Netherlands

Michael J. Davis, Ph.D., Texas A&M University, Health Science Center, College Station, TX 77843, USA

Jo G.R. De Mey, Vascular Biology Laboratory, Department of Pharmacology and, Cardiovascular Research Institute Maastricht, University of Limburg, The Netherlands

Andrew S. Douglas, Department of Biomedical Engineering, Johns Hopkins University, Baltimore, MD, USA

Gijs Elzinga, M.D., Ph.D., Laboratory for Physiology and, Institute for Cardiovascular Research, Free University of Amsterdam, 1081 BT, Amsterdam, The Netherlands

Gregorio Fazzi, Vascular Biology Laboratory, Department of Pharmacology and, Cardiovascular Research Institute Maastricht, University of Limburg, The Netherlands

Eric O. Feigl, M.D., Departments of Physiology and Biophysics, University of Washington, Medical School, SJ–40, Seattle, WA 98195, USA

Gadi Fibich, Courant Institute, New York University, New York, NY, 10012, USA

Lincoln E. Ford, M.D., Cardiology Section, University of Chicago, Chicago, IL 60637, USA

Wei Dong Gao, Ph.D., Postdoctoral Fellow, Division of Cardiology, Department of Medicine, The Johns Hopkins University, 844 Ross Building, Baltimore, MD 21205, USA

Thierry C. Gillebert, M.D., Ph.D., Department of Physiology and Medicine, University of Antwerp, Groenenborgerlaan 171, 2020 Antwerp, Belgium

Dan Gilon, M.D., Department of Cardiology, Hadassah University Hospital, Jerusalem, Israel

Masami Goto, M.D., Department of Medical Engineering and Systems Cardiology, Kawasaki Medical School, 577 Matsushima, Kurashiki, 701–01 Japan

Mervyn S. Gotsman, M.D., Department of Cardiology, Hadassah University Hospital, Jerusalem, Israel

Henry R. Halperin, M.D., Peter Bolfer Cardiac Mechanics Laboratory, Department of Medicine, The Johns Hopkins Medical Institutions, Baltimore, MD, USA

Gerd Hasenfuss, M.D., Universität Freiburg, Medizinische Klinik III, Hugstetter Strasse 55, 7800 Freiburg, FRG

Herbert H. Himmel, M.D., Department of Pharmacology, Duke University Medical Center, Durham, NC 27710 USA

Osamu Hiramatsu, C.E., B.Sc., Department of Medical Engineering and Systems Cardiology, Kawasaki Medical School, 577 Matsushima, Kurashiki, 701–01 Japan

Eric A. Hoffman, Ph.D., Department of Radiology, University of Iowa College of Medicine, 200 Hawkins Drive, Iowa City, IA, 52242–1077, USA

Christian Holubarsch, M.D., Universität Freiburg, Medizinische Klinik III, Hugstetter Strasse 55, 7800 Freiburg, FRG

William C. Hunter, Ph.D., Department of Biomedical Engineering, Johns Hopkins University, Baltimore, MD, USA

Yuho Ito, M.D., Hiroshima University of Medicine, 2nd Department of Internal Medicine, 1–2–3 Kasumi Minami–Ku, 734 Japan

Joseph S. Janicki, Ph.D., Cardiology 1E65, University of Missouri, One Hospital Drive, Columbia, MO 65212, USA

Ger Janssen, Vascular Biology Laboratory, Department of Pharmacology and, Cardiovascular Research Institute Maastricht, University of Limburg, The Netherlands

Christopher J. H. Jones, M.B.B.S., Department of Cardiology, University of Wales College of Medicine, Cardiff, UK

Michael Jones, M.D., SLAMS, NHLBI, NIH, Bethesda, MD, USA
Robert M. Judd, Ph.D., Departments of Mechanical and Aerospace Engineering and Medicine, 337 Jarvis Hall, SUNY at Buffalo, Buffalo, NY 14260, USA
Hanjörg Just, M.D., Universität Freiburg, Medizinische Klinik III, Hugstetter Strasse 55, 7800 Freiburg, FRG
Ameer Kabour, M.D., Cardiology 1E65, University of Missouri, One Hospital Drive, Columbia, MO 65212, USA
David A. Kass, M.D., Associate Professor of Medicine, The Johns Hopkins Medical Institutions, Baltimore, MD 21205
Fumihiko Kajiya, M.D., Ph.D., Department of Medical Engineering and Systems Cardiology, Kawasaki Medical School, 577 Matsushima, Kurashiki, 701–01 Japan
Kenneth M. Kempner, M.Sc., Division of Computer Resources and Technology, NIH, Bethesda, MD, USA
Akihiro Kimura, M.D., Department of Medical Engineering and Systems Cardiology, Kawasaki Medical School, 577 Matsushima, Kurashiki, 701–01 Japan
J. Yasha Kresh, Ph.D., Likoff Cardiovascular Inst., Departments of Cardiothoracic Surgery and Medicine, Philadelphia, PA 19067, USA
Lih Kuo, Ph.D., Texas A&M University, Health Science Center, College Station, TX 77843, USA
Gervasio A. Lamas, M.D., Cardiovascular Division, Department of Medicine, Brigham and Women's Hospital, Harvard Medical School, Boston, MA, USA
Amir Landesberg, M.D., Department of Biomedical Engineering, Technion–IIT, Haifa, 32000, Israel
Giora Landesberg, M.D., Department of Cardiology, Hadassah University Hospital, Jerusalem, Israel
John A. Lee, MB, BS, Ph.D., Department of Pathology, University of Sheffield Medical School, Sheffield S10 2UL, UK
John K–J. Li, Ph.D., Professor and Director, Cardiovascular Research Laboratory, Department of Biomedical Engineering, Rutgers University, Piscataway, NJ 08855–0909 USA
Nadav Liron, Department of Mathematics, Department of Biomedical Engineering, Technion–Israel Institute of Technology, Haifa, 32000, Israel
Julie Z. Livingston, Peter Bolfer Cardiac Mechanics Laboratory, Department of Medicine, The Johns Hopkins Medical Institutions, Baltimore, MD, USA
Chaim Lotan, M.D., Department of Cardiology, Hadassah University Hospital, Jerusalem, Israel
Ching–hsing Luo, Ph.D., Department of Biomedical Engineering, Case Western Reserve University, 505 Wickenden Bldg., Cleveland, OH 44106–7207, USA
Robert T. Mallet, Ph.D., Department of Physiology, Texas College of Osteopathic Medicine, Fort Worth, TX 76107–2699, USA
Dante E. Manyari, M.D., Departments of Medicine and Medical Physiology, The University of Calgary, 1667 Health Sciences Center, 3330 Hospital Drive NW, Calgary, Alberta, T2N 4N1, Canada
Eduardo Marban, M.D., Ph.D., Robert L. Levy Professor of Cardiology, Dircetor of Molecular and Cellular Cardiology, Division of Cardiology, Department of Medicine, The Johns Hopkins University, 844 Ross Building, Baltimore, MD 21205, USA
Robert E. Mates, Ph.D., Departments of Mechanical and Aerospace Engineering and Medicine, 337 Jarvis Hall, SUNY at Buffalo, Buffalo, NY 14260, USA
Beatriz B. Matsubara, M.D., Universidade Estadual Paulista–Botucatu, Brasil
Gary F. Mitchell, M.D., Cardiovascular Division, Department of Medicine, Brigham and Women's Hospital, Harvard Medical School, Boston, MA, USA
Morris Mosseri, M.D., Department of Cardiology, Hadassah University Hospital, Jerusalem, Israel
Arno M.M. Muijtjens, Cardiovascular Research Institute Maastricht, University of Limburg, Maastricht, The Netherlands

Louis A. Mulieri, Ph.D., Departments of Physiology and Biophysics, University of Vermont, Burlington, Vermont, USA
Yasuo Ogasawara, Ph.D., Department of Medical Engineering and Systems Cardiology, Kawasaki Medical School, 577 Matsushima, Kurashiki, 701–01 Japan
Jacques Ohayon, Ph.D., Laboratoire de Mécanique Physique, Université Paris Val de Marne, 94010 Créteil Cedex, France
Marc A. Pfeffer, M.D., Ph.D., Cardiovascular Division, Department of Medicine, Brigham and Women's Hospital, Harvard Medical School, Boston, MA, USA
Burkert Pieske M.D., Universität Freiburg, Medizinische Klinik III, Hugstetter Strasse 55, 7800 Freiburg, FRG
Frits W. Prinzen, Ph.D., Departments of Physiology and Biophysics, Cardiovascular Research Institute Maastricht, University of Limburg, P.O. Box 616, 6200 MD Maastricht, The Netherlands
Yusheng Qu, Ph.D., Department of Pharmacology, Duke University Medical Center, Durham, NC 27710, USA
Barry K. Rayburn, Peter Bolfer Cardiac Mechanics Laboratory, Department of Medicine, The Johns Hopkins Medical Institutions, Baltimore, MD, USA
Robert S. Reneman, M.D., Ph.D., Departments of Physiology and Biophysics, Cardiovascular Research Institute Maastricht, University of Limburg, P.O. Box 616, 6200 MD Maastricht, The Netherlands
Jon R. Resar, M.D., Peter Bolfer Cardiac Mechanics Laboratory, Department of Medicine, The Johns Hopkins Medical Institutions, Baltimore, MD, USA
Erik L. Ritman, M.D., Ph.D., Department of Physiology and Biophysics, Mayo Clinic, Rochester, MN 55905, USA
Yoseph Rozenman, M.D., Department of Cardiology, Hadassah University Hospital, Jerusalem, Israel
Yoram Rudy, Ph.D., Department of Biomedical Engineering, Case Western Reserve University, 505 Wickenden Bldg., Cleveland, OH 44106–7207, USA
Dan Sapoznikov, Ph.D., Department of Cardiology, Hadassah University Hospital, Jerusalem, Israel
Nairne W. Scott–Douglas, M.D., Ph.D., Departments of Medicine and Medical Physiology, The University of Calgary, 1667 Health Sciences Center, 3330 Hospital Drive NW, Calgary, Alberta, T2N 4N1, Canada
Richard P. Shannon, M.D., Cardiovascular Division, Beth Israel Hospital and the New England Regional Primate Research Center, One Pine Hill Drive, P.O. Box 9102, Southborough, MA 01772–9102, USA
Samuel Sideman, D.Sc., Heart System Research Center, The Julius Silver Institute, Department of Biomedical Engineering, Technion–IIT, Haifa, 32000, Israel
Avril V. Somlyo, Ph.D., Professor of Pathology and Molecular Physiology and Biological Physics, University of Virginia School of Medicine, Department of Molecular Physiology and Biological Physics, Charlottesville, VA, USA
Andrew P. Somlyo, M.D., Chairman and Charles Slaughter Professor of Molecular Physiology and Biological Physics Professor of Medicine (Cardiology), University of Virginia School of Medicine, Department of Molecular Physiology and Biological Physics, Charlottesville, VA, USA
Jos A.E. Spaan, Department of Medical Physics and Informatics, University of Amsterdam AMC, Meibergdreef 15, 1105 AZ Amsterdam, The Netherlands
Harold C. Strauss, M.D., Departments of Medicine and Pharmacology, Duke University Medical Center, Durham, NC 27710, USA
Stanislas U. Sys, M.D., Ph.D., Department of Physiology and Medicine, University of Antwerp, Groenenborgerlaan 171, 2020 Antwerp, Belgium

Joshua E. Tsitlik, M.D., Peter Bolfer Cardiac Mechanics Laboratory, Department of Medicine, The Johns Hopkins Medical Institutions, Baltimore, MD, USA

Katsuhiko Tsujioka, M.D., Department of Medical Engineering and Systems Cardiology, Kawasaki Medical School, 577 Matsushima, Kurashiki, 701-01 Japan

Eben E. Tucker, M.D., Cardiology Branch, NHLBI, NIH, Bethesda, MD, USA

Stuart E. Turvey, B.Sc. (Med), Department of Physiology, University of Sydney, NSW 2006, Australia

John V. Tyberg, M.D., Ph.D., Departments of Medicine and Medical Physiology, The University of Calgary, 1667 Health Sciences Center, 3330 Hospital Drive NW, Calgary, Alberta, T2N 4N1, Canada

Harry Van Der Heijden, Vascular Biology Laboratory, Department of Pharmacology and, Cardiovascular Research Institute Maastricht, University of Limburg, Maastricht, The Netherlands

Mark A. Vivino, M.Sc., Division of Computer Resources and Technology, NIH, Bethesda, MD, USA

Yudi Wang, M.D., Ph.D., Departments of Medicine and Medical Physiology, The University of Calgary, 1667 Health Sciences Center, 3330 Hospital Drive NW, Calgary, Alberta, T2N 4N1, Canada

Sima Welber, M.Sc., Department of Cardiology, Hadassah University Hospital, Jerusalem, Israel

Walter Welkowitz, Ph.D., Department of Biomedical Engineering, Rutgers University, Piscataway, NJ 08855, USA

Nicolaas Westerhof, Ph.D., Laboratory for Physiology and, Institute for Cardiovascular Research, Free University of Amsterdam, 1081 BT, Amsterdam, The Netherlands

Toyotaka Yada, M.D., Department of Medical Engineering and Systems Cardiology, Kawasaki Medical School, 577 Matsushima, Kurashiki, 701-01, Japan

Frank C.P. Yin, M.D., Ph.D., Peter Bolfer Cardiac Mechanics Laboratory, Department of Medicine, The Johns Hopkins Medical Institutions, Baltimore, MD, USA

Daniel Zinemanas, D.Sc., Heart System Research Center, The Julius Silver Institute, Department of Biomedical Engineering, Technion-IIT, Haifa, 32000, Israel

INDEX

A1 receptors 11, 13
Acetoxymethyl ester 7
Acetylcholine 17
Acidosis 19, 20, 22–24, 26, 28, 39, 48, 71, 73, 182, 234, 240
Actin 44, 60, 61, 279, 281, 377, 404
  striation 53
Action potential 11, 16, 20, 79, 82–84, 86–89, 403
  duration 6, 12, 27, 55, 56, 80, 84, 86, 89
  threshold 12
Activation 9, 15, 16, 35, 39–45, 47, 48, 54, 59, 60, 62, 65–70, 72–75, 84–87, 91, 92, 96, 184, 185, 199, 200, 203, 257–259, 261–263, 284, 287, 292, 303, 344, 349, 376, 401, 402, 406
Active bridges 40
Adenosine 11, 13, 14, 16, 35, 106, 114, 121, 155, 157, 159, 160, 169, 182, 194, 202–204, 234, 235, 238, 252, 401
  hypothesis 199, 200, 203, 204
  diphosphate, see ADP
  monophosphate, see AMP
  triphosphate, see ATP
Adenylate 233, 235, 237, 239
Adolescent hypertrophy 166
ADP 32, 35, 44, 47, 199, 233–235, 237, 239
Adrenergic blockade 114, 199, 200
Adrenergic receptor 11, 184, 185, 199, 200, 203
Adrenergic–adenosine interaction 203
Adults hypertrophy 166
Adventia 278
Aequorin 7, 8, 22, 53, 91, 93–98, 339
Afterdepolarizations 79
Afterload 113–115, 128, 129, 132, 303, 331, 332, 350, 351, 353, 361
Albumin 160, 186, 227, 228
Aldosterone 293
Alpha-adrenergic 184, 185, 204, 317
Alpha-receptor 200
Alpha1-agonist 54
Altered loading 337, 339
Alternans 79, 84, 87, 88
Alveolar expansion 358, 361
Alveolar vessels 361
AMP 7, 126, 203, 233–235, 237, 239
Analog models 325
Anesthetics 160
Aneurysm 273, 274, 291
Angina 19, 280, 281
Angiography 266, 280, 394
Angiotensin 54, 293, 296, 316, 317, 344, 366
Anionic sites 55
ANOVA 109
ANP, see Atrial natriuretic peptide
ANS, see Autonomic nervous system
Ansae subclaviae 11
Anticoagulant 279
Aorta 135, 174, 175, 305–310, 321–323, 327, 331, 332
Aortic pressure 126, 127, 234, 236, 238, 262, 306, 310, 319, 326–330, 332, 351, 391
Aortic valve 127, 310, 325, 345, 390, 391
ApEn 214
Apical descent 349, 350
Apnea 353, 354, 360
Arachidonic acid 16, 35–37
Arrested heart 116, 144, 177, 225, 226, 292
Arrhythmia 11, 12, 19, 20, 23, 79, 87, 89, 209, 214, 215, 402
Arrhythmogenesis 88
Arterial
  compliance 289, 306, 307, 319, 320, 325, 328, 330
  load 301–305, 309, 327, 328
  resistance 191, 303, 306, 307, 331, 365
  system 244, 303, 313, 319–322, 325, 326, 328, 330–333
  tree 186, 193, 325, 357

Arteries 19, 21, 133, 136, 145, 171, 173, 175, 183, 186, 193, 223, 273, 278, 280, 282–288, 315, 319, 321, 323, 327, 330, 332, 352, 361, 394, 395, 397
Arterio–ventricular 325, 330
Arteriolar diameter 133, 177, 251
Aspirin 279
Asymmetric deformation 383, 386–388
Asynchronous electrical activation 257, 262
Asynchrony of contraction 257
Atherectomy 278, 279, 281
Atheroma 19, 278, 280, 281, 370, 405
ATP 11–17, 20, 23, 27, 28, 32–35, 44, 47, 61, 68, 93, 95, 182, 194, 199, 204, 233–235, 237–239, 401–403
  binding 11, 44
  hydrolysis 23, 47, 61, 68
  inhibition 11
ATPase 7, 28, 34, 47, 61, 71, 92, 93, 95–97, 238, 239
Atrial
  baffles 351
  natriuretic peptide (ANP) 54
  septal defects 374
  stiffness 350, 351, 361
Atrioventricular canal 374
Atrophy 261
Atropine 200
Attractor 208–211, 213, 215
Autocorrelation 209, 210, 212
Autonomic nervous system (ANS) 11, 365, 366, 370
Autoregulation 51, 52, 121, 139, 182, 184, 185, 189, 190, 193, 194, 210, 234, 353
  capacity 138

Back pressure 153, 191, 313
Baffle 351
Balloon angioplasty 278
Barium contractures 43
Basal metabolism 302, 305
Beeler–Reuter 5, 80, 168
Benzofuran isophthalate 24
Beta–adrenergic 184, 200
  blockade 114
  receptors 184
Beta
  agonist isoproterenol 114
  agonists 52
  blocker 114
  escin 32
  receptor 199–203
Bifurcation 88, 209, 214, 215, 305, 393, 405
Biomechanical model 373, 375–377, 379
Biplane circumference 265, 267, 269
Biplane left ventriculography 265, 266
Blood content 163, 170, 228
Blood flow 52, 114–117, 138, 164, 166, 181, 182, 184, 189–193, 199–201, 203, 204, 219, 220, 223, 224, 228–230, 258, 261–263, 279, 305, 319, 325, 328, 339, 341–343, 351, 353, 354–358, 360, 361, 365, 370, 371, 393, 394
Blood volume 163–170, 221, 223, 226, 306, 314, 315, 355, 358, 361, 393
Body mass 234, 320, 321, 323
Boundedness 208
Box dimension 212, 213
BR *see* Beeler–Reuter
Brain 36, 252, 253, 319, 365, 371
Branches 135, 247–249, 284, 292, 357
Brownian motion 210
Butanedione –2,3, monoxime 92
Bypass 19, 92, 113, 121, 278, 306

Caffeine 23, 32, 33, 96
Calcium 3, 4, 6–9, 19, 26–28, 31–37, 45, 47, 56, 59–67, 69–76, 89, 91, 92–98, 217, 234, 238, 239, 240, 284, 289, 305, 310, 340, 343, 401, 402, 406
  activation 41, 48, 96
  channel 12, 15, 16, 20, 27, 92, 96
    antagonist 116
  current 11, 13
  cycling 91, 94–97
  detector 21
  –Fluo–3 34
  homeostasis 339, 342
  metabolism 17
  phosphate 32
  pumps 93
  release 33, 34
  sensitization 34
  transient 6, 9, 11, 12, 20–24, 43, 48, 69, 70, 73, 80, 88, 345, 403
Calmodulin 8, 32, 34
Capacitive flow 157
Capillary 53, 137–149, 161, 170, 193, 219, 223–226, 228–230, 244–249, 361
  augmentation 253
  blood pressure 224
  enhancement 248, 249, 251–253
  flow 137, 138, 144, 146, 147, 246, 253
  length 137–139, 145, 147, 149
  perfusion 153, 244, 245
  pressure 158, 159, 220, 224
  recruitment 245, 252
  tethering 147, 148
Captopril 266, 274
Carbachol 33
Carbon dioxide 200, 244

Cardiac
cell 3, 73, 79
mechanics 103, 125, 135, 347, 352, 353, 383
output 52, 307, 313–316, 320, 322, 332, 344, 345, 353, 361, 362
rhythm 209, 216
Cardiomyocyte 51, 52, 54, 199
Cardiomyopathy 91, 92, 95, 96, 98, 262, 292, 337, 342
Cardioplegia 92, 105
Cardiovascular
interaction 301
regulation 366, 370
Carotid 175, 200, 353, 368–371, 395, 396, 405
declamping 369
endarterectomy 365, 368, 370
Catecholamines 37, 239, 251
Catheterization 266, 268–270, 272, 374, 377
Cation channels 16
Caudal shift 354
Cavity
pressure 126, 128, 129, 132, 222, 227, 259, 263, 375, 376
volume 225, 259, 263, 264, 383, 384, 386–389
CBF *see* Coronary blood flow
Cellular responses 79
Centerline
method 266
wall motion 268, 269, 271
Chamber stiffness 103, 296, 308, 340
Chaos 88, 207, 208, 211, 213, 215, 216
Chaotic
activity 79, 86, 87
attractors 209, 211
cycling 215
dynamics 208, 215, 216
Chemical energy 39
Chemomechanical transduction 302, 305
Circulation 16, 51, 54, 113, 116, 119, 127, 128, 133, 135, 137, 153, 154, 158, 160, 164, 170, 171, 173, 174, 178, 191, 193, 219, 223, 224, 229, 253, 313, 314, 316, 323, 325, 331, 354, 365
Circulatory filling pressure 314, 315
Circumferential shortening 302, 386
Clamp 12, 15, 89, 96
Collagen 113, 114, 116–120, 125, 129–132, 135–137, 139, 147, 148, 219–222, 279, 281, 288, 291, 292, 293–297, 340, 343, 344, 373, 376, 404
Collagenase 292, 295
Collapse 114, 176, 178
Collapsible vessels 114
Color Doppler flow 396
Compliance 106, 127, 132, 133, 135, 138, 154, 160, 193, 221, 226, 228, 247, 272, 273, 289, 291, 292, 293–296, 302, 303, 305–308, 315, 317, 319, 320, 323, 325, 326, 328–330
Compressive stress 117
Concavity 268, 270, 271
Concentric hypertrophy 259
Conductance 80, 82, 305, 307, 310, 354, 355, 357
Conduction velocity 22
Confocal 52
Congenital heart disease 351, 373
Congestive heart failure 266, 313, 315, 339, 342
Connective tissue 52, 53, 120, 221, 291, 292
Constant perfusion pressure 114, 115, 121, 127, 128
Continuum mechanics 137, 138
Contractile 27, 35, 39–41, 45, 47, 60, 63, 69–72, 75, 95, 221, 233, 234, 265–274, 283, 284, 286–288, 306, 307, 343, 378–380, 402, 403
dysfunction 342
efficiency 39
elements 40, 41, 43, 74, 288, 380
performance 20, 114, 301, 302, 304, 305, 325
proteins 40, 41, 55, 91–93, 96, 378
regulatory apparatus 31
segment 265, 267, 269–273
state 31, 52, 310, 322, 337
work 257–259, 261–263
Contractility 17, 31, 35, 36, 43, 47, 103, 104, 106, 114, 125, 127, 129, 131, 132, 135, 157, 204, 273, 288, 302, 307, 308, 337, 343, 373, 374, 376–379
Contraction 3, 7, 8, 17, 23, 24, 31–35, 39, 44, 45, 47, 48, 54–56, 59, 60, 63, 66, 68–75, 88, 89, 91, 92, 93–95, 97, 104–111, 113, 116, 119–121, 127–129, 132, 135, 138, 149, 157, 173, 174, 177, 191, 230, 257, 270, 272, 273, 288, 289, 304, 319, 351, 353, 384, 402, 403, 406
Contracture 20, 117, 118, 121, 234
Contrast
agent 167, 357, 360, 361
dilution 168, 351
Control mechanism 59, 60, 69, 70, 73–75, 132, 192, 243
Convexity 268
Coronary
blood flow (CBF) 114–118, 181, 182, 184, 189–193, 199–201, 203, 204, 219, 223, 325, 328, 339, 341–343

Coronary *(cont'd)*
  circulation 16, 51, 54, 113, 119, 127, 133, 135, 137, 153, 154, 158, 160, 164, 170, 173, 191, 223, 229, 253
  compression 125, 127–129, 132
  endothelium 51, 52
  flow 19, 115, 117–121, 125–129, 132, 135, 138, 144, 145, 149, 153, 158, 185, 194, 220–222, 224, 225, 227–230, 233–235, 237, 238, 307, 309, 310, 330, 331
  hemodynamics 125, 135
  perfusion 104, 106, 109, 110, 114, 116, 117, 121, 125, 135, 154, 182, 221, 225, 226, 228, 229, 238, 307, 309, 311, 319, 321, 328, 330, 331
    pressure (CPP) 114, 116, 117, 121, 125, 135, 154, 182, 221, 225, 228, 229, 330
  reserve 138
  volume 138
Correlation dimension 209, 211, 212
Coupling 3, 8, 9, 14, 16, 31–34, 36, 55, 59–62, 70, 72, 73, 88, 89, 91–95, 97, 104, 115, 116, 119, 120, 121, 125, 193, 288, 302, 305, 358, 361, 403
Coupling function 115
Covalent crosslinks 292
CPP 114–117
Creatine phosphate 234, 236, 240
Crimp 291, 292
Crossbridge 20, 27, 31, 40, 41, 47, 59–66, 72–74, 76, 91, 93–96, 98, 403
  cycle 3, 34, 35, 44, 45, 47, 59–65, 68, 69, 72, 73, 93, 94, 96
Crosslinking 291
CrP 234, 236, 238
CT scanners 164
Curvature 103, 110, 267, 270–274, 375
  analysis 265, 272
  plots 268, 270, 273
Cytoplasmic Ca 32
Cytosol 3, 7, 8, 96

Decay time 319–321, 323
Deformation 113, 119, 120, 135, 263, 380, 383–390
Denervation sensitivity 11
Deoxyglucose-2, 234, 238
Depolarization 12, 34, 79, 403
Detached phase 45
Detached state 44
Dextran 53, 116
Diacylglycerol 16
Diaphragm 305, 323, 353, 354, 357, 358, 361
Diastasis 114
Diastolic
  abnormalities 337, 343
  aortic pressure 330
  dysfunction 291, 293–295, 337, 339, 343, 344
  filling 129, 147, 148, 387
  flow 114, 119, 126, 146, 147, 308, 309
  function 92, 291, 293, 294, 337, 339–343, 345
  motion 388
  pressure 20, 157, 292, 310, 311, 316, 319–321
    decay 319, 320
  rapid filling 137
Dicrotic notch 328
Dihydropyridine 96
Dilatation 121, 181–185, 279, 280, 296, 297, 343, 344

Dilated
  cardiomyopathy 91, 92, 95, 96, 98, 337, 342
  ventricle 291, 294, 295
Dilation 19, 157, 159, 166, 193, 268, 292
Dilution method 165, 167, 170
Dimension 209, 211–215, 217, 355, 406
Dimensionality 211, 212
Dispersion 167, 210
Distensibility 120, 139, 140, 145
Doppler 173, 374, 377, 393–397
Drills 278
DSR *see* Dynamic spatial reconstructor
DTNB 117–119, 295
Ductus arteriosus 374
Duration of diastole 319–321
Dynamic spatial reconstructor (DSR) 164, 348, 350–353, 358, 362
Dynamic transverse stiffness 103, 105, 109

Early ejection 326
Ebihara–Johnson 81
E–C *see* Excitation–contraction
Eccentric hypertrophy 259, 273
Echo 348, 371, 380, 394–397
ECP *see* Extravacular compressive pressure
Edema 106, 116, 119, 121, 160, 219, 221, 227, 228, 245, 291, 294, 295, 344
EE *see* Endocardial epithelium
EGF *see* Epidermal growth factor
EIPA 24–26
Ejecting beats 303, 304, 310
Ejection
  fraction 266, 269, 270, 301, 302, 304, 307, 309, 327, 340, 353, 390
  parameters 302

Elastance 135, 178, 301, 308–310, 325–328, 351, 365, 380, 402
Elastic theory 115, 120
Elasticity 74, 137, 140, 144–147, 159, 292, 294, 321
Electrocardiogram 320, 327
Electromechanical coupling 31
Electron
  beam 347, 353–358, 360, 361
    scanner 357
  microscopy 52, 53, 117
Ellipsoidal model 266, 267, 384
Ellipticalization 383–388
Embedding 212–214, 217
Embolization 106, 109, 165, 166, 293
Enalaprilat 316
End–stage cardiomyopathy 342
End–systolic pressure–thickness relationship (ESPTR) 131
End–systolic pressure–volume relationship (ESPVR) 302–308
Endarterectomy 278, 365, 368, 370
Endo/epi ratio 342
Endocardial 115, 133, 139, 144, 165, 169, 170, 173, 175, 176, 178, 259, 260, 265, 267, 268, 269, 270, 272, 342, 374, 375, 380, 390, 402
  epithelium (EE) 51–56, 127
Endocardium 51–54, 56, 115, 120, 143, 145, 170, 176, 178, 263, 390
Endomysium 292
Endothelial cells 16, 28, 51–54, 56, 149, 158, 393, 403
Endothelial control 183
Endothelin 54, 279
Endothelium 16, 17, 28, 51–56, 149, 158, 181–185, 278, 279, 281, 288, 393, 398, 402, 403
Energetic
  contraction 39
  efficiency 301, 302, 305–307, 309
  performance 301, 302
Energy 3, 23, 39, 44, 47, 48, 93–97, 115, 129, 186, 194, 200, 228, 233–236, 239, 240, 316, 327, 328–330, 332, 333, 384, 403
  demand 243
Entropy calculations 213, 214
Epidermal growth factor (EGF) 279
Epifluorescence 4
Epimysium 292
Esmolol 114
Esophageal 394
ESPTR *see* End–systolic pressure–thickness relationship
ESPVR *see* End–systolic pressure–volume relationshio
Essential hypertension 305
Ethylisopropylamiloride 24
Excitability 79–87, 288
Excitation 3–5, 31, 59, 60, 70, 72, 75, 87–89, 91–95, 97, 215, 288, 403
Excitation–contraction (E–C) 3, 31, 60, 72, 88, 91–95, 97, 288, 302–305, 403
  coupling 3, 31, 60, 72, 88, 91–95, 97, 288
Exercise performance 19
Exogenous energy 233
External work 47, 233, 302, 327
Extrasystolic 41, 43, 44, 52, 88, 257
Extrasystolic beats 257
Extravascular (interstitial) compartment 116
Extravascular compressive pressure (ECP) 125, 127–132, 135, 136

Fast CT 166, 167
Fatigue 45, 47
Feedback 51, 59–61, 64–66, 69, 70, 72, 73, 75, 76, 158, 159, 186, 192, 193, 199, 207, 325, 330, 379
Ferret 3, 4, 6, 12–17, 21, 22, 53, 54
Ferritin 239
Fetal heart 295, 347
Fiber
  diameter 291
  disorganization 373, 376–380
  strain 257, 258, 261, 262, 384, 385
  volume 223, 224
Fibril 291
Fibrillation 79, 88, 350, 351
Fibrinolysis 278
Fibronectin 279
Fibrosis 293, 343
Flow 19–21, 39, 48, 51, 52, 56, 65, 109, 113–121, 132, 137–141, 143–149, 153, 154, 157–161, 164–166, 170, 171, 173, 174, 181–186, 189–194, 199–201, 203, 210, 233–240, 243–253, 258, 261–263, 278, 279, 283–285, 288, 301, 303, 305–311, 314–317, 319–322, 326, 327–332, 339, 341–343, 345, 351, 353–358, 360, 361, 365, 370, 371, 390, 395, 404, 405
  3D 394
  dynamics 115, 120, 125, 127, 129, 133
  impediment 114, 119
  pulse 115, 325
  regulation 158, 160, 204
  signal 125–128
  velocity 393, 394, 396–398
Fluid transport 125, 134, 135, 219–230
Fluorescence 4–6, 12, 14, 25
Fluorescence ratio 6, 12, 14, 25
Fluorine 21

Fluorocarbon 105, 106
Fluorochromes 53
Fontan procedure 352
Force 3–9, 20–22, 27, 32–35, 40–47, 52, 53, 56, 59–62, 65–76, 91–94, 96–98, 105, 107, 110, 125, 132, 135, 157, 158, 178, 191, 220–222, 224, 225, 230, 263, 264, 284, 285, 287, 288, 291, 302, 304, 323, 388, 401–403
  frequency 91, 93, 96, 97
  generation 3, 62, 70, 71, 113, 229, 310, 391
  production 20, 93, 94, 98
  velocity 40–44, 59, 66, 67, 72
Fourier 375
  analysis 371
  transform 366, 371
Fractal
  analysis 166
  characterization 211
  dimension 212, 213
Fractional luminescence 339, 340
Free acid 3, 7, 9
Freewall 350
Functional residual capacity 359
Functional residual capacity (FRC) 357–359, 361
Fura–5, 7–9, 12, 14, 15, 33, 96, 97

G–protein 8, 16, 31, 32, 34–36
Gas perfusion 22
Geometric distortion 266
Geometry 109–111, 114, 125, 135, 163, 222, 259, 262, 265, 266, 268, 270–273, 333, 343, 352, 357, 358, 360, 374, 376, 380, 396
Glibenclamide 182, 204
Glucose 4, 22, 234, 236–239
Glycolysis 20, 22, 210, 234
Golgi complex 55
Graft 113, 121, 278, 305
Great vessels 327, 374
Gregg phenomenon 106, 109, 110
Growth factor 279–281

Haemoglobin 191
Heart
  human 91, 96, 97
  period 320, 321
  rate 136, 155, 157, 159, 160, 207, 228, 234–236, 319–323, 339–341, 343–345, 350, 351, 353, 362, 368, 369, 372
    variability 214, 365, 366, 371
  volume 226, 322, 347, 348, 350–353, 361
Heat 91, 93–98, 401, 403
Heparin 32, 33, 36, 279
Heterogeneity 166, 185, 186, 192–194, 253, 380
Heterometric autoregulation 51
Hibernation 323
High risk patients 366
Hilum 355
HLHS 351
Hodgkin–Huxley 80
Homeodynamics 207
Homeometric autoregulation 51, 52
Homeostasis 207, 339, 342
Homeostatic mechanisms 16
Hounsfield number 355
Hydralazine 293, 316
Hydraulic
  conductivity 224
  resistance 244, 246
Hydrolysis 23, 44, 47, 61, 68, 93–96, 403
Hydrostatic pressure 138
Hydroxyproline 294, 340
Hypercalcemia 238
Hypertension 36, 283, 287, 289, 293, 295, 296, 302, 305, 309, 374
Hypertensive rats 283, 293, 296
Hypertrophy 166, 167, 259, 261–263, 272–274, 283, 284, 287, 293–296, 344, 374, 378, 379, 405
Hypocontractile myocardium 273
Hypoplastic left heart syndrome 351
Hypoplastic left heart syndrome (HLHS) 351
Hypoxia 17, 39, 45, 47, 97, 98, 182, 199, 200, 202–204
Hypoxic response 201

Imaging 163, 165, 169, 171, 179, 347, 352, 353, 357, 380, 393–395, 397
IMP *see* Intramyocardial pressure
Impaired contractility 337, 343
Impedance 155, 303, 305, 320, 326, 327, 332
Impediment 113–115, 119, 133, 220
Impulse
  conduction 257
  propagation 262, 263
In situ 5, 32, 303, 305, 307
In vitro 52–54, 182, 284, 289, 337, 339, 343, 345, 377, 390
In vivo 27, 35, 52–54, 104, 114, 121, 163, 166, 174, 178, 182, 184, 234, 239, 240, 292, 301, 307, 360, 377, 378
Incompressibility 221, 225
Indentation
  probe 103, 104, 111
  strain 103–105, 107, 109, 111

Indentation *(cont'd)*
  stress 103–107, 109, 111
Indicator dilution 165, 167, 170
Indo–1 8
Infarct expansion 265, 272, 273
Infarction 11, 12, 259, 265–274
Inosine 234, 235
Inositol phosphates 15, 16
Inotropic 52–56, 107, 109, 237–239
  agent 17, 39, 43, 45, 234
  alterations 39
  effect 7, 17
  infusions 353
  interventions 41, 43, 47, 233, 238, 239
  mechanisms 39, 41
  state 7, 43, 52, 114, 115
Inovar 350
InsP3 32–34, 36
Instability 207, 215
Intact heart 3, 8, 9, 34–37, 41, 43, 52–54, 56, 60, 65, 70, 75, 76, 92, 98, 103, 104, 106, 108–112, 157, 159, 183, 184, 186, 199, 200, 203, 279, 289, 301, 303, 304, 339, 347, 351, 352, 374, 378, 402, 403
Integrated model 221, 222, 228–230
Intercellular 53, 55, 72, 74, 98, 193
Interleukin I 279
Internal load 42, 46, 47, 65, 67–69, 120
Interstitial 53, 113–117, 143, 144, 200, 219–230, 251, 291, 292, 294, 373
  fluid 114, 120, 125, 128, 129, 140, 219–221, 223–225, 228–230
    transport 220, 224
  space 113, 116, 119, 135, 136, 199, 230
Interstitium 113, 114, 119, 121
Intima 278, 279, 281
Intracavitary irradiation 52
Intracellular 3–7, 9, 11, 15–17, 22–25, 28, 31–34, 36, 47, 59, 60, 71–74, 113, 120, 234–236, 240
  calcium 3, 12, 19–21, 27, 93, 96, 98, 339, 342, 343, 402
Intracyclic changes 163
Intramyocardial 113–117, 119–121, 128, 133–135, 137, 140, 142, 157, 163–170, 174, 219
  blood volume 163–168, 170
  capacitance 127, 153, 154
  compartments 113
  compliance 127, 133
  pressure (IMP) 114–121, 125, 128–130, 133, 136, 220, 225, 229, 230
  pump 121, 133, 146, 153, 154, 161
  structure 113, 119
Intrathoracic pressure 332, 362
Inverse problem 376, 380

Ionic
  channel 79
  currents 80
  pumps 80
Iontophoresis 4, 7, 9
Ischemia 17, 19–23, 25–28, 48, 71, 106, 111, 174, 204, 234–237, 239, 240, 266, 292, 330, 342, 343, 378, 379, 402
Isolated
  heart 111, 121, 240, 301, 303, 305, 307, 310, 337
  muscle 52, 55, 56, 91, 301
Isometric
  force 40–42, 45, 52, 53, 91, 288
  tension 32, 54, 94, 98, 378
  twitch 52, 53, 94–96
Isoperfusion 258
Isoproterenol 7, 114, 293
Isostrain 258
Isotonic force 41, 42
Isovolumic
  contraction 115, 120, 127, 132, 257, 303, 304
  relaxation 127, 129, 130, 148, 340, 341, 389
Jet ventilation 353, 362

K+ channels 182
Ketamine 175
Kinematic model 383, 385
Kinking 176, 177
Kolmogorov–Smirnov (K–S) test 367–369, 370
Krebs–Hensleit 175, 176
Krebs–Ringer 92, 97

L–arginine 183, 185
Lactate 21, 23–28, 234, 236–238, 240
Lactic acid 23, 25
Langendorff 12, 20, 114
Laplace's law 285, 321
Late systolic flow 126
Late ventricular enlargement 265, 266, 268, 272, 273
Lead marker 168, 169
Left bundle branch block 262
Left ventricle *ventricular* (LV) 11, 21, 52, 56, 92, 98, 106, 110, 114–116, 120, 125–133, 135, 137, 139, 141–145, 148, 155, 157, 166, 167, 173–178, 200, 219, 221–223, 225–230, 233, 234, 237, 238, 258–262, 265–270, 272, 292–294, 301, 302, 304, 316, 325–330, 332, 337, 339–342, 345, 349–353, 362, 373–376, 378, 379, 383–388, 394, 404, 405

Left ventricle *ventricular* (LV) *(cont'd)*
  shape 267, 273
  pressure 113–119, 126, 128–132, 169, 221, 225, 329
Lesions 278, 280, 281
Leukotrienes 16
Lidocaine 132
Light emission 91, 94
Loading 4, 5, 7, 68, 69, 72, 73, 75, 103, 108, 125, 127, 132, 135, 139, 157, 240, 259, 301–309, 316, 325, 330, 337, 339–341, 345, 373–377, 379, 380, 386
Lumped interaction model 326
Lung 17, 88, 160, 186, 313, 347, 348, 350, 352–362, 389
  capacity 359
  expansion 354, 358, 360
  inflation 352–354, 362
LVP *see* Left ventricular pressure
Lymphatic
  circulation 219
  flow 135, 226, 227, 229
  outflow blockage 221
Lysis 117, 119, 278, 279

Markers 104, 105, 165, 167, 170, 281, 383, 385, 388–390, 404
Maximal enhancement 249
MBF *see* Myocardial blood flow
Mean circulatory pressure 314
Mean resistance 301–306, 309
Mechanical
  energy 384
  force 40
  impediment 113, 119
  performance 9, 19, 20, 53, 54, 60, 70, 72, 74, 75, 93, 402
Media 132, 135, 278, 279, 283, 285–288, 395
Membrane 8, 16, 23, 32, 33, 36, 55, 56, 79–83, 87, 88, 104, 120, 147, 148, 182, 224, 279, 281
  action potential 79
  excitability 79, 81–83
  potential 4, 9, 22, 81–83, 217
  reactivation 81
Metabolic
  control 182, 183
  demand 159, 181, 183–185, 243
  flow 190
  inhibition 22
  regulation 258
  vasodilation 157
Metabolism 17, 35, 37, 181, 194, 199, 200, 233, 302, 305, 321, 402
Methoxamine 327, 331
Michaelis–Menten 11, 12, 14
Microcirculation 113, 117, 119, 138, 142, 146, 153, 160, 163, 165, 173–177, 181–186, 243, 245, 252, 291, 313
Microsphere 170, 355
Microspheres 106, 165, 166, 168, 316, 339
Microstructure 129, 246, 251
Microvascular 53, 120, 163–165, 169, 181–185, 249, 251
  bed 243
  patency 163, 164
  resistance 116, 181, 183–185
  tone 181, 182
Microvasculature 113, 119, 138, 163, 169, 246, 247, 250, 251
Microvessels 138, 166, 170, 174, 175, 178, 181–186, 252
Mid-systolic flow 126, 127
Millar transducers 126
Minimum energy 384
Mitochondria 32, 92, 193
Models 9, 48, 59, 74, 84, 88, 98, 110, 111, 132, 133, 138, 148, 153, 154, 160, 169, 178, 221–224, 228, 229, 243, 244, 253, 272, 284, 293, 315, 325, 332, 337, 340, 389, 401, 402–406
Modulus of elasticity 292, 321
Morbidity 274, 302
Mortality 274, 302
mRNA 96
Multiresolution 365, 366, 368
Muscarinic blockade 366
Muscle 3–6, 8, 9, 22, 23, 28, 31–37, 39–45, 47, 48, 51–56, 59, 60, 62, 63, 65, 66, 69–75, 91–93, 96–98, 104, 109–111, 113–115, 119–121, 129, 131, 135, 136, 138, 139, 140, 143, 157–159, 166, 168, 170, 174, 179, 182, 183, 199, 211, 217, 246, 247, 252, 257, 259, 260, 264, 274, 278, 279, 281, 283–285, 287, 288, 292–294, 301, 304, 339, 344, 349, 373, 374, 376, 388, 389, 402–404
  damage 19, 20
  mechanics 219–222, 228–230
  paralysis 132, 226
Mustard 352
MVO_2 191, 194, 200, 302–308, 351
Myocardial
  blood flow (MBF) 164, 258, 319, 339, 342, 351, 353, 361
  deformation 135
  energetics 39, 303
  function 19, 52, 54, 97, 125, 135
  metabolism 181, 200
  performance 51–55, 91
  perfusion 103, 113, 114, 165–167, 192, 341–343

Myocardial *(cont'd)*
pump 125, 160
stiffness 293, 295, 340, 341, 345
Myocardium 3, 16, 17, 19, 20, 28, 43, 47, 52–56, 72, 91–98, 113–115, 119, 120, 125–127, 129, 131, 132, 133, 135, 139, 144, 154, 157, 164–170, 173, 174, 178, 182, 186, 187, 191, 193, 203, 204, 219–222, 226, 228, 229, 233, 234, 237, 239, 243, 252, 259, 272, 273, 291, 292, 294–296, 308, 319, 325, 337, 340, 343, 348, 349, 406
Myocyte 13, 15, 20, 24, 25, 28, 98, 120, 138, 144, 148, 204, 279, 293, 294, 343, 378, 402, 403
Myocytes 11–17, 23, 24, 26–28, 37, 96, 97, 121, 129, 137, 139, 147–149, 169, 170, 193, 194, 199, 200, 204, 221, 278, 279, 281, 291–294, 337, 379
Myofibrillar Ca^{++} sensitivity 53
Myofibrillar proteins 19–21, 24
Myofilament 7, 8, 45, 303, 310
Myogenic 153, 158–160, 181–185
control 182, 183
mechanism 159
regulation 158
Myoplasm 80
Myoplasmic Ca^{2+} 11
Myosin 32–35, 37, 40, 44, 60, 61, 63, 71, 98, 279, 281, 404
heads 32
isoform 43
light chain phosphatase 31, 32, 34
phosphatase 35
Myothermal 91, 93, 96, 97

Na^+/Ca^{2+} exchanger 7, 19, 23, 25, 26
Na/H exchanger 19, 23, 24, 26
NADH 233, 235, 239
Negative pressure 347
Neomycin 32
Nervous system 11, 17, 160, 246, 365, 366, 370 (*see also* Autonomic nervous system)
Neurohumoral control 51, 184
Nitric oxide 183–186
synthase 183
Nitrogen-breathing 200
Nitroglycerin 184, 316, 317
Nitroprusside 284, 327, 328
Nitrous oxide 350
Nitrovasodilator 183
NMR 8, 21, 27
Noncontractile segment 265, 267–272
Noninvasive imaging 347
Norepinephrine 184, 234, 238
Normothermia 114
Nutrients 228, 243, 244

OFA *see* Oscillatory flow amplitude
Opacification 166
Orthogonal wavelet 367
Orthonormal bases 366, 367
Oscillatory flow amplitude (OFA) 127–129, 227
Osmium ferrocyanide 32, 33
Osmotic pressure 116, 137, 138, 140, 141, 144, 221, 225
transient 116
Oubain 52, 215, 216
Oxygen 43, 233, 240, 243–246, 252, 302–305, 402
consumption 181, 182, 184, 189–194, 200, 203, 204, 264, 302, 304, 305, 307, 311
control 190, 192
demand 244, 251, 258
metabolism 199
pressure 189–193
saturation 191
supply 190, 191, 199, 245, 251
tension 97, 199, 200, 203, 204, 246, 251
Oxygenation potential 273

P2Y receptor 11, 14
PA 13, 113, 138, 141–144, 146–148, 158, 374, 378
Pacing 79, 159, 182, 257–263, 315, 337, 339–345, 350, 351, 361
Papaverine 181
Papillary muscle 3, 4, 6, 7, 9, 22, 27, 43, 52, 54, 56, 97, 259, 260, 264, 292, 380, 388
stiffness 293
Paracellular diffusion 53
permeability 53
Paradise protocol 92
Parenchyma 182, 355
Parenchymal volume 164, 361
Passive
elasticity 294
elements 42
stresses 117
Peak twitch tension 91, 93–96
PEEP ventilation 362
Pentobarbital 175, 226, 229, 230, 339
Perfusion dynamics 113
Perfusion pressure 47, 106, 109, 111, 114–117, 120, 121, 125, 127, 128, 135, 154, 159, 182, 190, 191, 192, 220, 221, 225, 228–230, 244, 245, 248, 301, 308, 330

Pericardial
  cradle 175, 200
  sac 348, 357, 358
Perimysium 292
Perinephritis 293
Periodic stimulation 79, 80, 84
Peripheral
  circulation 313, 314
  resistance 305, 319, 320, 323
Permeability 53, 55, 185, 186, 246
  coefficient 244
Permeabilization 32
pH 4, 21, 24, 26, 27, 45–47, 71, 234–237, 239, 240
Pharmacological 11, 52
  mechanisms 14
Pharmacomechanical coupling 31–34, 36
Phase space 210, 211, 215
Phasic fluctuations 159
Phasic IMP 119
Phenotype 279, 281
Phenoxybenzamine 200
Phenylephrine 33, 34, 54
Phosphate 19, 21, 27, 32, 39, 47, 234, 236, 240, 402
  bonds 93, 200
  hydrolysis 93–96
Phospholipase C 16, 32
Phosphorylation 7, 21, 32–35, 37, 199, 233, 235, 237, 239, 240
Physiological messenger 33
Pinching 176, 177
Placebo 266, 274
Plaque 278, 280, 281
Plasmin 279
Plasminogen 279
Platelet 16, 17, 54, 279, 282, 393
Poiseuille's law 164, 170, 171, 405
Positive pressure ventilation 353, 362
Post dilatation stenosis 280
Post–extrasystolic potentiation 41, 43, 44, 52
Post–infarction 11, 12, 265
Potassium 27, 28, 33, 55, 80, 82, 84, 85, 87, 93, 105, 204, 284
Potential work 302
Potentiation 41, 43, 44, 52, 88
Power density spectrum 210
Power output 39, 40, 44, 323
Power stroke 44, 46
Precapillary sphincters 246, 251, 253
Preload 72, 73, 75, 106, 114, 115, 128–130, 233, 234, 303, 308, 313, 331, 332, 353
Premature stimulation 79, 87
Pressure
  distribution 244, 245, 247

Pressure *(cont'd)*
  regulator 153, 154, 158–161, 253
  inflow 153–155
  thickness relationship 131
  volume 110, 135, 287, 292, 295, 296, 302–310, 313–317, 351, 386
    area (PVA) 302–308
    loop 303, 306, 309, 351
    relation 110, 295, 304, 307, 310, 315
Probability density function 209, 210, 213
Prolate ellipsoid 384
Prone 355–360
Propidium iodide 53
Prostaglandin 16, 183
Prostaglandins 16, 182
Protein
  G 8, 16, 31, 32, 34, 35
  kinase 15, 16
Proteoglycans 279
Protons 19, 21, 348
PTCA 278–281
Pulmonary 33, 316, 327, 331, 347, 360–362, 379
  atresia 374
  blood flow 354–358, 360, 361
Pulsatile 119, 121, 177, 289
  energy 327–330, 332, 333
  load 301, 302, 305–309
  work 327
Pulse
  amplitude 117, 119
  wave velocity 321, 322
Pump model 133, 153, 154
Pumping LV 115
Purine 233–235, 237, 239
Purkinje system 257
PVA *see* Pressure volume area
Pyruvate 194, 233–240

QRS 320, 368

Radial
  stress 131, 132
  stretching 131
Radiolabeled myocardium 165
Radiopaque markers 165, 167, 383, 385, 388
Radius 110, 138–140, 170, 268, 321, 375
Randomicity 207, 208
Reactive hyperemia 159, 244, 245
Recoil 278, 281, 282, 389
Reconstruction 394, 397
Recovery 20, 22–24, 26, 79–85, 87, 93, 97, 237–240, 268, 272
Recruitment 166, 169, 170, 184, 245, 252,

Recruitment *(cont'd)* 253, 316
Reentrant 79, 88
Reference state 224, 225, 376, 385
Reflected waves 326, 327, 330
Reflection coefficient 322, 327, 332
Reflections 302, 303, 325, 326, 328, 330–333
Regional 110, 119, 120, 137, 138, 143, 145, 164, 210, 257–260, 262–268, 283, 292, 337, 339, 352, 355, 358–361, 379, 390
  function 103, 132, 265
  hypertrophy 262
  intramyocardial blood volume 163
  lung expansion 354, 358
  shape 267
  wall
    motion 267, 268, 270, 348
    strain 104
    stress 104, 272, 273
Regression 266, 278, 280, 282, 293, 296, 320, 355
Relaxation 6, 7, 35, 52–54, 60, 63, 68–70, 73–75, 93, 95, 113, 120, 126–130, 148, 182, 310, 339, 389
  time 126, 127, 340, 341
Remodeling 113, 119, 259, 265, 266, 269, 271, 273, 274, 279, 283, 284, 287, 288, 291, 293, 294, 373, 374
Renin 344, 366
Renovascular hypertension 293
Reperfusion 19, 20, 22, 23, 26, 106, 111, 233, 234, 237–240
Repolarization 12, 27, 56, 79, 80, 82, 83, 87–89
Resistance 46, 113, 116, 119, 120, 127, 132–135, 139, 147, 149, 153, 154, 158–161, 165, 170, 177, 178, 181–185, 190–194, 223, 244–246, 283, 301–307, 309, 311, 313–316, 319, 320, 323, 326, 331, 362, 365
  distribution of 182
Respirator 327, 353
Respiratory gated ventilation 361
Responsiveness 19, 20, 87, 182, 183, 287
Restenosis 279–282, 404
Resting tension 293
Restoration 20, 233, 238
Retrograde flow 137, 147
Right ventricle 4, 54, 260, 303, 344, 351, 379, 385
Rigor 34, 292
Risk factors 278, 282
Rotation 357, 383–385
Rupture 278, 280, 281, 291
Ryanodine 23, 32, 92, 96, 106, 118
Saddle bifurcation 215
Sarcolemmal receptor 91
Sarcomere length 3, 5, 7, 9, 64–66, 69–71, 139, 228, 258, 264, 377, 390
Sarcoplasmic reticulum (SR) 7, 20, 23, 32, 33, 48, 65, 80, 88, 92, 93, 95–97, 238, 240, 350, 351, 403
Scaffolding effect 119
Scan, 3D 167
Scanning transducers 394
Scintigraphy 316
Senning 352, 374
Shape 55, 72, 75, 148, 194, 267–271, 273, 274, 278, 292, 306, 332, 357, 358, 360, 373, 375, 377, 379, 384, 386, 389–391, 394, 397, 404
  factor 373, 375, 390
Shear stress 52, 55, 158, 183, 185, 186, 279, 287, 288, 393
Shortening 9, 12, 16, 24, 34, 41, 44–47, 52, 53, 56, 60, 63–67, 69, 72–75, 120, 132, 179, 245, 271, 302, 303, 304, 351, 386, 389–391
Signal analysis 366
Single cell 9, 27, 88, 89, 243, 245, 403
Sinus
  pressure 365
  rhythm 234, 257, 350, 351, 374
Skeletal muscle 39, 41, 43, 47, 65, 138, 139
Skinned 9, 41–43, 60, 72, 76, 402, 403
  fibers 8, 21, 41
Slow electrical activation 257
Slow recovery 24, 79–82, 87
Sodium 19, 27, 80–84, 88, 93, 240
  current 80, 83
  pentobarbital 175, 230
  pump 28, 215
SPAMM 348, 349, 352
Spatial distribution 163
SPECT 163–165, 168–170
Sphericalization 292
Sphericity index 265, 267–270
Sphincter 246, 253
SR *see* Sarcoplasmic reticulum
Staged repair 352
Starling 51, 140, 244, 263
Starling's law 51, 140
Stearic hinderance 40
Stenosis 165, 280, 281, 284, 289, 393, 394
Stent 278, 281
Stiffening 120, 273, 305, 309, 310
Stone heart 20
Strain 46, 103–105, 107–111, 132, 135, 140, 257, 258, 261, 262, 283, 285, 288, 358, 376, 380, 384, 385, 388, 389
Strength–interval 82–84, 86, 87

Stress 37, 52, 55, 103–111, 113–115, 117, 119, 120, 131, 158, 183, 185, 186, 233, 234, 235, 237, 240, 258, 259, 263, 272, 273, 279, 283, 285–288, 292, 302, 304, 307, 308, 317, 321, 339, 340, 342, 343, 378, 379, 384, 388, 393, 404, 405
  tensor 220, 222, 376
  strain 104, 108, 132, 135
Stretch 46, 73, 108, 110, 129, 132, 139, 182, 289, 365
Stretch receptors 365
Stretching 75, 105, 108, 120, 129, 131, 139, 176, 257, 278
Stroke work 302
Stroke-work 302
Structural adaptation 257, 259
Struts 114, 117, 139, 292, 294
Stunned myocardium 273
Stunning 20, 238
Subendocardial microcirculation 173–175
Subendocardial vessels 133, 173, 176–178
Subintima 279
Supernormality 82–86
Supine 355–361, 389
Synchronous activation 75, 259
Systemic filling pressure 314
Systolic
  function 302, 303, 340
  hypertension 302, 309
  properties 302

Tagging 348, 349, 352, 380
Takens' theorem 210
Temporal resolution 165
Tensile
  strength 291, 292
  stress 117
Tension 22, 26, 27, 32, 53, 54, 72, 75, 76, 91, 93–98, 104, 148, 157, 158, 199, 200, 203, 204, 217, 246, 251, 265, 272, 273, 283–288, 293, 339, 340, 342, 343, 375, 376, 378, 380, 403
  transients 45, 46
Tetralogy of Fallot 374
TGV 374, 377, 378
Thermoregulation 366
Thickening 129, 131, 132, 179, 239, 293, 294
Thoracic aorta 305
Thorax 347, 351, 355, 357, 358, 389
Thrombolysis 279
Thrombolytic agents 19
Thromboxanes 16
Thrombus 19, 54, 278, 279
Tidal volume 362
Tight junctions 53, 55
Tissue 20, 27, 52–54, 56, 89, 92, 98, 103, 106, 109, 110, 117, 149, 174–176, 219, 221, 234, 243–245, 253, 262, 271–273, 281, 291, 292, 295, 380, 393, 396, 398, 403
  oxygen 189–193
  plasminogen activator 279
  pressure 113, 116, 119–121, 135, 137–140, 142–144, 147, 191, 193, 376
TOF 374, 378
Tomography 164, 168
Tonic 33, 35, 54, 366
Torsion 383–390
  axis 383, 385, 386, 388, 389
Tortuosity 139
Total heart volume 347, 348, 350, 351, 353
Trabeculae 3, 4, 9, 337, 339, 342, 343
Traction 113–115
Transcapillary exchange 244, 245
Transducer 4, 32, 46, 104, 130, 259, 284, 327, 374, 393–396, 398, 404
Transduction
  efficiency 302, 305
  mechanism 3, 48
Transendothelial 51
  physicochemical control 55
Transforming growth factor beta 279, 281
Transition thickness 131, 132
Translation 4, 383–385
Transmission efficiency 327–330, 332
Transmural blood flow 133, 341
Transposition 352, 374
Transverse stiffness 103–111
Triton X-100 52, 53
Tropomyosin 40, 45, 61
Troponin 3, 9, 27, 40, 45, 59–66, 70–75, 403
Troponin-C 3, 27, 60, 92
Turbulence 207, 279
Twist 350, 389
Twitch 41–43, 52–56, 74, 91–98
  force 6, 42, 52, 53, 92

Ultrafiltration 137, 138, 140, 141, 144
Ultrasonic probe 353, 397
Ultrasound 52, 53, 164, 259, 393–397
Unpredictability 207, 208
Unstressed volume 315–317
Untwists 348, 349
Urate 234, 235
Uterus 292, 347

Vagal tone 366
van Willebrand factor 279

Vascular
compliance 138, 305
compression 173, 177, 357
flow 223, 393
loading 301, 302, 306
network 219, 301
patency 117
resistance 149, 159, 165, 181, 193, 314–316, 362
surgery 366
tone 114, 155, 157–159
Vasoactive
agents 316
therapies 302
Vasoconstriction 158, 185, 190
Vasodilatation 128, 158, 182, 184
Vasodilation 121, 153, 155–159, 165, 166, 186, 199, 200, 203, 244, 245
Vasodilator therapy 305
Vasodilators 186, 316
Vasodilatory metabolites 182
Vasomotion 170, 211, 213, 245, 246
Vasomotor tone 366
Velocity 22, 40–47, 59–61, 63, 64, 66–69, 80, 173, 174, 179, 210, 303, 321–323, 374, 393, 394, 396–398
of shortening 52, 53, 67, 69, 72, 390
Venoconstriction 313, 315
Venous
capacitance 313, 315, 316
compliance 315
reservoir 313, 314
resistance 159, 313
return 128, 137, 219, 313
system 313, 314
vasculature 316
Ventilation 353–355, 358, 360–362
Ventricular
afterload 350, 351
enlargement 265, 266, 268, 269, 272–274
geometry 265, 266, 270, 272, 343
pacing 257–262, 337, 339, 340, 342–345
septal defect 374
structure 125, 291
topography 266
Ventriculography 265, 266
Venular diameter 133, 177
Verapamil 117, 121, 229, 345
Vessel
diameter 157–159, 285
elasticity 159
Video–microscope 173–178
Viscosity 139, 186, 253
Voltage–clamp techniques 96
Volume
enlargement 272–274
Volume *(cont'd)*
overload 259, 263, 295, 331, 373, 374, 378, 379
pump 302, 361
Volumetric image 351, 359
von Willebrand factor 55

Wall
elasticity 137, 144, 147
mass 257, 259–262, 287
motion 262, 266–271, 273, 348, 353, 377
stress 104, 105, 109–111, 113, 259, 272, 273, 283, 285–288, 302, 308, 321, 339, 340, 342, 343
thickness 103, 131, 226, 259, 262–264, 274, 321, 373, 384
volume 219, 221–225, 227–230, 263, 264, 340, 383, 386–388
Wash–out 182
Water content 119
Waterfall 125, 133, 153, 154, 178
Wave
propagation 326
reflections 302, 303, 325, 328, 330, 331, 333
velocity 303, 321, 322
Waveform morphology 114
Wavelet transform 366, 368, 370, 371
Wenckebach
patterns 79
periodicity 80, 88
Whale 323
White noise 210
Windkessel 302, 303, 320, 326
Willebrand, von 55
Wolfe–Parkinson–White syndrome 262
Work 8, 17, 20, 22, 26, 28, 31, 36, 39–41, 43, 45, 47, 75, 114, 143, 160, 169, 178, 182, 184, 186, 193, 207, 233, 257–259, 261–264, 280, 288, 294, 302, 304, 311, 327, 331, 332, 337, 343, 345, 347, 351, 358, 361, 372, 373, 379, 389, 390, 401, 406
Workload 258, 262

X–ray 360, 389, 394
CT 163, 164, 167, 169, 347, 353
Xanthine 234, 235
Xylocain 350

Zero
flow 109, 116, 138, 153, 154, 157, 159
load 303
pressure 315, 351